Bathing in Public
in the Roman World

Bathing in Public
in the Roman World

Garrett G. Fagan

Ann Arbor

THE UNIVERSITY OF MICHIGAN PRESS

Copyright © by the University of Michigan 1999
All rights reserved
Published in the United States of America by
The University of Michigan Press
Manufactured in the United States of America
♾ Printed on acid-free paper

2002   2001   2000   1999   4   3   2   1

A CIP catalog record for this book is available from the British Library.

Library of Congress Cataloging-in-Publication Data

Fagan, Garrett G., 1963–
    Bathing in public in the Roman world / Garrett G. Fagan.
        p.   cm.
    Includes bibliographical references and index.
    ISBN 0-472-10819-0 (cloth : alk. paper)
    1. Public baths—Rome. 2. Rome—Antiquities. 3. Rome—Social
life and customs. 4. Inscriptions—Rome.   I. Title.
DG97.F34   1999
391.6′4—dc21   98-51147
                                                    CIP

D. M. matris optimae
optimoque patri

Acknowledgments

This book is the product of a truly international effort that has seen work progress in Canada, the United States, Germany, Ireland, England, Italy, and Tunisia. On my travels, I have encountered many individuals who helped the project reach completion. I shall try to remember as many as I can, but if I miss any names, it is through human frailty and not purposeful omission.

My first debt is to the Killam Trust at the University of British Columbia, whose generous financial support provided me with the time to prepare the manuscript in 1995–96. James Russell, my sponsor at UBC, offered many invaluable insights and deployed his oracular knowledge to my benefit, thus saving me from several gaffes, oversights, or misconceptions. Fikret Yegül and Janet DeLaine read the entire manuscript and offered many helpful criticisms. I thank also David Engel, Philip Harding, and Harry Edinger for looking over my translations of the inscriptions, and I thank Simon Weber-Brown for checking the original texts. Kim Stabler and Celia Schultz proof-read the entire manuscript and did much of the checking, respectively. Richard J.A. Talbert is to be thanked for suggesting the topic in the first place and seeing it through an earlier manifestation, as did George Paul and Daniel Geagan.

Various individuals assisted at other stages of production, directly or indirectly. F. Yegül, C. Parslow, R.J.A. Wilson, and A. Koloski-Ostrow provided or offered to provide original illustrations; J.J. Rossiter hosted me on an extended visit to Carthage; H.-J. Schalles provided an enlightening tour of the reconstructed *balneum* attached to the guest house in the Archaeological Park at Xanten; D. Candilio provided access to otherwise closed-off areas of the Baths of Diocletian; J. Boersma, C. Bruun, and J. DeLaine gave me offprints of their work on the baths; and conversations and correspondence with all of the above as well as with A. Corbeill, D. Gargola, E. Haley, C.H.

Hallett, P.B. Harvey, A. Trevor Hodge, M. McDonnell, M.F. Trundle, and C.J. Simpson have required me to crystallize, revise, or abandon my arguments at various points. Naturally, none of the preceding should be held accountable for any remaining errors or for the opinions I express. A great debt of gratitude also goes to my editor at the University of Michigan Press, Ellen Bauerle, without whose patience, support, and levelheadedness this book would never have been finished. My wife, Katherine, has offered vital emotional support on a sometimes rocky road, and I thank her deeply for it.

My final acknowledgment is to Michael Shiels, S.J., who long ago wrote on a schoolboy's Latin homework, "Stay with the Roman world; it has a lot to offer," and who thereby set me on the path that has led me here.

Contents

x   *Contents*

Abbreviations

Abbreviations for ancient authors used throughout this book follow those in *The Oxford Classical Dictionary*[3]; abbreviations for journals and periodicals follow those listed in the *American Journal of Archaeology* 95 (1991): 1–16; for items not listed there, I have followed the form in *L'Année Philologique* (Paris, 1927–). Abbreviations of epigraphic collections follow those in F. Bérard et al., *Guide de l'épigraphiste: Bibliographie choisie des épigraphies antiques et médiévales*[2] (Paris, 1989), 16–17; such collections that have been used in the composition of this book are listed below, pp. 229–30. Included here are works cited in the notes only by author's name or by an acronym, as well as those works not found in any of the above sources. For works cited occasionally in the notes but not frequently enough to warrant inclusion here, a short form of the title is used that is readily traceable in the main bibliography at the back of the book.

CGL	G. Goetz, ed. *Corpus Glossariorum Latinorum.* 7 vols. Leipzig, 1888–1923.
Curchin	L.A. Curchin. *The Local Magistrates of Roman Spain.* Toronto, 1990.
Degrassi	A. Degrassi. *I fasti consolari dell'impero romano dal 30 avanti Cristo al 613 dopo Cristo.* Rome, 1952.
Duncan-Jones, *Economy*	R. Duncan-Jones. *The Economy of the Roman Empire: Quantitative Studies*[2]. Cambridge, 1982.
Duncan-Jones, *Structure*	R. Duncan-Jones. *Structure and Scale in the Roman Economy.* Cambridge, 1990.
FTUR	G. Lugli. *Fontes ad Topographiam Veteris Urbis Romae Pertinentes.* 7 vols. Rome, 1952–69.
FUR	Carettoni, G., A.M. Colini, L. Cozza, and G. Gatti, eds. *La pianta marmorea di Roma antica, Forma Urbis Romae.* 2 vols. Rome, 1960.

Heinz

W. Heinz. *Römische Thermen: Badewesen und Badeluxus im römischen Reich*. Munich, 1983.

Jackson

R. Jackson. *Doctors and Diseases in the Roman Empire*. Norman, 1988.

Koloski-Ostrow

A.O. Koloski-Ostrow. *The Sarno Bath Complex*. Rome, 1990.

Laurence

R. Laurence. *Roman Pompeii: Space and Society*. London, 1994.

LTUR

E.M. Steinby, ed. *Lexicon Topographicum Urbis Romae*. Vols. 1 and 2. Rome, 1992, 1995.

Manderscheid

H. Manderscheid. *Bibliographie zum römischen Badewesen unter besonderer Berücksichtigung der öffentlichen Thermen*. Munich, 1988.

Manderscheid, *Skulpturenausstattung*

H. Manderscheid. *Die Skulpturenausstattung der kaiserzeitlichen Thermenanlagen*. Berlin, 1981.

Meiggs

R. Meiggs. *Roman Ostia*[2]. Oxford, 1973.

Merten

E.W. Merten. *Bäder und Badegepflogenheiten in der Darstellung der Historia Augusta*. Bonn, 1983.

MRR

T.R.S. Broughton. *The Magistrates of the Roman Republic*. 2 vols. Baltimore, 1951, 1952. Supplement, 1960.

Nielsen

I. Nielsen. Thermae et Balnea: *The Architecture and Cultural History of Roman Public Baths*[2]. 2 vols. Århus, 1993.

OLD

P.G.W. Glare, ed. *The Oxford Latin Dictionary*. Oxford, 1982.

Pasquinucci

M. Pasquinucci, ed. *Terme romane e vita quotidiana*. Modena, 1987.

PECS

R. Stillwell, ed. *The Princeton Encyclopedia of Classical Sites*. Princeton, 1976.

PGM[2]

H.D. Betz, ed. *The Greek Magical Papyri in Translation*[2]. Chicago, 1992.

PLRE

A.H.M. Jones, J.R. Martindale, and J. Morris. *The Prosopography of the Later Roman Empire*. Vols. 1 and 2. Cambridge, 1971, 1980.

RE	*Paulys Realencyclopädie der classischen Altertumswissenschaft.* Stuttgart, 1894–1980.
Richardson, *Dictionary*	L. Richardson jr. *A New Topographical Dictionary of Ancient Rome.* Baltimore, 1992.
Richardson, *Pompeii*	L. Richardson jr. *Pompeii: An Architectural History.* Baltimore, 1988.
Scarborough	J. Scarborough. *Roman Medicine.* Ithaca, 1969.
Solin	H. Solin. *Die griechischen Personennamen in Rom: Ein Namenbuch.* 3 vols. Berlin, 1982.
Sullivan	J.P. Sullivan. *Martial: The Unexpected Classic.* Cambridge, 1991.
Syll.	M. Rostovtzeff. *Tesserarum Urbis Romae et Suburbi Plumbearum Sylloge.* St. Petersburg, 1903.
Tab. Sulis	R.S.O. Tomlin. "*Tabellae Sulis:* Roman Inscribed Tablets of Tin and Lead from the Sacred Spring at Bath." In *The Temple of Sulis Minerva at Bath,* vol. 2, *The Finds from the Sacred Spring,* edited by B. Cunliffe, 59–277. Oxford, 1988.
Thermes	M. Lenoir, ed. *Les thermes romains: Actes de la table ronde organisée par l'École française de Rome.* Rome, 1991.
Thomasson	B.E. Thomasson. *Laterculi Praesidum.* 3 vols. Göteborg, 1972–90.
Toner	J.P. Toner. *Leisure and Ancient Rome.* Cambridge, 1995.
Veyne	P. Veyne. *Le pain et le cirque: Sociologie historique d'un pluralisme politique.* Paris, 1976.
Weber	M. Weber. *Antike Badekultur.* Munich, 1996.
Wesch-Klein	G. Wesch-Klein. Liberalitas in Rem Publicam: *Private Aufwendungen zugunsten von Gemeinden im römischen Afrika bis 284 n. Chr.* Bonn, 1990.
Yegül	F. Yegül. *Baths and Bathing in Classical Antiquity.* Cambridge, MA, 1992.

Introduction

For the Romans, bathing was a social event. The abundant physical remains of public baths stand in eloquent testimony to this fact and are found in almost every type of Roman settlement, from cities, towns, and hamlets to religious sanctuaries and frontier forts. Even Roman baths dubbed "private" by modern scholars—those located in domestic settings—were hardly so by the standards of today. Except for the very earliest examples, such baths were habitually designed to accommodate more than one bather, and written testimony makes it clear that they were used for such social purposes as welcoming visitors or extending dinner parties. We are clearly in the presence of a deeply rooted communal bathing habit, where the act of getting clean has become a social process, to be shared not only with invited guests (in private baths) but with everyone (in public ones).[1]

To most modern Western sensibilities, communal bathing is an alien concept. Public bathhouses are today generally associated with licentiousness and sexual promiscuity. Due in part to the thorough dissemination of efficient hydraulic and heating systems and also to a long-standing Christian heritage of abhorrence of bodily functions and public nudity, most Westerners bathe privately in their own homes. The same is not true the world over, however, and perhaps it will be useful to preface our examination of the now defunct Roman bathing culture by briefly surveying communal bathing habits that survive to this day, albeit often under siege from Western-influenced, private alternatives.

In western Europe, only the Finns still practice a truly public bathing habit. Their saunas are found all over the country, in private homes, attached

---

1. Some houses have two sets of "private" baths, one large and one small (an example is the Casa del Criptoportico at Pompeii [located at 1.6.2/4]). The best explanation for this arrangement is that the grander suite was for the use of the host and guests, while the smaller one was for everyday purposes. Roman private baths are in need of greater study. For preliminary work on the subject, see N. de Haan, "Privatbäder in Pompeji und Herkulaneum und die städtische Wasserleitung," *Mitteilungen des Leichtweiss-instituts für Wasserbau der Technischen Universität Braunschweig* 117 (1992): 423–45; id., "Dekoration und Funktion in den Privatbädern von Pompeji und Herculaneum," in E. M. Moormann, ed., *Functional and Spatial Analysis of Wall Painting,* (Leiden, 1993), 34–37; id., "Roman Private Baths," *Balnearia* 2, no. 2 (1994): 8–9. See also Pasquinucci, 77–78 (by M. Cerri).

to commercial premises, or as community services. As recently as 1970, 85 percent of the country's households were without a fixed bath or shower facility, despite piped water in 47 percent of households.[2] Nonetheless, most saunas today are of the domestic kind, and public facilities are in rapid decline as more and more people are able to afford their own installations. (It is important to note that public saunas are being replaced by private ones, not by showers or bathtubs.) In earlier times, when Finns built a homestead, the sauna was often the first structure erected; in fact, some families lived in the sauna rather than construct a separate dwelling.[3] The sauna ritual is complex and involves perspiration, sponging, and mild whisking with birch leaves dipped in hot water. Often beer, soft drinks, and snacks are consumed during breaks between bouts in the sauna chamber. Throughout, the company of other bathers is a vital component of the whole experience, even if the sauna is in a domestic setting. Finns prefer to take their saunas in the company of family members and friends rather than alone. Business conferences and even government cabinet meetings can convene there.[4] Finally, it is widely believed that the sauna has healing qualities. At one time, births used to take place in the sauna, and the ill would be treated there. In fact, research into the curative value of the sauna is still ongoing.[5]

Among the Japanese, bathing is so central an activity that it features in the opening scenes of their creation legend. Urban public baths were introduced to Japan only in the Edo period (1603–1868), but antecedents are known to have operated in association with Buddhist temples. More recently, under Western influence, public baths have declined sharply in popularity, and the spread of piped water and heating systems has enabled many people to enjoy a bath at home.[6] Nevertheless, the bathing customs of the temple, public,

---

2. See C.M. Sutyla, *The Finnish Sauna in Manitoba* (Ottawa, 1977), 25.

3. See C. Bremer and A. Raevuori, *The World of the Sauna* (Helsinki, 1986), 153–61 (public saunas), 9 (homestead).

4. Various groups—be they families, coworkers, schoolchildren, or friends—habitually take saunas together: see, e.g., Bremer and Raevuori, *World of the Sauna*, 23–33, 85–93 (families); 15–21, 115–29 (coworkers); 35–45 (schoolchildren); 73–83 (musicians in an orchestra); 131–37, 173–84 (friends). See also Sutyla, *Finnish Sauna*, 40 (cabinet meetings). Most companies and banks have "representation saunas" in which important negotiations with representatives from other companies take place. In fact, businesses compete with each other to boast the best-appointed "representation sauna"; see A. Paasilinna and T. Ovaska, *A Businessman's Guide to the Finnish Sauna* (Helsinki, 1984).

5. See Bremer and Raevuori, *World of the Sauna*, 12. The Finnish Sauna Society sponsors research into the medical aspects of sauna culture.

6. See P. Grilli and D. Levy, *Furo: The Japanese Bath* (Tokyo, 1985), esp. 22–26, 44–57 (religious associations); 73–83, 87–107 (public baths); 87–90, 165–66 (modern decline). The medieval Japanese association of baths with monasteries and charity is analogous to the situation in Europe in the early Middle Ages; see Yegül, 319.

and domestic bath have remained largely unchanged over the centuries and bear resemblance, in some respects, to documented ancient Roman practice. Like the Romans, the Japanese bathe communally in hot water; nudity is an accepted facet of the public bathing process; and the bath, despite its deep religious roots and associations, has evolved into a sensual, rather than a spiritual, experience. In their heyday, the public baths of Kyoto, Edo, and Osaka were social centers, where lovers met, philosophers debated, and commoners gossiped. In fact, some modern commentators are of the opinion that the decline of the *sento,* the neighborhood public bath, has led to a concomitant decline in community spirit, so that despite baths at home, some Japanese still take an occasional trip to the local public bathhouse. The Japanese, like the Finns, are also convinced that bathing, especially in hot springs, is medically beneficial in both a preventive and a remedial capacity.[7]

The Islamic bath *(hammam)* offers the closest parallels to ancient Roman practice. Unlike the Finnish sauna or the Japanese *sento,* it is a direct descendant of the once ubiquitous Roman *balneum.*[8] The public baths of modern countries like Tunisia or Turkey are also in decline as Western bathing habits spread through the urban areas, but there are still sixty-seven registered public baths in Istanbul, and it is unlikely that they will disappear altogether. In Tunisia, *hammam*s are still a thriving enterprise and are found all over the country. While medieval Westerners were espousing the principle of "going unwashed" *(alousia)* to prove the dominance of the soul over corporeal weakness, Islamic civilization was adhering to the public bathing habits of the ancients and preserving them for the modern age.[9] The similarities between Roman baths and the *hammam* are marked. Both feature a series of rooms through which one progresses, and specific procedures are restricted to the appropriate rooms. Both processes involve sweating, washing, and massage, all undertaken in a specified order. (Breach of this order at the *hammam* garners reprimands from other bathers, as I discovered from expe-

---

7. See Grilli and Levy, *Furo,* 90 (public bath and the community); 55–56, 132–41 (medicinal value).

8. For the links between ancient Roman and modern Islamic baths, see Pasquinucci, 110–11 (by P. Spinesi); Yegül, 339–49. The handbook for a Turkish bath in Montreal is entitled *The Modern Turkish or Roman Bath, St. Monique Street* (Ottawa, 1984). The public baths of the Arab world, of course, partly owe their continued existence to the purificatory requirements of Islam. However, the intensity of religious feeling varies from place to place, so that in a place like Tunisia the religious aspect of the process is less pronounced than in it would be in Iran, for instance.

9. On *alousia,* see Yegül, 318. On Islamic baths, see M. Ecochard and C. Le Coeur, *Les bains de Damas: Monographies architecturales,* 2 vols. (Beirut, 1942–43); H. Grotzfeld, *Das Bad im arabischen-islamischen Mittelalter: Eine kulturgeschichtliche Studie* (Wiesbaden, 1970).

rience.) In addition, both feature bath attendants available for hire, as well as separate facilities, sections, and/or bathing hours for men and women. The main differences are the replacement of communal immersion in the Roman bath with individual washing in buckets or at basins in the *hammam;* the nonacceptance of open nudity at the latter, in which individual cubicles are provided for those desiring a complete wash; and the substitution of a rub-down with an abrasive mitten in place of the Roman practice of anointing and strigiling. Also, for the most part, the ancient medium-hot room *(tepidarium)* has been abandoned, although I was told that some facilities still employ it.

Despite these procedural similarities and differences, a trip to the *hammam* is very similar to the Roman experience in its social nature. On one visit I made, for instance, a new entrant to the hottest room was expected to shake hands with everyone else present. The *hammam* is one of the chief places where friends meet and relax, chat, laugh, and spend time together. For women especially, it is the only public space where they can congregate and socialize together away from men. A visit to the *hammam* is not quite a leap back in time to ancient Rome, but it is a step in the right direction.

Some general observations can be made that appear to apply equally to Finnish, Japanese, and Islamic bathing customs. First, it seems that bathing in public can be more than just a bodily necessity—it can be a cultural choice. Second, the corporeal pleasures of bathing, when shared, tend to promote a sociability that in turn transforms essentially pragmatic public baths into meeting places and venues for social interaction. Third, the bathing ritual is often felt to be medically beneficial, not just for generating a sense of well-being, but also for curing illnesses. Finally, regular bathing is often associated with civilized living and spiritual purity. Too much reliance should not, however, be placed on raw comparisons between existing public bathing cultures and that of ancient Rome: we cannot expect to find accurate answers to Roman questions in the Japanese *sento,* the Finnish sauna, or even the Islamic *hammam.*[10] In the pages that follow, the references to surviving or better-documented bathing habits should be seen not as hard evidence for Roman conditions but as suggestive possibilities for ill-illumined aspects of Roman practice. A good example is provided by the question of spiritual purity and bathing, a feature shared by all of the modern bathing cultures just outlined. There is little evidence that the Romans, at least in pagan times, associated their local bathhouses with spiritual purifica-tion, even if they did appreciate the relaxing effects of taking a hot bath (see,

10. See M. Golden, "The Uses of Cross-Cultural Comparison in Ancient Social History," *EchCl* 11 (1992): 309–31.

e.g., Ter. *Phorm.* 339–40; Suet. *Vesp.* 21). Certainly, baths that stood in sanctuaries served as places for ritual cleansing, as well as offering more mundane services, and baths of all kinds carried divine associations with deities, such as Venus (for pleasure) and Asclepius (for health). But these associations do not appear to have had a specifically spiritual or cultic character, and they reflect more the physical pleasures and benefits of bathing rather than a religious or metaphysical desire for purity.[11] Definitive conclusions drawn from bald comparisons between certain aspects of modern public bathing cultures and their ancient counterparts should therefore be avoided.

Setting the Parameters of the Study

It would be impossible in the space provided by a study such as this one to review every aspect of Roman public bathing culture in all areas of the empire at all periods. Nevertheless, the organization of this work is largely thematic, asking several broad sociohistorical questions pertaining to the baths' operation: What was a trip to the baths like? When and why did they become popular? Who built and maintained them? Who used them? What sort of social function(s) did they serve? Given the mass of material that could be brought to bear on these questions, a sharper focus is essential. First, the ambiguity surrounding the term *public* requires clarification.[12] In the present context, there are two—by no means mutually exclusive— connotations for this word: "publicly owned" and "publicly accessible." Throughout this book, the latter connotation is preferred, so that the phrase *public bath* denotes those establishments that were open to the public, whether publicly or privately owned. Given this preference, rather arbitrary limits need to be placed on the sorts of facilities to be considered, if we are to avoid being swamped by the primary evidence or risking major distortions. Therefore, the main focus of what follows is first and foremost on those public baths that served the urban communities of the empire. As a result, several types of bathing establishment that undoubtedly served a communal function are excluded from the main thrust of the inquiry. Baths in a domes-

---

11. This is the position of Patriarch Gamaliel II, who, when accused of idolatry for visiting baths adorned with a statue of Aphrodite, replied that the statue was for decoration, not worship; see *m. Abod. Zar.* 3:4. In contrast, Jews are permitted in the Mishnah to help gentiles build bathhouses but must desist when construction reaches "the vaulting on which they set up an idol"; see *m. Abod. Zar.* 1:7.

12. On the difficulty of determining public from private in the Roman context, see A.M. Riggsby, " 'Public' and 'Private' in Roman Culture: The Case of the *Cubiculum*," *JRA* 10 (1997): 36–56. (Riggsby refers amply to important prior work on the subject.)

tic setting, despite their social character, are a good example. More openly accessible baths at locations that suggest peculiarities of function or of clientele are similarly best left to one side. Two examples are military baths and those in religious sanctuaries.[13] Both types are usually typologically indistinguishable from "normal" public baths and appear not to have excluded the general public entirely—as the discovery of children's teeth and women's accoutrements at the fortress bathhouse at Caerleon proves conclusively, at least for that facility.[14] But presumably both catered chiefly to the needs of rather restricted categories of bathers, soldiers in one case and pilgrims in the other. To be sure, the operation of military and sanctuary baths raises interesting questions: Did officers and men bathe together (see HA *Pesc. Nig.* 3.10)? What proportion of military baths were open to the public? If civilians were permitted, were all comers or only members of soldiers' families welcome? Did soldiers and civilians bathe simultaneously? Did sanctuary baths serve a primarily religious or secular purpose? Regrettably, such questions cannot be meaningfully addressed here without diverting the inquiry considerably. Another type of facility it seems advisable to pass over is the Greek gymnasium of Roman date or the hybrid bath-gymnasium found so plentifully in the Greek East.[15] Gymnasia played a particular role in the Greek tradition, and it remains unclear to what extent that role continued into Roman times; in any case, their social function appears to have been quite different from that of the urban public baths that interest us, even if there were significant overlaps.[16] However, should any of these excluded catego-

---

13. *Mansio* baths, facilities attached to imperial road-stations, are a related type. They seem to have been open to the local population, while also serving traveling imperial officials; see the examples at Chelmsford in Britain (N. Wickenden, *Caesaromagus: A History and Description of Roman Chelmsford* [Chelmsford, 1991], 10–13), Valesio in Italy (J. Boersma, "Le terme tardoromane di Valesio (Salento)," in *Thermes*, 161–73; id., Mutatio Valentia: *The Late Roman Baths at Valesio, Salento* [Amsterdam, 1995]), and Ad Quintum in Macedonia (Nielsen, 2.43 [C.352]). Many such *mansiones* may have formed the core of the small towns of Roman Britain, with the baths perhaps serving as a stimulus for the rise of a community spirit; see B.C. Burnham and J. Wacher, *The "Small Towns" of Roman Britain* (Berkeley, 1990), 4–5, 12–14.

14. See J.D. Zienkiewicz, *The Legionary Fortress Baths at Caerleon*, vol. 2, *The Finds* (Cardiff, 1986), 223 (teeth), 146–55 (R.J. Brewer on beads from necklaces), 196–202 (S.J. Greep on pins and needles).

15. On these structures, see A. Farrington, "Imperial Bath Buildings in South-West Asia Minor," in S. Macready and F.H. Thompson, eds., *Roman Architecture in the Greek World*, (London, 1987), 50–59; Nielsen, 1.104–11; Yegül, 250–313, and id., *The Bath-Gymnasium Complex at Sardis* (Cambridge, MA, 1986).

16. On gymnasia, see J. Delorme, *Gymnasion: Étude sur les monuments consacrés à l'éducation en Grèce* (Paris, 1960). On the continuance of their traditional role, see Farrington, "Imperial Bath Buildings."

ries of building offer evidence relevant to conditions at the Roman urban public bath, it will be mentioned, albeit suitably qualified.

Next, there is the issue of geographic and chronological parameters. Certain chapters, by their content, set their own limits. The inquiry into the growth and spread of the bathing habit focuses perforce on Rome and Italy in the late Republic and early Empire. For the more thematic chapters, the establishment of limits is more difficult. Over its thousand-year history, Roman bathing culture must have displayed regional variations and undergone change over time.[17] But certain conditions (such as the prevalent social atmosphere or the taking of snacks) must have been all but universal. Since the evidence derives from all parts of the empire and from all times, it seems unnecessarily restrictive to exclude a particularly illuminating item by setting strict geographic and chronological limits for the thematic chapters. Throughout this study, the main focus is on the western empire in the era sometimes termed the "central period" (ca. 200 B.C. to A.D. 200), but instructive material from the East and from the late Empire will not be passed over in silence.[18]

The Sources

I may as well insert, as I might at almost every point in this essay, my sense of frustration in describing matters taken for granted among the contemporaries of the Empire and therefore little reported—matters which (as the ancients would have said) were undignified, contributed nothing to their sense of what counted, and therefore were seldom mentioned in their proper works of literature. We catch only random hints. At best they are suggestive.[19]

The student of Roman bathing culture can fully identify with Ramsay Mac-Mullen's frustration: no ancient writer provides a detailed account of life at

---

17. Certain features of some Roman baths in the Greek East, for instance, suggest regional variations in the procedures of bathing. Some establishments have central galleries that allow the bather to pick and choose between rooms, rather than being channeled purposefully from one to the other; examples are Bath II 7A at Anemurium in Cilicia, Baths I 2A at Antiochea-ad-Cragum in Cilicia, and the Baths of Trajan and Hadrian at Cyrene (for all of these examples, see the appropriate plans in A. Farrington, *The Roman Baths of Lycia: An Architectural Study* [Ankara, 1995], esp. 7–15).

18. For the "central period," see K.R. Bradley, *Slavery and Society at Rome* (Cambridge, 1994), 6.

19. R. MacMullen, *Roman Social Relations, 50 B.C. to A.D. 284* (New Haven, 1974), 41.

the baths, and most refer to it allusively, providing the modern investigator with mere glimmers and glimpses. Despite their volume, therefore, deploying and interpreting the sources in pursuit of answers to specific sociohistorical questions proves challenging and, on occasion, fruitless. As a result, the nature of the evidence and strategies for approaching it deserve consideration.[20]

Prodigious quantities of material—archaeological, epigraphic, and literary—pertain to Roman baths. It would take several lifetimes to sift through and master it all, so I make no claim here to comprehensiveness in citing it. Of the urban public bathhouse alone, the remains of more than one thousand examples must be known from the empire, most not fully published. Hundreds of inscriptions attest the existence of baths and record the actions of their benefactors. In addition, scores of literary references mention baths and bathing in a wide variety of contexts. As if this were not enough, new material is constantly coming to light. I have been as thorough as possible in presenting the available evidence, while at the same time not wishing to overburden the notes with an unnecessary proliferation of repetitive supporting citations. The notes, therefore, present a representative sample of evidence and should not be viewed as offering the final word on the matters they address. It is hoped that new evidence will illuminate, rather than undermine, the thrust of my presentation.

In general, two chief problems exist in assessing the ancient sources for bathing culture. The first is the difficulty of tying the varying types of evidence together. Archaeology has revealed scores of bath buildings in varying states of preservation. These remains allow detailed study of their architecture and technology but reveal little about the actual experience of the bathers. For this experience, the written evidence is crucial. There is also an abundance of this material, but it too is of varying quality. Inscriptions, for instance, tend to be highly formulaic, recording constructional activity or bath-related benefactions, such as gifts of free bathing and/or oil; far less frequently do they throw light on the bathers themselves. The literary material is the most useful for reconstructing the bathing experience, since it helps to illuminate attitudes toward baths and frequently offers vignettes of Roman bathers in action. But rarely do any of these classes of evidence interconnect directly. The continued widespread confusion over ancient bath-related terminology serves as an illustration. Since so few inscriptions and even

---

20. For a fuller discussion of the nature of the sources and problems of interpretation, see G.G. Fagan, "Interpreting the Evidence," in D.E. Johnston and J. DeLaine, eds., *Roman Baths and Bathing,* (Portsmouth, RI, forthcoming).

fewer literary allusions can be securely associated with surviving remains, putting written and archaeological sources together proves difficult, if not impossible in many cases. Ball courts *(sphaeristeria)* are an apt example. Despite the huge volume of physical remains of baths and numerous written references to them, few ball courts can be securely identified in the archaeological record. In fact, it remains unclear if such courts were covered rooms, open areas, or both. The same uncertainty surrounds the nature of many other rooms alluded to in the written sources, such as entrance halls *(atria* or *basilica thermarum)* or scraping-off rooms *(destrictaria).*[21] Indeed, the function of many nonheated rooms in surviving ruins, especially in the larger facilities, stands open to question.[22] One aim of this book is to try to take into account all the available types of evidence in pursuing certain questions, but we must avoid forcing the often incompatible material into offering answers that it is not equipped to yield.

The second major difficulty with the sources is that of typicality. It is highly unlikely that Roman bathing habits were constant and unchanging over their thousand-year history and throughout the length and breadth of the empire. So how can we be sure that any piece of data—which is, after all, the product of a specific time and place—illustrates a general norm rather than a local variation? There is no secure way out of this quandary, but perhaps the best way forward is to look for instances where data from a variety of times and places point in the same direction. Such a coincidence cannot offer complete peace of mind, but it does mollify concern to some degree. Uncertainty over typicality also requires that the ancient evidence be treated with critical respect. At the same time, it would be tedious and repetitious to lay out all of the options every time uncertainty exists. Therefore, where the problem is acute, detailed discussion can be found in the footnotes; otherwise, the issue of typicality is to be borne in mind by the reader at all times when assessing the evidence. It limits our conclusions but hopefully does not obviate them.

---

21. A list of parts of baths mentioned in the epigraphic sample is provided in appendix 3. For *sphaeristeria,* see nos. 54 and 55; Pliny *Ep.* 2.17.11, 5.6.27; *Dig.* 17.1.16. A part of the palaestra in the Stabian Baths has been proposed as a *sphaeristerium;* see H. Eschebach, *Die Stabianer Thermen in Pompeji* (Berlin, 1979), 17, 61, 70. For the uncertainty over *atria* and *basilica thermarum* and *destrictaria,* see Nielsen, 1.162 (s.v. "basilica thermarum") and 165 (s.v. "destrictarium"). For a recent attempt (not entirely conclusive) to make sense of some of these terms, see R. Rebuffat, "Vocabulaire thermal: Documents sur le bain romain," in *Thermes,* 1–34.

22. This was brought home to me on a visit to the Thermae of Diocletian in 1989, when Dott.ssa D. Candilio of the Museo Nazionale in Rome could offer no explanation for the function(s) of several huge vaulted chambers adjacent to the Basilica Santa Maria degli Angeli.

The Bathing Ritual

The Roman bathing ritual was complicated, combining what in modern terms would be considered a visit to the gymnasium, bathroom, and massage parlor.[23] The bather entered the establishment, disrobed, was anointed with oils, and then exercised, usually by playing ball games of one sort or another (see, e.g., Mart. 7.32). Once a good sweat had been worked up, the bathing process proper was embarked on. A series of variously heated rooms confronted the customer, and it was largely a matter of choice which rooms were visited and in what order. The most basic bath required a visit to the medium-heated room, then the hottest room, and then back through the medium-heated room to the cold room. Depending on the size and luxury of the establishment, all of these rooms could have pools, heated to the appropriate degree. Optional amenities could also be on offer, such as very hot sweat chambers or open-air swimming pools. Despite the volume of ancient evidence pertaining to the baths, it is not clear at what stage the main wash took place—a vivid illustration of the limitations of our sources. At some point along the route, often in the medium-heated room, the bather enjoyed a strigiling—scraping with specially designed instruments called *strigiles*— to remove the oil and sweat and dirt that had accumulated while exercising. Finally, the bather dried off and, for those who could afford it, was anointed with perfumes; the bather then changed into fresh clothes and went home.

Even with the possibility of taking a quick bath, the full process was complex and demanded a considerable amount of time to complete, so it was almost inevitable that a trip to the baths became a social event. Given what we have seen of other bathing cultures that are comparably sociable and leisurely, it is hardly surprising that Roman baths became community centers of sorts, places where a variety of people could meet, bathe, chat, snack, drink, and relax. The majority of this book is primarily concerned with these "secondary" aspects of the bathing ritual, although, given the relative apportioning of space in later baths as compared to earlier ones, one begins to wonder whether it was the bathing itself that ultimately became secondary.[24]

---

23. For ancient outlines of the process, see, e.g., Pliny *HN* 28.55; Mart. 6.42; Petron. *Sat.* 28. For modern accounts, see Heinz, 142–56; Pasquinucci, 22–39, 48–60, esp. 22–24 (by D. Alessi); Weber, 54–67; Yegül, 33–40.

24. Thus the heated areas—i.e., for those "practical" bathing purposes—account for 33 percent of the total area of early baths (e.g., the Forum Baths, Pompeii) but much less (between 21 and 29 percent) of later baths of comparable size (e.g., North Baths, Cemelenum; Silchester; Weissenburg). In the large "imperial" establishments at Rome, the functional area was even smaller, comprising only 18 percent of the total area of the Baths of Trajan, for instance; see J. DeLaine, "New Models, Old Modes: Continuity and Change in the Design of Public Baths," in

Throughout this book, the focus is on the people who used the baths and those who provided and maintained them, rather than on the buildings themselves. Surveys of apparently well-worn subjects aim not to recap the work of others but to put that work into a broader sociohistorical perspective. Thus, when we look at the baths of Rome, we are interested not in the physical remains and the myriad interpretative difficulties they present but in who was responsible for this construction, under what circumstances they acted, and why. This investigation starts with an assessment of what a visit to the baths was like, as can be reconstructed primarily from the *Epigrams* of Martial, one of our most informative sources on the everyday workings of Roman bathing culture. The inquiry then adopts a quasi-diachronic form, as it turns to the issue of when and why the baths became popular at Rome and in Italy. An attempt to account for that popularity follows. This attempt leads to consideration of the connection between baths and medicine and, more particularly, to the possibility that the eminent doctor Asclepiades of Bithynia played a role in promoting regular bathing among the Romans in the late second and early first centuries B.C.

The focus of this study then shifts to the issue of responsibility for bath construction, which is investigated in two parts, the first covering Rome, the second covering Italy and the provinces. For the latter, inscriptional evidence proves vital. The epigraphic sample included in this book presents pertinent Latin inscriptions that record not only acts of constructional benefaction (i.e., the erection, repair, extension, and adornment of baths) but also non-constructional activities (e.g., offers of free bathing and provisions of oil); there are also nonbenefactory texts (e.g., advertisements for baths and bathroom-wall graffiti) and a sample of Greek texts for purposes of comparison.[25] (Throughout the book, entries in the epigraphic sample are referred to by number alone, in the form "no. 1" or "nos. 1, 2, 3," etc.) As a preface to the topic of the baths as social centers, a brief consideration of the physical environment at the baths follows the study of benefactors. Finally, the bathers themselves are examined in detail, to learn their social identities and the degree of their social mixing and interaction at the baths, and thereby to discern something of the broad social function of the urban bathhouse in Roman civilization.

H.-J. Schalles, H. von Hesberg, and P. Zanker, eds., *Die römische Stadt im 2. Jahrhundert n. Chr.: Der Funktionswandel des öffentlichen Raumes* (Bonn, 1992), 257–75.

25. For a fuller explanation of the criteria employed in selecting the inscriptions and of the organizational principles behind the epigraphic sample, see the introduction to the sample.

Chapter 1

A Visit to the Baths with Martial

There are very few ancient descriptions of what a visit to the baths was like. Some sources recount the physical surroundings that confronted the bather (usually positively), and a variety of others provide informative, if allusive, details, but only a handful actually describe a visit to the baths in any coherent fashion.[1] Three examples stand out. The first is the schoolbooks *(colloquia),* usually of late Imperial date, that were designed to acquaint the pupil with the vocabulary and protocols of daily life.[2] In addition to the baths, they cover such mundanities as getting up, eating lunch, visiting the forum, and bedtime. While the style may not be high literature, these schoolbooks offer an unusually candid glimpse into the bathing process, albeit in a somewhat detached and clinical fashion as imposed by their didactic purpose. The second noteworthy source is the lengthy complaint in Seneca's *Epistles* about how annoying it was for him to live over a bathhouse at Baiae.[3] He lists at length the noises that emanated from the baths: the slaps

Throughout, all dates are A.D. unless otherwise stated. Unless otherwise indicated, the text and translation of Martial used throughout this book are the most recent available, those of D.R. Shackleton Bailey in the Loeb Classical Library (1993), the text of which largely reproduces his Teubner edition (1990).

1. For surroundings, see Mart. 6.42; Stat. *Silv.* 1.5; Vitr. 5.10; Sen. *Ep.* 86.4–13; Pliny *Ep.* 2.17.11, 5.6.25–27; Luc. *Hipp.* For other allusions to the pleasures of the baths, often expressed in terms of the presence there of Eros, nymphs, and the Graces, see L. Robert, "Épigrammes relatives à des gouverneurs," *Hellenica* 4 (1948): 76–84; K.M.D. Dunbabin, "*Baiarum Grata Voluptas:* Pleasures and Dangers of the Baths," *BSR* 57 (1989): 12–32.

2. See A.C. Dionisotti, "From Ausonius's Schooldays? A Schoolbook and Its Relatives," *JRS* 72 (1982): 83–125. Other informative schoolbooks include the *Colloquia Monacensia* (*CGL* 3.644–54) and the *Colloquium Montepessulanum* (*CGL* 3.654–59). Most such schoolbooks date to the third century or later.

3. Sen. *Ep.* 56.1–2. Seneca writes that he lived *supra ipsum balneum,* which would seem to mean, as translated in the Loeb Classical Library edition (R.M. Gummere, 1917), "right over a bathing establishment" (for a *cenaculum* over a bathhouse in Pompeii, see no. 258). Another possibility, however, is that the phrase means "right up the road from a bathhouse," in which case the din Seneca describes must have been considerable to disturb his musings. Physical remains, even from the same site, support both interpretations. Some of the smaller baths at Ostia, such as the Baths of the Philosopher, are built on the lower floors of larger *insulae* and can feature apartments above; see J. Boersma, Amoenissima Civitas: *Block V.ii at Ostia—*

of the masseur, the song of the loud bather, the roars of the food-stall owners, the rumpus accompanying the arrest of a thief. The passage nicely captures the voluble social atmosphere that was no doubt a regular feature of a visit to any of the empire's public baths. Finally, there is the instructive *Life of Aesop,* an anonymous first-century Egyptian composition that is concerned with the often unbearably childish relationship between a cunning slave and his frequently fooled owner and so is replete with vignettes of daily life among those levels of society habitually neglected in more formal tracts. Although set in a Greek context, the *Life* clearly reflects the norms and habits of the early Imperial Roman period, and bathing features heavily.[4]

All of these sources, then, are useful in their own way (and so will be referred to again below), but they offer only glimpses into the social atmosphere that prevailed at the baths, and they allow little to be said about the salient features of the broader bathing culture in its social context. For this sort of information, the *Epigrams* of the satiric poet M. Valerius Martialis are of unparalleled usefulness.

By the time Martial left Rome for his native Bilbilis in Spain in 98, he had lived in the imperial capital for some thirty-four years.[5] During this extended sojourn, he subsisted on patronage, inheritances, and favors given in return for writing poetry on commission for the wealthy and the vain. He did well over the years and ended up living in a townhouse, owning a small farm at Nomentum, and earning equestrian status.[6] He himself asserts that the focus of his poetry was not the mythological achievements of legendary heroes but the humdrum of humanity he observed around him (10.4.8–12). Although the pages of Martial may not be reliable for determining precise historical details—such as the true identities behind the pseudonyms he lends some of his characters—the effectiveness of his satiric verse rests on reference to the

---

Description and Analysis of Its Visible Remains (Assen, 1985), 131–32. Many baths stand in close proximity to living quarters: see Meiggs, 416–17; J.E. Packer, *The Insulae of Imperial Ostia* (Rome, 1971), 74.

4. For the date, composition, and nature of this work, see B.E. Perry's Loeb Classical Library edition of *Baebrius and Phaedrus* (1965), xxxv–xlvi; L.W. Daly, *Aesop without Morals* (New York, 1961), 19–23. Future references are to the text of Perry's edition, *Aesopica* (Urbana, 1952).

5. Two references in book 10—published originally in 95 and in a revised form in 98—provide essential biographical details: 10.24 was composed for Martial's fifty-seventh birthday, and 10.103.7–9, composed close to his departure in 98, states that he had been in Rome for thirty-four years; see Sullivan, 1–6, 44–55.

6. See Mart. 9.18.2 and 9.97.8 (townhouse), 2.38 (farm), 3.95.9–10 (equestrian status); Pliny *Ep.* 3.21.3 (poetry on commission). For a recent overview of Martial's life and work, see Sullivan, 6–55, esp. 26–30.

shared cultural and social experiences of its audience.[7] The value of Martial's allusions to baths and bathing, therefore, is precisely that they play on the audience's acquaintance and familiarity with the situations the poet describes or remarks on. As a result, Martial presents the modern reader with a particularly clear window onto the social operation of public baths at Rome in the late first century A.D.[8] At the same time, however, it must be appreciated that Martial's evidence is tied to a specific time and place. It is therefore subject to the problem of typicality discussed above in the introduction, and it remains very possible, if not likely, that Martial's portrayal of Roman bathing culture will prove misleading if applied wholesale to the wider Roman world. That is why below, where possible, Martial's testimony is compared with other sources from different times and occasionally from different places, so that alternatives to his depictions are also presented, and so that the wider operation of the baths can be glimpsed. Nevertheless, the richness and unusual candidness of Martial's evidence remains remarkable, and with its limitations realized, it can function as a prism through which we can observe the poet's contemporaries as they bathed. We can, in effect, visit the baths with Martial as our guide.

Thermae and Balnea

On numerous occasions, Martial differentiates between the two types of baths at Rome: the *thermae* and *balnea*.[9] The ancient evidence for the meanings of these terms is so contradictory that trying to disentangle it has proven an intractable problem for modern scholarship.[10] Logical efforts at rationalization are confounded by the evidence. For instance, a conceivable solution

---

7. On the relationship of poetry, albeit principally of the Augustan period, to real life, see J. Griffin, *Latin Poets and Roman Life* (London, 1985), 48–64; on Martial in particular, see Sullivan, esp. xxii–xxiv. On the general usefulness of anecdotal material for deducing this sort of information, see R.P. Saller, "Anecdotes as Historical Evidence for the Principate," *GaR* 27 (1980): 69–83.

8. Martial refers expressly to baths and bathing dozens of times and alludes to the practice on several other occasions.

9. See Mart. 2.14.11–13, 2.48, 3.20.15–16, 7.34.10, 9.75, 12.82.1–2. Martial is not alone: the late Imperial Regionaries also draw the distinction, the *balnea* far outweighing the *thermae* in number, 856 to 11 (*Notitia Urbis Regionum* 14 = *FTUR* 1.1.5). The distinction extended beyond Rome: a glance through the texts collected in the epigraphic sample reveals *thermae* and *balnea* in abundance, sometimes in clear distinction (see, e.g., nos. 102, 215; *CIL* 13.1132).

10. So, for instance, the Baths of Sura in Rome are listed as *thermae* in the Regionaries (*FTUR* 1.1.5) but as *Bal(nea)* on the Marble Map: see *FUR* fr. 21 (pl. XXIII); E. Rodríguez Almeida, Forma Urbis Marmorea: *Aggiornamento generale, 1980* (Rome, 1981), fr. 21 (pl. XV). Contradictions like this lead Heinz (27–29) and Nielsen (1.3) to despair of ever distinguishing the ancient definitions of the terms.

is to follow etymological reasoning and conclude that *thermae* were heated baths and that *balnea* were thus unheated. But the clear and abundant evidence for heated *balnea* renders this suggestion untenable.[11] Modern scholars have proposed distinguishing the buildings by virtue of their relative size—*balnea* occupied part of a city block; *thermae* were much larger—or have suggested that *thermae* were publicly owned, *balnea* privately so.[12] A recent attempt to define the two types of building by modern typological classifications (primarily by the presence or absence of an exercise court, a palaestra) is inherently flawed and has met with little acceptance.[13] Since ancient evidence can be adduced in support of all but the last of these possibilities, confusion prevails.[14]

The search for firm and universally applicable definitions that take into account and accord with all the ancient material is therefore unrealistic for these terms. Instead, it has to be accepted that usage often varies from writer to writer and even within the works of individual authors. Martial is a case in point. He speaks of the city's "three *thermae*" in obvious reference to the large-scale public establishments of Agrippa, Nero, and Titus (which he consistently labels *thermae* when he names them individually), but he then applies the word to private bath suites in people's villas.[15] Since it is unlikely that the private *thermae* he mentions were on the huge scale of the imperial establishments, size cannot be his chief criterion of distinction; nor can ownership, since he applies the term *thermae* to private and public facilities alike. What, if anything, lies behind the differentiation in Martial's eyes? In several

11. Thus the Loeb translation of Seneca (J.W. Basore, 1932) translates *balnearia et thermas* (*Dial.* 9.9.7) as "cold baths and hot baths." Note also that D.R. Shackleton Bailey's recent Loeb Classical Library edition of Martial (1993) frequently renders *thermae* as "warm baths" (e.g., at *Spect.* 2.5–7; *Ep.* 2.14.11–13, 2.78, 3.25). For heated *balnea*, however, see, e.g., Petron. *Sat.* 41; Sen. *Ep.* 86.10; Pliny *HN* 11.99, 23.54, 25.77, 31.40, 31.102; Pliny *Ep.* 3.14; Plut. *Mar.* 12.4. Inscriptions also describe heated baths (with hypocausts) as *balnea* or *balneum*; see, e.g., nos. 50 and 239.

12. For size, see, e.g., Meiggs, 416; F. Yegül, "The Small City Bath in Classical Antiquity and a Reconstruction Study of Lucian's 'Baths of Hippias,'" *ArchCl* 31 (1979): 108–31. For ownership, see, e.g., Shackleton Bailey's Loeb Classical Library edition of Martial (1993), vol. 1, p. 14, note b. For ownership and size in combination, see Richardson, *Dictionary*, 385–86, s.v. "Thermae, Balineum, Lavacrum"; Yegül, 43.

13. See Nielsen, esp. 1.3, and the reviews of J. DeLaine ("Roman Baths and Bathing," *JRA* 6 [1993]: 348–58); G.G. Fagan (*Hermathena* 152 [1992]: 100–105); and F. Yegül (*AJA* 97 [1993]: 185–86).

14. For size, see, e.g., no. 102, where *balneae* at Lanuvium are replaced with *thermae, ampliatis locis et cellis*. For ownership, see, e.g., CGL 3.651.10, where the question *ad thermas aut in privato?* implies that *thermae* were publicly owned.

15. Mart. 2.14.13, 10.51.12 (three *thermae*); 2.48.8, 3.20.15–16, 3.36.1–6, 7.34 (individually named *thermae*); 2.78, 9.75, 10.79.3–4, 11.51 (private *thermae*). The link between public *thermae* and large villa baths is currently being investigated by J. DeLaine.

passages, the poet seems to indicate that, for him, the defining feature of *thermae* was luxury of environment, especially as manifested in elaborate decoration.

> Non silice duro structilive caemento
> nec latere cocto, quo Samiramis longam
> Babylona cinxit, Tucca balneum fecit:
> sed strage nemorum pineaque compage,
> ut navigare Tucca balneo possit.
> idem beatas lautus extruit thermas
> de marmore omni, quod Carystos invenit,
> quod Phrygia Synnas, Afra quod Nomas misit
> et quod virenti fonte lavit Eurotas.
> sed ligna desunt: subice balneum thermis.
>
>   (9.75)

[Tucca did not make his *balneum* of hard stone or concrete or burnt brick, with which Samiramis girdled the length of Babylon, but with the wreckage of woods and a framework of pine, so that Tucca could go to sea in his *balneum*. The same luxurious Tucca constructed fine *thermae* of every marble that Carystus discovered, that Phrygian Synnas or African Numidia exported, that Eurotas laved with his verdant stream. But wood is lacking: put the *balneum* under the *thermae*. (trans. adapted)]

For the sake of effect, the juxtaposition here—a wooden *balneum* contrasted to a stone and finely marbled *thermae,* which, admittedly, may be a public bath of some size—is particularly stark. But the basic point is clear enough: the *thermae* were luxuriously appointed; the *balneum* was not. (The joke lies in Martial's suggestion that the *balneum* be used to heat the *thermae,* when he recommends that the former be burnt in the hypocaust under the latter.) Comparable is the poem about one Torquatus who builds (apparently private) *thermae* "of varied marble" *(vario de marmore),* in contrast to his poor neighbor, who can only build a cooking pot (10.79). The most extensive description of a *thermae*-style bathhouse in Martial is that of the Baths of Etruscus, which were lavishly appointed and featured a myriad of marbles and other stones, fine lighting, and excellent water quality (6.42). It may seem significant at first glance that Martial calls these baths *thermulae,* "little *thermae,*" possibly implying that size did in some way feature in his definition of *thermae*. It could be argued that Martial thought that the lavish decoration had earned Etruscus' baths the label *thermae,* but the building was on a smaller scale than he would normally associate with *thermae* proper. The requirements of poetic meter, however, cannot be ignored here. *Thermulae* is a rare word in Latin,[16] so it is quite possible that Martial used it primarily out of metrical considerations, with only secondary concern for its semantics. As a reminder of the inconsistency across the sources, it should be noted that Statius denotes Etruscus' facility with the word *balnea* (*Silv.* 1.5.13).

Altogether, Martial can be seen to apply the term *thermae* to buildings that were lavishly and luxuriously decorated, whether they were large-scale imperial facilities or finely furnished and presumably smaller private establishments. *Balnea,* in contrast, appear as simpler, more run-of-the-mill bathhouses. Scrutiny of the appearance of the two terms in a variety of sources points to a broad chronological distinction that may have influenced Martial's use of them in these passages. No Republican source applies the word *thermae* to a bathhouse; rather, *balneum, balnea,* and *balneae* are preferred.[17] In fact, the term *thermae* does not appear until the first century A.D., and then it is used only in reference to a private facility.[18] In Martial's day, it seems that *balnea* was (widely?) used to denote baths of the older Republican type. It can therefore be postulated that calling baths *thermae* came into fashion only in the first century A.D., when bathing luxury was on the rise, and when bath decoration, in particular, was getting increasingly lavish (see Sen. *Ep.* 86.6–7, 90.25). Given the splendor of the imperial *thermae,* it is hardly surprising that they were thus called and that, given their size, scale also came to be associated with the word (see no. 102). But truly magnificent private baths, although on a smaller scale than the imperial facilities, could also earn the title; indeed, it seems initially to have been applied only to

16. It is also found in an inscription from Lugudunum advertising *thermulae salutares,* which were probably fed by hot springs; see no. 255.

17. See, e.g., Varro *Ling.* 9.68; Cic. *Cael.* 61–67. (The Republican written evidence is treated in more detail in chapter 2.) This detail is also noted by Richardson, *Dictionary,* 385–86, s.v. "Thermae, Balineum, Lavacrum."

18. It is used in reference to the *thermae* of Cn. Domitius Ahenobarbus, consul in 32 (*PIR*[2] D 127). Seneca the Elder (*Controv.* 9.4.18) reports the words of Vallius Syriacus, a contemporary of Domitius (on whom, see *RE* 8A.2391, sv. "Vallius 5" [Helm]). Note that Seneca the Younger also applies the term only to private baths, on the two occasions when he uses it (*Dial.* 9.9.7 and *Ep.* 122.8). Exactly when the word came to denote large-scale public facilities is unclear. An inscription from Spain commemorating the construction of *thermae* (no. 158) has been dated by letterform to the Augustan period, but it may stem from any time in the first century A.D.

private baths.[19] From this perspective, whether baths were termed *thermae* or *balnea* approaches a value judgment, rendering all but futile the search for defining characteristics of either "type" in the scale or form of surviving remains. In all likelihood, there was a wide latitude of personal choice in what one called a bathhouse—hence the confusion and contradiction in the sources—and one suspects that a tendency to grandiloquence could prevail, in that calling an establishment *thermae* added an air of sophistication to an otherwise nondescript facility. A parallel is provided by a change in the nomenclature of places where gladiatorial spectacles were staged, from *spectaculum* to *amphitheatrum*. As with *balneum* and its variants, *spectaculum* was a plainer term that denoted both the activity and its locus, whereas *amphitheatrum*, like *thermae*, had a sophisticated Greek sound to it.[20] So although Martial does not definitively solve the semantic problem of *thermae* and *balnea*, he does offer a thread that may assist in making future headway through the terminological labyrinth.

Martial provides little information about *balnea*. He names them occasionally, mentioning the Balnea of Stephanus near his house, the Balnea of Charinus, the Balnea of Lupus, Gryllus, Faustus, and Fortunatus (which may have been known as "The Four Baths"), and the Balnea of Tigellinus—the latter apparently quite splendid, since they find mention in the same breath as the Thermae of Titus and Agrippa.[21] Many of these establishments appear to have been situated in the Campus Martius: Martial reports that when Selius is out hunting dinner invitations, he spends his day in that part of the city, at the Thermae of Agrippa, at the Balnea of Lupus, Gryllus, Faustus, and

---

19. Privately owned *thermae* are known at Rome from various sources, but it is often unclear whether or not they were open to the public: e.g., known from Regio VI are the *Thermae Novati, Olympiadis, Sallustianae, Tiberianae,* and *Timothei* (listed sequentially in *FTUR* 4.13.421–43). Known from Regio V are the *Thermae Helenianae*, probably a part of an Imperial-era villa complex (*FTUR* 4.12.290–91; Yegül, 86).

20. *Spectaculum* is amply attested in Republican sources as denoting the place for the staging of spectacles: see, e.g., Plaut. *Curc.* 647; Cic. *Har. resp.* 22 and *Sest.* 124; *CIL* 10.852 = *ILS* 5627 (Pompeii; ca. 80 B.C.). In contrast, *amphitheatrum* only appears in the Augustan period: see Vitr. 1.7.1; *RG* 22.3; *AE* 1938.110 (Luceria; ca. 2 B.C.). See R. Étienne, "La naissance de l'amphithéâtre: Le mot et la chose," *REL* 43 (1966): 213–20.

21. See Mart. 11.52.4, 14.60 (Stephanus); 7.34 (Charinus); 1.59.3, 2.14.12 (Lupus and Gryllus); 2.14.11 (Faustus and Fortunatus); 5.70.4 ("Four Baths"); 3.20.16 (Tigellinus). It should be noted that reference to a *balnea* of Charinus might be a joke: the name *Charinus* is attested only three times at Rome (see Solin, 3.1298, s.v.), and seems to have denoted "pervert," in much the same way that the names *Don Juan* and *Casanova* denote a romantic lover today; see *RE* 3.2143–44, s.v. "Charinos 7" (Stein). In all, dozens of *balnea* can be named from Rome, though hardly a trace of any survives (or, at least, few have been published); see appendix 2.

Fortunatus, and at various other public landmarks.[22] Likewise, Martial's house was located on a spur of the Quirinal Hill overlooking the Campus, so that the Balnea of Stephanus can be located in much the same vicinity. No doubt, however, *balnea* of varying quality could be found all over Martial's Rome, as the Regionaries make clear for a later age (see appendix 2). What architectural features distinguished the older *balnea*-type of bathhouse from *thermae* can no longer be ascertained with certainty in every case, since the two terms were so liberally applied to baths of various types. But if we can draw reliable implications from the relatively few Republican baths that have been investigated and published (often incompletely)—for example, those in Campania at Pompeii, Herculaneum, Cumae, and Cales—*balnea* were rather functional, poorly lit facilities sporting stucco, rather than marble, decoration and lacking statuary and other ornate refinements (see figs. 2–5, 9, 10).[23] When commenting on the gloomy and windy baths in Rome, Martial is probably referring to older baths of this sort, and he calls them *balnea,* not *thermae* (1.59, 2.14.11–13).

Fashionable and Unfashionable Baths

Martial liked to go to the Thermae of Titus. The demands placed on him by the duties of *clientela,* however, forced him on occasion to frequent the Thermae of Agrippa, the preferred facility of one of his patrons. The Thermae of Nero, renowned for their luxury, appear to have been too hot for his liking, although he was not unfamiliar with them. As an alternative to these monumental establishments, Martial used the Balnea of Stephanus, where he would meet dinner guests invited to his townhouse, which was nearby. But above the lot stood the Thermulae of Etruscus, so luxurious that the poet

---

22. Mart. 2.14.11–13; see Sullivan, 151–53. Graffiti from Pompeii's basilica expresses the hopes of Campanian counterparts to Selius: "Whoever invites me to dinner—let him prosper" *(quisque me ad cenam vocarit valeat)* (CIL 4.1937); "Hey, L. Isticadius—whoever does not invite me to dinner is, as far as I'm concerned, a barbarian" *(L. Isticadi, at quem non ceno, barbarus ille mihi est)* (CIL 4.1880).

23. The stucco decorative schemes of the Stabian Baths, retained even after the earthquake of 62, are a good model of Republican modesty; see Eschebach, *Stabianer Thermen,* 74–95 (a section on decoration by A. De Vos and M. De Vos). Stucco per se could be lavish and refined (as in this case), but when compared to the marble paneling, mosaics, metal fittings, and statuary of later baths, it surely appeared less impressive to the ancient visitor; on stucco, see J.-P. Adam, *Roman Building: Materials and Techniques* (Bloomington, IN, 1994), 224–27. The first baths associated with decorative statuary are the Thermae of Agrippa at Rome; see Pliny *HN* 34.62. Pliny also lists these baths as equipped with marbles and paintings (35.26), but he notes that they were conservatively decorated when compared to later excesses (36.189). Similar sentiments about simple Republican baths are expressed by Seneca (*Ep.* 86.4–5).

could claim, "if you don't bathe in the little *thermae* of Etruscus, Oppianus, you will die unwashed."[24] Canius Rufus, a friend and patron of Martial's, could be found at the Thermae of Agrippa or the Balnea of Tigellinus (3.20.15–16), while one Fabianus apparently frequented the Thermae of Nero (12.83).

These passages clearly reflect personal preferences for particular facilities, but they also point to a deeper social circumstance: a broad differentiation between baths considered fashionable and unfashionable. Clearly Etruscus' baths were the height of luxury, and Martial's poem seems to act as a sort of advertisement for them, perhaps designed to attract customers from among those who read it (although it is unclear whether these baths were open to the public or not). Seneca (*Ep.* 86.8) caustically comments that once popular baths would be quickly abandoned if a newer establishment sporting some novel luxury started doing business, and Ammianus Marcellinus (28.4.10) notes that it was common in polite society to inquire of a stranger what baths he used. That these notices are centuries apart seems to reflect a long-standing tradition in Rome whereby it was chic to be seen in certain baths rather than in others, perhaps analogous to the rating of nightclubs or restaurants among modern socialites. Indeed, Seneca's comment, even if no doubt exaggerated, suggests a faddish pattern of behavior more commonly associated with modern popular culture.

Martial is even more instructive when he provides evidence for the other side of the coin. Of Selius, who roots out dinner invitations from among the city's public haunts, he writes:

Nec Fortunati spernit nec balnea Fausti
    nec Grylli tenebras Aeoliamque Lupi:
nam thermis iterum ternis iterumque lavatur.

(2.14.11–13)

[Nor does he scorn the *balnea* of Fortunatus nor those of Faustus, not yet the gloom of Gryllus and Lupus' Aeolian cavern. As for the three *thermae*, he uses them again and again. (trans. adapted)]

The joke is partly on the quality of the dinner Selius could expect from the users of such dingy baths, but Martial appears to assume that his audience

---

24. Mart. 3.36.5–6 (Thermae of Titus vs. Agrippa); 3.25 (Thermae of Nero), 10.48.3–4 (too hot); 2.48, 7.34.4–5 (luxurious); 12.83 (familiar); 11.52.4, 14.60 (Baths of Stephanus); 6.42 (Baths of Etruscus: *Etrusci nisi thermulis lavaris, / illotus morieris, Oppiane*). See also Stat. *Silv.* 1.5.

would pick up on the names of the places and so identify with his characterization of their facilities. If this supposition is correct, these places were apparently baths of proverbial grubbiness, at least in the circles in which Martial moved. A similar assumption can be seen to stand behind a poem written from Baiae.

Dat mihi Baiana quadrantes sportula centum.
    inter delicias quid facit ista fames?
redde Lupi nobis tenebrosaque balnea Grylli:
    tam male cum cenem, cur bene, Flacce, laver?

(1.59)

[The dole at Baiae presents me with a hundred farthings. What is such poverty doing amid luxury? give me back the murky baths of Lupus and Gryllus. When my dinner's this bad, why should my bath be so good?]

Just as the baths at Baiae are presented as a byword for splendor, so the Balnea of Lupus and Gryllus are presented as their antitheses.[25] What these baths were really like can only be guessed at. Martial's references, when coupled with the remains of Republican baths in Campania or the small corner bathhouse depicted in a fragment of the Severan Marble Map, offer clues that such baths were small, dark (Gryllus), drafty (Lupus), and generally unpleasant.[26] It is clear that, as far as Martial was concerned, they were below serious consideration and used only by the desperate.

The evidence seems clear enough that a sense of fashion surrounded what baths were "in" and what baths were not. If, like Selius, you visited a lesser facility, you were open to the sort of ridicule from which Martial made his living. The details of this fashion are lost to us, and any attempt to reconstruct it must be speculative,[27] but its very existence, as alluded to in the sources presented above, is noteworthy and suggests something of the vitality of bath culture in Martial's Rome.

---

25. For Baiae's reputation for luxury and excellent baths, see P. Howell, *A Commentary on Book One of the* Epigrams *of Martial* (London, 1980), 245–46; Dunbabin, "*Baiarum Grata Voluptas*"; Pasquinucci, 87–92 (by M.A. Vaggioli); Yegül, 93–94; id., "The Thermo-Mineral Complex at Baiae and *De Balneis Puteolanis,*" *ArtB* 78 (1996): 137–61.

26. See figs. 2–4, 10. For the corner bath on the Marble Map, see *FUR* fr. 25 [pl. XXV]; Rodríguez Almeida, *Forma Urbis Marmorea,* fr. 25 [pl. XVIII].

27. For instance, did the modest *balneum* depicted on the Marble Map (see previous note) as standing near the Horrea Lolliana alongside the Tiber in Regio XIII cater mainly to dockworkers? Unfortunately, the mere location of a bath is not the most secure basis for drawing conclusions about the nature of its clientele; see below, chapter 5, pp. 118–19.

Dinner Parties and Invitations

One of the salient social functions of baths in Martial's writings and elsewhere is that they act as meeting places for dinner guests. Given the shape of the Roman day, this function is not surprising. The working day usually ended at about noon, and the main meal of the day was not taken until the late afternoon or early evening. The baths were therefore an excellent way to fill in the intervening period, and in any case, bathing conditions were best in the early and middle parts of the afternoon.[28] Bathing after a meal was not unknown, although it was not recommended: Juvenal (1.139–46) alludes to the bather who meets a sudden end after entering the bath with a stomach full of undigested peacock; the combination, it seems, proved lethal.[29]

Martial frequently alludes to friends meeting in the baths before adjourning to the dining couch. The examples are too repetitive to enumerate in detail, but two examples will be illustrative. Julius Cerealis is encouraged to meet Martial at the Balnea of Stephanus before enjoying a modest but pleasant meal at the poet's house, which is nearby. Elsewhere, Martial counts his dinner guests as he waits for them to assemble at the baths; he realizes there is room for one more and adds Lupus to his list.[30] Presumably, Lupus would only learn of his belated invitation when he showed up at the baths, a circumstance that provides Martial with a subject for several cutting poems: the unpopular or indigent dinner-hunter who scours the baths and harasses the bathers in search of dinner invitations. We have already met Selius, who stoops from the fine *thermae* to notoriously disagreeable establishments in search of the desired invitation. But none appears more annoying than Men-

---

28. For the shape of the day, see Mart. 4.8; Cic. *Deiot.* 17 and *Vat.* 31; J.P.V.D. Balsdon, *Life and Leisure in Ancient Rome* (London, 1969), 17–26; F. Dupont, *Daily Life in Ancient Rome* (Oxford, 1992), 188–90; Laurence, 122–32. The eighth hour, the exact time of which varied according to the season (see E.J. Bickerman, *Chronology of the Ancient World*[2] [London, 1980], 13–16), was optimal for bathing, as is clear from references in Martial (in some cases when he complains about bathing late, at the tenth hour): 3.36.1–6 (tenth hour), 4.8, 10.48.1–6, 10.70.13–14 (tenth hour), 11.52.1–4. The habit of bathing before a meal is abundantly attested in other sources spanning the Imperial period: e.g., Val. Max. 9.5.3; Petron. *Sat.* 130; Pliny *HN* 14.139; Pliny *Ep.* 3.1.7–8, 3.5.9–11; Juv. 6.419–26; Anon. *Life of Aesop* 2, 3, 38–39, 67; Apul. *Met.* 5.2–3, 8.7, 8.29, 10.13; Ath. 1.5e; Luc. *Gall.* 9; Lib. *Or.* 1.85, 1.108, 1.174, 1.183. See also no. 216 (the Lanuvium burial club meets at the baths before dining together); compare the *Acta Fratrum Arvalium,* s.v. *annis* 218 and 241 (*CIL* 6.2114.10, *CIL* 6.2114.14–18 = G. Henzen, *Acta Fratrum Arvalium Quae Supersunt* [Berlin, 1874], 203 and 225, respectively). For the time of the best bathing conditions, see Mart. 10.48.1–6; Vitr. 5.10.1.

29. For nonfatal postprandial bathing, see Hor. *Epist.* 1.6.61; Petron. *Sat.* 72–73; Persius 3.96–99. Eating too soon after bathing could also be perilous; see Pliny *HN* 7.183.

30. Mart. 11.52.1–4 (Cerealis), 10.48.1–6 (Lupus). For other predinner baths, see 2.14.11–13, 2.40, 3.44.12–15, 6.53, 9.19, 12.87 (?).

ogenes, the sycophant who, leechlike, attaches himself to his victim and torments him with inane praise until the invitation is reluctantly proffered.

Effugere in thermis et circa balnea non est
 Menogenen, omni tu licet arte velis.
captabit tepidum dextra laevaque trigonem,
 imputet exceptas ut tibi saepe pilas.
colliget et referet laxum de pulvere follem,
 etsi iam lotus, iam soleatus erit.
lintea si sumes, nive candidiora loquetur,
 sint licet infantis sordidiora sinu.
exiguos secto comentem dente capillos
 dicet Achilleas disposuisse comas.
fumosae feret ipse propin de faece lagonae
 frontis et umorem colliget usque tuae.
omnia laudabit, mirabitur omnia, donec
 perpessus dicas taedia mille "Veni!"

(12.82)

[To escape Menogenes in the *thermae* and around the *balnea* is not possible, try what device you will. He will grab at the warm trigon-ball with right and left so that he can often score a point to you for the balls he catches. He'll collect from the dust and bring back the loose follis-ball, even if he has already bathed and already put on his slippers. If you take your towels, he'll say they are whiter than snow, though they be dirtier than a baby's bib. As you comb your scanty hair with the split ivory, he'll say you have arranged the locks of Achilles. He'll fetch you an aperitif with his own hands from the dregs of a smoky flagon and continually wipe the moisture from your forehead. He'll praise every-thing, admire everything, until after enduring a thousand annoyances you say: "Come to dinner." (trans. adapted)]

It is a sign of how desperate and how annoying Menogenes is that, although washed, dried, and dressed, he returns to the palaestra and interferes with Martial's ball games at the start of the poet's bathing ritual. At the other end of the spectrum is Dento, formerly a regular at Martial's dinner table, who now avoids the poet in the baths and refuses his invitations—because he has found a better class of dinner host (5.44.1–8). The dinner-invitation custom was, of course, a two-way street. Certain bathers would only choose their dinner guests from those they met at the baths, giving Martial the opportunity to imply that, in at least one case, selection was made on the basis of homosexual attraction (1.23).

Other sources provide often amusing vignettes that play on the social custom of bathing before the day's main meal. Plutarch (*Mor.* 707E) evokes the predicament of the "shadow," the man secondarily invited to a dinner party by one of the guests: he cannot go directly to the meal without his sponsor, nor does he want to play the part of the man's bath attendant. Petronius (*Sat.* 26–28) portrays the tasteless vulgarity of Trimalchio's bath before his even more vulgar dinner party. Trimalchio, whose guests are gathering at a public bathing facility, is first encountered by Petronius' heroes as he plays ball games with attractive boys in the palaestra. Later he is depicted bathing luxuriously with fine accoutrements as he is attended by slaves who drink and squabble. The *Life of Aesop* illustrates yet another possibility: the unplanned dinner party that grows out of a chance meeting of friends in the public baths. One of the pet motifs of the *Life* is the slave Aesop outwitting his master, Xanthus. When Aesop is ordered to do exactly as he is told following a period of rebelliousness, he takes to doing tasks precisely as asked of him and no more (a practice analogous to what would be termed in modern union circles "working to rule"). When Xanthus sets out for the baths and orders Aesop to bring along the towels and oil flask, Aesop complies. At the baths, Xanthus asks for oil and is handed an empty oil flask. Xanthus, Aesop points out, had only ordered that the oil flask, not the oil, be brought to the baths. Xanthus' fury abates when he spots some of his friends in the establishment and spontaneously decides to invite them home for dinner. He orders Aesop to return home and "prepare lentil," with predictable results (Anon. *Life of Aesop* 38–41). While such puerility may debar the *Life of Aesop* from inclusion in the classical canon, it provides unusually direct testimony for daily life among the less-vaunted inhabitants of the ancient world. Xanthus' spontaneous dinner invitation to friends encountered in the baths is portrayed here in intimate detail and yet in a casual manner, as it was such an everyday occurrence. It also provides another detail for the overall association of baths and dinner parties discernible so clearly through Martial's verses.

Nudity and Male/Female Mixed Bathing

Martial and a chorus of other sources strongly imply that nudity was the norm in the baths.[31] In most of these sources, the word used to denote the

---

31. See, e.g., Mart. 1.23, 3.3, 3.51, 3.68, 3.72, 6.93.7–10, 9.33, 11.22, 11.51, 11.63, 12.83;

unclothed state is *nudus*. This term, however, did not necessarily mean absolute nakedness but applied also to situations where people were stripped of
their usual clothing and were thus improperly or scantily dressed.[32] To what
extent bathers wore clothes at all remains, then, a debated issue among
modern scholars, but one we need not delve into here in any detail.[33] To be
sure, some sources mention bathing robes (e.g., Dio 77[78].4.3; HA *Alex.
Sev.* 42.1), but they appear to have been worn in the palaestra or on the way
home from the baths, not in the interior of the establishment. States of
improper dress in the baths, if not complete nudity, stand behind the conservative prohibition on fathers bathing with adolescent sons or on sons-in-law
bathing with fathers-in-law.[34]

On Martial's part, absolute nakedness is clearly attested in his portrayal of
life at the baths, such as when he suggests to a friend that if he hears applause
in the bathing rooms, it is probably a response to the appearance there of
Maro's member (9.33). In fact, in Martial's eyes, to use the baths clothed,
even partially, was to draw attention to oneself.

> Menophili penem tam grandis fibula vestit
>   ut sit comoedis omnibus una satis.
> hunc ego credideram—nam saepe lavamur in unum—
>   sollicitum voci parcere, Flacce, suae:
> dum ludit media populo spectante palaestra,
>   delapsa est misero fibula: verpus erat.

(7.82)

[So large a sheath covers Menophilus' penis that it would be enough by
itself for all our comic actors. I had supposed (we often bathe together)
that he was anxious to spare his voice, Flaccus. But while he was in a
game in the middle of the sportsground with everybody watching, the
sheath slipped off the poor soul: he was circumcised.]

Cic. *Cael.* 62 and *Fam.* 9.22.4 (= SB 189); Sen. *Ep.* 122.6; Juv. 11.156–58; Petron. *Sat.* 30, 73,
92; Suet. *Aug.* 94.4; HA *Heliogab.* 8.6. The practice may have been picked up from Greek
gymnasia; see Plut. *Cat. Maj.* 20.8.

32. For instance, soldiers or gladiators stripped of their weapons were described as *nudi;*
see, e.g., Caes. *B Gall.* 1.25.4; Sen. *Controv.* 9.6.2.

33. The issue is discussed in most modern treatments of Roman bathing: see, e.g., Merten,
87–88; Nielsen, 1.140–44; Yegül, 34–35. A recent study suggests that total nudity may have
prevailed only during the act of cleaning itself, but the evidence presented for clothed bathers
appears to be restricted to the palaestra—the situation in the interior of the baths is far less clear;
see C.H. Hallett, "The Roman Heroic Portrait" (Ph.D. dissertation, University of California at
Berkeley, 1993), 90–99. Note that in a mosaic from Piazza Armerina (fig. 30), a completely
naked bather is being oiled by two naked attendants.

34. For references, see chapter 2, n. 28.

Given the prevailing atmosphere of nakedness at the baths—be it complete or partial—the attested bathing together of men and women comes as a shock to many modern sensibilities, as well as to some ancient ones (see, e.g., Pliny *HN* 33.153; Quint. *Inst.* 5.9.14). Of the few social issues raised by the baths' functioning that have attracted prior scholarly attention, that of mixed bathing has proven among the most divisive and resistant to resolution. That mixed bathing was practiced is hardly in doubt, but disagreement has arisen over its prevalence. As is the case with so many details of the baths' operation—the application of the terms *thermae* and *balnea,* for instance, or the "typical" degree of nudity—the sources are contradictory. On the one hand, there is testimony for separate bathing wings in Republican baths (possibly even entire establishments reserved for women) or for separate bathing times for men and women; on the other, there is the absence of bathing wings for women in baths of the Imperial period and the reported imperial edicts that banned or permitted mixed bathing, which would imply that it was a widespread habit.[35] Modern reactions to this material have been understandably diverse. It has been suggested that mixed bathing took place only in less respectable establishments, that only prostitutes and lowly women practiced it, or that the habit varied from place to place, with the imperial *thermae* being reserved solely for men. Another view holds that the fashion changed over time: it was unpopular in the Republic, accepted in the early Empire, but unacceptable again after Hadrian's ban. Combinations of these possibilities can also be found in the modern literature.[36] But the ancient evidence offers counterpoints to all of these blanket solutions. Women could use the Baths of Trajan, so imperial *thermae* were not off-limits to them; Clement of Alexandria comments that one could meet noble ladies naked in the baths, so less-respectable women were not the mixed

---

35. A sample of the evidence follows. For separate bathing wings, see the Stabian and Forum Baths at Pompeii (figs. 1, 6–8); or the Forum Baths at Herculaneum; Varr. *Ling.* 9.68; Vitr. 5.10.1. For separate bathing establishments (or possibly wings) for men and women, see nos. 46, 88, 151, 209; *Anth. Pal.* 9.620. See also *CIL* 9.1667 (Beneventum; no date); Gell. *NA* 10.3.3 (which may refer to separate wings or to separate baths). For separate bathing hours, see no. 282 (lines 20–21); *SEG* 26 (1976/77) 1043/44 (Arkades, Crete; Julio-Claudian). For unsegregated baths, see *Anth. Pal.* 9.783 or the remains of any of the imperial *thermae*, the Central Baths at Pompeii, or the Suburban Baths in Herculaneum. For imperial decrees, see Dio 69.8.2; HA *Hadr.* 18.10, *Marc.* 23.8, *Alex. Sev.* 24.2. The comments of Merten (79–100) are perceptive.

36. See Balsdon, *Life and Leisure,* 28 (lowly establishments and less respectable women); Hallett, "Roman Heroic Portrait," 103, and Yegül, 33 (less respectable women); H. Blümner, *Die römischen Privataltertümer* (Munich, 1911), 427–28, and J. Carcopino, *Daily Life in Ancient Rome* (London, 1956), 281–82 (imperial *thermae* for men only); Merten, 79–100 (variation over time); Nielsen, 1.147–48 (variation over time and less respectable women).

baths' only female patrons; and strict chronological boundaries between periods of acceptability (or not) for mixed bathing are hard to establish.[37]

The best solution to this problem is not to seek an umbrella solution at all but to accept that in all likelihood mixed bathing varied from region to region or even from establishment to establishment, much in the same way that nude sunbathing is variously practiced on the beaches of modern Europe. Whether one went to a mixed bath or not was a matter of personal choice, and the empire no doubt contained baths to suit the tastes of both the prude and the pervert.[38] Such a situation pertained in the Byzantine world, for instance, where written sources make it clear that baths with separate wings for men and women could be found, as could places where men and women bathed together. A striking illustration of the latter is the story told by John Moschus (ca. 550–619) about the lustful nun of Alexandria who, possessed by a demon, would enter baths and tempt laymen and even priests to perform sex acts with her. Aroused clerics were so obsessed with the seductive nun that their sleep was marred by nocturnal emissions.[39] Clearly, the context of mixed bathing is not clear-cut here, since there were opportunities for separate bathing or for mixed bathing, as one felt the need.

As far as Martial was concerned, bathing with women was a matter of course (2.52, 3.51, 3.72, 6.93, 7.35, 11.47.1–2, 11.75). In fact, he is amazed when women who express a sexual interest in him refuse to share a bath; in one instance he ruminates in graphic detail over the possible physical defects afflicting such a woman—and concludes that she may just be an idiot (3.72; compare 3.51). (This poem also leaves no doubt that men and women could bathe together completely naked.) Martial evidently thought it odd, even puzzling, for a woman *not* to bathe in the company of men. One recent view

---

37. See Chron. A. 354 = *FTUR* 3.10.463 (women in the Baths of Trajan); Clement *Paid.* 3.31–33 (Stählin). As to chronological boundaries, do the women who use public baths in Cicero (*Cael.* 62) or Ovid (*Ars Am.* 3.638–40) reflect Republican norms? Inscriptions for separate bathing hours date from the Imperial period and derive from very particular contexts; see chapter 1, n. 35.

38. R. Bowen Ward ("Women in Roman Baths," *HThR* 85 [1992]: 125–47) comes to similar conclusions, although perhaps overestimating the commonness of the mixed bathing habit. See also C.S. Sommer, "Waren Frauen in der Römerzeit schmutziger als Männer? Überlegungen zur Eintrittspreisgestaltung in römischen Thermen," *Fundberichte aus Baden-Württemberg* 21 (1996): 301–6; Weber, 150–58.

39. On the lustful nun, see John Moschus, *Pratum Spirituale*, (for text, see E. Mioni, "Il Pratum Spirituale di Giovanni Mosco: Gli episodi inediti del Cod. Marciano greco II, 21," *OCP* 17 [1951]: 92–93 [no. 11]). For an overview of Byzantine baths as represented in written sources, including references to segregated bathing of the sexes, see H.J. Magoulias, "Bathhouse, Inn, Tavern, Prostitution, and the Stage as Seen in the Lives of the Saints of the Sixth and Seventh Centuries," *EpetByz* 38 (1971): 233–38.

questions Martial's reliability in this regard by pointing out the satiric nature of his poetry. Since he is satirizing women who bathe with men, his statements cannot be taken at face value.[40] It is important, however, to be clear about what Martial is satirizing in these verses. He lampoons women at the baths, to be sure, but never for the mere fact of their presence there. Instead, he casts barbs at them for a variety of reasons: for not bathing with him (3.51, 3.72), for having large breasts (2.52), for being malodorous (6.93), or for bringing male slave attendants who are not completely naked, itself a suggestive comment on the degree of expected nudity at the baths Martial visited (7.35, 11.75). The context of the mixed baths appears in these poems as just that: an unremarkable backdrop for Martial's main jokes.[41] Nothing in these passages supports the view that the women in question were all prostitutes or of low social standing. Altogether, there can be little doubt that, for Martial, bathing with women was the norm.

Paradoxically, this conclusion does indeed raise a valid reason for hesitation in applying Martial's evidence to society at large, and it has nothing to do with the satirical purpose of his verses. Martial's sexual mores, so far as they can be reconstructed, were hardly monkish.[42] For such a man, and perhaps for his circle of friends, bathing with women was a regular occurrence. But for others, this need not have been the case. Pliny's objections to mixed baths (*HN* 33.153) have already been noted, but there are hints even in Martial's verses that mixed bathing was not to everyone's taste. Those women who refuse to bathe with the poet are a good example. So is Lattara, the man who avoids the "baths frequented by the feminine cohorts" (Mart. 11.47.1–2: *omnia femineis quare dilecta catervis / balnea devitat Lattara?*). Lattara and Martial's "prudish" women exercise a personal choice. Evidently, there were places they could go to bathe without running into the opposite sex. Martial also gives a hint that even in mixed baths there could be "women's recesses" (7.35.7: *feminei recessus*) of uncertain function, although the context leaves it unclear whether these rooms were to be found in the baths or elsewhere. At one point Martial also warns the upright Roman woman *(matrona)* to beware his verses, full of naked men at the baths (3.68.1–4). Presumably, Martial, who preferred to bathe with women, wrote about the environment he was familiar with and so gives the impression that

---

40. See Yegül, 33.

41. The suggestion that these poems reflect "numerous [bath] scandals in Domitian's reign" seems exaggerated; see J.C. Anderson Jr., "The Date of the *Thermae Traiani* and the Topography of the *Oppius Mons*," *AJA* 89 (1985): 502 n. 16.

42. See Sullivan, 185–210.

everyone shared his view, which is not necessarily the case.[43] It is impossible to say whether Martial represents the majority opinion. Certainly there is evidence that women and men (especially husbands and wives) did bathe together, imperial decrees against mixed bathing were issued by Hadrian and other emperors, and some church fathers felt compelled to proscribe it expressly, all of which leads to the conclusion that the habit was, if not widespread, at least noticeably popular.[44]

The final verdict on this knotty question must be that whether one bathed in mixed baths or not was a matter of choice: the city (and empire) contained establishments to suit every taste, and depending on the source one reads, the habit will appear unremarkable or objectionable, hence the overall contradictory nature of the evidence. There is no question of a simple or universal solution, but we must rather think in terms of regional, chronological, and even facility-by-facility variation. Roman bathing culture was more varied and vibrant than blanket solutions to such thorny questions have tended to assume.

Irritating Bathers

Martial refers occasionally to irritating fellow-bathers, of whom the dinner-hunting Menogenes is a prime example (above, chapter 1, p. 23). But there are other types.[45] Before he became rich, Aper used to harangue drinkers at the baths, demanding that the cups be smashed and the wine poured away (12.70.5–6); Fabianus was in the habit of making fun of bathers with hernias, until he got one himself (12.83); and some bathers displayed objectionable habits that made life for their fellows less than agreeable (e.g., 2.42, 2.70; 6.81). Martial, being a well-known poet around town, was subject to a unique irritation in the form of the aspirant poet Ligurinus, who hounded him relentlessly with his atrocious verse.

Et stanti legis et legis sedenti,
currenti legis et legis cacanti.
in thermas fugio: sonas ad aurem.
piscinam peto: non licet natare.

---

43. This caveat hardly applies to all of Martial's evidence for the social functioning of baths, since, as shown above, abundant evidence often corroborates his allusions. In the case of women at the baths, however, where other evidence is contradictory, Martial's personal proclivities have to be given serious consideration.

44. For husbands and wives at the baths, see below, chapter 8, p. 197. On decrees, see above, chapter 1, n. 35. For the church fathers, see Bowen Ward, "Women," 142–46.

45. See Plut. *Mor.* 61C–D, 62A, for flatterers who hang about the baths.

ad cenam propero: tenes euntem.
ad cenam venio: fugas edentem.

(3.44.10–15; see also 3.45, 3.50)

[You read to me as I stand, you read to me as I sit, you read to me as I
run, you read to me as I shit. I flee to the baths: you boom in my ear. I
head for the pool: I'm not allowed to swim. I hurry to dinner, you stop
me in my tracks. I arrive at dinner, you drive me away as I eat.]

Petronius offers corroboration for this particular vignette when Trimalchio,
having gotten drunk and moved the party into his private bathing suite,
begins to murder some songs at high volume (*Sat.* 73) and when another
character almost gets beaten up for inconveniencing the bathers with his
poetry as they languish in the pools (*Sat.* 91–92). Seneca, it will be remembered, was able to pick out the voice of the singing bather amidst the general
cacophony generated in the baths (*Ep.* 56.2). It seems that then, as now,
some bathers liked the sound of their own voices and were not averse to
sharing their (often unwelcome) vocal talents with the public.

Violence, Eating, Drinking, Sex, and Thieves: Some Oversights in Martial

Despite his value, Martial should not be thought of as a complete source for
the bathing experience. There are some bath-related attitudes and customs
that Martial either only perfunctorily alludes to or does not mention at all.
For example, it seems from other sources that bathers could get hit as they
went about their business. Pliny the Younger records the indignity suffered
by Larcius Macedo, a man of praetorian rank but slave ancestry. Macedo
was making his way through the crowd at an unspecified public bath in
Rome when he was inadvertently slapped by an equestrian, whom one of
Macedo's slaves had asked to make way. The blow was so severe that Macedo nearly fell over (*Ep.* 3.14.6–8). Similarly, Seneca, to illustrate the virtue
of forgiveness, offers the probably apocryphal story of Cato the Elder being
punched while he was at the baths. Afterward, as the perpetrator was apolo-
gizing profusely, Cato magnanimously replied, "I don't recall being hit"
(*Dial.* 4.32.2). Centuries later, Libanius records an assault on his bathing
companions in Athens, apparently the result of rivalry between schools in the
city (*Or.* 1.21). That these incidents were not isolated is suggested by Seneca's comment in comparing the circumstances of life to those in a bathhouse, a crowd, or a roadway: "some things will be thrown at you, some

things will hit you" (*Ep.* 107.2: *quaedam in te mittentur, quaedam incident*). The situation behind these incidents is, simply, the crowding at the baths. People would be jostling and milling about, especially at the peak hours, and close contact with others was unavoidable. This problem of crowding is why Macedo had a slave with him to clear a path through the mob. And for this same reason, in the *Life of Aesop* (65–67), Xanthus sends Aesop ahead to check on the crowds at the baths before he decides whether or not to venture out himself. The propensity for violence displayed by Romans in such close social interactions is particularly interesting—they appear to have had no hesitation in hitting first and asking questions later, especially when the offender was of lower social status (indeed, Macedo's equestrian assailant had aimed his blow at the offending slave but struck Macedo by mistake). A visit to the baths, it seems, could be more than metaphysically dangerous.[46]

Martial is not particularly informative about other bath-related circumstances as well. He rarely makes it explicit, for instance, that he regards baths as a key element in daily life. He does drop occasional hints, however, such as when he produces a stripped-down list of life's necessities.

Coponem laniumque balneumque,
tonsorem tabulamque calculosque
et paucos, sed ut eligam, libellos:
unum non nimium rudem sodalem
et grandem puerum diuque levem
et caram puero meo puellam:
haec praesta mihi, Rufe, vel Butuntis,
et thermas tibi habe Neronianas.

(2.48)

[An innkeeper, a butcher, a *balneum,* a barber, a board and pieces, and a few little books (but I must choose them), one friend not too new, a large boy smooth-cheeked for a long time to come, and a girl of whom my boy is fond: give me these, Rufus, even at Butunti, and keep Nero's *thermae.* (trans. adapted)]

(Note, by the way, the implied distinction between *balneum,* meaning here something like "a simple bath," and the luxury and sophistication of Nero's

---

46. One wonders, in fact, to what degree Romans enjoyed "comparatively pacific day-to-day relations with each other," as has recently been claimed; see J.E. Lendon, "Social Control at Rome," *CJ* 93 (1997): 87. For the evil eye and other supernatural perils at the baths, see Dunbabin, "*Baiarum Grata Voluptas,*" 33–46.

thermae.) Elsewhere, baths feature in Martial's daily routine (4.8, 7.76) and in that of others (3.30.4), and the essentially social nature of the habit stands behind his disparaging comments on people who bathe alone (11.51, 12.50.1–3). The baths are also presented as the haunts of commoners and are included among the places where Martial, musing on the unsophisticated life, would spend his day if he were not required to move among the wealthy and influential (5.20). While these mentions of baths are little more than inferences, other sources provide more explicit testimony of the centrality of baths in the daily routine.[47] One of the quaintest is the forlorn epitaph of C. Domitius Primus, who longs for his earthly pleasures, baths among them, in the afterlife (no. 262). This simple but eloquent testimony to the central place of baths among the pleasures of the Romans is mirrored in the more famous epitaph of Ti. Claudius Secundus, who declares, "baths, wine, and sex ruin our bodies, but they are the essence of life."[48]

Gravestones like these raise other questions when they associate baths, drinking, and sex. It is clear that the latter two joys could be found at the baths. Martial explicitly refers to drinking in the bathhouse only once: Aper, a formerly strident critic of bathing drinkers, after inheriting some money, "doesn't know how to go home from the baths sober" (12.70.8: *sobrius a thermis nescit abire domum*). This solitary quip is insufficient to assume that consumption of alcohol was a familiar feature of the bathing experience, but it should be noted that other sources comment on the capacity of the heat, humidity, and exercising at the baths to raise a thirst.[49] What tends to draw the attention of the moralists (and satirists) are those bathers whose drinking they deemed inappropriate. Thus, Petronius reports that Trimalchio is accompanied by slaves who drink wine, and both Seneca and Pliny the Elder comment with evident distaste on the habit.[50] Broad generalizations, however, should be avoided. It is doubtful that all bathers or even a majority of them would go home the worse for wear from alcohol, but the opportunity was there if one had the means and inclination to avail oneself of it.[51]

---

47. See, e.g., Cic. *Fam.* 14.20.1 (= SB 173; baths are necessary to life and health); Pliny *Ep.* 9.36.4 (baths in Pliny's daily routine).

48. No. 261. Similar sentiments accompany a gaming board etched into the pavement of the forum at Timgad (no. 275).

49. See Ael. Arist. 25.311; Anon. *Life of Aesop* 39; Celsus 1.3.6–7; Pliny *HN* 14.140.

50. Petron. *Sat.* 28; Sen. *Ep.* 122.6; Pliny *HN* 14.139–40. See also Quint. *Inst.* 1.6.44.

51. Note also that drinking shops are often located near bathhouses, as at Pompeii, where taverns and cookshops are found in close proximity to all three major establishments: 6.8.8, 6.8.9, and 7.4.4 near the entrances to the Forum Baths; 9.1.6, 9.1.8, 9.1.15–16 (on the Strada Stabiana), 8.4.12 (on the Via dell'Abbondanza), and 7.1.1, 7.62 (on the corner of the Via dell'Abbondanza and the Vicolo del Lupanare) near the Stabian Baths; 5.1.1, 5.1.32, and 7.2.15

Eating at the baths is another activity for which Martial gives only a single hint but that is otherwise attested as quite common. Martial portrays Aemilius as eating eggs, lettuce, and fish at the *thermae* (12.19). Since bathing normally took place before dinner, this sort of snack food appears the most commonly consumed at the baths. There would be little point in eating a large meal at the baths only to face the day's main repast on arrival at dinner *(cena)*. So snacks were the order of the day. Direct and striking physical evidence for eating and drinking in baths comes from Caerleon, where the drains of the baths have yielded glass plates, jugs, cups, and fragments of animal bones, presumably remnants of light snacks.[52] A podium outside the entrance to the Sarno Baths in Pompeii appears to have been an egg seller's stand, and a graffito price list or tally from a room near the vestibule of the Suburban Baths in Herculaneum reads, "Nuts, drinks— 14; hog's fat—2; bread—3; cutlets, for 3—12; sausage, for 4—8; 51."[53] The numbers are prices in *asses* for each item, with the final figure probably a price for an unspecified combination of goods and services. This text painted onto the wall indicates the location of a temporary stall or booth, of a sort attested by inscriptions near the amphitheater at Pompeii.[54] This evidence of a vendor's booth echoes Seneca's complaint about the noises emanating from the baths at Baiae: "Then there are the varied calls of the cake seller, and the sausageman, and the confectioner and all the peddlers of snacks selling their commodities, each with his own characteristic intonation."[55] Other graffiti from the Suburban Baths in Herculaneum make it clear that the food could be eaten on the premises, but one of the schoolbooks suggests that the snacks

near the Central Baths. For the identification and location of all these taverns, see the appropriate entries in L. Eschebach and J. Müller-Trollius, eds., *Gebäudeverzeichnis und Stadtplan der antiken Stadt Pompeji* (Cologne, 1993). A *caupona* opened onto the Palaestra Baths at Pompeii (fig. 20), and the entrance to the Suburban Baths yielded evidence of trade in liquids (probably wine); see L. Jacobelli, "Die Suburbanen Thermen in Pompei: Architektur, Raumfunktion und Ausstattung," *ArchKorrBl* 23 (1993): 327–29. Written evidence offers corroboration. Fragmentary inscriptions associate *tabernae* and *balnea,* suggesting that the two stood in the same vicinity, if not in the same complex (see *CIL* 9.1667, 10.3161; see also no. 97). Martial depicts Syriscus as frittering away an inheritance of ten million sesterces in the *popinae* "near the Four Baths" (5.70.4: *circa balnea quattuor*), while Nero, on the day his grand *thermae* were dedicated, sang almost naked in a tavern near the new establishment (Phil. *VA* 4.42). For taverns and cookshops in Roman towns, see below, chapter 3, p. 77.

52. See Zienkiewicz, *Legionary Fortress Baths,* 98–116 (D. Allen on glass), 225–41 (T.P. O'Connor on animal bones).

53. See nos. 276 (eggs), 277 (list).

54. See *CIL* 4.1096 = *ILS* 5921a, *CIL* 4.1096a, *CIL* 4.1097a, *CIL* 4.1097b, *CIL* 4.1115. Like modern street vendors, operators of such booths had to procure licenses from the local authorities; see *Dig.* 18.1.32.

55. Sen. *Ep.* 56.2: *iam biberari varias exclamationes et botularium et crustularium et omnes popinarum institores mercem sua quadam et insignita modulatione vendentis.*

were purchased on leaving, presumably to be eaten on the way home.[56] Altogether, we must imagine stalls or even strolling vendors at or near the entrances to baths, calling out to attract customers, and selling their goods to people as they entered or left the facility. All this evidence demonstrates that eating and drinking could take place at the baths, albeit usually on a small scale.

What can we determine about the occurrence at the baths of sex, the third pleasure listed in the epitaphs of Primus and Secundus? Martial gives no direct indication that sex took place at the baths, though at several junctures he associates bathing with sexual activity, as when, for instance, he wants women who like him to bathe with him, when he comments that some fellow bathers went to the baths to ogle genitals, or when he surmises that a certain Lattara avoids women's baths to avoid the temptation of sex.[57] In most of these vignettes, the baths appear more as a prelude or accessory to sexual trysts than as an actual setting for them. The poem about Laevina is illustrative. She was a virtuous wife until she went on a tour of Italy and, at Baiae, ran off with a younger man; Martial plays on the image of her being inflamed simultaneously by the heat of the baths and by the heat of passion (1.62). While it is true that the inference partly indicts Baiae, a community reputed for dissolute behavior, the degenerating sexual effect of baths on Laevina cannot be ignored. Clearer is the suggestion offered to Laecania when she comes to the baths with a covered slave to wash her in the pool: that she go away and enjoy the hidden member in private (7.35). The *Life of Aesop* (32) offers a similar vignette. Aesop entices the mistress of the house to buy a handsome slave who can tend to her bathing needs and to her personal ones afterward. In these passages, then, the baths appear to act as an appetizer for the main course.

Other sources, however, leave little doubt that sex could take place in the baths themselves. Ovid depicts the *balnea* of Augustan Rome as favorite meeting places for young lovers, where the girl's chaperone could be left outside (*Ars Am.* 3.638–40), while Ulpian includes baths among the places where adultery could take place (*Dig.* 48.5.10[9].1; compare Quint. *Inst.* 5.9.14). The allegedly depraved dips of the aged Tiberius were infamous (see Suet. *Tib.* 44.1). The changing room of the Suburban Baths at Pompeii has

---

56. No. 278 (eating at the baths). See also *Colloquia Monacensia* (CGL 3.652.10): "buy for us as we leave the bath minces, lupin seeds, and bitter beans" (*emite nobis a balneo minutalia et lupinos ⟨et⟩ fabas acetatas*).

57. For women, see above, chapter 1, pp. 26–29. See also Mart. 1.96.11–13, 9.33, 11.22.7–10 (voyeurs; compare Petron. *Sat.* 92), 11.47 (Lattara). Martial's tryst with Lydia *in piscina marina* (11.21) cannot with certainty be set in a bathhouse.

yielded several erotic frescoes depicting various sex acts, apparently making explicit the association of baths with sexual pleasures.[58] Greek magical papyri contain useful tips on how to attract partners at the baths, not all of which appear particularly promising on the surface: "To get a certain lover at the baths: rub a tick from a dead dog on the loins"; "Love spell of attraction: . . . Take a pure papyrus and with blood of an ass write the following names and figure, and put in the magical material from the woman you desire. Smear the strip of papyrus with moistened vinegar gum and glue it to the dry vaulted vapor room of a bath, and you will marvel."[59] For strong testimony of sex at the baths, graffiti from the Suburban Baths at Herculaneum appear incontrovertible: "Apelles, chamberlain of the emperor, and Dexter had lunch here most pleasantly and fucked at the same time" (no. 278). More vigorous still was the visit by the same duo recorded in the following graffito: "We, Apelles the Mouse and his brother Dexter, lovingly fucked two women twice" (no. 279). Assuming that these comments record actual events and are not just lewd fantasies—after all, Roman bathroom graffiti cannot be taken at face value any more than their modern counterparts—these texts leave little doubt that sex took place in the bath building. A less crude graffito records that a man called Hermeros had been waiting for his lover Primigenia at the baths until he gave up and set out for Puteoli, but not before leaving her a message: "Hermeros to his mistress Primigenia: come to Puteoli and in the Timinian district ask the banker Messius for Hermeros, son (or slave) of Phoebus" (no. 280). The room where these graffiti appear is immediately adjacent to the vestibule, suggesting that the activities they record were restricted to a particular part of the bathhouse and were not performed elsewhere in the establishment. It is therefore unlikely that other bathers would have to step over copulating couples to use the facilities.

The status of the women involved in these trysts is unclear, but they may have been prostitutes. Certainly, prostitution was not uncommon at baths. Again from the Suburban Baths at Herculaneum comes this graffito: "Two companions were here and, since they had a thoroughly terrible attendant called Epaphroditus, threw him out onto the street not a moment too soon. They then spent 105½ sesterces most agreeably while they fucked" (no. 281). The money, not by any means an inconsiderable sum, was apparently

---

58. See L. Jacobelli, *Le pitture erotiche delle Terme Suburbane di Pompei* (Rome, 1995), esp. 92–97.

59. *PGM*² 127.1–12 (dead dog), 36.69–75 (vapor room). It is not immediately clear from the latter spell, however, whether the woman was to be attracted while at the baths. For other bath-related spells, see *PGM*² 2.44–51, 7.467–77 (casting spells into a furnace of a bathhouse), 36.333 (a spell to be put on the flat stone of a bath), 38.1–26 (a spell to be deposited [?] in baths).

paid to prostitutes. Other sources fill out the sordid picture somewhat. A text from Ephesos makes mention of a brothel (παιδισκεῖον) located at the Varius Baths, and the upper level of the Suburban Baths at Pompeii may also have served as such. Evidence that such places existed raises the possibility that some of the rooms of indeterminate function in the remains of larger baths may have served as brothels or prostitute's cells. In any case, even for baths without specific areas for sex, brothels could be located nearby.[60] So when Ammianus (28.4.9) reports that late Imperial aristocrats would go to the baths expecting to meet their favorite courtesans there, it is unclear whether the sex would take place at the baths (a definite possibility), at a nearby brothel, at some other location supplied by the courtesan, or at the customer's house. In most cases when prostitutes are said to be active at the baths, it is probably safest to assume that they plied their trade in the establishment itself. As a result, the Jewish Midrash recommends avoiding baths because they are places of prostitution, and Ulpian describes a scam practiced among certain bathmen *(balneatores)* in the provinces who kept slaves attached to their baths ostensibly as clothes guards but really as prostitutes.[61]

Mention of clothes guards raises another facet of life at the baths that Martial only vaguely alludes to: thievery.[62] This feature of the baths recurs in

---

60. See no. 309 (Varius Baths). The possible location of a brothel over the Suburban Baths is suggested by a wall grafitto advertising sex inside (*CIL* 4.1751); see Jacobelli, *Pitture erotiche,* 97. Recently, it has been suggested that the cubicles attached to the Sarno Baths at Pompeii may have been used for sex: see Koloski-Ostrow, 94–95; for a contrary view, see G. Ioppolo, *Le Terme del Sarno a Pompei* (Rome, 1992), 72. The brothels of Pompeii, including the famous example at 7.12.18–20, are all within a short walk from the town's major baths; see Laurence, 70–78, esp. map 5.1 on p. 77.

61. A.J. Wertheimer, *Batei Midrashot*² (Jerusalem, 1954), 2.143 (I am indebted to E. Dvorjetski for this reference); *Dig.* 3.2.4.2. Prostitutes appear to have been common at or near baths in Byzantine Palestine; see C. Dauphin, "Brothels, Baths, and Babes: Prostitution in the Byzantine Holy Land," *Classics Ireland* 3 (1996): 47–72; . On Jewish attitudes toward Roman baths, see M. Goodman, *State and Society in Roman Galilee, A.D. 132–212* (Totowa, 1983), 81–84. Note that the records of the baths at Apollinopolis in Egypt include the name of a servant girl who worked there, Sempremakis; see H.C. Youtie, "Records of a Roman Bath in Upper Egypt," *AJA* 53 (1949): 268–70 (= id., *Scriptiunculae,* vol. 2 [Amsterdam, 1973], 990–93). A parallel situation pertained in medieval Germany, where *Badmädchen,* supposedly employed to wash and massage customers and to tend to the customers' other bathing needs, often doubled as prostitutes: see M.E. Wiesner, *Working Women in Renaissance Germany* (New Brunswick, 1986), 95–97; S. Stolz, *Die Handwerke des Körpers: Bader, Barbier, Perückenmacher, Friseur Folge und Ausdruck historischen Körperverständnisses* (Marburg, 1992), 104–10. Similarly, a great volume of legislation sought to distinguish Japanese public baths from brothels and to limit the possibility of moral lassitude at the baths; see Grilli and Levy, *Furo,* 76–78.

62. E.g., Aper brings a one-eyed old woman to watch his shabby robe (Mart. 12.70.2). The only other place where Martial may possibly allude to this phenomenon is at 12.87, where Cotta

the sources from Plautus to the *Digest* and so must have been an endemic problem for the baths' owners and customers alike. A wide variety of sources from the intervening period testify to the problem from different perspectives, on one occasion even from that of the thief.[63] The most direct and poignant evidence, however, comes from the victims themselves who, finding themselves bereft of clothing on emerging wet from their ablutions, wrote curse tablets to bring divine retribution down on the perpetrators. The most eloquent curses come from the huge haul of curse tablets *(defixionum tabellae)* from the spring at Bath in England.[64] One example reads: "Solinus to the goddess Sulis Minerva. I give to your divinity and majesty [my] bathing tunic and cloak. Do not allow sleep or health to him who has done me wrong, whether man or woman, whether slave or free, unless he reveals himself and brings those goods to your temple."[65] In the absence of a police force, the purpose of such tablets was to call on supernatural assistance to retrieve the stolen articles or at least to punish the thief. One common method of seeking retrieval was to transfer ownership of the stolen item to the deity, thus entrusting the detective work to divine agency. It may seem unlikely that such an approach could be effective, but in a superstitious world, results could be surprising. One remarkable text from Kavak in Turkey records the actions of a contrite thief who returned a stolen cloak, which had probably been lifted from a bathhouse: "The god was vexed with the

---

loses his sandals twice and so goes to dinner barefoot. It is not clear where the sandals were lost, but the predinner bath is a good candidate for the location.

63. See Plaut. *Rud.* 382–85; *Dig.* 47.17.1 (a whole section given over to "thieves who lurk about the baths"). Other sources are, e.g., Cat. 33.1; Sen. *Ep.* 56.2; Petron. *Sat.* 30.7–11; Ath. 3.97c. The thief's (fictional) perspective is presented in Apul. *Met.* 4.8, 9.21. Apuleius satirically presents bath thieves as occupying the lowest level in the hierarchy of larceny (*Met.* 4.8).

64. These tablets are collected in *Tab. Sulis.* Some 130 such tablets have been recovered from the Sacred Spring, many fragmentary; most deal with acts of theft. Not all the stolen goods, however, were pilfered from the baths (compare the theft of a ploughshare in *Tab. Sulis* 31 and a theft from a house in *Tab. Sulis* 99), but they seem the most likely context for disappearances of articles of clothing (compare *TAM* 5.1.159, where a cloak is stolen from the bathhouse and the thief cursed) and perhaps also for disappearances of sums of money and jewelry; see Tomlin's comments, *Tab. Sulis,* pp. 80–81. For other such thefts, see *Tab. Sulis* 8, 34, 54, 98 (money); 5, 6, 20, 43, 49, 55, 61–65 (clothing and blankets); 15, 97 (jewelry). On curse tablets in general, see J.G. Gager, *Curse Tablets and Binding Spells from the Ancient World* (Oxford, 1992). A tablet from Valencia may record the thievery of a tunic from a set of baths; see J. Corell, "Drei *defixionum tabellae* aus Sagunt (Valencia)," *ZPE* 101 (1994): 282–85.

65. *Tab. Sulis* 32 (trans. Tomlin): *deae Suli Minerv(a)e Solinus dono numini tuo maliestati paxsa(m) ba(ln)earum et [pal]lleum [nec p]ermitta[s so]mnum | nec san[ita]tem⟨.⟩ei qui mihi fr(a)u\dem [f]ecit si vir si femi[na] si servus | s[i] l[ib]er nissi [⟨s⟩s]e retegens istas | s[p]ecies ad [te]mplum tuum detulerit . . .* (the rest of the text is fragmentary, apparently calling down misfortune on the thief's family and children). The "bathing tunic" appears to have been a garment worn on the way home from the baths (like a modern bathrobe); see HA *Alex. Sev.* 42.1. See also D.R. Jordan, "Curses from the Waters of Sulis," *JRA* 3 (1990): 437–38.

man and after some time had him bring the cloak to the god, and he openly confessed his guilt." Other tablets record pleas and protestations of innocence, apparently offered by those who had learned a curse had been placed on their heads.[66] In such an environment as this, curse tablets may have been an effective way of dealing with the sort of petty thievery endemic at the baths.

Prevention is preferable to remedy, and bathers naturally attempted to protect their belongings before they were forced to resort to curse tablets to retrieve them. There were various means of effecting this protection. The changing rooms in many baths feature niches for storing utensils and clothes, though it is not clear that these niches were originally fitted with doors and locks to make their use secure.[67] The affluent could bring to the baths a slave whose sole purpose was to watch the owner's clothes during the bathing process. On entering the bath, the schoolboy of the *colloquia* instructs his accompanying slave, "Do not fall asleep, on account of the thieves" (*CGL* 3.651.10: *ne addormias propter fures*). Alternatively, a slave attached to the bathhouse could be hired to watch clothes; such slaves were called *capsarii*. Of course, there was no guarantee that a *capsarius* would not be crooked, a fact that generated a specific law governing such individuals.[68] It seems that where there were baths, there were thieves. This situation is an indirect testament to the popular and crowded nature of bathing establishments.

The evidence of Martial, in conjunction with a wide variety of other written sources, allows us to get a feel for the vitality of the Roman bathing experience. It is safe to suggest that, despite regional and chronological variations in aspects of the bathing culture (for instance, with regard to terminology and mixed bathing), the main characteristics of the baths' atmosphere were likely reproduced in almost any bathhouse in the empire. The broad picture is one of a noisy, vibrant place, with dinner parties meeting; bathers eating,

66. See Gager, *Curse Tablets*, 176 (which includes the cited text from Kavak).

67. See the *Tosefta* (*t. Toh.* 8:7, 8:8), which reports that niches in baths can be either "open from one to another"—so that "the utensils were detached from them (i.e., hanging out)"—or "locked and sealed"; even in the latter case, however, one can return to the niche to find "the lock open and the seal spoiled."

68. See *Dig.* 1.15.3.5 (crooked *capsarii*), 3.2.4.2 (slaves as clothes guards and prostitutes), 16.3.1.8 (a *balneator* can act as a *capsarius*). Diocletian's price edict includes a maximum charge for a *capsarius*; see no. 286. Another text mentions a *capsararius (sic) de Antonianas (sic)*, apparently attached to the Baths of Caracalla (no. 273). They could also be found among the *familia* of private citizens; see *CIL* 6.7368 = *ILS* 7413, where a slave doubles as a *capsarius* and *a cubiculo*. Such private *capsarii* were probably the personnel who accompanied their owners to the baths, as attested in several sources—e.g., Mart. 12.70; Anon. *Life of Aesop* 38–39; Petron. *Sat.* 30.7–11.

drinking, and singing; vendors shouting; prostitutes strutting; and thieves prowling. In addition to these particular vignettes offered by the sources, we should imagine there an everyday, timeless social environment characteristic of places of human congress everywhere, with friends meeting and observing the world go by, and with people gossiping, catching up on news, or negotiating business informally. Where Romans gathered in numbers, one can expect much activity, and the baths were where Romans met informally at close quarters on a daily basis. Martial has made it clear that to visit the baths was not only to touch a nerve center of ancient urban life but to participate in a complex social convention defined by fashion. He has proven an instructive guide.

Chapter 2

The Growth of the Bathing Habit

The marked growth in the popularity of the bathing habit among the Romans of the late Republic and early Empire has caught the attention of several scholars but has been largely unstudied in detail.[1] In this chapter, the disparate and varying evidence is surveyed in an attempt to chart the rise of the popularity of baths at Rome and in Italy in the first centuries B.C. and A.D. These limits are imposed by the evidence, which indicates that Roman-style baths emanated from the Italian peninsula out into the empire and that they did so most markedly in the second century A.D. Since the Romans presumably first took to the bathing habit themselves before exporting it, the inquiry that follows concentrates perforce on Rome and Italy and does not extend beyond ca. A.D. 100. At Rome at about this time, construction of the biggest set of baths the city had yet seen (the Thermae of Trajan) was underway, and the period of greatest dissemination of baths into the provinces was just beginning. Both are sure signs that public bathing had come to occupy a central place in the daily routine of the Romans by the early second century.

The clearest way to trace the growth of the bathing habit would be to chart the numbers of baths at Rome and in Italy in successive waves. Unfortunately, such a procedure is not possible, given the inconsistency of the physical record.[2] Sporadic, incomplete, and/or poorly published archaeological investigation precludes a comprehensive comparison of bath sites across the Italian peninsula that would afford a complete picture of growth.[3]

---

1. See, e.g., Heinz, 10 (assigning it, too specifically, to the second quarter of the first century B.C.); Nielsen, 1.43 (an increased dispersion of baths outside Latium and Campania in first centuries B.C. and A.D.); Yegül, 30, 48 (general expansion in the late Republic and early Empire).

2. Nielsen, for instance, catalogues some sixty-seven bath sites from Italy. Of these, thirty-eight are at Rome, Ostia, or Pompeii.

3. The results of Nielsen's Italian survey are worth noting, although her catalogue is selective and is to be used only with caution for quantitative analysis. She lists seven public baths of the first century B.C. (C.1, 35, 40–42, 52, 62); a possible eighth would be the Forum Baths in Herculaneum (C.38), which she dates variously to the first century A.D. or to the first century B.C. (at 1.39 and 2.7 [C.38, F.], respectively). In contrast, Nielsen lists seventeen public facilities of the first century A.D. (C.2, 3, 15, 18, 28, 39, 43–47, 53, 57, 59–61, 63).

At Rome, for instance, despite the evidence of the Regionaries, only a hand-ful of *balnea* have been excavated and adequately published, although one suspects that others must have been discovered over the years but have gone unreported.[4] What is more, the vast majority of the known *balnea* at Rome appear to be of Imperial date, which leads to the distressing realization that no early baths are (officially) known from the city.[5] However, the remarkable remains at Pompeii provide evidence precisely for the period under study here and are given due consideration below.[6] Unfortunately, since Pompeii is unique in preserving a number of Republican structures side by side with early Imperial ones, productive comparison with sites elsewhere in Italy is not currently possible.

The written sources provide few precise figures for baths in any ancient city. Most authors who refer to the volume of baths in a given community do so in vague terms. Typical is the comment of Aelius Aristides that second-century A.D. Smyrna had "so many baths that you would be at a loss to know where to bathe."[7] Similarly, for Rome, only one statement clearly enumerat-ing the city's baths survives, the entry in the *Notitia Urbis Regionum* that records 11 *thermae* and 856 *balnea* (an exact figure not above suspicion).[8]

---

4. The most fully described *balneum* at Rome is the Severan establishment published in A. Cassatella and I. Iacopi, "Il balneum presso le Scalae Caci sul Palatino," in *Thermes,* 129–38. Others are less satisfactorily reported—as are the so-called *Balneum Nereatii Cerealis* (Richardson, *Dictionary,* 49, s.v.) or the *Thermae Lateranenses* (ibid., 393, s.v.)—or they garner bare mention in general reports, such as A.M. Colini et al., "Notiziario di scavi e scoperte in Roma e Suburbio, 1946–60," part 2, *BullCom* 90 (1985): 307–440, where baths at the Piazza dei Cinquecento are reported in a single sentence at 322; another set may lurk among the structures unearthed on the Via Giovanni Giolitti (see ibid., 325). The situation has not im-proved in recent years—a recent guidebook notes that "extraordinarily few examples [of the city's small baths] have been found"; see A. Claridge, *Rome* (Oxford, 1998), 54.

5. Note, however, that M. Medri is soon to publish a private Republican *balneum* in the vicinity of the Palatine.

6. Even the Pompeian evidence is not without its problems: sporadic publication, com-partmentalization of the evidence, and uncontextualized interpretation abound; see A. Wallace-Hadrill, *Houses and Society in Pompeii and Herculaneum* (Princeton, 1994), 66–72, or, more forcefully, id., "Public Honour and Private Shame: The Urban Texture of Pompeii," in T.J. Cornell and K. Lomas, eds., *Urban Society in Roman Italy* (New York, 1995), 40–43.

7. Ael. Arist. 15.232 (Jebb; trans. Behr): λουτρὰ μέν γε τοσαῦτα ὥστε ἀπορήσαις ἂν οὐ λούσαιο. The rhetorical context of the statement (a speech to a visiting governor) may justifiably raise doubts as to its reliability. Note also the colorful apocryphal story that when the Arabs arrived at Alexandria, they used the books of the celebrated library to keep the city's four thousand baths heated for six months; see A.J. Butler, *The Arab Conquest of Egypt*[2] (Oxford, 1978), 401–26.

8. *Notitia* 14 (= *FTUR* 1.1.5). When, however, the region-by-region figures for *balnea* are added up, the total reaches 967 in the *Notitia* and 942 in the *Curiosum* (these totals supersede those erroneously cited in my "Pliny *Natural History* 36.121 and the Number of *Balnea* in Early Augustan Rome," *CP* 88 [1993]: 333). The reason for the disparity is unclear; see Ch. Bruun,

Though this information is noteworthy, the Constantinian date of the notice renders it all but useless for the current inquiry. A comment of Pliny the Elder appears pertinent. Drawing explicitly from the memoirs of M. Agrippa's aedileship (33 B.C.), Pliny records that Agrippa, during his year in office, staged games and offered 170 *balinea gratuita* in the city, adding that "the number has since grown at Rome without limit."[9] At first glance the passage might be taken (as it often has) to show that early Augustan Rome had 170 *balnea* and that the number grew sharply between 33 B.C. and the mid–first century A.D., when Pliny was writing. The shortcomings of Pliny's wording in this passage need to be appreciated, however. Analysis of the epigraphic record reveals that the phrase *balneum gratuitum* was a synonym for *gratuita lavatio,* or "free bathing." The notice, then, shows only Agrippa's generosity in offering free bathing opportunities to the masses. Neither Pliny nor Agrippa gives any indication as to how the benefaction was effected— the "170 free baths" could conceivably have been offered in one bathhouse over 170 days.[10] As a result, the notice offers no concrete numbers for Rome's *balnea*. Nevertheless, Pliny's observation about the subsequent rise in the number of free baths offered in the city can reasonably be taken to reflect a concurrent escalation in the bathing habit during the Augustan and early Imperial periods. An increase in the number of the city's baths would have been an obvious corollary of this situation, but Pliny does not expressly mention such an increase, and there is no direct evidence that there was one. As a result, Pliny's notice does indeed provide evidence for growth in the public bathing habit at Rome in the Julio-Claudian period, but it does so in a vague and oblique manner. As we shall see, comparably indirect and allusive written material is what constitutes our chief evidence for charting the rise in the popularity of baths, so reaching firm conclusions is a difficult and risky task.

Given these difficulties, my procedure in what follows is to present the written material and then the archaeological evidence for baths in the late

---

The Water Supply of Ancient Rome: A Study of Roman Imperial Administration (Helsinki, 1991), 74 n. 48. Despite this disparity, the overall impression left by the *Notitia* that imperial Rome had hundreds of bathhouses should not be questioned—nineteenth-century Edo featured more than 550 public baths (see Grilli and Levy, *Furo,* 78).

9. Pliny *HN* 36.121: *adicit [sc. Agrippa] ipse aedilitatis suae commemoratione et ludos diebus undesexaginta factos et gratuita praebita balinea CLXX, quae nunc Romae ad infinitum auxere numerum.* Pliny's *Natural History* was completed by A.D. 77 (see *praef.* 3) but was evidently many years in the writing; see *RE* 21.271–439, s.v. "Plinius 5" (Kroll), esp. 299–300. The notice does not show, as Nielsen (1.35 and n. 79) claims, that Agrippa increased the number of Rome's *balnea.* Dio (49.43.3) corroborates this notice, but without the precise figures.

10. For a fuller discussion, see Fagan, "Pliny *Naturalis Historia* 36.121."

Republic and early Empire, to see what information can be gleaned about the process of growth in these years. The evidence is often difficult to interpret, but there is enough to suggest that in the first century B.C. Romans began bathing in public more frequently and in greater numbers than before and that this led to a greater prominence of baths in their daily life. In the first century A.D., the time of the early emperors, bathing appears to have become noticeably more popular, a process that elicited the sort of observation made by Pliny above. In the following century, the momentum of this early Imperial phase of growth carried over into the provinces, so that the second century is now rightly considered the golden age of baths in the Roman world, a time when hundreds of communities empire-wide were building their first facilities.[11]

Before setting forth the evidence for growth, the question of the baths' origins needs to be addressed. In this field of study, theories abound amid a dearth of evidence, and the matter is too involved and troubled to delve into profitably here; to pass over it in silence, however, would be inadvisable.[12] Public baths are known from various Hellenistic sites around the Mediterranean, including places in south Italy and Sicily, such as Gela, Syracuse,

---

11. An indication of this golden age is provided in H. Jouffroy, *La construction publique en Italie et dans l'Afrique romaine* (Strasbourg, 1986), 125–29, where "le siècle des Antonins" sees more bath constructions than any other period. Note also that of the 387 baths catalogued by Nielsen, some 152 (40 percent) are dated to the second century A.D. in their initial phases. Naturally, some pre-second-century baths are known from the provinces, but none before the first century B.C., and the absolute figures are very low (see below). Totals for early public bath sites outside Italy, arranged into Nielsen's four province groups, are provided below. Note that the dates have been assigned according to the catalogue entries in Nielsen, since Manderscheid does not provide dates for the individual buildings he catalogues; and only urban public baths are counted, excluding military, sanctuary, private, and gymnasia baths.

Province Group	First Century B.C.	First Century A.D.
Western	6	18
Northern Frontier	1	10
North African	—	1
Eastern	—	9

References (to Nielsen's catalogue entries): Western, B.C.: C.98–100, 110, 112, 135; A.D.: C.75–77, 84, 85, 90, 105, 109, 111, 113, 114, 116, 124–28, 130 (two Augustan baths [C.101, 115], which may be either first century B.C. or A.D., are excluded). Northern Frontier, B.C.: C.189; A.D.: C.138, 147, 154, 156, 158, 164, 185, 197, 198, 200 (the low totals here are mainly due to the large number of military baths in these provinces). N. African, A.D.: C.212 (most baths in this region were built in the second century A.D., the period of its greatest prosperity). Eastern, A.D.: C.254, 276, 282, 285, 296, 304, 305, 327, 360 (the Augustan baths at Pergamum [C.307] are excluded).

12. For an overview of the modern literature on the origins of Roman baths, see J. DeLaine, "Recent Research on Roman Baths," *JRA* 1 (1988): 14–17, and DeLaine's more recent observations in "Roman Baths and Bathing," *JRA* 6 (1993): 354–55.

Megara Hyblaea, and Velia. These baths, however, are of the Greek type, in that they accommodated bathing in individuated hip-baths and their rooms are marked by a rather haphazard internal arrangement with respect to each other. Nevertheless, the bald fact of their existence indicates that public bathing was not, in itself, a Roman invention.[13] For the genesis of Roman-style baths—marked by their communal pools and clear sequence of rooms—the evidence points to Campania. Here can be found the oldest near-intact set of Roman baths (the Stabian Baths at Pompeii, ca. 140 B.C.), as well as the earliest remains so far known (at Cumae, ca. 180 B.C.), even if the latter are poorly preserved and ill understood. Written evidence also converges in and around Campania in the third and second centuries B.C., so that, although the paltry quantity of material counsels caution in drawing hard-and-fast conclusions, what is available indicates that Campania was the wellspring of Roman baths, at least in their developed form.[14] The region is a good candidate for the nursery of the Roman-style bath. It lay at a confluence of cultures (Etruscan, central Italian, Greek, and Roman) and was a prosperous, vibrant, and architecturally innovative place in the third century B.C., the very time when Roman-style baths appear to have emerged under combined Greek and local influences.[15] Once established in Campania and central Italy, the bathing habit reached Rome sometime in the third century B.C., certainly before Plautus, whose plays offer a starting point for our investigation into the growth of the habit.[16]

---

13. On Greek baths, see R. Ginouvès, *Balaneutikè: Recherches sur le bain dans l'antiquité grecque* (Paris, 1962). On their possible influence on Roman forms, see J. DeLaine, "Some Observations on the Transition from Greek to Roman Baths in Hellenistic Italy," *MeditArch* 2 (1989): 111–25.

14. For the remains of the Stabian Baths, see Eschebach, *Stabianer Thermen,* esp. 8–25. For the place of the structure in the early development of Roman baths, see the differing assessments of Heinz (53–57), Nielsen (1.25–36), and Yegül (57–66). Other early Campanian baths are attested at Capua (216 B.C.; see Livy 23.7.3) and at Teanum Sidicinum, Cales, and Ferentinum (ca. 130–21 B.C.; see Gell. *NA* 10.3.3). Dio (15.57.30) and Valerius Maximus (9.6 ext. 2) transfer the Capuan story told by Livy (loc. cit.) to Nuceria, which may raise suspicions as to its accuracy. Nevertheless, all three sources locate these early baths in Campania. But note also the early baths at Aletrium in Central Italy (no. 157) and at Musarna in Etruria (late second century B.C.; see further H. Broise and V. Jolivet, "Le bain en Étrurie à l'époque Hellénistique," in *Thermes,* 79–95).

15. Assuming that the Roman baths at Cumae were not the first ever built, a date in the third century B.C. can reasonably be postulated for the emergence of Roman-style baths. On Campania in this period, see M. Frederiksen, *Campania,* ed. N. Purcell (Rome, 1984), 221–84; Nielsen, 1.25–26; Yegül, 48–55 (the latter prefers a central Italian origin).

16. Varro is clear that baths were "introduced into the city" from elsewhere (*Ling.* 9.68: *primum balneum . . . cum introiit in urbem*).

The Written Evidence: Plautus to Martial

In several passages, Plautus—whose plays constitute the earliest body of extant Latin literature—refers to baths and bathing as habitual elements in the day-to-day life of Rome. The playwright alludes to slaves waiting for their masters to return from the baths, the danger of thievery at the baths, and renegade slaves squandering their master's money on bathing; he also makes passing mention of *balneatores* connected with the administration of the facilities.[17] Plautus' tone in these passages is reminiscent of Martial's, in that the baths are presented as unremarkable and everyday facets of urban living. Various inferences about the nature of these early baths can be drawn from Plautus' passages. They were crowded places, so thieves could operate successfully there; they charged for their services, so money could be spent there; and women used them, so when a courtesan spent a long time in the bath, an impatient client could complain, "If women could be loved for as long as they bathed, all lovers would be bathmen."[18] It seems that Plautus was familiar with baths.

Since Plautus' theater was rooted in the models of Greek New Comedy, the chief difficulty in interpreting his evidence lies in determining to what extent he elicits Greek, rather than Roman, conditions. It is conceivable that Plautus' bath-related passages use Greek culture as their frame of reference and so are imperfect determinants of contemporary Roman bathing practice, such as it was. Two considerations suggest otherwise. First, Plautus was not a mere translator of Greek originals but an adapter who lent his Greek situations a distinctly Roman flavor, drawing on specifically Roman circumstances to do so.[19] Second, given Plautus' comedic purpose, it would make little sense for him to portray situations completely alien to his audience. Rather, like Martial, Plautus assumed that his audience would know what he

---

17. Plaut. *Asin.* 356–57 and *Persa* 90–91 (waiting slaves); *Rud.* 382–85 (thievery); *Trin.* 405–8 (squandering of money); *Poen.* 703 and *Truc.* 322–25 *(balneatores)*.

18. Plaut. *Truc.* 324–25: *si proinde amentur, mulieres diu quam lavant, / omnes amantes balneatores sient.*

19. Many commentators have appreciated this aspect of Plautus' art: see W.S. Anderson, *Barbarian Play: Plautus' Roman Comedy* (Toronto, 1993), 133–51; R.C. Beacham, *The Roman Theatre and Its Audience* (Cambridge, MA, 1992), esp. 29–31; G.B. Conte, *Latin Literature: A History* (Baltimore, 1994), 49–64; G.E. Duckworth, *The Nature of Roman Comedy: A Study in Popular Entertainment* (Princeton, 1952), esp. 384–95; K. Gaiser, "Zur Eigenart der römischen Komödie: Plautus und Terenz gegenüber ihren griechischen Vorbildern," *ANRW* 1.2 (1972): 1079–95; A.S. Gratwick, "Drama," in E.J. Kenney, ed., *The Cambridge History of Classical Literature*, vol. 2, *Latin Literature* (Cambridge, 1982), 103–15.

was talking about. It is true that people can identify and relate to facets of foreign cultures without firsthand experience of them, but it would make little sense for Plautus to comment in detail on the conditions inside a bathhouse—as he does, for example, in *Rudens* 382–85—if the audience had not experienced such a facility, especially in an age lacking mass communication and offering very limited opportunities for travel abroad (excepting the travel of soldiers).[20] On the whole, therefore, Plautus should be seen as the first source to testify to the popularity of public bathing at Rome, even if the precise nature of the facilities themselves cannot be securely determined.[21] How widespread and common the bathing practice was among the Romans in Plautus' day is also not crystal clear, but he consistently presents baths as an unremarkable feature of the urban scene.

Other second-century B.C. evidence is scarce. Terence refers to baths on several occasions, but since he was more concerned than Plautus was with preserving the Greek flavor of his models, his testimony must be treated with more caution.[22] A fragment (98R) of the playwright Caecilius Statius (d. ca. 168 B.C.) mentions a bath, but it is not particularly informative. An obscure reference in Nonius Marcellus has been taken to suggest that baths were a rarity in third-century B.C. Rome, since the comment has been mistakenly accredited to Cato the Censor: "When I was a boy I had an ordinary tunic and toga, shoes without puttees, a horse without a riding blanket; I did not

---

20. For recent use of Plautus as a reliable source for social conditions in the Roman world of his day, see K.R. Bradley, *Slavery and Rebellion in the Roman World, 140 B.C.–70 B.C.* (Bloomington, 1989), 27–30. Note also the comment of O. F. Robinson ("Baths: An Aspect of Roman Local Government Law," *Sodalitas* 3 [1984]: 1065) that "there are references in Plautus which, although they may stem from his Greek sources, suggest that Roman audiences would not find public baths unfamiliar." Plautus also refers to the peculiarly Greek institutions of gymnasia and palaestrae, the existence of which at Rome is not otherwise attested for this period: see *Amph.* 1011; *Epid.* 197–98; *Bacch.* 66–67 (note Varro's rejection of the need of gymnasia for Romans, at *Rust.* 2 *praef.* 2). But it is noteworthy that Plautus' characters do not interact with these buildings as intimately as they do with the *balnea*. Instead, gymnasia and palaestrae appear as remote elements in Plautus' generalized cityscape. On one occasion (*Bacch.* 419–34), Plautus does describe activities at the gymnasium, but his purpose in doing so is to attack the new Greek-influenced education that was growing in popularity among the elite, so his reference to gymnasia in this instance is more topical and satirical than presumptive of any direct experience of gymnasia on the part of his audience.

21. Nielsen's claim (1.27 n. 13) that Plautus portrays Greek-style βαλανεῖα (with hip-baths), not Roman-style baths, is tenuous. Plautus' references are too vague to determine the typology of the structures to which he refers.

22. Many of the studies cited above (chapter 2, n. 19) include consideration of Terence's works. What importance, if any, can be placed on Terence's use of the supine form *lavatum* for a bath (see *Haut.* 655; *Eun.* 592, 596, 600), as opposed to *balineum* (which he uses only once, at *Phorm.* 339), is far from clear.

bathe daily, and the gaming board was scarce."[23] In fact, the notice should be disregarded as evidence for early bathing at Rome for two reasons. First, the provenance of the remark is far from certain. Nonius is here citing Varro's lost work "Catus on Bringing Up Children," in which Cato the Censor no doubt featured prominently. Nonius, however, does not make it clear whether the speaker is Varro, Catus, or Cato. The chronological point of reference for the notice is therefore unclear—it could be the late third century B.C. (Cato), the second century (Catus?), or the first (Varro). Second, the implications of the notice are ambiguous. The speaker (whoever he is) may indeed be saying that baths were generally rare in his youth, but equally, he could be vaunting his own temperate behavior over that of more luxuriously inclined contemporaries. If the latter is the case, a very different inference can be drawn: that though baths were common, not rare, in the speaker's world, he avoided them out of exemplary modesty.[24] Finally, even if the remark is attributed to Cato, he spent his boyhood in Tusculum, not Rome, so the comment is irrelevant as to the status of bathing in the capital. These uncertainties make the passage too troublesome for consideration in the current context.

Later sources can provide some information about this early period, but it must be remembered that such notices may either be mistaken or misleading, insofar as these authors could retroject contemporary bathing habits into the past. Despite these concerns, the passages are worth noting. Varro, writing in the first century B.C., states that when baths were initially introduced into the city of Rome, they had two sections, one for men and one for women. Interestingly, this observation coincides with the archaeological evidence, which shows that Republican baths frequently (but not invariably) featured such an architectural division.[25] The main point to note here is that the baths are seen as arriving at Rome from elsewhere with an already established architectural form, which would be logical if they had originated in Campania and had come to Rome subsequently. The Augustan historian Pompeius Trogus, as epitomized by Justin in the third century A.D., comments that the Romans introduced hot-water bathing to Spain after the Second

---

23. Non. 108M (155L), s.v. "ephippium": *mihi puero modica una fuit tunica et toga, sine fasceis calciamenta, ecus sine ephippio, balneum non cotidianum, alveus rarus.* For the attribution to Cato, see, e.g., Z. Mari, *Tibur*, vol. 4 (Florence, 1991), 46; Nielsen, 1.29. Nonius (194M [285L], s.v. "balneae") also preserves the fragment of Caecilius Statius (98R) just alluded to.

24. On Varro's *Catus de liberis educandis*, see *RE* Suppl. 6.1172–277, s.v. "Terentius 84" (Dahlmann), esp. 1264.

25. See Varro *Ling.* 9.68. Many of the Campanian baths had two sets of rooms (Stabian and Forum Baths at Pompeii; Forum Baths at Herculaneum), but the early baths at Cumae only had one.

Punic War (Justin *Epit.* 44.2.6). If this notice is accurate, it provides corroboration for the evidence of Plautus and the proposed appearance of baths in the capital sometime in the third century B.C.[26] For the following century, Plutarch reports that when Fulvius Flaccus was fleeing his pursuers during the bloody aftermath of C. Gracchus' death in 121 B.C., he hid in a disused bathhouse but was discovered and killed along with his eldest son (*C. Gracch.* 16.4). Plutarch also tells how Jugurtha, incarcerated in the Tullianum in 104 B.C., quipped, "Goodness, how cold your bath is!" The historicity of the remark is impossible to establish, and caution is certainly advisable, since the story has the "famous-last-words" feel of a later invention.[27]

Cicero, by far the most prolific and extant of our Republican sources, provides the most detailed information about baths and bathing in the Republic, for both the second and the first centuries B.C. In two passages illustrating the wit of his forensic and oratorical hero, L. Licinius Crassus, Cicero throws light on second-century B.C. bathing culture. He reports how Crassus, to humiliate his opponent M. Junius Brutus in court, made disparaging and suggestive comments concerning a bathhouse Brutus had inherited from his father and subsequently sold; Crassus made lewd allusions to father and son bathing together, a custom considered improper by Romans of the time.[28] That these were public baths is indicated by a nicety of Ciceronian Latin. Cicero is consistent in using the form *balneae* for public baths and *balneum* for private ones; he uses the former to denote Brutus' baths.[29] Brutus' father, therefore, seems to have bought or built a public bath as an investment sometime in the second century B.C. That senators should be involved in catering to the public bathing habit is a fair indication that it had become sufficiently widespread and popular for them to do so. Cicero

---

26. The earliest physical remains of baths in Spain, however, date to the first century B.C.; see Nielsen, 2.16 (C.110[?] and 112; both in Hispania Tarraconensis).

27. Plut. *Mar.* 12.4: Ἡράκλεις, εἶπεν, ὡς ψυχρὸν ὑμῶν τὸ βαλανεῖον. On the unreliability of such "last-words" motifs (as exemplified in Tacitus), see V. Hunink, "Lucan's Last Words," in C. Deroux, ed., *Studies in Latin Literature and Roman History,* vol. 6 (Brussels, 1992), 390–407.

28. The two passages, *De or.* 2.223–24 and *Clu.* 141, refer to the same incident. For Licinius Crassus (consul in 95 B.C.), see *MRR* 2.11, 579 (Licinius, no. 55); for Brutus, see ibid., 2.40, 576 (Junius, no. 51). On the prohibition of father/son joint bathing, see Cic. *Off.* 1.129; Plut. *Cat. Maj.* 20.7–8; HA *Gord.* 6.4.

29. For *balneum* used for private baths in villas, see *Att.* 2.3.4 (= SB 23), 13.52.1 (= SB 353), 14.13a.1 (= SB 367); *Fam.* 9.16.9 (= SB 190), 14.20.1 (= SB 173). For *balneae* used for public baths, see *Cael.* 61–67; *Rosc. Am.* 18. In this regard, Cicero seems to follow the grammatical prescripts laid out by Varro (*Ling.* 9.68), and he is one of our only sources to do so consistently.

(or Crassus, as reported by Cicero) in no way comments that it was improper or unusual for members of the senatorial order to own such a building.[30]

Cicero continues to be informative for the first century B.C. He reports in the *pro Roscio* (delivered in 80 B.C.) that the elder Roscius was murdered in the vicinity of the Pallacine Baths.[31] Cicero orients the senatorial jurors to the scene of the murder by reference to this establishment. The jurors, therefore, appear to have been familiar with these baths, at least by repute. Some twenty-four years later, Cicero had cause to refer again to another of the city's bathing facilities, this time in more detail. When defending M. Caelius in 56 B.C., he sets part of his presentation inside the Senian Baths, which had been portrayed by the prosecution as a rendezvous for an alleged conspiracy to poison the infamous Clodia, sister of Cicero's archenemy, P. Clodius Pulcher.[32] Cicero makes a farce out of the prosecution's alleged conspiracy, with its cabal of slaves and *amici* of Clodia waiting in the crowded baths to ambush Caelius' friend P. Licinius as he accepted the vial of poison. In doing so, Cicero presents the interior of these baths as an unremarkable backdrop for a comedy of errors, a neutral context requiring little elaboration for the jurors to picture. Once more, the assumption is that the elite jurors would know what he was talking about. In fact, in this instance, Cicero takes it for granted that the jurors would know what life was like *inside* the Senian Baths. This assumption on Cicero's part suggests not that the jurors had visited this particular establishment but rather that Cicero evidently thought they were familiar with comparable facilities; otherwise he would have had

---

30. His suggestive comment on father/son joint bathing can hardly be seen as disparaging the bare fact of bath ownership by the Bruti. Although officially frowned on as unseemly, senators did indulge in speculative business ventures, with real estate large among them: see P. Garnsey, "Urban Property Investment," in M.I. Finley, ed., *Studies in Roman Property* (Cambridge, 1976), 123–36; I. Shatzman, *Senatorial Wealth and Roman Politics* (Brussels, 1975), 11–46. M. Licinius Crassus, for instance, who was held up as a paragon of greed, earned his vast fortune from property, mining, renting skilled slaves, agriculture, and inheritances; see A.M. Ward, *Marcus Crassus and the Late Roman Republic* (Columbia, MO, 1977), 68–77. Even the virtuous Cicero had property interests in Rome; see *Att.* 11.2.2–3 (= SB 212), 14.9.1 (= SB 363). Plutarch presents Cato the Elder, in many ways the model of a Roman Republican man, as having money unashamedly invested in various ventures he considered safe and sure; see *Cat. Maj.* 21.5–6. Interestingly "hot waters" (ὕδατα θερμὰ) are among Cato's properties, but the reference here is probably to developed springs rather than artificially heated urban public baths; on such springs, see Heinz, 157–75; Weber, 118–29; Yegül, 92–127. The renting of bathhouses for profit as a matter of course is attested in later sources, such as the Jewish Mishnah: see *m. B. Bat.* 5:3; *m. Abod. Zar.* 1:9. See also no. 282.

31. Cic. *Rosc. Am.* 18. They appear to have been named after the street on which they stood; see *RE* 18.3.156–57, s.v. "Pallacinae vicus" (Welin).

32. Cic. *Cael.* 61–67. These baths may have been named after their builder, but their location is not traceable. The establishment may have been the property of the senatorial family of the Saenii; see appendix 2, under "Named Baths of Uncertain Location."

to provide them with more contextualizing information. That such aristocratic young men as Licinius or the *amici* of Clodia could be portrayed at the Senian Baths without comment goes a long way to discredit the recent claim that Rome's Republican baths were "definitely not places of much social respectability."[33]

The only other contemporary testimony is provided by Catullus, who likens the rapacity of Vibennius to that of "the cleverest clothes-thief at the baths" (33.1–2: *O furum optime balneariorum, / Vibenni pater et cinaede fili*). As with Plautus, the phenomenon of thievery at the baths is assumed as something the reader will identify with, suggesting a familiarity with the experience of public bathing among Catullus' audience.

It seems from the foregoing testimonies that by the mid–first century B.C., baths had become a familiar fact of life at Rome, so accepted a part of the urban landscape that they could be used as landmarks and backdrops in forensic speeches delivered to juries drawn from the elite and in allusions penned by poets and playwrights. Evidence of the attitudes that generated this situation is to be found in Cicero's letters, such as when he writes to his wife and includes bathing among "the necessities for life and health" or when he looks forward to a visit of Atticus and promises to have the bath heated in anticipation. Indeed, by Cicero's day, offering a bath to an arriving guest appears to have been a common courtesy; Cicero asks it of his host Paetus and also of his wife in preparation for his own advent. In other passages, Cicero presents taking a bath as a nondescript part of the daily routine.[34] Reference in all of these instances appears to have been to private baths attached to houses or villas, but there is no reason to suppose that similar attitudes were not extended to public facilities.

Some noncontemporary writers also throw light on this period, but they are subject to the caveats already raised for such secondary material (above, chapter 2, p. 47). Dio relates that in 60 B.C. Faustus Sulla, son of the dictator, furnished the Roman people with free baths and oil (among other benefactions), and similar largess is credited to Augustus and Agrippa.[35] Dio de-

---

33. J. Carter, "Civic and Other Buildings," in I.M. Barton, ed., *Roman Public Buildings*[2] (Exeter, 1995), 47.

34. Cic. *Att.* 2.3.4 (= SB 23; bath prepared for Atticus' arrival; 60 B.C.); *Fam.* 14.20.1 (= SB 173; baths as a necessity, wife to prepare bath; 47 B.C.); *Fam.* 9.16.9 (= SB 190; Paetus; 46 B.C.). For daily baths, see *Att.* 13.52.1 (= SB 353), 14.13a.1 (= SB 367). Note also Val. Max. 9.5.3, where Pompey is accosted leaving a bath.

35. See Dio 37.51.4 (Faustus Sulla); Dio 49.43.3 and Pliny *HN* 36.121 (Agrippa in 33 B.C.); Dio 54.25.4 (Augustus in 13 B.C.). Likewise, Nero provided free oil to senators and *equites* at the dedication of his baths in Rome (see Suet. *Ner.* 12.3), and inscriptions attest analogous benefactions in various towns (see nos. 214–21, 331–36).

scribes Sulla's benefaction as "brilliant" (λαμπρῶς), which tends to suggest that the baths of the city were numerous. Suetonius records that when Augustus' mother, Atia, was pregnant with the future emperor (in 63 B.C.), she was afflicted with a mark on her body in the form of a serpent that caused her to avoid public baths for the rest of her life (*Aug.* 94.4). In this case, however, there is reason for pause, since Suetonius identifies his source as the *Theologumena* of Asclepiades of Mendes, a grammarian possibly of Tiberian date.[36] Such an omen story is, in any case, more likely to have arisen after Augustus achieved greatness, and so it may reflect later attitudes toward bathing in public. Nonetheless, it implies that for an upper-class woman of childbearing age to avoid public baths for the rest of her life was a notable act of self-denial.

For the early Imperial period, more contemporary evidence becomes available. The Augustan poets Horace and Ovid provide useful information. For Horace, baths were regularly encountered facilities, characteristic of urban living. They charged entrance fees and were part of the poet's daily routine.[37] Ovid portrays the city's "many baths" as meeting places for furtive lovers, where a young woman's chaperone could be left outside while she cavorted inside (*Ars Am.* 3.638–40). Besides providing an indication of the practice of mixed bathing in Augustan Rome, the reference illustrates the habitually vague but suggestive nature of written evidence for the number of baths in any given city. A further indication of their prevalence at this time is suggested by Vitruvius, who devotes an entire chapter of his architectural handbook to describing them.[38] It is evident that Vitruvius was drawing on a store of accumulated knowledge about how to erect such buildings, which points to a long tradition of familiarity with the type among prior Roman architects. The medical writer Celsus, of Tiberian date, can also be noted here. He frequently includes bathing, in all probability in public facilities, as part of his treatments.[39]

Perhaps the most instructive evidence comes from a man who, in his public pronouncements at least, claims to have despised baths and bathing.

---

36. For Asclepiades, see *RE* 2.1627, s.v. "Asklepiades 26" (Schwartz). Here Asclepiades is seen as a possible contemporary of Seleukos, an astrologer and grammarian known to Tiberius; see *RE* 2A.1248, s.v. "Seleukos 28" (Stählin).

37. See Hor. *Epist.* 1.11.11–14 (baths in general), 1.14.14–15 (urban feature); *Sat.* 1.3.137–39 (cheap bath), 1.6.125–26 (regular element of daily routine). For a survey of bathing references in the Augustan poets, see Griffin, *Latin Poets,* 88–111.

38. Vitr. 5.10. The date of Vitruvius' work is disputed, but he claims to have been known to Caesar the Dictator (1 *praef.* 2), which might place the work in the thirties or early twenties; for a recent discussion, see B. Baldwin, "The Date, Identity, and Career of Vitruvius," *Latomus* 49 (1990): 425–34.

39. Celsus is treated in detail below, at chapter 4, p. 86.

In numerous passages, the mid-first-century A.D. philosopher L. Annaeus Seneca voices his abhorrence of the contemporary bathing culture and, in doing so, provides many useful insights into the practice.⁴⁰ His most sustained diatribe is stimulated by a visit to the villa of Scipio Africanus, where he sees the great man's private bath. The raw simplicity of the small, dark place conjures in Seneca romantic images of old Republican virtue, which he contrasts to the luxury of current bathing habits (*Ep.* 86.4–13). Seneca's diatribe speaks volumes as to the growth in the baths' popularity. At one point, he expressly says that "once" *(olim)* there were a few modestly appointed baths in the city, clearly implying that in his own day such was not the case. He also comments on the fickleness of contemporary bathers, who abandon a once popular establishment as an antique when a new luxury appears elsewhere.⁴¹ This would imply that in Seneca's Rome, new baths were opening with some frequency. Seneca's heavy-handed moralizing cannot be taken at face value: he had an ax to grind, and he no doubt exaggerated for effect.⁴² But his general portrayal of a sharp rise in the baths' popularity and of a concomitant increase in their luxury coincides with the similar and more-or-less contemporary observations of Pliny the Elder, which suggests that Seneca was not making it all up.⁴³ From another perspective, it would make little sense for Seneca to devote so much time and energy to denouncing widespread bathing luxury if the baths were not sufficiently common and popular to earn such vocal disapproval.

---

40. Sen. *Dial.* 7.7.3 (pleasure lurks in the baths), 10.12.7 (pampered people at the baths); *Ep.* 56.1–2 (dreadful noises emanating from a bath), 86.4–13 and 90.25 (deplorable growth in bath luxury; see 122.8), 108.16 (baths emaciate the body), 122.6 (excessive drinking at the baths).

41. Sen. *Ep.* 86.8–9. Note that in Japan, novelty baths of all sorts have arisen in mutual competition. They are associated with hot-spring resorts and offer a wide variety of out-of-the-ordinary bathing experiences: bathing in milk, in a golden tub, in glass-bottomed tubs set in rivers, or even in suspended gondolas affording scenic coastal views (see Grilli and Levy, *Furo,* 157–59).

42. Public moralizers often fall short of their own standards, as was the case even with the archetypal Cato the Elder (see, e.g., Plut. *Cat. Maj.* 19.4–8). Seneca can be shown to exaggerate in at least one instance. He swears he shunned hot baths all his life and only bathed in cold or sun-warmed water; see *Ep.* 108.16 and 123.4 (shuns baths), 83.5 (cold water). Yet he died by suffocation in a steam bath, presumably attached to his villa (see Tac. *Ann.* 15.64.4–5). For one who avoided baths, he demonstrates a suspicious familiarity with conditions there (in one passage, he lists types of marbles found in baths; see *Ep.* 86.6–7). Dio (61.10.2–4) is especially scathing on the contrast between Seneca's words and deeds. Despite this evidence to the contrary, one recent biography accepts that Seneca avoided hot baths for medical reasons; see M.T. Griffin, *Seneca: A Philosopher in Politics* (Oxford, 1976), 41–42.

43. See Pliny *HN* 36.121 (rise in free baths); see also 33.153 (rise in bath luxury since the Republic), 36.189 (rise in bath luxury since Agrippa's day).

In the surviving segment of the *Satyricon,* by the Neronian novelist Petronius, baths appear as common elements in daily life. Characters meet at the baths, lose clothes and companions, sing poetry, revel, and complain about overly enthusiastic masseurs.[44] Such a situation is also reflected in Juvenal and Martial, whose works date to the very end of the period under consideration here. In both authors, baths and bathing feature regularly, making it clear that by then the bathing habit was well established as a common, frequent, and popular pastime.[45]

Finally, a comment in Pliny the Younger, writing toward the end of the first century, is particularly noteworthy. When describing his villa at Laurentium, Pliny reports that the nearby *vicus* (village) housed no less than three public baths, which he was not averse to using if his private suite was unavailable.[46] It is immediately surprising that a place so small as a *vicus* should have at least three baths sufficiently comfortable for Pliny to visit, and there may have been more, since Pliny only mentions the ones he would use.[47] But we should not extrapolate too much from this passage. The proximity of the town to the large population centers of Ostia and Rome may have generated a greater number of bathhouses here than was typical for such a small place.[48]

As evidence for growth, inscriptions are barely informative and are vitiated by some interpretative difficulties. For the entire Republican period, there are only nine bath-related inscriptions in the epigraphic sample, as well

---

44. Petron. *Sat.* 26–28 (meeting dinner party), 30 (clothes lost), 42 (massage), 72–73 (a private bath at end of a party), 91 and 92 (poetry), 97 (slave lost), 130 (a private bath?); see also 53 and fr. 2. The Petronian authorship and Neronian date of this work have been most cogently argued for by K.F.C. Rose, *The Date and Author of the* Satyricon (Leiden, 1971).

45. The evidence of Martial is fully treated in the previous chapter. For baths in Juvenal, see 1.142–43, 2.149–52, 6.374–76, 6.419–25, 7.1–5, 7.232–33, 11.3–5.

46. Pliny *Ep.* 2.17.26. The remains of this humble town, Vicus Augustanus Laurentium (see *CIL* 14.2045), have been partially excavated, but no public baths datable to Pliny's time have been uncovered: see A. Claridge, "Il vicus di epoca imperiale nella tenuta presidenziale di Castelporziano: Indagini archeologiche 1984," in *Castelporziano,* vol. 1, *Campagna di scavo e restauro 1985* (Rome, 1985), 71–78; id., "Il Vicus di epoca imperiale: Indagini archeologiche nel 1985 e 1986," in *Castelporziano,* vol. 2, *Campagna di scavo e restauro 1985–1986* (Rome, 1988), 61–73; C. Pavolini, *Ostia* (Bari, 1983), 249. See also Meiggs, 69–70; A.N. Sherwin-White, *The Letters of Pliny: A Historical and Social Commentary* (Oxford, 1966), 199.

47. Pliny's fastidious bathing tastes are suggested by what he expected from his private facilities; see *Ep.* 2.17.11 (in his Laurentine villa), 5.6.25–27 (in his Tuscan villa).

48. *Castella* and *vici* could have baths, as written evidence and archaeology make clear: see Apul. *Met.* 8.29; nos. 82, 107, 120, 167. The numerous baths attached to military installations appear also to have served local communities.

as two other, possibly Republican texts.[49] In contrast, early Imperial texts (including Augustan examples) number thirty-nine.[50] Not too much store can be placed on this slight numerical increase, however, since the overall number of Imperial inscriptions far outweighs that of Republican ones. As a result, there is little room for firm conclusions based on quantitative analysis. Nevertheless, one noticeable feature of the material is its geographic distribution. All but two of the Republican texts are of Italian origin, but for the early Imperial period, many other regions are represented: Spain, Gaul, and North Africa in the West; Thrace, Asia, and Lycia in the East. The geographical dispersion of Roman bathing culture, so dramatically attested for the second century A.D., had already begun in the first. Within Italy, the early Imperial inscriptions testify to the continuing spread of baths throughout the peninsula (most are commemorations of bath construction). Particularly informative are the stipulations at Pisa for mourning the death of Augustus' son C. Caesar in A.D. 4: the town's temples, public baths, and taverns were to be closed for a prescribed period.[51] Pisa apparently had several sets of *balnea* at this time, although—typically—firm figures cannot be adduced.

All of this written evidence, when viewed cumulatively, suggests a steady growth in the popularity of baths in the first century B.C., followed by a sharper increase in the bathing habit in the early Imperial period, from Augustus to Martial. Beginning with the vague allusions in Plautus, baths had grown to become necessities of life for Cicero, as well as familiar urban landmarks and part of the daily routine for many of his contemporaries. Most of this written testimony is indirect, so the perception of growth for this period is perforce based more on impression than on solid data. For the

---

49. Nos. 21, 61–67, 157 (Republican); nos. 204, 205 (possibly Republican or Augustan). Note also some possibly bath-related inscriptions recording work on *piscinae*, CIL 1².1693 = ILLRP 521 (Acerantia; post–Social War) and CIL 1².1714 = ILS 5729 = ILLRP 542 (Lacedonia; post–Social War). *Solaria* are also mentioned in CIL 1².1236 = ILS 5392 = ILLRP 116 (Nola; post-Sullan), CIL 1².1719 = ILS 5621 = ILLRP 600 (modern Frigento; uncertain date), and CIL 1².779 = ILLRP 766 (Tolosa; uncertain date). In relation to the latter, note the sundial found in the Stabian Baths (see Eschebach, *Stabianer Thermen,* 17). In addition, a bilingual inscription of Republican date from Delos (*ILS* 9366 = *ILLRP* 755) records work on the *laconicum* there, but it appears not to refer to a Roman-style bath.

50. Nos. 1–4, 68–78, 158–68, 204–9, 215, 226, 250, 257, 258, 261, 269. Note also CIL 11.3010 (Ager Viterbiensis; *balneum* mentioned; dated by Nielsen [1.40 n. 25] to the first century); 14.4711 (Ostia; *balneum* mentioned; dated by Nielsen [loc. cit.] to the early Augustan period); see also citation in next note (n. 51).

51. See CIL 11.1421 = ILS 140, lines 20–24.

following century, the evidence is somewhat more explicit. Comments made by Pliny the Elder and Seneca on the rise of the luxury and popularity of baths in their lifetime are reflected in suggestive passages in other authors. Despite the absence of numerical precision, most of the sources reviewed above, including the inscriptions, reflect a process of growth covering the first century B.C. and continuing into the next.

One (admittedly crude) method of illustrating this process is to trace the occurrence of bath-related word stems (i.e., *therm-*, *baln-*, *balin-*) in authors of the periods surveyed.[52] The figures should be treated with caution, since there are many reasons why one author refers to baths and another does not. Low totals for bath references do not necessarily require a lack of experience with baths on the part of specific authors or their audiences, nor do high totals imply the opposite. Cicero's letters, for instance, are generally less focused on the sort of materialistic concerns that preoccupied Pliny the Younger, and so it is not surprising that they feature fewer references to baths and bathing, while Celsus and Pliny the Elder, both writers very much concerned with medicine and health, are more likely to allude to baths. Authors of the two periods who wrote in similar genres or set their works in similar social contexts do, however, show a divergence in the frequency of their allusions to baths and bathing (as with Horace and Catullus as opposed to Martial or Juvenal). Altogether, the first-century A.D. authors, as a group, refer to baths more consistently and frequently than do the earlier writers. This broad feature of the figures may reflect the increased prominence and popularity of baths in the world of the first-century A.D. authors as against those of the previous century. This increased prominence would suggest that the already rising popularity of baths received an impetus from the establishment of the Principate. Certainly, the early emperors increased the architectural development of the capital and, in particular, oversaw the construction of the Thermae of Agrippa, Nero, and Titus.[53] An examination of the archaeological evidence is called for to see what it can contribute to the discussion.

---

52. The search was conducted using the Packard Humanities Institute's database of Latin texts. Adjectival uses of *therm-* or references to personal names and places have been excluded. The figures are as follows. For the Republic: Plautus, 10; Catullus, 1; Cicero, 36; Terence, 1. For the early Empire: Horace, 4; Celsus, 101; Juvenal, 12; Seneca, 37; Pliny the Elder, 71; Pliny the Younger, 32; Petronius, 18; Martial, 50.

53. See the early chapters of J.B. Ward-Perkins, *Roman Imperial Architecture* (London, 1981), or W.L. MacDonald, *The Architecture of the Roman Empire,* vol. 1² (New Haven, 1982). Bath building at Rome is surveyed below, in chapter 5.

The Archaeological Evidence: The Public Baths of Pompeii

Despite the great volume of archaeological evidence for baths, the physical record displays many shortcomings that limit its usefulness for tracing the historical development of the bathing habit. Most urban sites, including Rome itself, afford an incomplete picture of growth, since many contain only one or two bathing establishments, which are frequently ill investigated, or which, even when more fully explored, often date to a period subsequent to that under consideration here.[54] Some sites are, however, instructive in themselves. The evidence for a wooden bathhouse associated with an as yet unpublished Tiberian fort at Velsen in Holland suggests how deeply ingrained the bathing habit had become by that date: the soldiers on campaign would rather erect a temporary facility than do without.[55] But by and large, as matters stand, a full picture of growth cannot be reconstructed from archaeological evidence alone.[56] As with the written material, we are forced to rely on impressions gained from specific loci, usually (for Italy) Ostia, Herculaneum, and Pompeii. The latter is the most informative with regard to baths, since it contains side-by-side at the one place bathhouses datable to the Republican and early Imperial eras. Pompeii can therefore be used as an archaeological testing ground for the process of growth we have discerned in the written testimony.[57] In documenting the city's baths, we are interested less in the minutiae of their architecture and technology (which, in any case, have been published more fully elsewhere) and more in any indications of

---

54. The barely published bathhouse at Cales (90–70 B.C.) provides a good example of scant investigation: see W. Johannowsky, "Relazione preliminare sugli scavi di Cales," *BdA* 46 (1961): 258–68; S. de Caro and A. Greco, *Campania* (Bari, 1981), 242. The earliest baths at Ostia are Julio-Claudian: see Meiggs, 406; Nielsen, 2.6 (C.28) (on the Baths of Invidiosus); however, a fragmentary inscription (*CIL* 14.4711) attests to the existence of a late Republican or early Imperial bathhouse there.

55. The evidence for the bathhouse comprises postholes for a putative clay-lined wooden hypocaust, strigils, and wooden sandals *(sculponea)* worn by bathers. The whole complex appears to have been associated with the campaigns of A.D. 16–25. I am indebted to A.V.A.J. Bosman for this information, gained in conversation with him at the First International Conference on Roman Baths (Bath, April 1992). By way of comparison, Mr. Bosman, an ex–United Nations soldier, told me how Finnish troops posted in Lebanon insisted on taking saunas, regardless of how high the ambient temperature was. Similarly, the 1948 Finnish Olympic team brought to London its own sauna, which it bequeathed to a local sports center when the games were over (see W.R. Mead, *An Experience of Finland* [London, 1993], 28–30).

56. The same is true also for other subjects of archaeological investigation in Italy; see T.W. Potter, *Roman Italy* (Berkeley, 1987), 63.

57. The issue of the typicality of the city's evidence for Roman Italy is thorny, but several recent studies have made cases for its usefulness in this regard: see Laurence, 133–41; Richardson, *Pompeii,* esp. xv–xvi; Wallace-Hadrill, *Houses and Society,* 14–16, 174.

growth they exhibit, both in the development of the buildings themselves and within the context of their wider urban setting.

The oldest baths at Pompeii—indeed the oldest near intact set anywhere—are the Stabian Baths (see figs. 1–5). By 80 B.C., when Pompeii became a Roman colony, this facility was already a substantial complex, occupying half an *insula* (city block) in the city's center, and boasting a palaestra, two sets of bathing rooms, and a latrine.[58] The establishment of the Sullan colony heralded an extension of the building's facilities. As recorded in an inscription (no. 61), the city's authorities renovated the palaestra and added two new rooms: a *laconicum* for sweating and a *destrictarium* for scraping off with strigils. In the century-and-a-half between these alterations and the destruction of the city in 79, the Stabian Baths grew further. Specifically, a house to the west of the palaestra was demolished to make room for a recreation wing featuring an outside pool with flanking rooms (which functioned either as shallow pools or open loggias), a second changing room, and a ball court. In the north wing, open rooms off the palaestra were added, probably exedrae for relaxation. Most of these alterations, especially the addition of the open-air pool, likely coincided with the introduction into Pompeii of a conduit from the Serino aqueduct in the Augustan period.[59] Taken as a whole, the building's facilities expanded

---

58. The baths occupy the southern half of *insula* 7.1, with entrances at 8, 14, 15–17, 48, 50, and 51 (see map 1). The fullest description of the building is in Eschebach, *Stabianer Thermen.* For full bibliography, see Manderscheid, 175, s.v. "Terme Stabiane." Now add Eschebach and Müller-Trollius, *Gebäudeverzeichnis,* 242–43; Nielsen, 1.25–33 (see 2.7 [C. 40]); Richardson, *Pompeii,* 100–105; Weber, 34–39; Yegül, 61–63. The early history of the building was reconstructed by Eschebach as an evolution from a fifth-century B.C. Greek bathhouse to a Roman-style facility by the second century B.C. Eschebach's scheme has been widely accepted, but it is not without its problems (see, for instance, Richardson, *Pompeii,* loc. cit.).

59. See H. Eschebach, "Die innerstädtische Gebrauchswasserversorgung dargestellt am Beispiel Pompejis," in J.-P. Boucher, ed., *Journées d'études sur les aqueducs romains* (Paris, 1983), 86–88, where construction techniques suggest an Augustan date for the aqueduct; an inscription appears to name it as the *Fontis Augustei Aquaeductus:* see I. Sgobbo, "L'acquedotto romano della Campania: 'Fontis Augustei Aquaeductus,'" *NSc,* 1938, 75–97. Agrippa may have had a villa in Campania (see Dio 54.28.2). He had been responsible for much hydraulic work at Rome, and his links to the region could have stimulated the aqueduct's construction. Although aqueducts were not a prerequisite for baths (a well had fed the Stabian Baths for many years before the arrival of the aqueduct water), there must have come a time when the expansion of facilities demanded one, especially when large open pools were added. More work needs to be done on this issue, but see H.B. Evans, "Water Distribution: *Quorsum et cui bono?*" in A.T. Hodge, ed., *Future Currents in Aqueduct Studies* (Leeds, 1991), 21–27, and now see also id., *Water Distribution in Ancient Rome: The Evidence of Frontinus* (Ann Arbor, 1994). For a summary and extensive bibliography of recent work on the water supply of Roman towns, see A.O. Koloski-Ostrow et al., "Water in the Roman Town: New Research from *Cura Aquarum* and the *Frontinus Society,*" *JRA* 10 (1997): 181–91.

steadily in the Republic but more rapidly under the early Principate. The change in the nature of the alterations is also noteworthy. Whereas the Republican authorities had added mostly operational rooms, in the form of a sweat bath and a strigiling room, their Augustan and early Imperial counterparts preferred amenities more for recreation than function—open-air pools, a ball court, and exedrae. This divergence testifies to the changing priorities of those who used the baths and reflects the advent of the sort of luxurious habits that so irked Seneca.

That the Augustan renovations in the Stabian Baths were stimulated solely by the introduction of the aqueduct cannot be the whole story. After all, there were other uses to which the Pompeians could (and did) put their aqueduct water—feeding public basins, troughs, fountains, and private residences. That they chose to assign some of the new water to an expansion of their main bathing facility suggests not only that the popularity of bathing was generally on the rise but also that the Pompeians were trying to keep up with current bathing fashions.[60] By the Augustan period, the Stabian Baths must have had the appearance of an antique, an establishment built in and for a bygone age. By adding more and luxurious facilities, the people of Pompeii were in all likelihood imitating models that they had heard of or seen. Certainty is impossible, but the construction at Rome of the great Thermae of Agrippa may have been exerting an influence on the form of the peninsula's bathhouses, and this influence may be reflected in the "modernization" of the Stabian Baths.[61]

The foundation of the Sullan colony in 80 B.C. saw not only the implementation of the alterations to the Stabian Baths but also the construction of an entirely new facility just north of the forum. The so-called Forum Baths are smaller than the Stabian Baths, but their construction attests a desire on the part of the new authorities to lend their colony greater dignity (see figs. 6–

---

60. A conduit from the aqueduct led straight to the (enlarged) reservoir in the baths; see Eschebach, *Stabianer Thermen,* 34.

61. To be sure, a general shift in the design of baths from the first century B.C. to the first century A.D. is traceable in Italy and elsewhere. The "newer" baths usually lack bathing wings for women, are more roomy, have more and bigger windows, and display increased decorative refinement. The type may start with the Thermae of Agrippa, themselves not very well understood due to the scrappy physical remains. On bath development, see Nielsen, 1.43–49; Yegül, 57–91. For the Thermae of Agrippa, see below, chapter 5, pp. 107–10. Outside Rome, the changes are attested, for instance, by a comparison of the Republican-era Forum Baths at Herculaneum with the Julio-Claudian Suburban Baths; I will show that the "new baths" make their appearance at Pompeii also.

12).[62] These baths were later extended, probably in the Augustan period, by the addition of the women's section, which was rather inexpertly crammed into the northwest corner, so that it encroached onto the street (see figs. 7, 8).[63] If it is accurate to date this addition to the Augustan period, the first-century B.C. construction and subsequent extension of this building keeps step with contemporary developments in the Stabian Baths, and the changes in the internal arrangements of both buildings can in turn be read as reflecting a general growth in the bathing habit at Pompeii and elsewhere.

Still more suggestive was the discovery in 1950 of yet another public bathhouse of Republican date, since labeled, somewhat unimaginatively, the Republican Baths (see figs. 13, 14).[64] Like the city's other two facilities, it was a double building with a palaestra, but on a much smaller scale, occupying only a section of the *insula* in which it stood. Looking at the building materials and the primitive form of the hypocaust—whereby the floor was raised not on pillars but on continuous walls broken by diagonal openings—the excavator, A. Maiuri, postulated a construction date of ca. 90–80 B.C. An earlier construction date has recently been proposed, chiefly on the basis

---

62. The baths occupy the center of *insula* 7.5, with entrances at 2, 7, 8, 10, 12, and 24. For a full bibliography, see Manderscheid, 173, s.v. "Pompei, Terme del Foro." Now add Eschebach and Müller-Trollius, *Gebäudeverzeichnis,* 286–87; Nielsen, 1.30–34 (see 2.7–8 [C.42]); Richardson, *Pompeii,* 147–53. It has recently been argued that these baths have their genesis in the Samnite period and were substantially refurbished, not initially constructed, in the Sullan period; see L. Eschebach, "Die Forumsthermen in Pompeji, Regio VII, Insula 5," *AntW* 22 (1991): 257–87. This reconstruction, however, is based on tenuous evidence and is explicitly modeled on H. Eschebach's scheme for the Stabian Baths, itself not above suspicion. It also contradicts the inscription (no. 62) dating the main construction to ca. 80 B.C.

63. That the women's section is a later addition is further suggested by its being equipped with a hypocausted *tepidarium,* whereas the men's section is not. This difference indicates that the women's *tepidarium* was built after the men's, at a time when hypocausts were habitual in such rooms; see Nielsen, 1.155–56, s.v. "tepidarium." Richardson (*Pompeii,* 151–52) dates the extension to the Augustan period, based on differences in construction techniques (clearly visible in fig. 8). Nielsen (2.7–8 [C.42, F.]) lists major rebuilding in the Augustan period but does not specify the nature of it. In contrast, Eschebach ("Forumsthermen," 271–72) would date the women's section to the "refurbishment" of ca. 80 B.C.

64. This small establishment occupies the southeast corner of *insula* 8.5, with an entrance at 36. It was advantageously sited near the entrance to the Triangular Forum and the theater (see fig. 14). The main publication remains A. Maiuri, "Scoperta di un edificio termale nella Regio VIII, Insula 5, Nr. 36," *NSc,* 1950, 116–36. See Manderscheid, 174, s.v. "Pompei, Terme Repubblicane." Now add Eschebach and Müller-Trollius, *Gebäudeverzeichnis,* 384–85; Nielsen, 1.32 (see 2.7 [C.41]); Yegül does not devote any space to the building. It has attracted little attention since Maiuri's excavations: a recent survey of Pompeii's public buildings (Laurence, 20–37) does not acknowledge its existence, and a major study of the city's architectural history mentions it once, and only then in connection with a well on the premises (Richardson, *Pompeii,* 52). Today, the site is overgrown and inaccessible.

of the hypocaust, but in the absence of any further investigation of the site, the excavator's date is preferred.[65] Thus, the Republican Baths were opened for business at about the same time as the Forum Baths, and they operated in close proximity to the Stabian Baths, which lie only one block north (see map 1). The small scale of the building and the circumstances of its later abandonment suggested to Maiuri that, unlike the city's two main public baths, it was a privately owned facility.[66] This proposition fits with the written testimony concerning people of substance investing in baths, and it offers an explanation for the building's abandonment in Augustan times.[67] The Augustan extension of the Stabian Baths, rendered more comfortable than ever with their new amenities, may have put this place out of business—the Republican Baths simply went out of fashion. If this hypothesis is correct, these small baths offer a fascinating glimpse into the rise and fall of a privately owned public bathing establishment, recalling Seneca's condemnation of a fickle public abandoning older baths as more luxurious ones became available.[68] As to evidence for growth, that an entrepreneur felt secure enough to open the Republican Baths even as the city was building (or had built) an entirely new establishment near the forum possibly reflects the proprietor's perception of a rise in the popularity of public bathing; that the facility operated for half a century suggests that this perception was not misplaced.

---

65. See DeLaine, "Some Observations," 120 n. 32. DeLaine views this hypocaust as intermediate between Greek protohypocausts in Magna Graecia and the fully developed Roman *suspensura* on pillars. Despite the plausibility of her scheme, the many gaps in the evidence for the early development of the hypocaust make it suspiciously neat. Also, other considerations could explain the unusual form of the hypocaust. For instance, perhaps it was less costly to construct than the more exacting requirements of a floor raised on individual pillars. Recent studies maintain the construction date proposed by Maiuri: see Nieslen, 2.7 (C.41); Yegül, 57.

66. That the Stabian and Forum Baths were publicly owned is suggested by inscriptions from both buildings recording the work of *duoviri* there: see nos. 61 (Stabian Baths); 62, 68 (Forum Baths). No inscriptions from the Republican Baths survive, if there were ever any in the first place.

67. The area occupied by the baths was cleared and converted into a peristyle/dining room attached to the neighboring Casa della Calce. Construction techniques in the new annex suggest an Augustan date for these operations; see Maiuri, "Scoperta," 130.

68. See Sen. *Ep.* 86.8–9. There are, of course, many other possibilities to explain the baths' abandonment and the extension of the neighboring house (e.g., perhaps the property changed hands and the new owner did not want the hassle of running a bathhouse, or perhaps the owner of the Casa della Calce set out to expand the house in this direction), but they can only be guessed at. In general, we should not be too hasty to compartmentalize periods of change in Roman towns—in many places, construction, reconstruction, alteration, and redecoration must have been all but constant; see J. DeLaine, "The Insula of the Paintings at Ostia I.4.2–4: Paradigm for a City in Flux," in Cornell and Lomas, *Urban Society,* 79–106. The abandonment of the Republican Baths may have been just another example of this almost perpetual pattern of construction.

In the early Imperial period, no new baths were built within the walls of Pompeii until the last years of the city's life. It might appear that this hiatus contravenes our impression of a sharp rise of the bathing habit under the Julio-Claudians, but we shall see shortly that this is not the case. Also, several establishments dating to these years can be identified outside the city's perimeter. Just outside the Porta Marina,[69] a large and well-appointed establishment was built in the Tiberian period, the Suburban Baths (see figs. 15, 16).[70] It has the hallmarks of the "new" design: a single set of rooms, large windows facing west to catch the afternoon sun, and a cold pool with an adjacent fountain display decorated with colorful mosaics. Seneca would have hated it.

A recent study of the Sarno Baths complex on the slopes south of the city has suggested that it too was operating in the early first century. The evidence for this proposition, however, is slim.[71] Further, as reconstructed for this period, the facilities are strangely antiquated. For instance, they have no hypocausts and are supposed to have been heated with braziers. Given that

---

69. Gateways appear to have been popular locations for baths, as urban sites, such as Ostia or Timgad, demonstrate (provided in parentheses are references to Nielsen's catalogue and dates). Ostia: the Porta Marina Baths (C.25; Trajanic/Hadrianic) and Sullan Wall Baths (C.19; Hadrianic) at the Porta Marina; the Pharos Baths (C.26; Trajanic) at the Porta Laurentina; and the Baths of the Drivers (C.23; Hadrianic) at the Porta Romana—for an overview, see Meiggs, 418 (fig. 30); Nielsen, 2.4–6 (C.15–31). Timgad: all four gates have baths in their immediate vicinity, the Large Baths (C.242; second century) and Small North Baths (C.244; uncertain date) at the North Gate; the Large East Baths (C.238; first half of second century) at the East Gate; the Large South Baths (C.239; first half second century) at the South Gate; and the "Sertius Market" Baths (C.247; uncertain date) at the West Gate—for an overview, see Nielsen, 2.75 (fig. 39). It is noteworthy that all the "gate baths" at Timgad are among the earliest at the site, indicating that gates were regarded as prime locations for such buildings.

70. The baths are located at 7.A.2. On this recently excavated building, see L. Jacobelli, "Lo scavo delle Terme Suburbane: Notizie preliminari," *RStPomp* 1 (1987): 151–54; id., "Terme Suburbane: Stato attuale delle conoscenze," *RStPomp* 2 (1988): 202–8; id., "Die Suburbanen Thermen"; id., *Pitture erotiche*, 13–23. Jacobelli deduces the Tiberian date from construction method; see also Nielsen, 2.8 (C.43). This building appears to have been privately owned, since two *cippi* found at the extremities of the site have single lines cut across their upper surfaces and are inscribed *L(ocus) P(ublicus) P(ompeianorum)* or *L(ocorum) P(ublicorum) P(ersequendorum)*. They served to demarcate the line between the public property outside the baths and the lot of the privately owned establishment; see Jacobelli, *Pitture erotiche*, 20–23.

71. See Koloski-Ostrow, 47–49; Ioppolo, *Terme del Sarno,* 118–22 (following Koloski-Ostrow). The building is treated in more detail below, at chapter 2, pp. 66–67. Its early operation is proposed primarily on the basis of construction materials and techniques and architectural alterations in the building, but without full excavation, all conclusions about this confused and complicated corner of the city must be tentative (as Koloski-Ostrow [46] concedes). The functional relationship between the Sarno Baths and the neighboring Palaestra Baths, which has been used to argue for the early operation of the Sarno complex, is not clearly understood and so is not probative either way; see below, chapter 2, n. 90.

the patrons of the establishment were allegedly the occupants of the spacious apartments located elsewhere in the complex, this feature seems odd.[72] One could well ask how likely it is that affluent bathers would have preferred and presumably paid more for such outmoded baths when more modern amenities were available in the town. Given these points, the part of the Sarno complex now occupied by the baths seems to have served a different function originally and to have undergone conversion into baths at some later date.

Another set of baths in the vicinity of Pompeii is attested in an inscription, found in 1749 near the Herculaneum Gate, advertising "the Thermae of M. Crassus Frugi with seawater and the Baln(eae?) with freshwater."[73] The location of these baths is not known, but the owner has frequently been identified with the M. Crassus Frugi (consul in A.D. 64) who, Pliny the Elder reports, owned hot springs that came from the sea itself, in the Bay of Baiae. The identification, however, is far from certain, and since the baths may have run in the family for some time before Pliny's Crassus, their construction may date as far back as the reign of Tiberius.[74] At the very least, the inscription and Pliny's comment, when taken together, attest the family's interest in baths in this region, adding further detail to the picture of senatorial bath owners attested in the written evidence. The ramifications of one feature of this inscription have yet to be fully appreciated. A clear distinction is drawn in the text between two modes of bathing, one in seawater and one in freshwater. The availability of both modes would require that there were either separate structures close at hand or, at least, distinct sections in a single building; both possibilities are attested elsewhere.[75] This observation raises

---

72. See Koloski-Ostrow, 37–42; see also 48 (braziers), 57–58 (wealthy patrons).

73. No. 257. An alternative reading is to understand *baln.* as *baln(eum)*, which could then translate as "bathing with freshwater."

74. See Pliny *HN* 31.5. Given the confusion surrounding the meanings of *thermae* (see above, chapter 1, pp. 14–19), the word cannot confidently be said to indicate here *heated* seawater, which weakens the common identification of this Crassus with the Neronian consul (as found in, e.g., Koloski-Ostrow, 58; Yegül, 93). For doubts, see J.H. D'Arms, *Romans on the Bay of Naples: A Social and Cultural Study of the Villas and Their Owners from 150 B.C. to A.D. 400* (Cambridge, MA, 1970), 215. In fact, three M. Crassi Frugi—the consuls of A.D. 14, 27, and 64—are candidates for the construction and/or ownership of this building (see *PIR*[2] L 189, 190, and 191, respectively). *PIR* postulates that perhaps the Neronian Crassus inherited the baths from his father. If so, the building(s) would be of Tiberian date.

75. See, e.g., *Anth. Pal.* 9.680. For baths combining freshwater and seawater facilities, see Stat. *Silv.* 2.2.17–19. For baths offering seawater facilities only, see Suet. *Aug.* 82.2 and *Ner.* 31.2; HA *Heliogab.* 23.7. Many so-called thermal baths fed by natural springs had wings for regular bathing as well as for thermal immersion; examples are the thermal baths at Bath (see B. Cunliffe, *Roman Bath Discovered*[2] [London, 1984]; Heinz, 165–67) and Badenweiler (see Heinz, 169–75). An inscription from Aquae Neri in Aquitania that mentions *fontes Nerii et thermae p[ublicae]* (no. 97) should probably be interpreted to refer to such baths.

acute doubts for the recently proposed identification of Crassus' establishment with the Suburban Baths, since there is neither any sign of separate sections in the Suburban Baths nor any indication of another building nearby (although the possibility that there was one cannot be ruled out entirely).[76] Regardless of this issue, the facility (or facilities) of M. Crassus Frugi as attested in this inscription featured a "regular" bathing establishment and so should be added to the list of public baths serving Pompeii at this time.

Another extramural inscription may refer to a third early Imperial bathhouse near Pompeii. A text found outside the Nucerian Gate simply reads, *balneus Agrippae* (*CIL* 4.3878). *Balneus* possibly refers to a bathhouse, although it could conceivably refer to a member of the staff attached to a bath building. The prince Agrippa Postumus owned a villa at Boscotrecase in the outskirts of Pompeii, and it is inviting to see here a reference to a private *balneator* attached to his household.[77] But this view is largely speculation. Since the text is a mere graffito (the rest is illegible), it should be noted but left aside.

It seems, then, that early Imperial Pompeii acquired only two new public baths, both outside the city's walls. This number is hardly an indication of a rapid growth in the bathing habit. A tempting explanation for the apparent inertia is that the high number of private baths in Pompeii reduced demand for public establishments.[78] But such an explanation will not hold water, since the written evidence is clear that private citizens used public facilities even when they had access to domestic ones;[79] moreover, for the majority of residents, even in a prosperous place like Campania, public baths would have been their only option. The slow progress of bath construction in early Imperial Pompeii may have been the result of other intangible factors, such

76. See Jacobelli, "Scavo delle Terme Suburbane," 154; Nielsen, 2.8 (C.43, G.). An earlier identification of Crassus' baths with a structure on the promontory of Uncino at Oplontis, which appears to have had underground reservoirs for seawater, had been postulated by A. Maiuri ("Note di topografia pompeiana," *RendNap* 34 [1959]: 73–79; see *PECS*, 652–53, s.v. "Oplontis" [De Franciscis]). The nature and function of this latter building, however, are most unclear.

77. The use of *balineus* for *balneum* is attested at least once (see no. 259). The Greek word βαλανεύς (bathman), which seems morphologically close to *balneus,* is usually Latinized as *balneator.* Such men are known to have been attached to affluent households: see, e.g., *CIL* 6.7601; see also *CIL* 6.8742, *CIL* 6.9102 c. 13, *CIL* 6.9216, *CIL* 6.9217, *CIL* 6.9395/96.

78. Pasquinucci (70–71 [fig. 56]) provides a map of the city with public and private baths indicated on it. In all, twenty townhouses have private baths, and two more are located in suburban villas. In contrast, only one private suite has been identified at Ostia (in the House of the Dioscuri); see Meiggs, 259–60 (including the plan at fig. 20), 420.

79. For instance, Trimalchio meets his dinner guests at the public baths, despite having a private suite at home (see Petron. *Sat.* 26–27, 72; see also Pliny *Ep.* 2.17.26). See below, chapter 8, pp. 192–96, for the elite at the baths.

as siting problems in the city center or economic considerations, such as high rents in the heart of the city. These possibilities seem to find support in the evidence from the third and final period of the city's history, that traditionally dated as stretching from the earthquake in 62 to the final destruction of 79.[80] It is, however, unsafe to date all the later construction and repair at Pompeii through automatic association with the well-documented tremors of 62. This earthquake, though severe, cannot shoulder the entire blame for all the changes Pompeii underwent from the mid–first century A.D. to the disaster of 79, particularly in the field of construction.[81] In all likelihood, the city experienced many seismic events as Vesuvius grew more and more unstable in the time leading up to the eruption, and constant alteration, extension, and reconstruction appear to have been part of the ancient urban scene in any case. Altogether, however, the evidence does suggest that the last decades of the city's life saw a dramatic rise in bath construction in the city, even if a chronological boundary cannot be drawn precisely at the earthquake of 62. Furthermore, many of the projects were still underway when they were permanently halted by the eruption of Vesuvius, which suggests a later, rather than an earlier, date for their inception.

The heating and hydraulic requirements of public baths would render them particularly susceptible to earthquake damage, and seismic activity in the last years appears to have shut down the Stabian and Forum Baths, but only temporarily. In 79 the men's section of the Forum Baths was in operation, while the status of the Stabian Baths remains unclear. Certainly, the Stabian and Suburban Baths were undergoing general repairs and renovations when the final disaster struck, and it appears that at least the men's section of the Stabian Baths was open for business, albeit in a reduced capacity.[82] Outside the Porta Marina, the renovation of the Suburban Baths

---

80. Seneca (*Q Nat.* 6.1.1–3) dates this disaster to 63, Tacitus (*Ann.* 15.22.3) to 62. For a convincing resolution in favor of the Tacitean date, see G.O. Onorato, "La data del terremoto di Pompei, 5 Febbraio 62 d. Cr.," *RendLinc,* 8th ser., 4 (1949): 644–61. On the impact of the earthquake on Pompeii's history, see, e.g., Laurence, 35–37; A. Maiuri, *L'ultima fase edilizia di Pompei* (Rome, 1942), 7–10; Richardson, *Pompeii,* 261–368; P. Zanker, *Pompei: Società, immagini e forme dell'abitare* (Turin, 1993), 139–46.

81. See, e.g., J. Andreau, "Histoire des séismes et histoire économique: Le tremblement de terre de Pompéi (62 ap. J.-C.)," *AnnEconSocCiv* 28 (1973): 369–95; Koloski-Ostrow, 50.

82. See Maiuri, *L'ultima fase,* 70–72 (Stabian Baths), 73–74 (Forum Baths); Jacobelli, "Die Suburbanen Thermen," 329, 332–34 (Suburban Baths). The operation of the Forum Baths is indicated by the rededication of the building and the commemoration of this event by the staging of games, as recorded in painted inscriptions found on and in the building; see *CIL* 4.1177 = *ILS* 5144, *CIL* 4.1178 (both mention Cn. Alleius Nigidius Maius, a prominent citizen of the mid–first century A.D.; see J.L. Franklin Jr., *Pompeii: The Electoral Programmata: Campaigns and Politics, A.D. 71–79* [Rome, 1980], 102). See also, Eschebach, *Stabianer Thermen,* 70–72.

included the addition of a heated pool *(calida piscina)* and adjacent rooms (one with a hypocaust) to the north end of the existing structure, almost an adjunct facility in itself.[83] Here again, Seneca's railings against the heightening luxury of first-century bathing habits find reflection in the physical record. Indeed, the authorities at Pompeii had their hearts set on an entirely new bath, one that would bring their town fully up to speed with contemporary bathing fashions. Slightly north of the Stabian Baths, they were building the largest set of baths the city had seen to date, and it was very much in the "new" style. The Central Baths had a large palaestra with exedrae for relaxation, a single suite of spacious bathing rooms, large windows, an open-air pool *(natatio)*, and a latrine (see fig. 17).[84] Their unfinished state does not allow appreciation of their decoration, but given the tastes of the age, it was probably intended to be sumptuous. Had the Central Baths ever been completed, the Pompeians could have boasted that their city's center offered the most modern of facilities.

The authorities were not alone in building baths. Elsewhere in the city, private entrepreneurs were opening recreation centers that featured bathing suites; the baths could be used either independently or in conjunction with other facilities in these complexes. The most complete example of this sort of building is the Premises of Julia Felix *(Praedia Iuliae Felicis)*, thus named in a painted inscription (see figs. 18, 19).[85] The building is located around the corner from the amphitheater and presumably did a booming business during games. The bathing suite is named in the inscription as the *Balneum Venerium et Nongentum,* epithets of uncertain connotation but probably intended to promote the luxury and comfort of the establishment.[86] The

---

83. See Jacobelli, "Die Suburbanen Thermen," 332–33. The nearly contemporary Suburban Baths at Herculaneum are similarly appointed, with a separate hall featuring a heated swimming pool and open vistas of the sea: see Manderscheid, 121, s.v. "Herculaneum, Terme Suburbane"; Nielsen, 2.7 (C.39).

84. They occupy all of *insula* 9.4, with entrances at 5, 10, 15, 16, and 18. See Manderscheid, 172–73, s.v. "Pompei, Terme Centrali." Add also P. Bargellini, "Le Terme centrali di Pompei," in *Thermes,* 115–28; Eschebach and Müller-Trollius, *Gebäudeverzeichnis,* 420; Maiuri, *L'ultima fase,* 74–77; Nielsen, 1.47–48 and 2.8 (C.47); Richardson, *Pompeii,* 286–89 The size of the structure and its prime location strongly suggest that this bath was the work of the local authorities.

85. No. 258; compare nos. 254–56, 259. The complex of Julia Felix occupies all of *insula* 2.4, with the baths entered at 4 and 6. For a full description and analysis of the remains, see C.C. Parslow, "The *Praedia Iuliae Felicis* in Pompeii" (Ph.D. dissertation, Duke University, 1989). See also Eschebach and Müller-Trollius, *Gebäudeverzeichnis,* 92–93; Manderscheid, 173–74, s.v. "Pompei, Terme Praedia Iuliae Felicis;" Richardson, *Pompeii,* 292–98.

86. Several attempts have been made to explain the significance of the adjectives; see the notes to no. 258. That the vicinity of amphitheaters was a desirable location for bathhouses is reflected, perhaps, in the construction of the Thermae of Titus and Trajan adjacent to the

baths themselves were of moderate size and lacked a palaestra. Instead, just inside the entrance, there was a small peristyle with recesses for relaxation, giving the impression that the patrons tended more toward inactivity and socializing than strenuous exercise. The luxury of the surviving decoration and the large open-air swimming pool reinforce this impression. The other facilities in the complex (i.e., taverns, dining and reception rooms, gardens, and a *nymphaeum*) reveal the whole to be a sort of public recreation center accommodating a variety of leisure activities. The baths, however, remained the focal point, and that they underwent extensions even during their short period of operation suggests that they were a success.[87] Taken as a unit, the Premises of Julia Felix may represent an attempt to reproduce on a smaller scale the many amenities available in the large imperial baths in Rome, which had recently been enriched by the opening of the Thermae of Nero.[88]

At the other end of Pompeii, one or more private entrepreneurs erected similar facilities on the south slopes of the city, near the theater. The Palaestra Baths/Sarno Baths complex was a large, complicated, and unfinished laby- rinth featuring dining rooms, taverns, reception rooms, and two sets of baths on two levels (see figs. 20–22).[89] The relationship between the two wings of the building is unclear and will remain so until further study is carried out.[90] Until then, they ought to be treated separately. The Palaestra Baths were accessible through an entryway on the Via delle Scuole and feature the usual rooms, a small palaestra with three exedral rooms off it, and a balcony overlooking the scenic valley south of the city (fig. 20). As with the *Balneum Venerium et Nongentum*, the impression is of a facility catering more to the idler than to the athlete, though the decorative scheme in the palaestra— frescoes depicting athletes, wrestlers, and their trainers—may suggest other- wise. The establishment was functioning when the volcanic eruption of 79 occurred.

Colosseum. Note also the story that when Bishop Fructuosos was martyred by means of an ad hoc burning in the arena, the crowd built his pyre with wood from nearby workshops and baths; see H. Musurillo, *The Acts of the Christian Martyrs* (Oxford, 1972), s.v. "Fructuosos," 12.4–6.

87. For these alterations (namely, the addition of a *laconicum* and a *natatio*), see Parslow, "Praedia Juliae Felicis," 419–31.

88. Imperial *thermae*, however, did not feature set dining areas.

89. The complex is located at 8.2.17–24; the Palaestra Baths are entered at 22–24, the Sarno Baths at 17–20. For modern treatments, see Manderscheid, 174, s.v. "Pompei, Terme del Sarno e Palestra." Now add Ioppolo, *Terme del Sarno;* Koloski-Ostrow, passim; Nielsen, 1.45 and 2.8 (C.44, C.45); Richardson, *Pompeii*, 298–307.

90. Richardson (*Pompeii*, 298, 301) sees the two structures as undergoing alterations prior to amalgamation into one large facility; Koloski-Ostrow (27, 48, 55–58) inverts this order and reconstructs the buildings as having been originally integrated and only subsequently parti- tioned. The resolution rests on the dating of the blocking up of the communicating doors between the two complexes, but, on available evidence, no firm conclusions can be made on this key point.

In contrast, the Sarno Baths were still under construction when the end came (see figs. 21 and 22). They occupied the lowest level of a four-tiered complex that was comparable to the Premises of Julia Felix in its facilities and that was built on three terraces set against the natural gradient of the terrain. The baths were of modest dimensions, lacked a palaestra, and boasted large southward-facing windows offering a view of the valley below. Their accessibility directly from the street via a long corridor (entered at 8.2.17) demonstrates that they were intended as a public facility, even if also as an amenity at the disposal of the occupants of the apartments ranged on the three levels above. An unusual feature of the baths is the row of seven cubicles running east from the bathing suite. The function of these rooms is unclear. They may have been for thermal- or mineral-water bathing, similar to arrangements found in spas, such as Baiae or Badenweiler. No mineral springs, however, are located near the Sarno Baths, and the cubicles show no signs of plumbing. The analogously arranged cubicles in the Baths of Faustina at Miletus have been interpreted as changing rooms or chambers for instruction and conversation. At the Sarno Baths, however, a changing room (*apodyterium*) can be identified elsewhere in the complex (room A in fig. 21B), and it is difficult to see the point of hiding away instruction and/or conversation in such secluded cells.[91] In all likelihood, the cubicles served some other function (possibly prostitution, for which no archaeological evidence can be expected to remain), and they may have catered to a local quirk in the bathing habit (the Stabian Baths had a similar row of secluded cells, apparently to accommodate individual immersion in tubs).[92] The unfinished state of the building adds a further element of uncertainty to an already unclear situation.

Finally, it has been proposed that the small baths in the Casa di Giuseppe II, just down the street from the Palaestra/Sarno complex, comprised a "semi-public" facility that served both the apartment block and the general public (rather like the Sarno Baths).[93] However, these baths are extremely small and cramped even for an exclusive establishment, and they are not

---

91. See Koloski-Ostrow, 38 (on the identification of the *apodyterium*).

92. See Richardson, *Pompeii*, 305 (mineral bathing); see also Heinz, 162 (Baiae), 171 (Badenweiler). For the Baths of Faustina, see Manderscheid, 149–50, s.v. "Miletos, Thermen der Faustina"; Nielsen, 2.38 (C.306); Yegül, 291. A similar niche-lined corridor has been identified in the unexcavated Gymnasium Bath at Magnesia-on-the-Meander; see Farrington, *Roman Baths of Lycia*, 23–24. For the possible uses of the Sarno cubicles, see Ioppolo, *Terme del Sarno*, 72; Koloski-Ostrow, 94–95. The cells in the north wing of the Stabian Baths can be seen in the plan; see fig. 1. Comparable cubicles are found at the Maritime Baths at Tarracina: see F. Coarelli, *Lazio* (Bari, 1982), 324–25; Manderscheid, 205, s.v. "Terracina/ Tarracina, Grandi Terme alla Marina."

93. These small baths are located at 8.2.39. For their proposed "semi-public" function, see Parslow, "*Praedia Juliae Felicis*," 431–36; Richardson, *Pompeii*, 234–40.

accessible directly from the street. They may have served the tenants of the apartments, but if so, such an arrangement (i.e., an apartment block with a bathing facility reserved for use by the occupants) is a rarity.[94] It must be remembered that these baths, too, were unfinished in 79, so their intended final form remains a mystery.

The evidence of Pompeii provides physical corroboration for the impressions gained from the written evidence. At the start of the first century B.C., the city was equipped only with the Stabian Baths, but by the time the city's disastrous end came in 79, it had at least seven public establishments (excluding those in the Casa di Giuseppe II). Furthermore, the number of baths is seen to grow steadily in the first century B.C. (see map 1) and rapidly under the Julio-Claudians and Flavians (see map 2). The evidence for the Julio-Claudian growth is to be inferred chiefly from the sharp rise in bath construction in the years leading up to the destruction of the city. Damage caused by seismic disturbances may have allowed for greater real-estate speculation in the heart of the city than had previously been possible. The marked attention to bath construction at this time suggests that the Pompeians were reacting to external stimuli that had arisen elsewhere in the interim and that they were attempting to bring their city into step with the latest tastes, in which bathing evidently featured conspicuously. The implication, therefore, is that during the preceding decades, public bathing had come to enjoy a heightened profile in Roman life in general.

The extent of this trend can be roughly gauged by comparing the evidence for public baths in Italian communities in two periods, one covering the second and first centuries B.C., the other covering the period from Augustus to Trajan. When these data are mapped, it can be seen that baths proliferated across the peninsula most noticeably in the early Imperial period, although their numbers were also on the rise in the late Republic (see appendix 1). It is worth recalling that the first centuries B.C. and A.D. also saw the first dispersal of Roman baths outside of Italy, though the flood of the second century was yet to come. When taken together with the specific evidence from Pompeii, the growth of the bathing habit in Italy in the late Republic and early Empire seems very clear, with the greater proliferation falling in the latter period. What is the evidence for Rome itself?

---

94. Apartment *insulae* at Ostia, for instance, do not usually have baths built into them, but rather the baths are located close by; see Packer, *Insulae of Imperial Ostia,* 5–42, 72–74. The Baths of the Philosopher, integrated into *insula* 5.2 at Ostia, were either open to the public or reserved for a guild, but they were not used exclusively by the occupants of the *insula;* see Boersma, *Amoenissima Civitas,* 35–47, 120–37, 196–98.

Rome: The Evidence from the Aqueducts and Water Supply

The public baths of Rome are surveyed in more detail below (see chapter 5), but here we may note the remains of the large imperial establishments of the Augustan and early Imperial periods. Even if physical evidence for small baths is lacking, the Rome of the early Principate was equipped with successively large and elaborate, imperially funded bathing facilities: the Thermae of Agrippa, Nero, Titus, and Trajan. Today the remains of some of the imperial *thermae* stand as gaunt and imposing witness to their former splendor—and to the seriousness with which some emperors took the provision of baths for the populace. What is more, the construction of the first great baths in the city coincides with the evidence for growth we have seen in the written evidence and in the physical record at Pompeii.

In the absence of any useful physical remains of *balnea* from the city, a potentially fruitful approach for investigating the growth in the bathing habit at Rome would seem to be the water supply of the city, especially the figures supplied by Frontinus, who was the water commissioner *(curator aquarum)* in 97. Baths needed water; indeed, a recent monumental study of the Roman water supply asserts that aqueducts were built primarily to supply baths.[95] As a result, Frontinus' figures for water distribution in the city should bear witness to the growth in the bathing habit, all the more so since Frontinus was writing at the end of the first century A.D. and was thus looking back on the gathering wave of bath popularity. On the surface, Frontinus' evidence looks promising. He provides detailed figures for the urban distribution of the various aqueducts feeding the city (*Aq.* 78–86) and asserts that almost half the water reaching Rome (4,401 of 9,955 *quinariae*) was given over to public uses.[96] His figures (in *quinariae*) for the individual aqueducts feeding the city in his day are presented in table 1.[97]

---

95. See A.T. Hodge, *Roman Aqueducts and Water Supply* (London, 1992), 3, 5. Vitruvius (8.6.1–2) offers partial support for this view, when he specifies that one of the three conduits in a water-distribution center should be reserved for baths. For Frontinus, see Hodge, op. cit., 16–18; Evans, *Water Distribution,* passim.

96. The *quinaria* was a measurement of pipe width. Volume was calculated from the amount of water the pipe could convey in twenty-four hours (forty meters^3); see Hodge, *Water Supply,* 299–300. Evans can be confusing in his treatment of the figures. At one point (*Water Distribution,* 139 n. 6) he substitutes Frontinus' stated total for distribution within the city of 9,955 *quinariae* with a figure of 10,409½ *quinariae,* the sum reached by adding together Frontinus' figures for individual aqueducts. But shortly afterward (141) he uses the total of 9,955 without comment. I have therefore cited Frontinus' stated total here.

97. The most complete modern treatment of the aqueducts of Rome remains T. Ashby, *The Aqueducts of Ancient Rome* (Oxford, 1935); but see also, A.T. Hodge, "Aqueducts," in Barton, *Roman Public Buildings,* 127–49. Hodge's *Water Supply* focuses more on the provinces than on Rome. See also P.J.Aicher, *Guide to the Aqueducts of Ancient Rome* (Wauconda, 1995).

TABLE 1. Frontinus' Distribution of Water Use in Rome, Listed by Aqueduct

Aqueduct	Date	Total Capacity to City	In Caesar's Name	For Private Citizens	For Public Use	For Public Structures
Appia	312 B.C.	699	151	194	354	123 to 14 bldgs.
Anio Vetus	272 B.C.	1,106½	64½	490	552	196 to 19 bldgs.
Marcia	144 B.C.	1,102½	116	543	443½(?)	41 to 15 bldgs.
Tepula	125 B.C.	331	44	237	50	7 to 3 bldgs.
Julia	33 B.C.	597	18	196 (?)	383	181 to (10?) bldgs.
Virgo	19 B.C.	2,304	509	338	1,457	1,380 to 16 bldgs.
Claudia/Anio Novus	A.D. 38/52	3,498	816	1,567	1,115	374 to 18 bldgs.

Note: The figures (in *quinariae*) provided here are those given for the individual aqueducts in Evans, *Water Distribution.*

Other scholars have used these figures to estimate the various uses to which aqueduct water was put in the city, and at first sight such testimony does indeed appear compelling.[98] It is tempting to start calculating percentages. But unfortunately, Frontinus' evidence is so plagued with problems that it is all but useless for determining how much water went to baths; it cannot therefore be used in tracing the growth in the bathing habit. In the first place, the passage listing the figures for the aqueducts' capacity is in great confusion in the manuscripts, and drawing any statistical conclusions from it is at best perilous. Scholars have tried to emend the figures to make them arithmetically consistent, but such efforts are essentially guesswork, since it is not clear from the manuscripts which numbers are authentic and which are corrupt.[99] Also, in the cases of the figures for the Republican aqueducts, Frontinus provides those of his own time, so they do not reflect the aqueducts' original capacities. Aqueducts required heavy maintenance, and the capacities of the older lines were improved in later repairs, although how frequently is unclear.[100]

Even if Frontinus' figures for all the aqueducts were uncorrupted and reliable (which they are not), his method of categorizing the various uses to which the water was put is not helpful in determining what proportion went to the city's bathhouses. Frontinus does not mention baths explicitly, and establishing which of his categories they fall under proves impossible. Frontinus lists the aqueducts' distribution under three broad rubrics: "in Caesar's name" (nomine Caesaris), "for private citizens" (privatis), and "for public

---

98. See, e.g., R.J. Forbes, *Studies in Ancient Technology*[2] (Leiden, 1964), 1.173. Forbes' figures have subsequently been more heavily relied on than Frontinus' originals. For instance, Hodge (*Water Supply*, 267–68) quotes Forbes as reckoning that 17 percent of the water supply of Rome went to baths. Forbes actually says 17.1 percent went in Caesar's name, usage that *included* baths. Similarly, Yegül (393–94) reproduces Forbes' figures rather than Frontinus'. After careful and close consideration of Frontinus' evidence, Evans (*Water Distribution*, 140–44) comes to the general conclusion that aqueduct water was put to a wide variety of uses in the city and was not restricted to any particular use, e.g., only drinking or only bathing.

99. Thus the Loeb (trans. C.E. Bennett, 1925) and Budé (trans. P. Grimal, 1961) editions of Frontinus contain emended tables of figures. Evans (*Water Distribution*, 34–37) also uses emended figures. Despite the confusion about the figures, acknowledged by Evans at several junctures (e.g., at 2, 4–5, 80–81, 90–92, 101–2, 125, 135; see also id., "*Quorsum et cui bono,*" 21), he retains faith in their overall usefulness. But note the restrictions and uncertainties it imposes on his conclusions (see *Water Distribution*, 135–47).

100. For instance, Frontinus (*Aq.* 12.1) reports that Augustus improved the Marcia by adding a new source and conduit, and he alludes (at *Aq.* 87) to frequent repairs and improvements. In fact, the distribution of all of Rome's Republican aqueducts was much altered and expanded during the years between their construction and the composition of Frontinus' treatise; see Evans, *Water Distribution*, 70–71 (Appia), 78 (Anio Vetus), 89–90 (Marcia), 95–96 (Tepula).

use" *(usibus publicis)*. Under the last heading, he specifies figures "for public structures" *(operibus publicis)*. (These categories are used in table 1.) Since, also under "public use," he provides specific figures for public basins *(lacus)*, camps *(castra),* and ornamental fountains *(munera)*, the category of "public structures" cannot be taken to include such facilities. Does Frontinus' reference to public structures, then, denote the city's bathhouses? This seems unlikely. If all ninety-five public structures mentioned by Frontinus were baths, he would surely have listed them as such. Rather, his vague wording suggests that he had in mind various types of public building that required water (temples, circuses, amphitheaters, theaters, latrines, exedrae, etc.). Certainly, some bathhouses may lurk in the total of ninety-five "public structures,"[101] but surely not all of the city's bathing facilities are included there, since we would then have to accept that Rome contained fewer than ninety-five bathhouses at the end of the first century A.D.; given all that we have seen about growth so far, this is not likely.[102]

There is an added complication. It is entirely possible that figures for the water supply to privately owned but publicly accessible bathing facilities are included by Frontinus in the figures "for private citizens," insofar as these individuals put the water to commercial use.[103] Since it seems that Republican Rome did not feature any publicly owned bathhouses until the Thermae of Agrippa were bequeathed to the populace in 12 B.C.,[104] this consideration further vitiates the use of Frontinus' already suspect figures for this period, especially when it is remembered that such privately owned public baths continued to proliferate at Rome well into the late Empire. Because there is no way of knowing what forces drove private demands for water, we cannot tell what proportion of the figures for private uses went to privately owned, publicly accessible baths in the city. Only the figures given for the Aqua Virgo can be securely linked to bathing, since that aqueduct was opened along with the Thermae of Agrippa in 19 B.C. When Frontinus wrote, these baths were publicly owned, and this seems to explain the huge proportion of Virgo

---

101. Thus Frontinus (*Aq.* 84.2) specifies that, in the case of the Aqua Virgo, the *opera publica* total includes the Euripus, a pool associated with the Thermae of Agrippa but not a bathhouse in itself.

102. See Frontin. *Aq.* 78.3 for the total of ninety-five *opera publica*. Evans (*Water Distribution*, 8–12) acknowledges the difficulty of securely assigning *balnea* to any of Frontinus' categories, though he leans toward *opera publica* while admitting the unlikelihood of fewer than ninety-five baths in the city.

103. Frontinus (*Aq.* 91.5) reports that he found the exceptionally fine water from the Marcia being misused in baths, fullers' shops, and "other services disgusting to mention," which suggests that he viewed many baths as private commercial enterprises analogous to fullers' shops. For the commercial uses of water, see Hodge, *Water Supply,* 246–61.

104. See below, chapter 5, pp. 109–10.

water going to the *opera publica,* which shows that Frontinus included at
least one bathhouse in that category.[105] However, since the Thermae of
Agrippa were adjacent to the great pool, the Stagnum, it is unclear what
proportion of the water went to the bathing rooms proper. The figures for the
Claudia/Anio Novus, which fed the Thermae of Nero, might also be useful,
but here it is not clear whether the water was given "in Caesar's name" (since
the baths were imperial property) or "for public structures."

In light of all these uncertainties, we must conclude, disappointingly, that
Frontinus' figures are of little use for the current investigation. Nevertheless,
a glance at the raw data appears to raise an acute problem for our reconstruction of the process of growth in the first century B.C. It is curious that no new
aqueducts were built between 125 and 33 B.C., during the very period that
we have reconstructed as marked by a process of steady growth. Moreover,
the figures for private consumption in this period trail off, rather than increase. If baths were on the rise at Rome during these years, and if those
baths were privately owned but publicly accessible, we would expect more
aqueducts to be built to feed them. At the very least, would not more private
use be made of water, since in our scenario more private entrepreneurs would
be investing in baths as commercial enterprises? The misconception behind
this objection is that water for baths came mainly from aqueducts. While it
may be true that many aqueducts were built for baths, it is not the case that
many baths were built for aqueducts. This is especially true of the smaller
type of facility that appears to have predominated in Republican Rome. It is
clear that modest complexes could function perfectly well without a conduit.[106] Rome, equipped with an aqueduct water supply since the late fourth
century B.C., could have supported many small, modest Republican-style

---

105. Evans (*Water Distribution,* 9) would like to include all of the city's *thermae* among
Frontinus' *opera publica,* but since these baths were under direct imperial ownership and
control, they probably fall under the rubric *nomine Caesaris.* Indeed, Evans himself (loc. cit.)
comments that *nomine Caesaris* "could therefore include delivery to large structures under
imperial control, even if constructed for public benefit or entertainment."

106. The Stabian, Forum, and Republican Baths at Pompeii all operated, at least initially,
without an aqueduct, as did the first-century facility at Teate Marrucinorum (Regio IV), where
an extensive cistern complex fed the nearby baths: see J.P. Oleson, "Water-Lifting Devices at
Herculaneum and Pompeii in the Context of Roman Technology," in N. de Haan and G.C.M.
Jansen, eds., *Cura Aquarum in Campania* (Leiden, 1996), 67–77; F. Coarelli and A. La Regina,
Abruzzo, Molise (Bari, 1984), 150–51. For further examples, see Bruun, *Water,* 73 n. 43; Yegül,
390–95. A large number of baths that received their water from wells or cisterns are also known:
see B.D. Shaw, "The Noblest Monuments and the Smallest Things: Wells, Walls, and Aqueducts
in the Making of Roman Africa," in Hodge, *Future Currents* , 63–73; see also the numerous
references to waterwheels attached to baths in J.P. Oleson, *Greek and Roman Mechanical
Water-Lifting Devices: The History of a Technology* (Toronto, 1984); Hodge, *Water Supply,*
264–67.

baths supplied either by water concessions from the aqueducts or by privately owned wells or cisterns.[107] In such circumstances, establishments on the scale of the Thermae of Agrippa were not possible. It is hardly a coincidence that the latter facility, with its many pools and adjacent Stagnum, required its own aqueduct.

Given the uncertainty surrounding Frontinus' figures, the fact that smaller baths could operate without aqueducts, and the lack of evidence for exactly how privately owned baths were fed with water, it seems safer not to rely on arguments based on aqueducts and water supply to chart the growth of the bathing habit at Rome. Consideration of more recent water-consumption figures reinforces this conclusion. Data compiled in 1936 for the water consumption of various modern cities show that Rome (with 150 gallons per head per day) swamped places like London (at 35.5 gallons), Frankfurt (at 40 gallons), and Munich (at 55 gallons). In fact, Rome's closest competitor in the water-consumption stakes was New York, with 120 gallons.[108] By comparison, the Rome of 50 B.C. supplied more water per head per day (198 gallons) than any of the modern cities, including modern Rome. Apparently, high water consumption is a perennial feature of Roman life, with roots in ancient times. This observation further vitiates using ancient water supply as a barometer for measuring the popularity of the bathing habit, since even though public baths are not a prominent feature of the modern city, water consumption there remains on average higher than in most other major cities.

The evidence reviewed in this chapter, when assessed cumulatively, paints a picture of a growth in the bathing habit at Rome and in Italy in the first centuries B.C. and A.D. The process of growth appears to fall into two phases, one marked by steady—if unremarkable—progress (in the first century B.C.), and the other characterized by a more dramatic rise in bathing habit (in the first century A.D.). It is now time to seek explanations for these phenomena.

---

107. For wells at Rome, see Bruun, *Water,* 97 n. 2; Evans, *Water Distribution,* 135–36. Private conduits from public aqueducts were a rarity, and their relationship to baths is hard to interpret; see Bruun, op. cit., 63–76.

108. See Forbes, *Ancient Technology,* 1.171 (table 10). Things have not changed all that much: figures for the supply of drinking water show that the ancient Romans had at their disposal, on average, three times more per head per day than modern Germans; see H.-O. Lamprecht, *Opus Caementitium: Bautechnik der Römer*⁴ (Dusseldorf, 1993), 98 (fig. 53) (my thanks to A.T. Hodge for this reference).

Chapter 3

Accounting for the Popularity of
Public Baths

Not surprisingly, there is very little direct evidence as to why the Romans took to bathing in the periods reviewed in the previous chapter or, indeed, why public baths became such a core social institution in their culture at all. Perhaps on account of this general silence, modern students have not made any serious effort to get behind the mere fact of the baths' popularity and seek reasons for it. Ancient authors tend not to explain why they used baths, presumably because to do so would have been to state the obvious. Thus Pliny or Seneca can ponder the baths' great popularity, but they offer little by way of explanation for it. If Seneca implies anything, it is that a sheer love of luxury impelled people to bathe, a moralizing Stoic topos that cannot be taken at face value.[1] Archaeology is, for obvious reasons, a largely uninformative source for this topic, but it is not entirely useless. The nature of the evidence, then, precludes a straightforward explanation of the baths' popularity, which is clearly traceable and well documented. We must therefore resort to general considerations and observations, especially for the first period of growth (down to Augustus), since source material for this era is so meager. On the broadest perspective, we have already seen how public bathing, by its very nature, appears to promote a sociability among participants in whatever culture it is practiced (see above, introduction, p. 4). This intangible "social bathing" factor must have played a part in shaping Roman behavior as well. But can we be more specific as to why the Romans took to the public baths so enthusiastically and why they did so especially in the period stretching roughly from 100 B.C. to A.D. 100?

An immediate, almost facile reason is simply that the Romans liked bathing. Archaeology offers an instructive point of comparison between Greek and Roman practices that bears on this fact. Scholars have noted that

---

1. Sen. *Ep.* 86.6–13; *Dial.* 10.12.7. Such attitudes die hard: in 1761 the Protestant ministers of Philadelphia opposed a public bath in the city on the grounds that it would only promote the people's "Immoderate and Growing Fondness for Pleasure, Luxury, Gaming, Dissipation, and their concomitant Vices" (cited in M.T. Williams, *Washing "The Great Unwashed": Public Baths in Urban America, 1840–1920* [Columbus, 1991], 10).

the central difference between Greek palaestrae/gymnasia and Roman baths is that the latter subordinate facilities for sport and education to those for bathing and socializing. This distinction is clear from early in the history of Roman baths (witness the decommissioning of the *destrictarium* and the shrinking of the palaestra in the Augustan remodeling of the Stabian Baths in Pompeii) and becomes even more pronounced as the baths increased in size and complexity.[2] It is an important point to appreciate, since it shows that the Romans' conception and use of their baths appears to have been primarily as centers for relaxation and pleasure, not education and exercise. From later periods, too, there is ample evidence testifying to the pleasures of the bathing experience. To visit the baths was to step into the arms of *voluptas,* to enjoy pleasing and comfortable surroundings.[3] The result was to make one feel relaxed: Suetonius reports that the best time to ask an indulgence of the emperor Vespasian was immediately after his bath, and some baths displayed mosaic valedictions at their exits—for example, "You have washed well!" *(salvum lotum!).*[4] Inscriptions also attest the pleasures of baths in other ways. In one case, a benefactor's provision of water to a town's bathhouse was "so that the citizens of the town might not be deprived of its convenience" (no. 226). Verse inscriptions speak of a bath's "delight" (χάρις in Greek), as when the opening of the baths at Serdjilla in Syria in 473 resulted in the whole town enjoying its χάρις.[5] The reopening of the Baths of Faustina at Miletus was celebrated, since "all are relieved from their toils as they take their delights in the labor-lightening streams" (no. 315/16). Study of the surviving fabric of baths, both humble *balnea* and large-scale imperial *thermae,* has shown that over time, more and more space was devoted to nonfunctional purposes, that is, to ancillary recreational activities.[6] The pleasure of visiting the baths, then, is the most fundamental and direct reason

2. See Ginouvès, *Balaneutikè,* 9, 101–3, 145–50; Yegül, 21–24 (gymnasia); DeLaine, "New Models, Old Modes" (increase in complexity).

3. The diverse evidence has been assembled by Dunbabin, *"Baiarum Grata Voluptas,"* 12–32. Particularly illustrative are the praises of baths at *Anth. Pal.* 9.606–40, 9.680, 9.783–84, 9.814–15.

4. Suet. *Vesp.* 21 (Vespasian); *CIL* 5.4500 = *ILS* 5725 *(salvum lotum).* See also J. Russell, "Mosaic Inscriptions from the Palaestra at Anemurium," *AnatSt* 24 (1974): 95–102; id., *The Mosaic Inscriptions of Anemurium* (Vienna, 1987), 30–34 (no. 4). Such well-wishes were also inscribed on bathing equipment, such as strigils, as if the tools themselves were encouraging the bather to have a good time; see Zienkiewicz, *Fortress Baths at Caerleon,* 157–66 (G.C. Boon on an inscribed strigil). A macabre invocation of this phrase is recorded in the *Martyrdom of Perpetua and Felicitas* (21.2–3), where the crowd in the arena yells *Salvum lotum!* at Saturus after he has been bitten by a leopard and is bathed in blood.

5. No. 327. For comparanda, see Russell, *Mosaic Inscriptions of Anemurium,* 39–49 (no. 7).

6. See above, introduction, n. 24.

for their popularity. The Romans, however, enjoyed many other *voluptates* that were not put on offer to the general public on a daily basis.[7] What factors contributed to the widespread dispersal of baths in particular?

In general, it is safe to say that life in a Roman town was considerably more communal than is the case among Westerners today. Study of apartment blocks at Ostia and elsewhere reveals that the living quarters of the humble often lacked amenities considered absolutely fundamental in modern residences; many had no kitchens, latrines, or baths. As a consequence, many functions performed inside in private today were conducted by the Romans outdoors, in full public view.[8] For instance, in the absence of widespread private kitchens, Roman communities tended to have a plethora of taverns and public eating places, distributed so as to serve the populated parts of the town.[9] Public latrines, likewise, show a degree of openness that is shocking to modern sensibilities. Many are multiple-seaters, in which patrons would

---

7. Dinner parties, for example. They were an almost daily experience for the elite but were only offered to the masses as the occasional *epulum* (and even then, not always to the plebs); see, e.g., nos. 71, 72, 88, 95, 114. On dinner parties, see W.J. Slater, *Dining in a Classical Context* (Ann Arbor, 1991). On public banquets, see Duncan-Jones, *Economy,* 138–44; S. Mrozek, *Les distributions d'argent et de nourriture dans les villes italiennes du Haut-Empire romain* (Brussels, 1987). Note also J.F. Donahue, *"Epula Publica:* The Roman Community at Table during the Principate" (Ph.D. dissertation, University of North Carolina at Chapel Hill, 1996).

8. See Packer, *Insulae of Imperial Ostia,* 72–74; id., "Middle and Lower Class Housing in Pompeii and Herculaneum: A Preliminary Survey," in B. Andreae and H. Kyrieleis, eds., *Neue Forschungen in Pompeji* (Recklinghausen, 1975), 133–46. See also J.C. Anderson Jr., *Roman Architecture and Society* (Baltimore, 1997), 306–16; F. Pirson, "Rented Accommodation at Pompeii: The Evidence of the *Insula Arriana Polliana* VI.6," in R. Laurence and A. Wallace-Hadrill, eds., *Domestic Space in the Roman World: Pompeii and Beyond* (Portsmouth, RI, 1997), 165–81. It may be the case, however, that evidence for latrines and/or kitchens has not survived or was cleared away during earlier excavations; Packer, for instance, identifies a possible latrine and kitchen in the Insula of Jove and Ganymede at Ostia (*Insulae of Imperial Ostia,* 134–39). Nevertheless, the houses of the elite are often characterized, apart from their size, by the inclusion of precisely such amenities as baths, latrines, and well-defined kitchens; see Wallace-Hadrill, *Houses and Society,* 17–61.

9. Some cooking and eating undoubtedly took place in humbler dwellings, as the identification of kitchens, cookware, and food-related artifacts in such places confirms, but the situation in *pergulae* (mezzanines), *cenacula* (upper-level bedsits), and *tabernae* (habitable shops) remains unclear. For recent preliminary studies, see J. Berry, "Household Artefacts: Towards a Re-interpretation of Roman Domestic Space," in Laurence and Wallace-Hadrill, *Domestic Space in the Roman World,* 183–95; P.W. Foss, "Watchful *Lares:* Roman Household Organization and the Rituals of Cooking and Eating," ibid., 201–18. On cookshops and taverns, see, for Ostia, G. Hermansen, *Ostia: Aspects of Roman City Life* (Edmonton, 1981), 185–205; for Pompeii, Laurence, 70–87, esp. 82–83 (maps 5.2 and 5.3) on the wide distribution of *cauponae* and *popinae* throughout the city. On these facilities in general, see Anderson, *Roman Architecture,* 326–36; A. Dosi and F. Schnell, *A tavola con i Romani antichi* (Rome, 1984), 73–98; T. Kleberg, *Hôtels, restaurants et cabarets dans l'antiquité romaine* (Uppsala, 1957). Not surprisingly, such places were considered the haunts of the lowly; see Toner, 65–88.

attend to bodily functions, apparently in full view of others; and there is no indication of male/female segregation.[10] There could hardly be a better illustration of the communality of living in Roman towns.

Against this background, the popularity of baths becomes more understandable. Not only was bathing a pleasure; it was also a basic necessity. Without baths in their residences, the majority had access only to public facilities (unless they used the sea or rivers and streams, where available). Public baths therefore served a necessary function in much the same way as the snack bars and taverns did, and as necessities, they can be expected, once introduced, to have grown in popularity all but automatically. They became one more facet of living in a Roman community, so that entrepreneurs took advantage of the demand for them and invested in baths as businesses. To what extent the actions of bath-owning businessmen contributed to the popularity of baths per se remains open to question, since there is a risk here of putting the cart before the horse. Baths, however, could only be built by those who could afford to do so, and it can be surmised that the activities of entrepreneurs, such as Brutus or the owner(s) of the Republican Baths in Pompeii, may well have helped to disseminate the bathing habit still further. At Rome, as we shall see, all the public baths of the Republican era were privately built and owned.

These very general considerations lay the foundations for the popularity of baths, but there is still need to seek specific reasons why they became more popular in the first century B.C. Several observable trends in the late Republic combined to produce fertile grounds for the promotion of a popular bathing culture at Rome.[11] First, there was an increase in wealth and public ostenta-

---

10. On Roman latrines, a subject now enjoying the close attention of scholars, see J.W. Humphrey, "An Aspect of Roman Building Technology of the Empire: A Study of the Design, Construction, and Administration of Public Latrines," *ANRW* 2.37.6 (forthcoming); G.C.M. Jansen, "Private Toilets at Pompeii: Appearance and Operation," in S.E. Bon and R. Jones, eds., *Sequence and Space in Pompeii* (Oxford, 1997), 121–34; A.O. Koloski-Ostrow, "Finding Social Meaning in the Public Latrines of Pompeii," in De Haan and Jansen, *Cura Aquarum*, 79–86; R. Neudecker, *Die Pracht der Latrine: Zum Wandel öffentlicher Bedürfnisanstalten in der kaiserzeitlichen Stadt* (Munich, 1994). Note also F. Drexel, "Das Latrinenwesen in Rom und den Provinzen," in L. Friedländer, *Darstellungen aus der Sittengeschichte Roms*[10] (Leipzig 1922; reprint, Aalen, 1964), 4.310–11. For a lurid reconstruction of a visit to the Roman latrine (and the alternatives), see A. Scobie, "Slums, Sanitation, and Mortality in the Roman World," *Klio* 68 (1986): 407–18, 427–30.

11. The literature on the history and society of the late Republic is vast and cannot possibly be presented here; some of the more recent works that address the issues raised in the following pages include P.A. Brunt, *The Fall of the Roman Republic and Related Essays* (Oxford, 1988); Dupont, *Daily Life*; E.S. Gruen, *The Last Generation of the Roman Republic* (Berkeley, 1974); C. Nicolet, *The World of the Citizen in Republican Rome* (Berkeley, 1980); E. Rawson, *Intellectual Life in the Late Roman Republic* (London, 1985). Note also the second edition of the *Cambridge Ancient History*, vol. 9, *The Last Age of the Roman Republic* ed. J. A. Crook,

tion. The first century B.C. was the age of such rich dynasts as M. Licinius Crassus, L. Licinius Lucullus, C. Julius Caesar, and Cn. Pompeius Magnus, whose immense wealth far exceeded that of any of their predecessors.[12] These men and their ilk owned multiple properties in Italy and the provinces, and they were not averse to investing their wealth in construction, as illustrated by the number, luxury, and extent of their private dwellings.[13] A reflection of the increasing wealth of the period is that the number of villas owned by affluent Romans in Campania grew markedly between the time of Marius and that of Cicero.[14] A further indication of this trend is the increase in table luxury and in the consumption of exotic foods and wine, habits that, although they rose sharply in the early Imperial period, were clearly underway in the late Republic.[15] This taste for the lavish was not, however, confined to the private sphere. Through increased public patronage, displays of wealth in the form of games, spectacles, or public buildings were not uncommon. Pompey sponsored some of the most extravagant gladiatorial combats Rome had ever seen, and he built the city's first stone theater, surrounded by gardens and a portico decorated with famous Greek statuary and paintings.[16] Not to be outdone by his rival, Caesar is reported to have had an extensive building plan for the city (Suet. *Caes.* 44). Already in the previous

A. Lintott, and E. Rawson (Cambridge, 1994), and F. Millar's review of it, "The Last Century of the Republic: Whose History?" *JRS* 85 (1995): 236–43.

12. The wealth of Crassus in particular was proverbial (see, e.g., Cic. *Fin.* 3.75 and *Tusc.* 1.12; Sall. *Cat.* 48.5; Pliny *HN* 33.134; Plut. *Crass.* 2 and *Pomp.* 22.1), but the fortunes of Caesar and Pompey came to rival it; see E. Badian, *Roman Imperialism in the Late Republic*[2] (Ithaca, 1968), 81–83, 89–90.

13. See A. Boethius, *Etruscan and Early Roman Architecture*[2] (London, 1978), 183–95. At this time the Palatine Hill became the most exclusive residential area in Rome, with proprietors like Cicero, Crassus, Hortensius, and Catullus in residence: see F. Coarelli, *Roma*[7] (Bari, 1995), 149; T.P. Wiseman, *Catullus and His World: A Reappraisal* (Cambridge, 1985), 25–26.

14. See D'Arms, *Romans*, 18–72. In his catalogue 1 (pp. 171–201), D'Arms identifies some forty-four owners of villas or houses on the Bay of Naples for the period 75–31 B.C., compared to a mere handful from the second century B.C. (ibid., 1–17).

15. See Tac. *Ann.* 3.55 (early Imperial). For the late Republic, see Friedländer, *Sittengeschichte*, 2.285–315. On wine consumption, see N. Purcell, "Wine and Wealth in Ancient Italy," *JRS* 75 (1985): 6–9, 13–15.

16. See Boethius, *Early Roman Architecture*, 205–6; P. Greenhalgh, *Pompey: The Republican Prince* (London, 1981), 54–57 (theater), 58–61 (spectacles). Note also the luxurious wooden theater of M. Aemilius Scaurus, erected in 58 B.C., which Pliny (*HN* 36.114–15) claims was more extravagant than any permanent theater, and the novel wooden "double theater" of C. Scribonius Curio (52 B.C.), which pivoted to form an amphitheater even as the spectators remained seated (see Pliny *HN* 36.116–20). On the rise of public patronage in this era, see F. Millar, "Popular Politics at Rome in the Late Republic," in I. Malkin and Z.W. Rubinsohn, eds., *Leaders and Masses in the Roman World: Studies in Honour of Zvi Yavetz* (Leiden, 1995), 91–113; Rawson, *Intellectual Life*, 100–114; P.J.J. Vanderbroeck, *Popular Leadership and Collective Behavior in the Late Roman Republic (ca. 80–50 B.C.)* (Amsterdam, 1987), 81–86 (patronage), 97–99 (building programs).

century, marble had been introduced to Rome as a building material in public structures, but in the first century B.C., its use became widespread.[17] Pliny the Elder offers the opinion that the extravagance of the late Republican elite exceeded even that of his own generation.[18] The public, at least in the view of the rich, lapped all this luxury up and wanted their share of the splendor. Cicero could declare: "The Roman people hate private luxury but delight in public magnificence" (*Mur.* 76: *odit populus Romanus privatam luxuriam, publicam magnificentiam diligit*).

The first century B.C., then, was marked by increasing luxury and ostentation in both the public and the private domains. The growth of the public bathing habit finds a suitable backdrop amid such an atmosphere, where a society was growing more accustomed to the provision of luxuries. In particular, extravagant public building was on the rise, as was the willingness of ever richer leaders to spend large sums of money providing for such construction.[19] Here, however, a word of caution is required. There is no evidence that any of the powerful dynasts of the first century B.C. constructed and opened baths for public use, in the manner that the emperors later did.[20] Evidence we have surveyed elsewhere does suggest that senators and private people of substance participated in building baths, but it is noteworthy that neither Sulla, Crassus, Pompey, nor Caesar—the four most wealthy and powerful men of the first half of the century—are anywhere clearly attested as bath builders.[21] These men, however, belonged to the uppermost stratum of power and prestige, and neither Sulla nor Crassus were major builders in the first place (Sulla, in particular, displayed little interest in pandering to the

17. According to Roman tradition, Q. Caecilius Metellus Macedonicus was the first to use marble in a public building, a temple of Jupiter Stator, in 146 B.C. (Vell. Pat. 1.11.5); see also Anderson, *Roman Architecture*, 166–79; M.E. Blake, *Ancient Roman Construction in Italy from the Prehistoric Period to Augustus* (Washington, DC, 1947), 50–60, esp. 51.

18. Pliny *HN* 36.8 (luxury of L. Crassus' dwelling [95 B.C.] rare in Pliny's day), 36.114–15 (the temporary theater of M. Scaurus). As a gauge of the rapid slide into luxury, as Pliny saw it, he comments (*HN* 36.109–10) that M. Lepidus' house, reckoned the finest in Rome in 78 B.C., did not even make the top one hundred homes thirty-five years later.

19. See Veyne, 469–537. Crassus, the richest of the lot, is not representative, since he is reported to have said that men given to building need no enemies—they will ruin themselves (see Plut. *Crass.* 2.6). Not surprisingly, no public buildings at Rome are attributed to Crassus.

20. There are hints of bath-related activity by these men, such as Faustus Sulla's benefaction of free bathing to the populace in 60 B.C. (see Dio 37.51.4). L. Licinius Lucullus is reported to have erected "newfangled buildings" in his retirement, among them baths (see Plut. *Luc.* 39.2; compare *Mor.* 785F). Unfortunately, it is unsure whether these baths were open to the public: the passages can be interpreted either way (Plutarch includes them among collections of art, banquets, and ambulatories, all of which can be either public or private).

21. A *Balneum Caesaris* is attested in the *Forma Urbis Romae* (fr. 43), but it is more likely to have derived its name from some association with an emperor; it may even have been part of the imperial palace. See *LTUR* 1.157, s.v. "Balneum Caesaris" (E. Rodríguez Almeida).

masses). Rather, baths seem to have been built as businesses or investments by lesser individuals. Indeed, people further from the center of power may well have been stimulated to emulate the behavior of the more vaunted elite by constructing less extravagant public buildings, and small city baths, which also offered the possibility of financial return, were probably attractive propositions in this regard.[22] In general, though, the prevalent atmosphere of heightened materialism at this time can only have encouraged the growing tastes for luxury and leisure among the *principes* and populace and thus contributed to the spread of the public bathing habit.

A further and more direct contributing factor to the baths' popularity was the rise of the city's population in these years. Naturally, the more people there were, the greater would be the demand for public amenities, including baths—and the greater the chances for profit in providing them. The scrappy survival pattern of the sources precludes deduction of precise figures, but that the population of the city rose in the second and first centuries B.C. seems clear enough.[23] Given the living conditions of most of the city's population, it is also likely that they would have valued public spaces in which they could seek refuge from domestic squalor.[24] These two circumstances in conjunction probably contributed in some measure to the growth in the

---

22. Republican-style *balnea,* more functional and plainly decorated, were undoubtedly less costly propositions than the later "new" baths, with their marble paneling, statuary, mosaics, and architectural sophistication. On costs of baths, see below, chapter 6, pp. 173–75.

23. See Dio 38.1.2–3; Cic. *Att.* 2.3.4 (= SB 23). Note also Frontinus' comment (*Aq.* 7.2) that the Marcian aqueduct was built in 144 B.C. "because the growth of the city seemed to demand a greater water supply" *(quoniam incrementum urbis exigere videbatur ampliorem modum aquae).* Agrippa was responsible for two more aqueducts, in 33 and 19 B.C. (Frontin. *Aq.* 9 and 10), possibly in reaction to further population growth. Modern scholars generally agree on a rise in the city's population in the middle and late Republic, even if providing precise figures proves impossible: see J.P.V.D. Balsdon, *Romans and Aliens* (London, 1979), 12–13; P.A. Brunt, *Italian Manpower* (Oxford, 1971), 376–88, esp. 383–84; Gruen, *Last Generation,* 358–65; B. Kühnert, *Die Plebs Urbana der späten römischen Republik: Ihre ökonomische Situation und soziale Struktur* (Berlin, 1991), 27–29; O. F. Robinson, *Ancient Rome: City Planning and Administration* (London, 1992), 8–9. Overcrowding, generated by overpopulation, is the backdrop for the living conditions of the plebs described in Z. Yavetz, "The Living Conditions of the Urban Plebs in Republican Rome," *Latomus* 17 (1958): 500–517 (= R. Seager, comp., *The Crisis of the Roman Republic* [Cambridge, 1969], 162–79).

24. On living conditions, see Yavetz, "Living Conditions"; P.A. Brunt, "The Roman Mob," in M. I. Finley, ed., *Studies in Ancient Society* (London, 1974), 84–92. The comparative attractiveness of public spaces, especially baths, is emphasized by, e.g., MacMullen (*Roman Social Relations,* 63) and M. Marvin ("Freestanding Sculptures from the Baths of Caracalla," *AJA* 87 [1983]: 347). Scobie ("Slums, Sanitation, and Mortality," 431–32) denies this proposition on Marxist grounds, arguing that public opulence only bred resentment among the dispossessed, who were thereby reminded of their personal poverty. If this were the case, it must be said that there is no evidence to suggest it. Altogether, it seems more likely that the plebs would have enjoyed a trip to the baths and the brief brush with luxury that it entailed; even Toner (54) accepts this suggestion, and he is hardly an elitist (see ibid., 22).

popularity of baths as attractive public havens for the masses. This growing attractiveness of the baths requires not that all baths were immaculate and luxurious—Republican baths in particular seem to have been rather functional—but that staying at home was less preferable than going down the road to the local *balnea*. The general communality of urban living played a part here too, reinforcing with a social *mos* what may have been at heart a largely pragmatic choice.

Allied to the rise in the city's population was its increasingly hetero-geneous ethnic composition.[25] This factor is important, since many of the newcomers arrived from the eastern Mediterranean world, where, under Greek influence, public bathing was a long-established institution, be it in gymnasia or in the more lowly public baths (βαλανεῖα).[26] (Yet neither type of building was as popular among classical or Hellenistic Greek city-dwellers as public baths became among the Romans in the late Republic and early Empire.) As it is, the influence of Greek bathing habits on their Roman counterparts cannot be denied and finds reflection in the material record.[27] As a result, the arrival at Rome of larger numbers of people from regions where public bathing had long been practiced is surely significant and may well have contributed to the growing appreciation of baths among the lower orders.[28] At the upper levels of society, Hellenization had been in progress since the third century, but it would be unrealistic to limit the scope of this

---

25. For ethnic variety among the Roman population, see, e.g., Cic. *Comment. pet.* 54; App. *B Civ.* 2.120; Mart. 7.30. See also Balsdon, *Romans and Aliens,* 12–16; Gruen, *Last Genera-tion,* 359–61; Kühnert, *Plebs Urbana,* 29–32. The influx of foreigners is reflected in their sporadic expulsion from Rome, especially in the expulsion of Greeks. When Macedonians were expelled in 171 B.C., large numbers were affected: see Polyb. 27.6; Livy 42.48.3; App. *Mac.* 11.9–10. Other expulsions followed, sometimes broadly applied to *peregrini,* such as that stipulated by the *lex Papia* of 65 B.C. (see Dio 37.9.5; Cic. *Arch.* 10, *Att.* 4.18.4 [= SB 92], *Balb.* 52, *Off.* 3.47) and another (possibly confused with the *lex Papia*) mentioned by Pliny (*HN* 29.16). On expulsions from Rome, see Balsdon, *Romans and Aliens,* 98–102.

26. The definitive study of Greek baths remains Ginouvès, *Balaneutikè.* On gymnasia, see Delorme, *Gymnasion.* For a recent survey of both facilities and an assessment of their relation-ship to Roman baths, see Yegül, 6–29.

27. The issue is hotly debated, especially for the very earliest periods of development of Roman baths. The broad Greek influences, however, are clear. Greek baths had forms of hypo-caust long before Roman ones (see Gortys in Arcadia, as well as Gela, Megara Hyblaea, and Syracuse in Magna Graecia), and Roman baths feature areas designed to accommodate func-tions that were Greek in character, such as *destrictaria* for oiling, palaestrae for exercising, and *laconica* for intense sweating. I maintain not that the Romans derived their bathing habits directly from the Greeks (as Ginouvès and others have concluded) but that strong influences were at work.

28. In Hellenistic times, Greek gymnasia and public baths spread all over the eastern Medi-terranean, and in Egypt, Greek-style bathing appears to have survived even into the Roman period; see Nielsen, 1.95–104, esp. 101.

acculturation to the elite.[29] In the seething streets of the Subura and among the other haunts of the masses, new and interesting patterns of behavior (not all of them salubrious) must have been passing between foreigner and Roman. Overall, it is rarely possible to offer any clear documentation of these processes, since our written evidence derives overwhelmingly from the ruling class; but there are hints.[30]

A final factor that would have benefited the spread of baths and bathing was the concurrent improvement in building technology. Specifically, concrete (opus caementicium) increasingly came to be used to create ever larger and more complex structures.[31] The improvement in vaulting techniques, itself aided by increasing confidence with the medium of concrete, allowed larger interior spaces to be roofed without obstructive internal supports. These constructional developments gave Roman architects the means to erect larger and more complex baths, with their need for open spaces and vaulted roofs. Concrete was certainly not required for the construction of baths per se, and before the Thermae of Agrippa, there is no evidence to suggest the existence of a really magnificent establishment at Rome or anywhere else. Nonetheless, improvements in construction techniques enabled

---

29. As, for instance, do M. Beard and M.H. Crawford, in *Rome in the Late Republic* (London, 1985), 20: "The vast majority of Romans were excluded [from participation in this cultural explosion] (except as onlookers); they could neither read nor write, nor afford to decorate their homes. This restriction must constantly be borne in mind." Such a view seems unnecessarily restrictive in discounting informal contacts between foreigners and common Romans. For an overview of Hellenization in the Roman Republic, especially among the elite, see J.-L. Ferrary, *Philhellénisme et impérialisme: Aspects idéologiques de la conquête romaine du monde hellénistique* (Rome, 1988).

30. The periodic expulsions of Greek philosophers, such as that in 161 B.C. (see Ath. 12.547a) or that of Carneades and his disciples in 155 B.C. (see Plut. *Cat. Maj.* 22), seem to have been prompted by a fear among the senators of the effects their teachings might have on public behavior. Also suggestive is Juvenal's xenophobic metaphor (at 3.60–65) of the Orontes flowing into the Tiber to represent the influx of eastern Mediterranean manners into the city, albeit in reference to a later age. The presence of easterners is directly attested in the inscriptions from Rome bearing Greek names; see, e.g., *CIL* 1².1028 = *ILLRP* 877, *CIL* 1².1045 = *ILLRP* 880, *CIL* 1².1295 = *ILLRP* 965, *CIL* 1².1312 = *ILS* 7975 = *ILLRP* 925, *CIL* 1².1332 = *ILS* 7967 = *ILLRP* 928, *CIL* 1².1337 = *ILS* 1969 = *ILLRP* 828, *CIL* 1².1345 = *ILLRP* 963, *CIL* 1².1366 = *ILLRP* 931, and the numerous Greek names in the index of *ILLRP* (vol. 2, pp. 434–52). For such texts as indicators of ethnic and linguistic diversity in Rome, see I. Kajanto, *A Study of the Greek Epitaphs of Rome* (Helsinki, 1963), 1–6.

31. A spectacular example is the vast Sanctuary of Fortuna Primigenia at Praeneste, completed in ca. 100 B.C.; see Coarelli, *Lazio*, 137–48. For improvements in concrete construction, see Blake, *Roman Construction*, 324–52 and also the sections on concrete facings, 227–75 *(opus incertum* to *opus reticulatum)* and 282–307 (brick and tile). On concrete, see also, Adam, *Roman Building*, 79–81, 127–34; Anderson, *Roman Architecture*, 145–51; Lamprecht, *Opus Caementitium*; MacDonald, *Architecture of the Roman Empire*, 1.1–19.

the construction of more elaborate baths with a greater degree of ease than had previously been possible.

While such factors as those just discussed offer a context for the growth in the popularity of baths and no doubt contributed to it, they do not in themselves explain why baths became popular. Thus, while improved building technology made the construction of baths easier, it does not explain why that technology was used specifically on baths, as opposed to other buildings: the demand for the baths must already have been there when architects came to erect them. Likewise, increased ostentation may have heightened the people's expectations of the appearance of public structures, but it offers little insight into why baths in particular were built. Rather, all of the factors considered above must be seen as operating within a nexus of mutual effect, not in any simple or linear causal relationship. It is impossible to be sure, for instance, to what extent the construction of baths by rich individuals helped to stimulate the baths' popularity or to what extent it was a reaction to it. Instead, the processes outlined above influenced each other in ways that are often not clear, but the coincidence of their occurrence and their combined effect served to boost the prevalence of public bathing. A speculative reconstruction might be as follows: people's expectations of greater public comfort and their desire to avoid unnecessary and undesirable lingering indoors in cramped apartments led to a demand for public amenities; greater population growth only added to the demand, and cultural contact with increasing numbers of easterners in the city may have ignited ideas in the heads of some; simultaneously, improvements in construction techniques facilitated the erection of more elaborate baths. In this way, all four factors contributed to the rise in the popularity of baths, but not individually in any decisive way. It is their cumulative effect that is seen to be significant.

Still, a feeling of dissatisfaction lingers. Impersonal trends and general considerations are all very well, as far as they go. Beyond the simple enjoyment of the experience, can any more specific reason(s) be found as to why people visited baths in the first place? The answer that repeatedly comes back from the sources, and one that is shared by many other public bathing cultures, is that the Romans believed bathing was good for them. Indeed, baths and healthfulness were closely associated in the Roman medical consciousness. The association deserves consideration in its own right.

Chapter 4

Baths and Roman Medicine

For the average Roman, life was short. Modern estimates reckon ancient life expectancy at birth at around thirty years, partly due to the very high rate of infant mortality.[1] But even for adults, life could end at very short notice. Apparently healthy individuals could fall ill and die with bewildering suddenness, making understandable the frequency of passages in Roman letters that dwell on the state of the correspondents' health.[2] In such an environment, it is hardly surprising that medical treatises appeared, advising the reader to adopt a healthy regimen not only to cure illness once it had begun but to prevent it from starting in the first place.[3] In these tracts, baths feature heavily in both remedial and preventive capacities. The place of baths and bathing in the theory and practice of Roman medicine is a vast subject that

---

1. See Duncan-Jones, *Structure*, 93–104; these findings are largely in accord with those of K. Hopkins, *Death and Renewal* (Cambridge, 1983), 69–99, 146–49. See also S.L. Dyson, *Community and Society in Roman Italy* (Baltimore, 1992), 180–82; I. Morris, *Death-Ritual and Social Structure in Classical Antiquity* (Cambridge, 1992), 72–81 (the latter proposes an average of 38.8 years for men and 34.2 for women based on surviving skeletons from second-century Greece). For the horrendous (by modern standards) hygienic conditions in urban areas, see Scobie, "Slums, Sanitation, and Mortality." For the variety of ailments (often fatal) attested in skeletal remains, see Morris, op. cit., 92–96.

2. Concern for health lies behind the traditional opening formulae of Roman letters, cited by Pliny (*Ep.* 1.11.1): "If you are well, that is fine; I am well" *(si vales, bene est; ego valeo)*. To this opening Pliny adds, "That's good enough for me—it's all that matters" *(hoc mihi sufficit; est enim maximum)*. Elsewhere (*Ep.* 3.17) Pliny worries that a lengthy silence from a friend might be due to "one of those accidents that can befall mankind" *(quidquid accidere homini potest)*. Other health-related letters, frequently ending in fatality, can be found at Pliny *Ep.* 1.12, 1.22, 3.7.1–2, 4.1.7, 5.6.1–2, 5.16, 5.19, 5.21, 6.4, 7.1, 7.19.1–4, 7.21, 7.24.1, 7.26, 7.30.1, 8.1, 8.16.1, 8.19, 9.22.1. By way of comparison, Cicero sometimes signs off his letters with "Take care of your health" *(cura ut valeas* and variants); see e.g., *Att.* 2.11 (= SB 32), 2.23 (= SB 43), 2.25 (= SB 45), 3.7 (= SB 52), 4.8a (= SB 82), 5.11 (= SB 104), 6.3 (= SB 117), 12.4 (= SB 240), 16.16a (= SB 407a). (That he does so only occasionally suggests that it was more than an empty formula like "yours sincerely.") Note also Seneca's frequently expressed concerns over his health, outlined in Griffin, *Seneca*, 42–43.

3. On the ancient regimen and the reasoning behind it, see L. Edelstein, "The Dietetics of Antiquity," in O. Temkin and C.L. Temkin, eds., *Ancient Medicine: Selected Papers of Ludwig Edelstein* (Baltimore, 1967), 303–16; more recently, see Jackson, 32–55.

cannot possibly be covered in detail here.[4] For our current purpose—to explain the baths' popularity—the chief point to note is the strong and persistent connection between bathing and good health in Roman perceptions. It is important to this discussion not whether Roman baths served to promote health in actuality but rather that the Romans believed that the baths did so.[5] Four indicators make this belief most explicit.

Medical Writers. The prescription of baths in the works of medical writers is the most direct evidence of an ancient perceived connection between baths and health. The vast corpus of Galen's writings is peppered with references to baths and bathing for medical purposes, to be employed or avoided depending on the circumstances.[6] Galen was, of course, writing in the second century, when public bathing was already a well-established habit among the Romans, but early Imperial authors, such as Cornelius Celsus, Scribonius Largus, and Pliny the Elder, anticipate him in recommending baths for medical reasons. Celsus, writing during the reign of Tiberius, refers to remedial baths on dozens of occasions. The range of ailments for which either an increase or a decrease in the patient's bathing is prescribed is impressive, including fevers, inflamed intestines, liver complaints, small pustules, eye complaints, and, rather disturbingly, urinary and bowel problems, to take but a cross section.[7] Antonius Musa used cold bath treatments, with varying results, on members of the imperial house.[8] It is reported that Hadrian re-

---

4. For preliminary accounts, see M.-T. Fontanille, "Les bains dans la médecine gréco-romaine," in A. Pelletier, ed., *La Médecine en Gaule: Villes d'eaux, sanctuaires des eaux* (Paris, 1985), 15–24; R. Gros, "Les thermes dans la Rome antique," *HSMed* 21 (1987): 45–50; Jackson, 48–50; id., "Waters and Spas in the Classical World," in R. Porter, ed., *The Medical History of Waters and Spas* (London, 1990), 1–13; Scarborough, 76–93; Yegül, 352–55. For an assessment of the sophistication of ancient balneology, see W. Heinz, "Antike Balneologie in späthellenisticher und römischer Zeit: Zur medizinischen Wirkung römischer Bäder," *ANRW* 2.37.3 (1996): 2411–32.

5. For the less than salubrious conditions at some Roman baths, see chapter 7, p. 179–88.

6. The imposing volume of Galen's writings has so far deterred a collection of such references (see J. Kollesch and D. Nickel, "Bibliographia Galeniana, 1900–1993," *ANRW* 2.37.2 [1994]: 1351–1420), but baths feature particularly heavily in the *De Sanitate Tuenda* (6.1–452 Kühn; see also R.M. Green, *A Translation of Galen's Hygiene* (De Sanitate Tuenda) [Springfield, 1951]).

7. See Celsus 2.17.2–10, 3.6.13–14, 3.12.3–4 (fevers); 1.7.1 (inflamed intestine); 4.15.4 (liver complaints); 5.28.15d (small pustules); 6.6.17, 6.27b, 6.34b, 6.38 (complaints of the eye); 4.27.2 (urinary and bowel problems). For Celsus' date, see *RE* 4.1273–76, s.v. "Cornelius 82" (Wellmann).

8. He cured Augustus in 23 B.C. (see Pliny *HN* 25.77; Dio 53.30.3; Hor. *Epist.* 1.15) but was less successful with Marcellus a few months later (see Dio 53.30.4). For an account of Musa's life and practice, see M. Michler, "*Principis Medicus*: Antonius Musa," *ANRW* 2.37.1 (1993): 757–85.

served certain hours at the public baths at Rome for the ill, which at least reflects the popular perception of the baths' therapeutic value.[9]

Whatever the remedial benefits of baths, their perceived preventive value is of more immediate interest to the current inquiry, since it may have contributed to the regular use of baths by otherwise healthy persons. Celsus sketches the Roman gentleman's healthy regimen, or at least that which a doctor might prescribe: if, for some reason, a man has become fatigued, to maintain health he should rest a while, then take a bath or, in its absence, warm himself either by a fire or in the sun.[10] Bathing, in fact, was part of the dietetics of the classical world, which also included recommendations for diet and exercise. It had a heritage traceable to the Hippocratic school, although the role of bathing became far more prominent in the Roman period.[11]

Nonmedical Writers. Reference to medicinal baths and bathing among nonmedical writers is perhaps even more significant than the evidence of the medical treatises themselves, since it shows that medical precepts had entered people's general knowledge and could therefore influence their behavior. (Needless to say, most of our evidence in this regard pertains to the upper classes.) Plutarch, for instance, penned a lengthy discourse entitled "Precepts for Maintaining Health" (*De Tuenda Sanitate Praecepta* [= *Mor.* 122B– 37E]). More directly, Pliny the Elder reports how Charmis of Massilia, an advocate of cold-water bathing, became so influential at Rome that "we used to see old men, ex-consuls, frozen stiff in order to show off," because they adhered to Charmis' hydropathy even in the depths of winter.[12] Later, Pliny complains that unnamed Greek doctors have persuaded the Romans to anoint themselves and take boiling baths *(balineae ardentes)* when healthy (*HN* 29.26). The medicinal value of baths is further reflected in offhand and casual comments made by many other "lay" authors.[13] Pliny's health-related

---

9. See HA *Hadr.* 22.7. It is not clear to how many or to what sort of baths this regulation applied. The restriction indicates that sick people were attending the public baths in such numbers to justify the edict. There is no real reason to doubt the *Historia Augusta*'s trustworthiness in reporting this regulation, but note the comments of Merten (51, 71–72).

10. Celsus 1.2, 1.3.4–5, 1.3.9–10. Characters in Apuleius' *Metamorphosis,* as if following Celsus' strictures, take baths precisely to relieve fatigue; see *Met.* 1.23, 5.15, 8.7.

11. See above, chapter 4, n. 3. On baths in Hippocratic medicine, see L. Villard, "Le bain dans la médecine hippocratique," in R. Ginouvès et al., eds., *L'eau, la santé et la maladie dans le monde grec* (Paris, 1994), 41–60.

12. Pliny *HN* 29.10: *videbamus senes consulares usque in ostentationem rigentes.* For Charmis, a contemporary of Nero, see *RE* 3.2175, s.v. "Charmis" (Wellmann).

13. See, e.g., Cic. *Fam.* 14.20.1 (= SB 173; to his wife Terentia, 1 October 47 B.C.). The perceived value to health of hot water, sweating, and heat (all of which were obtained at the baths) is reflected in such passages as Suet. *Aug.* 82.2; Pliny *Ep.* 7.21.2; Plut. *Mor.* 42B, 122B–

letters include references to the sick man dreaming of baths and springs (*Ep.* 2.8.2, 7.26.2), and Pliny himself uses the baths to help tackle an eye problem (*Ep.* 7.21.2). Even someone as ostensibly inimical to baths on moral grounds as Seneca could appreciate their remedial qualities (*Ep.* 22.1, 68.7, 95.22). The importance of this apparently widespread perception of baths as a central element in the maintenance of health lies in its capacity to impel healthy people to make baths a regular part of their daily routine. It is noteworthy that the regimens of Spurinna and of Pliny himself conform almost exactly to that set out by Celsus.[14] (However, immoderate or over-zealous use of the bath was generally considered life endangering, by both medical and nonmedical writers alike.)[15] The association of bathing with health was long lived: in his fourth-century agricultural handbook, Palladius includes a section on bathing, which, he comments, "confers both great enjoyment and health," and the early church, confronted with the wide popularity and hedonistic pleasures of the baths, dared not ban usage altogether but preferred to justify visiting the baths on hygienic and medicinal grounds—as long as the bather did not enjoy it too much.[16]

Bath Decoration. From the physical remains of baths themselves come powerful visual associations of bathing with health. Putting aside the Roman exploitation of medicinal springs (such as Aquae Sulis, Aquae Sextiae, etc.) or the presence of baths in healing sanctuaries, ordinary "civic" baths often featured decorative motifs that affirmed for the visitor the healthy nature of bathing.[17] Of all the statues known to have once stood in the Thermae of Caracalla in Rome, the largest was a gilded colossus of Asclepius, of which only the head survives (see fig. 23), and which was probably accompanied by

---

37E, 956F; Ath. 2.45d; and HA *Tyr. Trig.* 12.7. Pliny's *Natural History* contains dozens of references to medicinal baths; see above, chapter 2, n. 52.

14. Compare Pliny *Ep.* 3.1.7–8 (Spurinna) and 9.36.3 (Pliny) with Celsus 1.2 and 1.3.4–5, 1.39–10.

15. See Celsus 1.3.6–7; Pliny *HN* 7.183 (eating after a bath); Sen. *Dial.* 6.22.6, 7.7.3; Pliny *HN* 29.26; Plut. *Mor.* 20A, 69B, and *Lyc.* 10.1–2 (immoderate bathing injurious to health and promotes weakness). The alleged effeminacy and enervation induced by warm bathing was a moralistic topos stretching back to fifth-century Greece: see, e.g., Ar. *Nub.* 1044–46; D.G. Kyle, *Athletics in Ancient Athens* (Leiden, 1987), 70–71. Romans familiar with these Greek attitudes perpetuated them: see, e.g., Livy 23.18.12; Plut. *Mor.* 785F and *Lyc.* 10.1–2; Dio 27.94.2, 62.6.4; HA *Comm.* 11.5, *Avid. Cass.* 5.5, *Pesc. Nig.* 3.10, *Alex. Sev.* 53.2.

16. See Pall. 1.39 (cited is §1: *quae res et voluptati plurimum conferat et saluti*). On the early church and baths, note the strictures of Clem. Al. *Paid.* 3.31–32, 3.46–48 (Stählin); see also Yegül, 315–18.

17. For Roman development of natural spa sites, see Heinz, 157–75; Jackson, "Waters and Spas," esp. 5–10; Yegül, 92–127.

an equally large statue of Hygieia, now entirely lost.[18] Further, a general survey of fragments of sculptures from bathhouses in Italy, North Africa, and Asia Minor reveals that representations of these two health-associated deities are the third most commonly found, after Bacchus and Venus.[19] More recently, Asclepius and Hygieia have been promoted to first place in the sculptural rankings.[20] Indeed, in many baths, the healing deities are found in multiple representations.[21] It seems that for many Romans who visited the baths, statues of these two deities would have reiterated, if subliminally, the healthy nature of what they were doing.[22]

There are hints of this association beyond the sculpture. In Lucian's description of a bath, Asclepius and Hygieia are the only named deities one expects to find there as part of the decoration (*Hipp.* 5). These divinities and others associated with health-promoting properties feature in mosaic decoration and epigrams from baths of the late Empire.[23] In addition, inscriptions record the setting up of statues of Asclepius and Hygieia in bathhouses or proclaim their part in ensuring that water healed thankful dedicators—one tells of the restoration of a bath to fulfill an oath to the healing god.[24] Other inscriptions attest the strong connection between bathing and health. One text advertises a facility as "healthy little baths"

18. See Marvin, "Freestanding Sculptures," 363–64. The head is forty-nine centimeters high, and the original statue is estimated at four meters.

19. See Manderscheid, *Skulpturenausstattung,* esp. the table between pp. 34 and 35: Bacchus and followers, seventy-one examples; Venus, Amor, etc., fifty-four examples; Asclepius and Hygieia, forty-three examples. Bacchus, the leading deity, represented pleasure and abandon; Venus, sensual satisfaction. Hygieia, the daughter of Asclepius, was long associated with her father, though she also enjoyed her own cult; see H. Sobel, *Hygieia: Die Göttin der Gesundheit* (Darmstadt, 1990), esp. 9–11.

20. See H. Manderscheid, "Römische Thermen: Aspekte von Architektur, Technik und Ausstattung," in *Geschichte der Wasserversorgung,* vol. 3, *Die Wasserversorgung antiker Städte* (Mainz, 1988), 120.

21. For example, the Hadrianic Baths at Lepcis Magna yielded six statues of Asclepius (see Manderscheid, *Skulpturenausstattung,* 104 [nos. 293–98]).

22. Most of this sculptural material dates to the second century, when sculpture became a regular feature of bath decoration; see Manderscheid, *Skulpturenausstattung,* 8–9 and the table between pp. 10 and 11. Manderscheid reports (9) that 70 percent of all known bath sculpture dates to the second century. Because he provides no dates for individual pieces, it is not possible to determine whether Asclepius and Hygieia were popular in baths from the outset or whether they became so at some later date; see ibid., 66–131.

23. See Dunbabin, *"Baiarum Grata Voluptas,"* 12–32.

24. See, e.g., nos. 90, 150 (statues set up); 119 (restoration as a vow). For dedications to these gods that include reference to curative water, see *CIL* 3.1561 = *ILS* 3846; *IGBulg* 3.1664; *Bull. ép.* 1961.805. Note especially *IGLS* 4.1685, where Ὑγία is present even in a Christian inscription. Another inscription, from Maxula in Africa, dedicates a thermal bath facility to Asclepius (*CIL* 8.997 = Wesch-Klein, 137–38 [no. 1]).

(thermulae salutares); another mentions the building of baths for the sake of the community's health; yet another asks, "What is the name of the bath?—Hygia"; and a further advises, "Be healthy and wash."[25] From Asia Minor comes an inscription recording the benefactions of two imperial freedpeople and dedicated to the emperors and to Artemis Augusta Baiana, a deity of healing (no. 306). It seems, then, that baths, no matter where they stood, regularly featured visual associations with health and healing, often in the form either of representations of Asclepius and Hygieia or of written recommendations and/or inducements to health.

Doctors Working at the Baths. Perhaps most suggestive of the connection between baths and health is the possibility that doctors worked at the baths. This topic is difficult and is not without its uncertainties, so caution is required before rushing to conclusions. It is known that medical masseurs *(iatraliptae)* could be found at baths,[26] as could other staff, but the literary and epigraphic sources contain no direct references to physicians actually working at the baths. Seneca, for instance, mentions various characters found there, including several with commercial interests *(Ep.* 56.1–2), but doctors are not among them, and the same is true of other written sources that give insight into who visited the baths. Although an argument from silence, it remains suspicious that, given the volume of references to baths and their clients, doctors do not appear among the crowd. Rather, the case for the presence of doctors at baths must be built on interpretations of specific archaeological finds and on inferences drawn from the broader problem of where doctors plied their trade. Typical of the archaeological evidence is the discovery of five medical instruments, including two scalpels, in a small room at Xanten's main bathhouse, in a deposit dated to the late third century. This evidence has been taken to indicate not only that a doctor was

---

25. See nos. 120 (baths built for health), 255 *(thermulae salutares).* For the bath named Hygeia (τί τὸ ὄνομα τοῦ λουτροῦ; Ὑγία), see Robert, "Épigrammes," 84 (an inscription over the entrance to a bath at Il Anderin in northern Syria; high Empire). For the invocation "Be healthy and wash" (ὑγιέ|νων | λοῦσε), see *SEG* 26 (1976/77) 438.3 (from baths at Hagios Taxiarchos, Argos; late fifth century). A similar wish—ὑγίενε, κύριε [Be healthy, sir]—is expressed in the closing lines of the Greek text of the schoolbook; see Dionisotti, "From Ausonius's Schooldays?" 103 (§63). Note also that the Baths of Julia Memmia at Bulla Regia were associated with the "health of the citizens" (see no. 187), as were fortress baths at Bu-Ngem in Tripolitania (see no. 285).

26. LSJ (s.v.) defines a ἰατραλείπτης as a "surgeon who practices by anointing, friction and the like." Pliny *(HN* 29.5) reports that such treatment was first devised by Prodicus, a disciple of Hippocrates. L. Robert *(Bull. ép.* 1976.661) connects the practice with gymnasia in fourth-century B.C. Greece, so its transference to the related environment of the Roman bath would seem natural enough. See further M. Wissemann, "Das Personal des antiken römischen Bades," *Glotta* 62 (1984): 88. Note also Merten, 126–29; Nielsen, 1.128–31.

present at the baths but that he performed complex operations there. Similar finds have been made at the Barbarathermen in Trier and at Weissberg in Bavaria.[27] The main problem with this entirely plausible conclusion is that many of the instruments in question could have served a cosmetic, rather than a surgical, purpose. Representing more clear-cut evidence is a *collyrium,* an oculist's unguent and instrument box, found at the Barbarathermen and inscribed with the name of its owner.[28] Such *collyria* are also known from several thermal sites in Gaul, indicating that at least eye doctors could be found at such places.[29] Teeth found in the legionary fortress baths at Caerleon may have been the handiwork of an ancient dentist, but this interpretation remains open to question.[30] The archaeological material, therefore, is not only sparse but open to alternative explanations. A few medical instruments in a small room in a bathhouse on the frontier and scattered remains from similar frontier sites hardly establish an empire-wide practice. Uncertainties as to whether some of the finds were surgical or cosmetic in function and as to how they came to be deposited in the baths in the first place leave drawing firm conclusions from this evidence risky at best.

The scant and ambiguous archaeological data for the presence of doctors at baths is bolstered somewhat by consideration of the question of where ancient practitioners saw their patients and performed complex operations. This problem has proven vexing. There were no civic hospitals on the modern model in the ancient world. That doctors operated on patients at home seems unlikely, since most people lived in small, cramped, and crowded apartments that lacked running water and abounded in possible distractions for the doctor; in addition, many people may not have been able to afford a "professional" doctor in the first place.[31] That treatment took place at doc-

27. See E. Künzl, "Operationsräume in römischen Thermen," *BJb* 186 (1986): 491–509 on medical instruments, see id., "Forschungsbericht zu den antiken medizinischen Instrumenten," *ANRW* 2.37.3 (1996): 2433–639.

28. See Künzl, "Operationsräume," 491–509 (the owner's name was C. Attius Victorinus).

29. See C. Salles, "Les cachets d'oculistes," in Pelletier, *Médecine en Gaule,* 89–102; see also C. Bourgeois and E. Sikora, "Médecine des yeux dans la sanctuaire de l'eau de Pouillé (Loir-et-Cher)," in ibid., 103–10.

30. Three of the teeth were from children (representing the first "milk" dentition), while two were from adults; they were found in deposits in the drain of the *frigidarium* covering three periods, from the first to the fourth centuries. According to the dentist who examined them, all may have been lost naturally, since none show definite signs of having been subjected to instruments; see Zienkiewicz, *Legionary Fortress Baths,* 223.

31. See Künzl, "Operationsräume," 491. In fairness, it must be said that the dimensions of the proposed operating room at the Xanten baths hardly compensate in terms of size for treatment at home, and the baths would scarcely be a quieter or less distracting environment in which the doctor could work. Künzl (495) says that the Hadrianic decree setting aside certain hours at the baths for the sick would clear the place of distractions: at these times doctors could

tors' houses is another possibility but is again unproved. Nothing in the groundplan of proposed doctors' houses at Pompeii (e.g., the Houses of the Surgeon, Apollo, Centaur, or Doctor) suggests treatment rooms; rather, the houses have the same layout as any other dwelling. Instead, the identification depends once more on finds of medical instruments on the premises.[32] Because, as will be seen below, medical knowledge was a standard (if not expected) element of a Roman gentleman's education, medical instruments found in apparently normal dwellings may be little more than part of Roman first-aid kits and so may not indicate the presence of a "professional" doctor.[33] That treatment in a doctor's house was not unknown is indicated by a reference in Plautus (*Men.* 946–50), but that it was a regular and widespread feature of Roman medical practice requires more evidence than is available at present. Finally, the *tabernae medicae* or *iatreia* that doctors used as workplaces appear from surviving testimony to have been little more than consultation rooms, not places for performing complicated operations.[34] Places of medical treatment cannot therefore be securely identified at the locations one would expect to find them, which brings us back to baths as a natural alternative. Not only was running water available there, but their prominence in Roman medical thinking would make them likely, if not obvious, theaters for medical activity.[35]

---

work in quiet. It is far from clear, however, that the regulation was empire-wide. On the absence of civic hospitals in the Roman world, see R. Harig, "Zum Problem 'Krankenhaus' in der Antike," *Klio* 53 (1971): 179–95. Doctors certainly could make house calls, as Martial (5.9) demonstrates, although no serious surgery was required in the case he mentions.

32. See H. Eschebach, *Die Arzthäuser in Pompeji* (*AntW* Special Issue 15, 1984). All the houses Eschebach lists as doctors' houses are identified by finds of medical (or, rather, possibly medical) instruments; see the catalogue at ibid., 6–66. For the examples cited above, see ibid., 6–10 (Surgeon), 10–14 (Apollo), 26–38 (Centaur), 38–41 (Doctor). Eschebach also proposes the existence of "Kliniken" at Pompeii, on the basis of certain medical finds in the House of the New Doctor I (ibid., 45–47) and the House of Acceptus and Euhodia (ibid., 48–50). That patients were treated at doctors' houses and, indeed, the means of identifying such houses, is doubted by Harig, "Zum Problem 'Krankenhaus,'" 186–87 (Eschebach himself admits these difficulties; see op. cit., 3, 6).

33. When I made this point in conversation with R. Jackson, he pointed out that many of the instruments were designed for use in serious surgery and so were less likely to be the property of the average household owner. This position, however, assumes that performing complex surgery was restricted to a "professional" class of doctors, which may not have been the case in the ancient world; see further below.

34. See Harig, "Zum Problem 'Krankenhaus,'" 182–86.

35. Thus argues Jackson, 48 (but see 65–67, where he omits baths from his discussion of places of treatment). See also his comments in "Roman Doctors and Their Instruments: Recent Research into Ancient Practice," *JRA* 3 (1990): 11, and in "Roman Medicine: The Practitioners and Their Practices," *ANRW* 2.37.1 (1993): 88, where baths are considered possible workplaces for ancient doctors; in "Waters and Spas" (9), he suggests that the crowds at baths would

At best, the proposition that doctors practiced at the baths is, given the current state of our knowledge, a possibility, albeit a sane and plausible one. A smattering of archaeological evidence backed by some general considerations makes this possibility somewhat stronger, but whether it was a regular and widespread practice remains open to question. It cannot be determined how likely it was that a Roman bather would run into a doctor or any medical practitioner "working the baths." Given that the evidence for medical activity at the baths lies primarily in finds of medical instruments—themselves often open to alternative interpretation—decisive proof in this regard cannot really be hoped for. It seems best to leave the matter of doctors at the baths open to debate, but we ought to note it here as a distinct possibility.

Nonetheless, the four factors outlined above combine to establish a clear and persistent link between bathing and health-consciousness in the Roman world. When did this association arise at Rome? Addressing this question leads to an intriguing possibility for the early popularity of baths in the city.

Asclepiades of Bithynia and the Growth of the Bathing Habit

It is stated in a recent study of baths in the classical world that the precepts of Greek Hippocratic medicine, including an appreciation of the role of bathing, were introduced to Rome primarily through Celsus and Galen, both writers of the Imperial period, when baths were already a fact of urban life. It is further noted that Celsus, the earlier of the two, used as a source the (now lost) works of Asclepiades of Bithynia, who lived in Rome at the end of the second and beginning of the first centuries B.C.[36] This is the very period when, according to our analysis, the baths were beginning to enjoy greater popularity. Given this coincidence and the widespread association of baths and medicine, the possible role of Asclepiades in promoting a perception of healthful bathing among the Romans deserves closer inspection.

In a scathing indictment of Greek medicine at Rome, Pliny the Elder asserts that the Roman people had lived for six hundred years without "professional" physicians until Greek-style medicine started to wreak its exorbitant havoc among them.[37] Traditional Roman medicine—as discernible elsewhere in the writings of Pliny as well as in Cato, Columella, and Varro—was marked by a self-help approach within the household, where the *pater-*

---

attract doctors looking for business. Yegül (355) considers baths natural places for doctors to practice but questions whether special rooms were reserved for them.

36. See Yegül, 353–54.

37. Pliny *HN* 29.1–28, esp. 29.11.

familias was required to have medical knowledge for curing the herds and members of his *familia*.[38] The main method of treatment was herbal remedy, often used in conjunction with magical and mystical elements intended to placate the supernatural forces seen as the causes of illness.[39] As contact with the Greek world increased in the third century B.C., the Romans encountered a medical system that had developed along very different lines to their own. Greek medicine, in addition to the mystical healing cult of Asclepius, also encompassed the Hippocratic system, which was based on rational analysis grounded in philosophy. The practitioners of this latter system operated on the bases of observation, diagnosis, and treatment. Given the magical pro-clivities of traditional Roman medicine, it is hardly surprising that the mysti-cal branch of Greek medicine was the first to gain acceptance at Rome, when a temple of Asclepius was built on the island in the Tiber River following a plague in 292 B.C.[40] After the establishment of the Asclepian cult, rep-resentatives of the Hippocratic system had to wait seventy-three years before arriving at Rome. In 219 B.C. the senate invited Archagathos the Pelopon-nesian to live in the city and provided him with Roman citizenship, a prac-tice, and a salary. Despite getting off to a good start, Archagathos' brutal methods and fondness for the knife and cautery earned him the nickname "The Executioner" *(carnifex),* and he left Rome in disgrace. Pliny notes that after these events, all physicians at Rome "became objects of loathing."[41] This statement is probably an exaggeration, since Pliny's account of Arch-agathos' career introduces a diatribe against Greek doctors in general, which

---

38. See Jackson, 9–11; Scarborough, 15–25; id., "Roman Medicine to Galen," *ANRW* 2.37.1 (1993): 3–48, esp. 3–22.

39. It seems that the large collection of herbal remedies assembled by Pliny (*HN* bks 20–27) reflects in no small measure aspects of this traditional Roman medical system. Pliny (*HN* 29.15) claims much of it derived from Cato the Censor's *commentarium* of recipes that Cato used to treat his son and other members of his household. A similar situation may pertain to parts of Scribonius Largus' pharmaceutical handbook, *Compositiones,* composed ca. 44–48, but the influence of Greek pharmaceutics on the *Compositiones* is not to be ignored. For the date of the *Compositiones,* see B. Baldwin, "The Career and Work of Scribonius Largus," *RhM* 135 (1992): 74–82, and S. Sconocchia's introduction to the Teubner edition of the *Compositiones* (1983), vi.

40. See Scarborough, 24–25. For the background of Greek medicine, see ibid., 26–37; Jackson, 12–31; E.D. Phillips, *Aspects of Greek Medicine* (New York, 1973). A temple of Hygieia also existed at Rome by the time of Cato the Elder's censorship (184 B.C.); see Plut. *Cat. Maj.* 19.4.

41. Pliny *HN* 29.12–13 (the career of Archagathos). The prejudice underlying Pliny's view of Greek doctors has been highlighted by V. Nutton in "The Perils of Patriotism: Pliny and Roman Medicine," in R. French and F. Greenaway, eds., *Science in the Early Roman Empire: Pliny the Elder, His Sources and Influence* (London, 1986), 38–39. See also J.H. Phillips, "The Emergence of the Greek Medical Profession in the Roman Republic," *Transactions and Studies of the College of Physicians of Philadelphia,* n.s., 3 (1980): 267–75.

is prefaced with an uncompromising quote from Cato the Censor (*HN* 29.14). Nevertheless, there is no explicit evidence for the presence of Greek doctors at Rome for most of the second century B.C.[42] This lack of evidence does not require that they were entirely absent, but it would imply that they maintained a low profile or at least that none among them earned any great fame.

With Asclepiades of Bithynia, the situation changed.[43] Because little of his biography can be reconstructed, much of his life is unclear or debatable, but an outline can be discerned. He probably hailed from Prusias-on-the-Sea, in Bithynia.[44] The question of his education is controversial. Pliny's hostile account of his life claims that he was initially a teacher of rhetoric and that, with no training whatsoever in medical matters, he turned to medicine out of a desire for profit.[45] At the other extreme is the view that he came from a medical family and had extensive training, gained in part by study in Athens and Parion.[46] The truth may lie somewhere in between. The nature of ancient medical education was radically different from its modern counterpart. It was far less specialized and more closely associated with general physical philosophy than with a specific medical science. Asclepiades' theory of physiology displays derivation from atomistic ideas, indicating an acquaintance with philosophy, and his attested eloquence points to a rhetorical element in

---

42. See Phillips, "Emergence of the Greek Medical Profession," 269, 271–72. Scarborough ("Roman Medicine to Galen," 25–26) reasonably suggests that doctors and medical theorists must have been among the various scholars and philosophers who flocked to Rome in this period.

43. A comprehensive study of the life and works of Asclepiades, with a collection of his fragments, is lacking. J.T. Vallance ("The Medical System of Asclepiades of Bithynia," *ANRW* 2.37.1 [1993]: 711–27) lists dozens of ancient writers (overwhelmingly medical) who mention Asclepiades by name. For his life, however, the main ancient source is Pliny (*HN* 26.12–20 and some passing references elsewhere in Pliny and in other authors). Modern treatments, aside from accounts in general books on Roman medicine, are R.M. Green, *Asclepiades: His Life and Writings* (New Haven, 1955); E. Rawson, "The Life and Death of Asclepiades of Bithynia," *CQ* 32 (1982): 358–70; J.T. Vallance, *The Lost Theory of Asclepiades of Bithynia* (Oxford, 1990); id., "Medical System"; *RE* 2.1632–33, s.v. "Asklepiades 39" (Wellmann); M. Wellmann, "Asklepiades aus Bithynien von einem herrschenden Vorurteil befreit," *NJbb* 21 (1908): 684–703.

44. Wellmann ("Asklepiades aus Bithynien," 691, and *RE* 2.1632) places him at Prusa or Kios, in Bithynia, but Rawson ("Life and Death," 359–60) argues convincingly for Prusias-on-the-Sea.

45. Pliny *HN* 26.12. This charge may be due in part to Pliny confusing Asclepiades the grammarian with Asclepiades the doctor; see below, chapter 4, n. 49. Recently, Scarborough ("Roman Medicine to Galen," 26 n. 96) has supported Pliny's assertions.

46. See Wellmann, "Asklepiades aus Bithynien," 689–91. Note the reservations of Rawson in "Life and Death," 365.

his education.[47] That he had some medical training is really not to be doubted, but it is impossible to say how broad and deep it was.

As is the case with the rest of his life, many details of Asclepiades' career at Rome remain uncertain. We do not know when he arrived, what brought him there, or how he came to be associated with the circle of L. Crassus, the leading jurist of the day. All this information would be revealing. It is, however, possible to make an informed guess as to the duration of his stay in the city. Pliny records that he died from a fall down stairs "in extreme old age" (*HN* 7.124: *suprema in senectute*), which, in Roman conditions, would mean, say, sometime in his seventies. The date of this event is firmly fixed by a reference in Cicero, where L. Licinius Crassus, Asclepiades' friend and probably his patron, is made to speak of him in the past tense in a passage set in 91 B.C.[48] There can be no doubt that Cicero's testimony is to be preferred above Pliny's vague statement that Asclepiades lived "in the time of Pompey the Great," which would place him maybe thirty years later, and which probably results from a confusion with Asclepiades the grammarian.[49] The earlier date also fits with Pliny's notice that Mithridates VI Eupator of Pontus invited Asclepiades to be his court physician but was turned down.[50] These events are more likely to have taken place before Mithridates' relations with Rome became irretrievably embittered ca. 90 B.C. and led to the First Mithridatic War (89–83 B.C.), and thus they fit the chronology of Cicero's comments concerning Asclepiades' death. If Asclepiades came to Rome as a youth, he may well have been there for the half century proposed by Cocchi

---

47. See Wellmann, "Asklepiades aus Bithynien," 684–87 (the philosophical background to Asclepiades' theories), 693–702 (Asclepiades' theories). For closer analysis of Asclepiades' philosophical influences, see G. Harig, "Die philosophischen Grundlagen des medizinischen Systems des Asklepiades von Bithynien," *Philologus* 127 (1983): 43–60; Vallance, *Lost Theory.* On his eloquence, see Pliny *HN* 26.12–13. Cicero (*De or.* 1.62) includes him among eloquent exponents of technical matters, commenting that "he used to overcome other doctors with his eloquence" *(eloquentia vincebat ceteros medicos).* On the connection between rhetoric and medicine, see G.W. Bowersock, *Greek Sophists in the Roman Empire* (Oxford, 1969), 67–68.

48. Cic. *De or.* 1.62. See Rawson, "Life and Death," 360–61. This observation had been made in the eighteenth century by A. Cocchi (translated in Green, *Asclepiades,* 8–10). See also D. Gourevitch, "Asclépiade de Bithynie dans Pline: Problèmes de chronologie," in J. Pigeaud and J. Oroz-Reta, eds., *Pline l'ancien: Temoin de son temps* Salamanca-Nantes, 1987), 67–81; Wellmann, "Asklepiades aus Bithynien," 691.

49. Pliny *HN* 26.12. For Asclepiades the grammarian, see *RE* 2.1628–31, s.v. "Asklepiades 28" (Wentzel). The later date has recently been supported, but mainly on the basis of this notice in Pliny; see C. Römer, "Ehrung für den Arzt Themison," *ZPE* 84 (1990): 83.

50. Pliny *HN* 7.124. The invitation should be set against the background of Mithridates' broader efforts to project an image of himself as a patron of the arts and sciences; see B.C. McGing, *The Foreign Policy of Mithridates VI Eupator, King of Pontus* (Leiden, 1986), 89–108.

in the eighteenth century,[51] but if he arrived relatively late in life, in his forties or early fifties, he can still be reckoned to have spent twenty or more years in the city. Thus, since his death occurred shortly before 91 B.C., Asclepiades may reasonably be placed at Rome in the decades between ca. 130 and 91 B.C.

In contrast to these uncertainties, some important salient facts about Asclepiades are recoverable. It seems that Asclepiades achieved tremendous fame at Rome in his lifetime and beyond. Pliny, for instance, claims that Asclepiades was chiefly responsible for the subversion of traditional Roman medicine and asserts, extravagantly, that this doctor "brought around to his view almost the entire human race, in a fashion no different than if he had arrived by dropping out of the skies."[52] This is strong testimony indeed. Even allowing for exaggeration, there can be little doubt that Pliny perceived Asclepiades' fame as towering. Corroboration is offered by Celsus, Scribonius Largus, and others who make mention of Asclepiades' fame and prominence among doctors at Rome. That his ideas were still being vilified centuries after his death is testimony to his lasting posthumous influence.[53] This influence was largely due to the prominence of Asclepiades' disciples after his death. Notable among them were Themison of Laodicea, who extended and radicalized his teacher's ideas to found the Methodist system, and Antonius Musa, whose fame at court I have already noted.[54]

Against this background of great fame, it is interesting to note that Asclepiades was an ardent advocate of baths as a remedial and a preventive measure against illness. Baths—where conditions were wet, dry, hot, and cold—aptly accommodated his corpuscular theory of physiology, which postulated a body comprised of small units (ὄγκοι) and spaces, or pores (πόροι). Health was maintained (or regained, if lost) by achieving the correct

---

51. See the translation of Cocchi's proposal in Green, *Asclepiades,* 27.

52. Pliny *HN* 26.13: *universum prope humanum genus circumegit in se non alio modo quam si caelo demissus advenisset.* Pliny (*HN* 7.124–25), in fact, considers Asclepiades the most famous doctor of all, indicating that his fame was not a short-lived phenomenon. Like Pliny, Celsus (*proem.* 11) considers Asclepiades and his disciple Themison to be the founders of "professional" Roman medicine.

53. See Celsus 4.9.2; Scribonius Largus *ep.* 7; Apul. *Flor.* 19 (where Asclepiades is said only to be superseded by Hippocrates himself). See also Asclepiades' contemporary Antiochos of Askalon, cited in Sext. Emp. *Math.* 1.201–2. See Rawson, "Life and Death," 358 (later vilification).

54. For Themison as a follower of Asclepiades, see Pliny *HN* 29.6; Cael. Aurel. *Morb. acut.* 2.233, 3.39, *Morb. chron.* 1.140, 3.78. For Musa, see above, chapter 4, n. 8. For Asclepiades' successors, see Rawson, *Intellectual Life,* 176–77; and on Themison, see J. Pigeaud, "L'introduction du Méthodisme à Rome," *ANRW* 2.37.1 (1993): 581–84.

balance between these elements through exercise, diet, drink, and bathing.[55] The plainest and most direct expression of Asclepiades' emphasis on baths in his treatments occurs in Celsus. After commenting on the usefulness of baths for treating fevers, Celsus adds: "The ancients used it [the bath] more timidly, Asclepiades more boldly."[56] Pliny elucidates this point of view, albeit with strong negative overtones. He avers that one of the reasons for Asclepiades' success at Rome was the pleasant nature of his therapies, among which featured "a system of hydropathy, which appeals to people's greedy love of baths, and many other things pleasant and delightful to speak of."[57] This hydropathy included cold-water treatment—indeed, Varro, quoted by Pliny, says Asclepiades liked to be called "Dr. Coldwater-Giver."[58] Asclepiades is also reported to have used *pensilia balnea* (discussed in the following paragraph), which Pliny labels "soothing to an infinite degree."[59]

Asclepiades' use of baths merits closer scrutiny. Precisely what the term *pensilia balnea* (literally, "hanging baths") refers to poses a difficult problem that brings into discussion the activities of Sergius Orata, the inventor of the device. Without delving into the details, it can be determined, at the very least, that the *pensilia balnea* were heated tanks of some sort.[60] This view would fit with what we know of Asclepiades' therapies, which involved hydropathy, sweating, and hot water—all elements of *balnea*.[61] But why, then, is Asclepiades mentioned in the sources as a giver of cold water, but not explicitly of hot water? The best explanation is that other medical writers do

---

55. The most complete accounts of his philosophy are Harig, "Philosophische Grundlagen"; Vallance, *Lost Theory;* id., "Medical System," 695–704. Note that among Asclepiades' writings was a work entitled *Salutaria Praecepta* (mentioned in Cael. Aurel. *Morb. acut.* 1.112). It would be interesting to know what Asclepiades had to say there with regard to the preventive qualities of bathing. Methodism, founded by Asclepiades' disciple Themison and most fully expounded by Soranus in the second century, placed a premium on bathing, in its regimens and remedies.

56. Celsus 2.17.3: *antiqui timidius* [sc. *balneo*] *utebantur, Asclepiades audacius.* That Celsus is here talking about hot baths is clear from the immediate context; see 2.17.1–2.

57. Pliny *HN* 26.14: *alia quoque blandimenta excogitabat . . . iam balneas avidissima hominum cupidine instituendo et alia multa dictu grata atque iucunda . . .* (Note, in passing, the revealing sentiment that people are considered inherently inclined toward baths.)

58. Pliny *HN* 26.14: *ipse cognominari se frigida danda praeferens, ut auctor est M. Varro.*

59. Pliny *HN* 26.16: *tum primum pensili balinearum usu ad infinitum blandiente.*

60. For my fuller thoughts on this issue, see G.G. Fagan, "Sergius Orata: Inventor of the Hypocaust?" *Phoenix* 50 (1996): 56–66. See also Rawson, "Life and Death," 361; Ö. Wikander, "Senators and Equites," part 6, "Caius Sergius Orata and the Invention of the Hypocaust," *OpRom* 20 (1996): 177–82.

61. As we saw above, Celsus expressly states that Asclepiades emphasized hot baths in his treatments; see above, chapter 4, n. 56. Asclepiadean remedial methods are reflected in some of Celsus' therapies; see, e.g., 1.3.9–10 (hot and cold bathing, wine drinking, sweating, and eating).

not associate Asclepiades with hot-water treatments, precisely because such treatments were generally accepted and in widespread use. Ancient medical authors were given to sharp polemic against both predecessors and contemporaries. If an author mentioned another doctor, it was usually to criticize him, and any prescribed remedies were presented in such a way that they appeared to be the author's own; there was no acknowledgment of contributions made to the field by others. Caelius Aurelianus (fl. ca. 450) is a good example. Caelius frequently prescribes Asclepiadean remedies (including hot baths) but never mentions their source. Instead, his references to Asclepiades come in the form of attacks against his other treatments, namely, methods Caelius himself would not use. As presented in Celsus, and despite the predominant silence of the sources, Asclepiades' remedies must have included as much hot as cold hydrotherapy.[62] To this essentially negative argument can be added positive evidence: Celsus' assertion that Asclepiades used baths more boldly than predecessors; Caelius Aurelianus' comments that Asclepiades was known as a heating and a cooling doctor; and the notice, also in Caelius, that his pupil, Themison, whom Caelius criticizes harshly, was not rid of his master's precepts, among which featured frequent recommendations of bathing.[63] In addition, that Pliny the Elder's notice of Asclepiades using "hanging baths" occurs in a context that implies immersion in hot water offers further corroboration that the Bithynian doctor used hot as well as cold baths extensively in his treatment system and was remembered for doing so. To be sure, the problem of the meaning of *pensilia balinea* must be taken into account, but in the case of Asclepiades' use of them, the best interpretation is that they were heated tanks of water, possibly in a terraced cascade arrangement. In fact, it is possible that Asclepiades, not their declared inventor Sergius Orata, first applied them to human bathing and, in doing so, added the element of heated water.

Asclepiades can therefore be shown to have lived at Rome at the cusp of the second and first centuries B.C., to have enjoyed high-society connections, to have advocated bathing in his treatment, and to have earned such huge fame in the city that many later writers ascribed to him the overthrow of traditional Roman medicine.[64] But is it likely that this one man helped

---

62. See J. Benedum, "Die *Balnea Pensilia* des Asklepiades von Prusa," *Gesnerus* 24 (1967): 102–6; id., "Der Badearzt Asklepiades und seine bithynische Heimat," *Gesnerus* 35 (1978): 20–43. For Caelius Aurelianus, see *RE* 3.1256–58, s.v. "Caelius 18" (Wellmann).

63. See above, chapter 4, n. 56 (Celsus); Cael. Aurel. *Morb. acut.* 2.231 (heating and cooling) and *Morb. chron.* 1.142, 1.179 (Themison).

64. For modern appraisals of his influence, see, e.g., H.M. Koebling, *Arzt und Patient in der Antiken Welt* (Zürich, 1977), 177–96; Phillips, "Emergence of the Greek Medical Profession,"

stimulate a popular interest in baths, especially in the absence of modern methods of mass communication? And can his precepts really have influenced the mass of the *populus,* especially the plebs, who would surely have had little or no understanding of Asclepiades' philosophical teachings? I believe that both of these questions can be answered in the affirmative.

In assessing the possibilities, a broad distinction ought to be borne in mind between the categories of ancient medicine that have been termed "high" and "low." "High" medicine was the rational, theoretical approach to treating patients, the supreme example of which was Galen. "Low" medicine, in contrast, was almost akin to folk medicine, of the sort found in abundance in Pliny's *Natural History,* and was characterized by a practical, cure-based approach to healing.[65] This latter system was undoubtedly more commonly found among the lower classes, who had neither the means to contract and pay for a "professional" doctor nor the education to practice "high" medicine themselves. Asclepiades' healing system appears to bridge the two traditions. While his corpuscular physiology and the composition of medical treatises locate him firmly among the theoretical "high" doctors, his remedial measures, employing popular and pleasurable treatments, bear the hallmark of cure-based, "low" medicine.[66] The public lecture, a practice common among Hellenistic doctors, would have provided a direct vehicle for the presentation of Asclepiades' ideas and treatments to the populace.[67] In fact, technical lectures by "experts" in specific fields were a feature of the cultural life of the city.[68] It is true that we have no way of knowing what strata of society attended such presentations, and detailed speculation about

---

273–74; Scarborough, 38–42; id., "Roman Medicine to Galen," 26–29. Rawson (*Intellectual Life,* viii) goes so far as to propose that "there is a case for arguing that the most influential Greek thinker at work in Rome in the first century B.C. was the doctor Asclepiades of Bithynia."

65. See J.M. Riddle, "High Medicine and Low Medicine in the Roman Empire," *ANRW* 2.37.1 (1993): 102–20.

66. On Asclepiades' "practical" treatments, see Scarborough, "Roman Medicine to Galen," 28–29.

67. Cicero (*De or.* 1.62) and Pliny (*HN* 26.12) refer to his eloquence displayed in lectures, see also Rawson, "Life and Death," 364. Typical of the Hellenistic precedents for such presentations is an inscription (*Bull. ép.* 1958.336) recording that an Istrian doctor, Diokles, on the strength of his public lectures at Cyzicus, was appointed public doctor there in the second century B.C. The itinerant life of the ancient doctor made such presentations essential, to attract patients and establish a practice: see Hdt. 3.125, 3.129–37 (Democedes, the earliest documented traveling doctor); Cic. *Clu.* 40 (L. Clodius, an itinerant doctor in early first-century B.C. Italy). See further Koebling, *Arzt und Patient,* 173–76; Phillips, *Greek Medicine,* 182–96. See also L. Robert, "Décret pour un médecin de Cos," *RPhil* 52 (1978): 242–51 (= id., *Opera Minora Selecta* 6.438–47).

68. For such lectures, see Plut. *Mor.* 71A; Dio Chrys. *Or.* 33.6; Ath. 3.98c; Lib. *Or.* 1.55. For modern views, see Rawson, *Intellectual Life,* 51–53; Scarborough, 27–28.

the composition of the audience would be fruitless, but that the plebs were entirely absent seems an unreasonable conclusion.[69] Even if Asclepiades influenced only the bathing habits of the elite, there is every possibility that such an influence spread to the lower orders through word-of-mouth report and behavioral imitation, all the more so when it was not social status or displays of wealth but health itself that was at stake.[70] Insofar as everyone, high and low, would have had a vested interest in new methods of maintaining health, Asclepiades' message concerning baths would have been as pertinent to the *plebs urbana* as to the senatorial elite. Also, it is clear from comparative research that methods of treatment based on complex theory can be practiced even by those unable to read, let alone comprehend, the original philosophical expositions.[71] In any case, the simple precept "Baths are good for you" hardly required an advanced education to understand. All of these considerations, when coupled with the known facts of Asclepiades' career, make his potential influence on Roman bathing customs a strong possibility.

Several general features of ancient medical practice strengthen the preceding argument. First, ancient medicine was extraordinarily open, and anyone who felt like trying could become a doctor. Second, medical education was unspecialized and lacked any set or even requisite curriculum of its own; rather, it was subsumed under the general rubric of philosophy. No diplomas or degrees attested to a doctor's competence, so anyone who wanted to could claim expertise.[72] Third, there were no controls for monitoring the compe-

69. Certainly, Galen's lectures at Rome were very much open affairs; see Galen *Libr. prop.* 1–11 (19.11–43 Kühn). Rawson (*Intellectual Life,* 53) imagines the Roman unemployed as having ample time to listen to academic arguments. Asclepiades would no doubt have spoken in Greek, but it is quite possible that, given the multiethnic composition of the plebs, his ideas could have moved quickly into that social stratum—Carneades' lectures in Rome in 155 b.c. caused quite a stir (see above, chapter 3, n. 30). Many nonelite Greek-speaking people no doubt lived at Rome, among them the Jews; see H.J. Leon, *The Jews of Ancient Rome* (Philadephia, 1960), 75–92. Such groups afforded a ready medium for the filtration of foreign ideas into the Roman plebs. On multilingualism at Rome, see Balsdon, *Romans and Aliens,* 116–45.

70. The imitation by the lower orders of upper-class fashions and behavior, while not to be overestimated, is clearly brought out in such passages as Cic. *Leg.* 3.30–31; Pliny *HN* 33.32–33, 33.152; Mart. 12.70. Social climbing has been traced through domestic interior decoration at Pompeii and Herculaneum; see Wallace-Hadrill, *Houses and Society,* 143–74.

71. See G. Karmi, "The Colonisation of Traditional Arabic Medicine," in R. Porter, ed., *Patients and Practitioners: Lay Perceptions of Medicine in Pre-Industrial Society* (Cambridge, 1985), 315–39. Karmi found that illiterate peasants in Syria-Jordan were still practicing classical Islamic medicine, with only vague notions of the theories that lay behind it.

72. Thessalos of Tralles, a practitioner of Nero's day, asserted that six months was sufficient training for a doctor; see Galen *Meth. med.* 1.2 (10.4–5 Kühn). On medical "education," see Jackson, 58–60; J. Kollesch, "Ärtzliche Ausbildung in der Antike," *Klio* 61 (1979): 507–13; Scarborough, 122–33.

tence of doctors, which left the door open to many forms of "popular" medicine, sometimes administered by quacks and tricksters.[73] Finally, medical knowledge was not restricted to any "professional" medical group (such did not exist on the modern model) but was widely disseminated, certainly among the upper classes, and probably also among the less privileged, who were no less concerned with medical matters than were their social betters.[74] All of these circumstances add greater scope to Asclepiades' possible influence. In a perilous world where medical knowledge was fluid, unregulated, and widely shared, the straightforward bathing precepts of the Bithynian physician could quite easily have spread throughout all levels of society. The high density of the urban population at Rome and their love of gossip only make the possibility stronger.[75] Swift oral transmission of information would have been relatively easy—all the more so if the information was uncomplicated and health-conducive in nature. In such an environment, a new and readily implementable tip on how to stay healthy was likely to get a wide audience.

Nonetheless, Asclepiades' influence should not be overstated. The evidence reviewed above makes it clear that he was responsible neither for introducing baths to Rome nor for initiating their popularity. He was indeed a clever man—that much comes through from the evidence—so he may have identified the nascent Roman penchant for baths and amplified it with a medical imprimatur. Such a tactic would have had the added benefit of expanding his popularity and fame and so increasing his roll of patients. If we take this view, Asclepiades is to be seen more as a catalyst in a trend rather

---

73. See Pliny's bitter comment (*HN* 29.17) on the openness of medicine, and see the *Digest's* noticeably lax definition of who can be considered a doctor (50.13.1.1–3). See further V. Nutton, "Murders and Miracles: Lay Attitudes towards Medicine in Classical Antiquity," in Porter, *Patients and Practitioners,* 23–53. Ancient quackery has yet to be fully investigated, but see F. Kudlien, "Schaustellerei und Heilmittelvertrieb in der Antike," *Gesnerus* 40 (1983): 91–98.

74. That the second-century doctor Rufus wrote a handbook called *Medicine for the Layman* reflects the dissemination of "high" medical knowledge among the upper class. Celsus appears to have been an encyclopedist, whose medical writings alone have survived extant (see *RE* 4.1273–76, s.v. "Cornelius 82" [Wellmann]). See also H.M. Koebling, "Le médecin dans la cité grecque," *Gesnerus* 46 (1989): 34–35; Nutton, "Murders and Miracles," 31–32.

75. See F. Castagnoli et al., *Topografia e urbanistica di Roma antica* (Bologna, 1958), 43–45; G. Hermansen, "The Population of Imperial Rome: The Regionaries," *Historia* 27 (1978): 129–68; K. Hopkins, *Conquerors and Slaves* (Cambridge, 1978), 96–98. Of course, precise numerical estimates are very uncertain, but the density of Rome's population in Cicero's day is clear enough; see Yavetz, "Living Conditions," 500–501 (= Seager, *Crisis,* 162–63); Scobie, "Slums, Sanitation, and Mortality." MacMullen (*Roman Social Relations,* 62–63) points out that Rome, with an estimated two hundred people per acre, was far more densely populated than would be considered acceptable today; see also Duncan-Jones, *Economy,* 276–77.

than an initiator of it. Also, we do not know whether he was alone in advocating baths. Other contemporary doctors, of whatever quality, may have been doing so at this time, but if so, Asclepiades is the only one of them to garner sustained attention in the sources. Given our current evidence, the notion that Asclepiades was merely the most eminent (and controversial) representative of a broader trend in medical thinking has to be admitted. But despite these uncertainties, Asclepiades' influence on Roman bathing habits appears to have been sustained and significant. The Rome of Asclepiades' day was a city in flux. It was experiencing rapid change not only in economics, politics, and social life but also in its intellectual and cultural atmosphere. The city's population was growing, Greek culture was becoming increasingly fashionable among the elite, and Greeks and other non-Romans were to be found among the plebs in ever greater numbers. Wealth, luxury, and ostentation were on the rise, in both the private and the public spheres. New construction technologies, especially ever more confident use of concrete, were being developed and would soon find expression in the building programs of Caesar, Augustus (despite his conservatism), and the emperors. Into this environment stepped the Bithynian doctor Asclepiades. His career and the context in which it is to be placed make it possible that his bath-related teachings, while perhaps initially gaining exposure only among the upper classes, filtered down to the less well-off. In the life-threatening conditions of the ancient city, everyone would have had an interest in new means of maintaining health. Whether or not it was part of a wider trend in medical thought at Rome, Asclepiades' simple message that baths, already available to the Romans at large, were not only pleasurable but healthy would have contributed to the growth of their popularity in the first century B.C. Even if the degree of Asclepiades' contribution cannot now be gauged precisely, it would seem rash to deny it altogether.

Chapter 5

Bath Benefactors 1: Rome

Who built Roman baths, and why? Such basic questions have been addressed only perfunctorily in previous studies.[1] An investigation of the social identity and motives of the baths' builders and maintainers throws light on several aspects of Roman society: the emperor as builder and public patron, the mechanics of local euergetism, the impulses that lay behind the construction and provision of amenities for the *populus,* and the symbolic significance of architecture in the Roman world. My inquiry into the builders of baths starts at Rome and initially serves two purposes: to complete the investigation into the growth of the popularity of baths and, simultaneously, to commence an inquiry into the social identity of bath builders. The appearance at Rome of the first large-scale baths (the so-called imperial *thermae*) and the subsequent dispersal of Roman-style baths into the provinces mark the culmination of the period of growth that started in the middle Republic (with Plautus); and that it was predominantly emperors who built the huge bathing complexes of the capital raises the issue of responsibility for bath construction, mainte-nance, and ownership that occupies this chapter and the next. My concern throughout this study lies less with the archaeological details of each com-plex and more with what light can be shed on the people and social processes that stand behind the buildings.[2] This chapter, therefore, is not a comprehen-sive reconsideration of the multifarious physical aspects of the baths of Rome but rather an overview that draws together archaeological and written mate-rial to identify the builders of the city's baths and to offer an assessment of their motives.

---

1. See, e.g., Nielsen, 1.119–22; Pasquinucci, 19–21; Yegül, 43–46, 322–23. Note also H. Meusel, *Die Verwaltung und Finanzierung der öffentlichen Bäder zur römischen Kaiserzeit* (Cologne, 1960), and Ch. Bruun's inconclusive investigation of bath ownership based on water-pipe stamps (*Water,* 72–76).

2. Our understanding of imperial-style *thermae* will be enhanced by J. DeLaine's forth-coming book on the subject.

The Republican Authorities and Emperors

Emperors were major builders of baths at Rome, but the Republican authorities are not attested in any source as providing public baths for the city. To be sure, our evidence for public construction in Republican Rome is limited, but the apparent disregard of baths by the authorities in the capital becomes more surprising when compared to the situation elsewhere in Italy. Here, inscriptions reveal that local councils and their officers were often responsible for erecting and maintaining public baths.[3] Yet, despite the existence of a mechanism for funding, contracting out, and supervising public construction, no bath can be identified as the product of official senatorial action at Rome in the Republican era.[4] Why this should be the case is not immediately apparent. Assuming that it is not due simply to a gap in our evidence, several possibilities present themselves. The conservative senators may have felt that subsidizing such vehicles of luxurious living as baths was an improper use of public funds.[5] An analogous situation pertained to permanent theaters, structures that met senatorial opposition as they were introduced into Rome with increasing frequency in the second and first centuries B.C.[6] Recent studies have highlighted the symbolic associations of Roman

---

3. The Stabian Baths at Pompeii have not left us an inscription commemorating their initial construction, but that they were at least publicly owned is indicated by the activities of *duoviri* in repairing and extending them; see no. 61. The Forum Baths are attested as built by the council (see no. 62) and adorned by local officials (see no. 68). Other inscriptions from elsewhere in Italy also state that baths were erected or restored "with public money" *(pecunia publica)* or by the agents of the local authorities; see nos. 63–67.

4. On the mechanisms of public construction, see D.E. Strong, "The Administration of Public Building in Rome during the Late Republic and Early Empire," *BICS* 15 (1968): 97–109. The absence of baths from the list of public buildings constructed at Rome between 200 and 78 B.C. compiled by F. Coarelli ("Public Building in Rome between the Second Punic War and Sulla," *BSR* 45 [1977]: 20–22) is noteworthy, if unsurprising. Coarelli's list comprises mostly buildings with literary attestation—that is, those that drew the attention of ancient authors and were therefore considered "important"—so, for instance, dozens of temple constructions find their way into Coarelli's catalogue. At the very least, however, the absence of baths from this list testifies to the "official" unimportance of baths in the Republic, in sharp contrast to the importance evidenced by the major bath projects undertaken in the capital by the emperors in the early Imperial period.

5. Note the comments of Cicero *(Off. 2.60)*: only strictly utilitarian buildings (e.g., walls, docks, aqueducts, etc.) are worthy of public patronage, whereas porticoes, theaters, and such are not (the absence of baths in Cicero's lists of "undesirable" buildings may be due to his dependence here on Greek sources). Hot-water baths were most likely viewed with suspicion by conservative Romans, as they certainly were by moralists of a later age (e.g., Seneca, at least in his public pronouncements; see above chapter 2, n. 40).

6. Particularly suggestive are the attitudes that lay behind the senate's decree of 151 B.C. stipulating that a permanent theater then under construction be dismantled and that the people thereafter watch plays standing up, since sitting induced effeminacy: see Livy *Per.* 48; Val. Max.

architecture, in which temples, fora, roads, and such were associated with virtue, while brothels, taverns, and other lowly structures were symbolic of vice. Baths occupied an ambiguous place on this scale, standing somewhere between useful public monuments and lowly havens of corporeal dissipation.[7] Such perceptions as these may have colored the Republican senators' view of the city's *balnea* and deterred them from spending public money on them (although they did not necessarily avoid them personally; see above, chapter 2, p. 49–50). This attitude may be reflected in the apportioning of the city's public water. Frontinus reports that "among the ancients," by which he means during the period of the Republic, all water entering the city in aqueducts was designated for specific public uses, but not for baths; instead, baths and fullers' shops were granted special dispensation to use runoff water from public troughs, and only then for a price.[8] This ordinance is hardly extraordinary, since the senate's chief concern was to provide the city with sufficient drinking water, but it shows that the baths of Republican Rome, like fullers' shops, were private commercial concerns and so were not entitled to use public water except by special license. Conservatism in architectural aesthetics can be added as a further factor. The baths, which employed a variety of new architectural techniques, may have been considered too "newfangled" for the sponsorship of the city's authorities, whose building activities tended toward traditional—and thus "virtuous"— monumental public edifices, such as temples, basilicas, and places of assembly, as well as toward more functional structures, such as aqueducts, bridges, roads, and walls; each of the two categories of building had its own architectural tradition, and the baths fitted neither neatly.[9] More practical reasons

---

2.4.1–2; Tac. *Ann.* 14.20. The situation with regard to theaters and baths, however, is not exactly parallel. For instance, elaborate theaters offered opportunities in a way that baths did not for political pandering to the mob, and conservative senators were bound to find that aspect of theaters especially objectionable. For a recent discussion of early Roman theaters, including early Italian examples, see Beacham, *Roman Theatre*, 56–85. See also Anderson, *Roman Architecture*, 282–87; Richardson, *Dictionary*, 380, s.v. "Theatrum."

7. See Sen. *Dial.* 7.7.3; see also ibid. 12.6.2. On the symbolic value of Roman architecture, see E. Gowers, "The Anatomy of Rome from Capitol to Cloaca," *JRS* 85 (1995): 23–32; E. Thomas and C. Witschel, "Constructing Reconstruction: Claim and Reality of Roman Rebuilding Inscriptions from the Latin West," *BSR* 60 (1992): 135–77; P. Zanker, *The Power of Images in the Age of Augustus* (Ann Arbor, 1988). On the place of baths, see Wallace-Hadrill, "Public Honour and Private Shame," 54–55.

8. Frontin. *Aq.* 94. Frontinus goes on to describe aediles and censors implementing water laws (95–98), thus providing a Republican context for the whole section.

9. See J.B. Ward-Perkins, "Taste, Tradition, and Technology: Some Aspects of the Architecture of Late Republican and Early Imperial Central Italy," in G. Kopcke and M.B. Moore, eds., *Studies in Classical Art and Archaeology: A Tribute to Peter Heinrich von Blanckenhagen* (New York, 1979), 197–204, esp. 202: "There was, then, in late Republican and early Imperial

may also have played a role. The activities of private benefactors were perhaps sufficient for the city's bathing needs. Rome's Republican baths were erected and maintained by people of substance; senators and *equites* were no doubt among them but were acting as private citizens.[10] Rome, the capital of a vast empire, was home to a greater proportion of wealthy families than were smaller Italian communities. As long as such people voluntarily built baths as business investments, there was simply no need for the authorities to do likewise, especially when only modest *balnea* were involved. For the Republic, then, the public baths of Rome were private enterprises rather than publicly provided services.

Agrippa dedicated his aqueduct, the Aqua Virgo, on 9 June 19 B.C. The aqueduct was associated with his baths, so, considering the hydraulic needs of the complex, this is also the earliest possible date for the opening of the entire facility.[11] At first glance, the Thermae of Agrippa, privately funded

---

Rome . . . two distinct canons of aesthetic values and proprieties, one of them felt to be applicable to the traditional categories of representative public architecture, the other to the more utilitarian and commercial types of building, both public and private." Ironically, according to Ward-Perkins (203–4), the baths later assisted in breaking down this aesthetic distinction, with the Thermae of Agrippa acting as a catalyst.

10. For Republican senators as bath owners (and probably bath builders), see above, chapter 2, pp. 48–49. Very few hints survive as to who built the privately owned *balnea* of Republican Rome; see Cicero's mention of the Pallacine Baths, named after a street, and of the Senian Baths, possibly named after their builder (see appendix 2).

11. See Frontin. *Aq.* 10; Dio 54.11.7 (dedication of Aqua Virgo). The construction date of the baths is unclear from the sources. Dio says Agrippa built a *laconicum* (which he also calls a *gymnasium*) in 25 B.C. (53.27.1) and dedicated the Aqua Virgo in 19 B.C. (54.11.7). The significance of these notices remains obscure: did Agrippa first build a Greek-style gymnasium, without baths, and only later add a bathing wing requiring its own water supply? The ruins of the original structure are too fragmentary to allow a firm resolution of this issue. The main publication of the remains is Ch. Hülsen, *Die Thermen des Agrippa in Rom: Ein Beitrag zur Topographie des Marsfeldes in Rom* (Rome, 1910). For a modern bibliography, see Manderscheid, 179–80, s.v. "Terme di Agrippa." Also add Nielsen, 1.43–45, 2.2 (C.1); Richardson, *Dictionary,* 386–87, s.v. "Thermae Agrippae"; J.-M. Roddaz, *Marcus Agrippa* (Rome, 1984), 278–82; F.W. Shipley, "Chronology of the Building Operations in Rome from the Death of Caesar to the Death of Augustus," *MAAR* 9 (1931): 50–51; id., *Agrippa's Building Activities in Rome* (St. Louis, 1933), 47–55; E. Tortorici, "L'attività edilizia di Agrippa a Roma," in *Il bimillenario di Agrippa* (Genoa, 1990), 47–52; Weber, 73–76; Yegül, 133–37. The dimensions of the building were ca. 100/120 meters by 80/100 meters (see Yegül, 133). The original name of the facility is also a matter of uncertainty. As just noted, Dio calls it variously τὸ πυριατήριον τὸ Λακωνικόν, γυμνάσιον (53.27.1) and τὸ βαλανεῖον του Ἀγρίππου (53, table of contents, i; see also 54.29.4). The earliest surviving references to it in literary sources occur with Pliny the Elder, who consistently uses *Thermae Agrippae* (HN 34.62, 35.26, 36.189); Martial also calls the building by this name (3.20.15, 3.36.5–6). The Severan Marble Map labels it *[Th]ermae [Agrip]pae* (FUR fr. 38). The *Historia Augusta* appears to describe it as *Lavacrum Agrippae* (Hadr. 19.10), while describing other imperial bath complexes as *thermae* (e.g., Sev. 19.5, Alex. Sev. 25.3, Prob. 2.1). (It is possible, however, that the *Historia Augusta* is here confusing with

and owned, seem to be fully in keeping with the pattern of Republican bath construction at Rome. Agrippa, on this level, can be seen as a prominent magnate who built a public bathhouse apparently as a commercial enterprise, because we know that the baths charged an entrance fee until his death in 12 B.C.[12] But two factors marked these baths as different from what had come before. First, there was the new political climate in which they were constructed and Agrippa's place in that climate. The private actions of individual senators during the era of the competitive oligarchy could be readily distinguished from their public actions: the latter were accompanied by all the formal signs and rituals of official sanction, whereas private undertakings were not. In particular, publicly funded construction was marked by the ritual of contract letting under censors sitting in state, the use of public funds for the work, and the final inspection and dedication by state officials. All of these actions were often acknowledged in an inscription placed on the finished product, which might also be named after the officials involved (e.g., Via Appia and Aqua Appia).[13] In contrast, a privately initiated construction project would display none of these features, except the association of the builder's name with the building. While these distinctions undoubtedly be-

Agrippa's establishment a bath building put up by one of the Agrippinas; see below, chapter 5, n. 23.) A restoration inscription of 344–45 (*CIL* 6.1165) describes the building as *termae (sic)*. Sidonius Apollinaris (*Carm.* 23.495–96) calls it *balnea*. The confusion over the building's name illustrates well the apparent chaos that reigns in ancient bath terminology.

12. Dio (54.29.4) reports that Agrippa bequeathed the baths to public ownership so that the people used them for free—implying that they had formerly paid—and also that he left estates from which to fund this benefaction. Nielsen's belief (1.45–46, 47 n. 78) that the baths were originally not open to the public must be rejected. She does not explain her reasoning, but it appears to be based on this statement in Dio. The passage, however, states only that Agrippa gave the baths over to public ownership; they had previously been his private property, which does not mean that they were for his exclusive use, as Nielsen seems to believe. It is clear from Dio's wording only that the transferal of the building to public ownership resulted in the people using the baths for free (τὸ βαλανεῖον τὸ ἐπώνυμον αὐτοῦ κατέλιπεν, ὥστε προῖκα αὐτοὺς λοῦσθαι); he does not say that they were then admitted for the first time. Finally, it is scarcely credible that Augustus, who placed great emphasis on ostensible moderation in the behavior of the ruling class, would have allowed his right-hand man to construct exclusively for his personal use such a vast and luxurious bathhouse, requiring its own aqueduct to function.

13. On the essential role of ceremony in defining state actions under the Republic, see D.J. Gargola, *Lands, Laws, and Gods: Magistrates and Ceremony in the Regulation of Public Lands in Republican Rome* (Chapel Hill, 1995), esp. 12–24. In the realm of public construction, for instance, note the activities of the censors Appius Claudius Caecus in 312 B.C. (*InscrIt* 13.3.79; Diod. Sic. 20.36.1–6) and Q. Fulvius Flaccus and A. Postumius Albinus in 174 B.C. (Livy 41.27). For the literary *testimonia* on the building activities of the censors in the period 199–70 B.C., see Coarelli, "Public Building," 3–7. Similar ritual surrounded the actions of local officials acting as representatives of municipal authorities; see, e.g., nos. 61 (contacts let), 64 (public money used).

gan to break down under the late Republican dynasts,[14] the new order of Augustus, where one family stood preeminent and monopolized political and military power, completed the transformation. Now the private actions of Augustus and of those close to him became, in effect, public actions, since the government *(res publica)* was all but incarnate in his person.[15] Agrippa, in undertaking the construction of his baths, can hardly be thought of as acting independently of Augustus and thus of the state, given that he enjoyed so many close ties to the imperial house.[16] Moreover, Augustus actively encouraged those around him to undertake public construction, and the Thermae of Agrippa was one of several edifices of public significance erected by Agrippa in the Campus Martius, along with the Diribitorium, the Saepta, and the Pantheon.[17]

The Thermae of Agrippa, therefore, represent the first instance whereby responsibility for building baths at Rome can be said unequivocally to fall within the ambit of the state. Whether or not it was actively recognized as such by contemporaries is all but impossible to gauge, since ancient popular perceptions are notoriously difficult to detect, but perhaps the second note-worthy aspect of the building played a key role here. In 12 B.C. Agrippa's will transferred ownership of the baths to the *populus*. Indeed, these were the only baths in Rome to undergo such "nationalization."[18] The public owner-

---

14. It is hard to see how, for instance, the constructional activities of Pompey or Caesar's reputed plans for the city were not viewed on some level as state actions.

15. For this view of the imperial order, see, e.g., Suet. *Aug.* 58.2 (Augustus' good fortune equated with the prosperity of the *res publica*). See also Veyne, 539–621; Thomas and Witschel, "Constructing Reconstruction," 165. For slightly contrasting, but not contradictory, views of the Augustan order, see F. Millar, *The Emperor in the Roman World* (London, 1977), esp. 611–20; E.S. Ramage, *The Nature and Purpose of Augustus's* Res Gestae (Stuttgart, 1987), 38–66.

16. In 23 B.C. Agrippa became Augustus' son-in-law and received *imperium proconsulare*, as an inscription attests (see E.V. Gray, "The *Imperium* of M. Agrippa," *ZPE* 6 [1970]: 227–38). In 21 B.C., when Augustus left Rome to tour the West, Agrippa was recalled from the East and left in charge of the city in Augustus' absence (see Dio 54.6.4–5; Suet. *Aug.* 63). In 18 B.C., the year following the baths' dedication, his *imperium* was renewed (and extended?), and he was granted *tribunicia potestas* (see Dio 54.12.4). Following these events, Agrippa is presented on coinage as Augustus' coregent: see C.H.V. Sutherland, *Coinage in Roman Imperial Policy* (London, 1951), 53–55; id., *The Roman Imperial Coinage,* vol. 1² (London, 1984), 51 and 73 (nos. 408, 409, 414). For an overview of Agrippa's position in the new order, see Roddaz, *Marcus Agrippa,* esp. 335–490.

17. See Suet. *Aug.* 29.4–5; Vell. Pat. 2.89.4. Augustus took his own building activities in the city very seriously: they occupy six chapters of his *Res Gestae* (19–24).

18. See above, chapter 5, n. 12. Claims that the Thermae of Agrippa were Rome's "first public baths" (see, e.g., Coarelli, *Roma,* 326; Yegül, 133) are therefore misguided on two counts: Rome demonstrably had publicly accessible baths long before Agrippa's complex was opened, and no other baths are known to have been publicly owned, so Agrippa's *thermae* represent a "first" in neither sense; see N.G.R. Brundrett and C.J. Simpson, "Innovation and the Baths of Agrippa," *Athenaeum* 85 (1997): 220–27.

ship of the complex, bequeathed by a man who was clearly established as Augustus' successor, could only have strengthened any already existing popular perception that the building was the product of a beneficent Augustan order dispensing favors to society at large. A related feature of the complex that deserves mention and that surely reinforced popular impressions of state involvement in its construction was its size and magnificence. Physical remains of the structure are too scrappy to support any concrete conclusions about its original appearance, but it is noteworthy that Agrippa's baths are the first baths known to feature monumental sculpture and that Pliny the Elder refers to them several times as a point of departure in artistic endeavor, implying that the building was perceived as groundbreaking in certain respects.[19] If, as the epigraphic evidence from the rest of Italy suggests, Republican Rome had before now lagged behind the Italian townships in building baths under state authority, the Thermae of Agrippa mark that moment when the capital seized the initiative and presented the world with a model to follow. I offer one final observation on these baths: if, as argued above, public baths had previously been considered below state sanction at Rome itself, the Thermae of Agrippa represent a reversal in official attitudes toward such facilities.[20]

Agrippa's lead was not followed until Nero opened his luxurious bathing complex, also in the Campus Martius, in the early or middle sixties.[21] Given

---

19. The Thermae of Agrippa are best attested in Renaissance drawings (esp. by Palladio) and from a fragment of the Marble Map, but both may record its later appearance following several restorations, some of which were extensive: see G. Zorzi, *I disegni della antichità di Andrea Palladio* (Venice, 1958), 71–72 with figs. 136–43; *FUR* fr. 38. Palladio's drawings are generally considered reliable, if not photographically accurate; see D. Lewis, *The Drawings of Andrea Palladio* (Washington, DC, 1981), 129–40. See also Pliny *HN* 34.62 (monumental sculpture outside entrance to baths; the piece, the Apoxyomenos of Lysippus, survives in copy in the Vatican Museum), 35.26 (paintings on marble surfaces in the baths), 36.189 (paintings and whitewash); Strabo 13.1.19 (another Lysippan sculpture near the Stagnum). Many modern scholars consider Agrippa's establishment to be the first in the long line of imperial *thermae*: see, e.g., Heinz, 60–67; Yegül, 133. Nielsen (1.45) prefers to see the Thermae of Nero as the first true model of the "imperial" type. Despite the clever arguments of Brundrett and Simpson ("Innovation"), there is no evidence that an establishment even approaching the size and magnificence of the Thermae of Agrippa existed in Republican Rome or anywhere else in the western empire at this time, so that these baths were indeed a largely novel structure.

20. Although there is no explicit evidence of any moral opposition to these baths among the conservative elements in the nobility, it may well be suspected (compare the situation in eighteenth-century Philadelphia described above, in chapter 3, n. 1). One wonders whether the association of the baths with Agrippa was also a shrewd move on the part of the *princeps*: if the baths gained acceptance and were successful (as they were to be), Augustus would earn kudos indirectly through Agrippa; if they failed, he could distance himself from the project.

21. There is some uncertainty as to the nature and precise date of this building, due in no small measure to contradictions in the sources: see Suet. *Ner.* 12.3 (*thermae* and gymnasium

the characters of the previous *principes,* it is not hard to see why no large baths were built in the intervening period: Tiberius was no great builder, Gaius' reign was too brief for meaningful construction projects to be undertaken, and Claudius was republican in his aesthetic tastes and not an extravagant builder in any case.[22] One of the Agrippinas, however, appears to have built a bath on the Viminal Hill, as attested by lead-pipe stamps and the evidence of later sources. This establishment may, however, have been private. No physical remains of the building are known.[23] In contrast to the inertia of his predecessors, Nero endowed the city with a bathing complex

dedicated in 60); Dio 61(62).21.1 (gymnasium dedicated in 60); Tac. *Ann.* 14.47.3 (Nero's gymnasium dedicated in 61); Hieron. *Chron., sub anno* 63 (p. 183 Helm; Nero's *thermae* built); Cassiod. *Chron., sub anno* 64 (p. 138 Mommsen; Nero's *thermae* built in 64); Philostr. *VA* 4.42 (Nero's gymnasium opened in 66). As a result of these notices, the exact nature of the building(s) has attracted scholarly speculation—did Nero build a gymnasium, *thermae,* or a combination of the two? (A good summary of the problem remains G. Lugli, *I monumenti antichi di Roma e Suburbio* [Rome, 1938], 3.212–18.) One solution is to argue that the same building enjoyed two designations, originally *gymnasium* under the philhellene Nero, later *thermae* under the Flavians; see B. Tamm, *Neros Gymnasium in Rom* (Stockholm, 1970), 11–13. Another view is that two separate buildings are denoted, the earlier of which, the gymnasium, burned down in 62 (see Tac. *Ann.* 15.22.3; this notice weakens the same-building theory) and was replaced with the *thermae* in 66; see A. Vassileiou, "Sur le date des thermes de Néron," *REA* 74 (1972): 94–106. Against the latter view is the evidence of Suetonius, Hieronymus, and Cassiodorus that the *thermae* were opened before 66. Yet another proposition is that the term *gymnasium* denotes a portion of the *thermae* given to exercise (two palaestrae and a *natatio*); see *LTUR* 2.372, s.v. "Gymnasium Neronis" (G. Ghini). Recent study of the physical remains cannot solve the problem and has revealed that most of the ruins date to the major reconstruction of Severus Alexander in 227, even if not much the same groundplan as Nero's original; see G. Ghini, "Le Terme Alessandrine nel Campo Marzio," *MonAnt,* occasional papers, 3, no. 4 (1988): 135–66. The building was generally referred to as the *Thermae Neronianae* (see, e.g., Mart. 2.48.8, 3.25.4, 12.83.5; no. 279; *CIL* 6.3052, *CIL* 6.8676) until it was renamed *Thermae Alexandrinae* following Severus Alexander's restoration (see, e.g., *FTUR* 1.1.5); Sidonius Apollinaris (*Carm.* 23.495–96) calls it *balnea.* For a full bibliography on this building, see Manderscheid, 185, s.v. "Terme di Nerone." Add also Ghini, "Terme Alessindrine"; *LTUR* 2.374, s.v. "Gymnasium Neronis" (G. Ghini); Nielsen, 1.45–46, 2.2 (C.2); Richardson, *Dictionary,* 393–95, s.v. "Thermae Neronianae"; Weber, 76–77; Yegül, 137–39. The dimensions are given by Heinz (68) as 190 meters by 120 meters.

22. See Lugli, *Monumenti antichi,* 2.44–53, where the building activities of Tiberius, Gaius, and Claudius occupy only the first three pages of a survey of the Julio-Claudian period. For Tiberius, see Suet. *Tib.* 47.1; F.C. Bourne, *The Public Works of the Julio-Claudians and Flavians* (Princeton, 1946), 31–37; B. Levick, *Tiberius the Politician* (London, 1976), 123. For Gaius (Caligula), see Suet. *Calig.* 21; A.A. Barrett, *Caligula: The Corruption of Power* (New Haven, 1989), 192–212; Bourne, op. cit., 38–41. For Claudius, see Suet. *Claud.* 20; Bourne, op. cit., 42–48; B. Levick, *Claudius* (New Haven, 1990), 108–11. The *Thermae Tiberianae,* however, are reported associated with the *Horti Sallustiani* in Medieval sources (see *FTUR* 4.13.439–42). Nothing is known of the building, and it is not recorded in ancient sources.

23. See the notes to no. 251; Richardson, *Dictionary,* 234, s.v. "Lavacrum Agrippinae." The bath finds no mention in a recent biography of Agrippina the Younger; see A.A. Barrett, *Agrippina: Sex, Power, and Politics in the Early Empire* (New Haven, 1996).

that was very much in keeping with the lavish tastes of the age and the popular bent of his reign. Very little of the building survives today, so secure conclusions about its original appearance cannot be drawn, but its luxuriousness is attested in Martial, who also hints that the baths were proverbially hot (see above, chapter 1, p. 19).

Titus was the next great provider of baths, but we should note in passing that the *Notitia* mentions a *Balneum Torquati et Vespasiani* in Regio I of the city (*FTUR* 3.8.3). It is conceivable that Vespasian had some interest in this building (or buildings) before his elevation to the purple, but that he erected it as emperor seems most unlikely: he was notoriously tightfisted and is unlikely to have graced a mere *balneum* with his imperial name, especially when the complexes of Agrippa and Nero already stood as precedents for the expected scale of imperial bath benefaction.[24] Vespasian's son, Titus, repaired the Thermae of Agrippa after a fire and erected his own public bathhouse, a structure somewhat smaller than the Thermae of Nero and reputedly thrown up in a hurry.[25] The haste was probably imposed by the impending dedication of the Flavian Amphitheater, which stood nearby. Titus appears to have wished that the bath complex and the amphitheater open at the same time, as indeed they did.[26] This concurrence would have had the advantage of drawing attention to Titus' own personal contribution (the baths) as separate from that of his father (the amphitheater), while

24. For a full discussion of the possibilities pertaining to this building, see below, chapter 5, p. 125.

25. See Dio 66.24 (repair of Agrippa's Thermae); Dio 66.25.1 and Suet. *Tit.* 7.3 (construction of new baths). For the haste, see Suet. loc. sit.; Mart. *Spect.* 2.7. For a modern bibliography on this building, of which little survives, see Manderscheid, 185–86, s.v. "Terme di Tito." Also add Heinz, 75–77; Nielsen, 1.46–47, 2.2 (C.3); Richardson, *Dictionary,* 396–97, s.v. "Thermae Titi"; Weber, 78–79; Yegül, 139–42. Recent excavation at the site revealed part of one of the aspidal *caldaria,* but insufficient Flavian remains survive to test the sources' claim that the structure was built in a hurry; see G. Caruso et al., "Scavi alle Terme di Tito," *ArchLaz* 10 (1990): 58–67. The building was termed *Thermae Titi* or *Thermae Titianae* into the later Empire (see, e.g., Mart. 3.20.15, 3.36.6; Hieron. *Chron., sub anno* 90 [p. 191 Helm]; no. 283; *FTUR* 1.1.5) and measured ca. 105 meters by 120 meters (Yegül, 139). F. Coarelli's suggestion (*Roma,* 211) that these baths were originally part of Nero's Golden House has not met with widespread acceptance (see esp. Richardson, loc. cit.), although Nielsen (1.46–47) presents it as a distinct possibility, albeit on a misguided analogy with the "private" Thermae of Agrippa.

26. Note the analogous holding of games and other benefactions at the dedication of baths elsewhere, as recorded in inscriptions. An example is the games given by Cn. Alleius Nigidius Maius at Pompeii, probably to mark the reopening of the Forum Baths after the earthquake of 62 (*CIL* 4.1177 = *ILS* 5144). See also nos. 10 (gladiatorial games?), 58 *(sportulae),* 71 (banquet and spectacles), 72 (banquet and *sportulae*), 101 and 165 (circus), 114 (theatrical games and banquet), 144 and 189 (banquet), 183 (games). Note also the fragmentary *AE* 1979.156 (circus and theatrical games given at Teanum Sidicinum in 151).

nonetheless advertising both at a single stroke in a masterful joint celebration of emperor and dynasty. Whatever the case, the Thermae of Titus quickly became a landmark in the city and were the favored facility of Martial (see above, chapter 1, p. 19).

Trajan erected the next large-scale set of baths at Rome. They were situated on top of the Oppian Hill and are the first to be sufficiently well preserved to allow serious archaeological study of original structures.[27] They were dedicated on 22 June 109.[28] They discretely (and symbolically) covered the last remnants of Nero's much resented *Domus Aurea* near the Colosseum and were by far the largest set of baths the city had seen to date. With their opening, Rome had acquired in just over fifty years three new large bathing complexes—those of Nero, Titus, and Trajan—the construction of which marks the last stage of the rise of public bathing that had begun almost two centuries before. It has been suggested, on the basis of their topographical proximity and their apparent conjunction in the Regionaries as *Thermae Titianae et Traianae,* that the Thermae of Titus and the Thermae of Trajan came to be assimilated into a single complex and even that the former acted as a vestibule for the latter.[29] This suggestion is surely mistaken. The Regionaries elsewhere refer to quite separate buildings in the same way (mentioning, e.g., *Thermae Alexandrinae et Agrippianae*), and the difference in elevation between the Thermae of Titus, themselves ill understood, and the Thermae of Trajan make their physical conjunction most unlikely.[30] Various sources also make mention of a bath called the *Balneum Surae* or *Thermae Surae* on

---

27. See Dio 69.4.1; Paus. 5.12.6. The main publications of this building are K. de Fine Licht, *Untersuchungen an den Trajansthermen zu Rom,* vols. 1 and 2 (Copenhagen, 1974; Rome, 1990). For a modern bibliography, see Manderscheid, 186–87, s.v. "Terme di Traiano." Now add Anderson, *Roman Architecture,* 272–76; Nielsen, 1.50–51, 2.2–3 (C.4); Richardson, *Dictionary,* 397–98, s.v. "Thermae Traiani"; Weber, 80–83; Yegül, 142–46. The building was called the *Thermae Traiani* or *Thermae Traianae,* see, e.g., no. 283; *CIL* 3.12336 (line 4), 6.1670 = 6.31889 = *ILS* 5716; *CIL* 6.8677–78; *FTUR* 1.1.5, 3.10.446–77. They measured 330 meters by 340 meters (Yegül, 144).

28. See *Fasti Ostienses,* A.D. 109 (= *FTUR* 3.10.461): X K(alendas) Iul(ias) imp(erator) Nerva Traianus Caes(ar) Aug(ustus) Germ(anicus) | Dacicus thermas suas dedicavit et publicavit. (*Publicavit* here means "opened to the public" rather than "made public property," since the baths are described as *thermas suas,* "his baths.") The main building is certainly Trajanic, even if parts of the substructures may date to Domitian's reign; see Hieron. *Chron.,* sub anno 90 (p. 191 Helm). The case for the Domitianic date of the building is forcefully argued by Anderson in "Date of the *Thermae Traiani,*" 505–9; but note the reservations of Yegül, 442–43 n. 41.

29. See, e.g., the *Notitia* and *Curiosum,* Regio III (= *FTUR* 3.10.1–2). For the vestibule argument, see Anderson, "Date of the *Thermae Traiani,*" 501.

30. See the *Notitia* and *Curiosum,* Regio IX; other later sources (e.g., no. 283) refer to the baths of Titus and Trajan as quite separate entities. See also Yegül, 442 n. 35.

the Aventine Hill.[31] This building appears to have been the responsibility of Trajan's favorite, L. Licinius Sura, although Aurelius Victor states that Trajan himself built the establishment to honor Sura.[32] Whatever the case, these baths can be included as an example of a person close to the emperor, if not the emperor himself, building a public bath on the Aventine Hill.

After the Thermae of Trajan, no new "imperial" sets are known at Rome until those of Caracalla, built between 211/12 and 215/16 at the southern end of the city, in Regio XII, near the Via Appia. Some ancillary bath construction by emperors and their associates is, however, attested in non-archaeological sources. Hadrian repaired the Thermae of Agrippa.[33] Cleander, the rich chamberlain of Commodus, put up baths in ca. 183, either in his own name or in that of the emperor, but no trace of the building survives.[34] The *Historia Augusta* also makes mention of the *Thermae Severianae* and the *Thermae Septimianae,* both the works of Septimius Severus, but little is known of the former structure (located in Regio I), and the latter (in Regio XIV) remains still more elusive: its very existence is predicated on a widely accepted emendation of the text of the *Historia Augusta,* and according to that source, some part of the building, possibly the water conduit that fed it, collapsed before the public could use the facilities. It is quite possible

---

31. *FUR* fr. 21 depicts a colonnaded courtyard with the inscription *bal[. . .] Surae;* a restoration of the structure by a Gordian is attested in an inscription (*AE* 1921.73). Another text from the area, dated to 414 (*CIL* 6.1703 = *ILS* 5715) records the restoration of the *cella tepidaria* of these baths or possibly of the nearby Thermae of Decius; see L.A. La Follette, "The Baths of Trajan Decius on the Aventine," in J.H. Humphrey, ed., *Rome Papers* (Ann Arbor, 1994), 85 (no. 15). Other sources term these baths variously: see *FTUR* 1.1.5 (called *Thermae Syranae* in the *Curiosum* and *Thermae Sures* in the *Notitia*), 3.8.177 (called *Thermae Suranae* in the *Notitia*), 1.1.6 (called *Thermae Suranae* in Polemius Silvius' fifth-century work *Quae sint Romae*); Dio 68.15.3[2] *(gymnasium).* See also E. Nash, *Pictorial Dictionary of Ancient Rome*[2] (London, 1968), 2.467–68, s.v. "Thermae Suranae"; Nielsen, 1.38–39 n. 15, 2.3 (C.5); Richardson, *Dictionary,* 395–96, s.v. "Thermae Surae."

32. Aur. Vict. *Caes.* 13.6; see also Dio, 68.15.3[2]. For Sura, see *PIR*[2] L 253. See also *RE* 13.471–85, s.v. "Licinius 167" (Groag), where it is suggested (481–82) that these baths became known as the *Thermae Decianae* after a restoration in the third century, a view now rendered untenable by a thorough study of Decius' baths; see La Follette, "Baths of Trajan Decius," esp. 59 n. 171. In any case, the appearance of *Thermae Suranae* (and variants) alongside *Thermae Decianae* in fourth-century sources (such as the Regionaries) strongly suggests separate structures.

33. See HA *Hadr.* 19.10. Few traces of the Hadrianic work survive in the meager remains of these baths; see M.T. Boatwright, *Hadrian and the City of Rome* (Princeton, 1987), 52–54.

34. See Dio 72(73).12.5; HA *Comm.* 17.5; Hdn. 1.12.4; Hieron. *Chron., sub anno* 183 (p. 208 Helm). Merten (20–23) argues that Cleander's baths are possibly to be identified with the *Thermae Commodianae* known from the sources: see, e.g., Hieron. *Chron.* loc. cit.; Cassiod. *Chron., sub anno* 184 (p. 144 Mommsen); *FTUR* 3.8.151–64; Richardson, *Dictionary,* 390, s.v. "Thermae Commodianae."

that the *Thermae Septimianae* are a fiction.[35] The Thermae of Caracalla, however, are very real. Since they are the most completely preserved set of imperial baths at Rome, they have understandably attracted sustained scholarly attention, the results of which need not be reproduced here.[36] Suffice it to say that the building followed the same general format as its predecessors, only on a still larger scale (see fig. 24). The penultimate imperially funded public baths built at Rome appeared under Diocletian and were erected between 298 and 305/6.[37] They were larger than any that had come before, and today they remain the largest Roman bathing establishment known anywhere in the empire. The immensity and luxurious appointment of these structures in their original state is hard to imagine (see fig. 25), but the Renaissance remodeling of the main hall *(frigidarium)* into the Basilica Santa Maria degli Angeli offers hints of their erstwhile splendor.

Miscellaneous information survives concerning bath projects initiated by emperors who reigned in the time between Caracalla and Diocletian. The Thermae of Decius (249–51), on the Aventine Hill, were on a much smaller

---

35. See HA *Sev.* 19.5 and the other sources cited by Merten, 24. Hieronymus' *Chronica* (*sub anno* 200 [p. 212 Helm]) dates the building to 200; Cassiodorus (*Chron.*, *sub anno* 201 [p. 144 Mommsen]) dates the baths to 201. See *FTUR* 3.8.2–3, 3.8.169–77, and *FTUR* 3.8.413–14 (*Thermae Severianae* in Regio I); Richardson, *Dictionary*, 395, s.v. "Thermae Septimianae" and "Thermae Severianae." E. Tortorici ("Terme Severiane, Terme 'Severianae' e Terme Septimianae," *BullCom* 95 [1993]: 161–72) argues that a preponderance of the evidence is in favor of the *Thermae Septimianae* as real; he also suggests a location for the *Thermae Severianae* immediately southeast of the Porta Capena. A recent assessment takes issue with Tortorici's location of the *Thermae Severianae* and remains cautious about accepting the existence of the *Thermae Septimianae*; see C.L. Gorrie, "The Building Programme of Septimius Severus in the City of Rome" (Ph.D. dissertation, University of British Columbia, 1997), 215–19 (*Thermae Severianae*) and 288–91 (*Thermae Septimianae*).

36. Hieronymus records their construction under the year 215 (*Chron.*, *sub anno* 215 [p. 213 Helm]); see HA *M. Ant.* 9.4–5 and *Heliogab.* 17.9. Heinz (124–41) devotes an entire chapter to them, and Manderscheid (180–82, s.v. "Terme di Caracalla") lists dozens of items for them. Add to the latter J. DeLaine, *The Baths of Caracalla: A Study in the Design, Construction, and Economics of Large-Scale Building Projects in Imperial Rome* (Portsmouth, RI, 1997); L. Lombardi and A. Corazza, *Le Terme di Caracalla* (Rome, 1995); Nielsen, 1.53–54, 2.3 (C.8); Richardson, *Dictionary*, 387–89, s.v. "Thermae Antoninianae"; Weber, 83–88; Yegül, 146–62. Their dimensions alone are impressive: the central building is 220 meters by 114 meters, while the outer enclosure *(peribolus)* stretches for 337 meters by 328 meters (see Lombardi and Corazza, op. cit., 46). In all, the entire complex covered almost thirty acres.

37. Their dedication, between 1 May 305 and 25 July 306, is recorded in an inscription; see *CIL* 6.1130 = *CIL* 6.31242 = *ILS* 646. See also HA *Prob.* 2.1; Hieron. *Chron.*, *sub anno* 302 (p. 227 Helm); *CIL* 6.1131; *FTUR* 1.1.5: in all these sources the complex is called *Thermae Diocletianae*. For a modern bibliography, see Manderscheid, 183–84, s.v. "Terme di Diocleziano." Also add Nielsen, 1.55–56, 2.3–4 (C.11); Richardson, *Dictionary*, 391–93, s.v. "Thermae Diocletiani"; Weber, 88–96; Yegül, 163–69. In its original state, the dimensions of the central building were 250 meters by 180 meters, and the *peribolus* ran for 380 meters by 370 meters (see Heinz, 112).

scale than the other imperial *thermae* and survive today only in very fragmentary form, save for a measured plan by Palladio.[38] But that a new, albeit
small, set of *thermae* was built at all in these troubled times is a testament to
the value placed on bathing culture by those who patronized it. Most of the
other evidence for this period derives from the *Historia Augusta* and is
therefore of dubious quality. Severus Alexander is reported not only to have
built *thermae* adjacent to the Thermae of Nero but to have added *balnea* to
any region of the city that lacked them. The passage does not make clear
whether Alexander's *thermae* denote an entirely new construction or the
well-attested major reconstruction and renaming of the Thermae of Nero;
and it is also unclear whether the alleged provision of *balnea* denotes only the
construction of new buildings or includes restorations, although the use of
the verb *addere* seems to suggest the former. Indeed, Merten, taking into
account the movement of imperial construction away from Rome to Constantinople in the years following Constantine's reign, as well as the continuance of private and church benefactions in Rome thereafter, argues that
the *Historia Augusta*'s report about Severus Alexander's *balnea* is little more
than a nostalgic evocation of the "the good old days" of imperial munificence.[39] There is also a curious notice that Gordian III restored the Thermae
of Titus and built *balneae* that were meant for private persons and fitted out
accordingly.[40] This odd statement is characteristic of the sort of obscurity
that pervades the *Historia Augusta,* and it seems to imply that Gordian built
baths that were to be used by a certain class of people and that were not open
to the general public. If so, why were they built, and who were the "private"
people? Merten argues that this passage reflects a restoration of the *Balneum
Surae* carried out by Gordian as attested in an inscription, but this argument

---

38. The main publication is now La Follette, "Baths of Trajan Decius." See also Manderscheid, 183, s.v., "Terme di Decio"; Richardson, *Dictionary,* 391, s.v. "Thermae Decianae";
Yegül, 162–63. These baths are well known from literary and epigraphic evidence, which attests
to their continued operation into the fifth century A.D.; see La Follette, op. cit., 83–85. They
measured a modest 44 meters by 70 meters (see ibid., 79).

39. See HA *Alex. Sev.* 25.3–4 (*thermae* built near Thermae of Nero) and 39.3–4 (*balnea
omnibus regionibus addidit, quae forte non habebant*); Hieron. *Chron.*, *sub anno* 227 (p. 215
Helm); Merten, 31–34. D. Palombi (*LTUR* 1.155–56, s.v. "Balnea Alexandri") accepts the
veracity of the notice about *balnea* and sees it as part of Severus' grand scheme for providing
public utilities to the people. In all probability, Severus Alexander's reported construction of
thermae is to be identified with the major overhaul of the Thermae of Nero, not with a separate
project; see Ghini, "Terme Alessandrine," 124–27. To date, no signs of a separate imperial
facility have been identified near the Thermae of Nero.

40. HA *Max. et Balb.* 1.4 (Titus) and *Gord.* 32.5: *opera Gordiani Romae nulla extant,
praeter quaedam nymfia et balneas. sed balneae privatis hominibus fuerunt et ab eo in usum
privatum exornatae sunt.*

does not fit with the *Historia Augusta*'s wording.[41] Another view is that the passage records Gordian equipping the baths of private individuals for his own personal use, but this view does not follow the sense of the passage, in which it seems clear that Gordian's *balneae* were built and fitted out for use by private persons.[42] Altogether, this notice remains cryptic and perhaps should not be taken seriously. Gordian is also reported to have planned a complex of *thermae aestivales et hiemales,* which never came to fruition. As with all reports concerning the unrealized intentions of emperors, this notice should be approached with extreme caution.[43] Finally, we read that Aurelian built *thermae hiemales* in the Transtiberine region and that the emperor Tacitus destroyed some of his own buildings to erect public baths. Little of this information can be checked against other sources, so it should be received with a healthy degree of skepticism.[44]

The last imperial set of baths erected at Rome was that of Constantine, opened in Regio VI, near the Quirinal Hill, in ca. 315, and executed on a much more modest scale than those of Caracalla or Diocletian: they occupy less than a quarter of the area of the latter.[45] Maxentius constructed *thermae* on the Palatine Hill, but they were part of the palace and were not open to the public.[46] An inscription reports that Constantine's mother, Helena, restored a set of baths that may have been part of the Palace of Heliogabalus on the Esquiline Hill; it is unclear, however, whether these baths were then open to the public.[47] The late Empire also saw many earlier baths restored (see immediately below).

---

41. Merten, 23 (esp. n. 41). For the inscription, see *AE* 1921.73, but it may commemorate a decoration of the building (as it is restored in *AE*).

42. See *LTUR* 1.160, s.v. "Balnea Gordiani" (D. Palombi).

43. See HA *Gord.* 32.7; Merten, 34–38; R.J. Rowland Jr., "Another Anachronism in the HA," *LCM* 2 (1977): 59. On summer and winter baths in general, see below, chapter 5, n. 49.

44. See, for Aurelian, HA *Aurel.* 45.2; Merten, 41–42. See, for Tacitus, HA *Tac.* 10.4; Merten, 11–15. Note, however, that a *balnea ex disciplina d. n. Aureliani* is mentioned in no. 190.

45. See Aur. Vict. *Caes.* 40.27. For a modern bibliography, see Manderscheid, 182–83, s.v. "Terme di Constantino." Also add Heinz, 122; Nielsen, 1.56, 2.4 (C.13); Richardson, *Dictionary,* 390–91, s.v. "Thermae Constantinianae"; Yegül, 169–72. See also *CIL* 6.1750 = *ILS* 5703; *CIL* 10.1126 (Abellinum; fourth century?); *FTUR* 1.1.5: in all these sources they are termed *Thermae Constantinianae.* Ammianus Marcellinus (27.3.8) calls the building *Constantinianum Lavacrum.*

46. On the remains, see G. Carettoni, "Terme di Settimio Severo e Terme di Massenzio in Palatio," *ArchCl* 24 (1972): 96–104; J.J. Hermann Jr., "Observations on the Baths of Maxentius in the Palace," *RM* 83 (1976): 403–24. See also Nielsen, 1.56, 2.4 (C.12); Richardson, *Dictionary,* 393, s.v. "Thermae Maxentii"; Yegül, 86.

47. See *CIL* 6.1136 = *CIL* 6.31244 and my fig. 26A. See also Nash, *Pictorial Dictionary,* 2.454–57, s.v. "Thermae Helenae"; Nielsen, 1.54–55; Richardson, *Dictionary,* 393, s.v. "Thermae Helenae"; Yegül, 86. Palladio provides a rough sketch of the building; modern remains are sparse: see Zorzi, *Disegni della antichità,* 72 and fig. 144; Coarelli, *Roma,* 238–39.

The foregoing evidence reveals that the emperors and their families displayed considerable munificence with regard to bath construction and maintenance at Rome, but, as in so many other areas of the emperors' activity, no systematic policy is detectable. Rather, the constructions were sporadic, with long intervening periods when emperors did not build baths in the capital at all. Nevertheless, the imperial *thermae,* once built, remained an imperial concern and were entrusted to the care of future emperors by those who erected them. Even the Thermae of Agrippa, the only imperial complex known to have been transferred to public ownership, remained in the care of the *princeps:* it is recorded as having been restored by Titus after a fire in 80, restored again by Hadrian, and yet again by Constantius and Constans in 344–45.[48] This record illustrates how the distinction between "public" and "imperial" spending at Rome is largely illusory, certainly by the time the Principate was well established.

In the absence of ancient testimony, what motivated individual emperors to construct particular bathing establishments, or for that matter *not* to construct them, remains largely a matter for conjecture, though it is hardly a reason for puzzlement, as most of the time emperors tended to act ad hoc.[49] Heinz suggests, for example, that Caracalla built his baths near a poor part of town in an attempt to "win the lower classes for himself."[50] While certainly plausible, such a claim is not verifiable on available evidence. These baths,

---

48. See Dio 66.24 (Titus); HA *Hadr.* 19.10 (Hadrian); *CIL* 6.1165 (Constantius and Constans). A restoration of the late second or early third century is also attested in the ruins; see Colini et al., "Notiziario di scavi," 372–73. Other imperial *thermae* are also on record as having been maintained by later emperors—the Thermae of Nero by Severus Alexander (HA *Alex. Sev.* 25.3–5) and the Thermae of Caracalla by Elagabalus and Severus Alexander (HA *Heliogab.* 17.8–9 and *Alex. Sev.* 25.3). In the late Empire, urban prefects often acted in the place of absent emperors; see the restoration of the Thermae of Decius in 414 (*CIL* 6.1703 = *ILS* 5715), the Thermae of Constantine in 443 (*CIL* 6.1750 = *ILS* 5703), and the Thermae of Trajan at some unspecified date in the later Empire (*CIL* 6.1670 = *CIL* 6.31889 = *ILS* 5716).

49. An apparent exception is the comment in the *Historia Augusta* (*Aurel.* 45.2) that Aurelian's plans to build winter baths in the Transtiberine region were "because there was a lack of adequately cold water there" *(quod aquae frigidioris copia illic deesset).* The precise meaning of the clause is a matter for dispute (see Merten, 38–42), but its main point is surely to explain why Aurelian planned to build specifically *winter* baths and not baths per se. On summer/winter baths, see Merten, 34–48; Nielsen, 1.138–40; Yegül, 43.

50. Heinz, 124. See the comments by La Follette ("Baths of Trajan Decius," 22) on the difficulty of applying such reasoning to the Thermae of Decius. She later states (81), however, that the late Imperial clientele was predominantly upper class, as suggested by the "gentrification" of the Aventine Hill and by epigraphic finds associated with these baths. Herodian (1.12.4) asserts that Cleander built his public baths to win the people over to him. Cleander's case, however, is rather special, since Herodian sets Cleander's motive for the bath construction against the background of his larger efforts to suborn popular support for himself in a bid for the purple.

being adjacent to the Via Appia, could also have been built for the benefit of suburbanites, travelers, or new arrivals to the city. In general, trying to deduce the social identity of an ancient building's clientele solely from its location has proven difficult and in most cases virtually impossible.[51]

Resort must therefore be had to general explanations. Claims that the Romans built baths out of a "concern for the general welfare of the public at large" appear exaggerated.[52] While the perceived therapeutic value of baths is not to be doubted, such claims give the impression that baths were part of a Roman "health plan" (which did not exist); in general, to credit that the central authorities undertook bath construction primarily out of an altruistic concern for public welfare is to take too narrow a focus and one informed more by modern assumptions than ancient realities. Rather, at the heart of the matter is the fact that public building was simply part of what the emperor did and was expected to do.[53] This expectation derived in part from the emperor's special relationship with the city's populace, whereby the inhabitants were, in effect, the emperor's immediate clients, his court.[54] Provision of amenities, such as baths for his people, was therefore a natural endeavor for the empire's preeminent patron. On the emperor's part, there was also, no doubt, an element of megalomania involved, as well as a desire for a sort of immortality, since buildings traditionally retained the builder's name. Thus Decius, by means of his baths, could ensure that his name would

---

51. See also DeLaine, "Recent Research," 29; id., "The *Balneum* of the Arval Brethren," *JRA* 3 (1990): 323–24. Such deduction is all the more difficult in the apparent absence of zoning in ancient cities.

52. See, e.g., Scarborough, 78–79, 94 (quote), 134. A.R. Hands (*Charities and Social Aid in Greece and Rome* [Ithaca, 1968], 144) likens the construction of Roman baths to similar programs in nineteenth-century London, where, as in America (for which, see Williams, *Washing "The Great Unwashed,"* 5–40), the authorities took the lead at both the national and local levels. Notions of "government sponsorship" still persist for the Roman period, albeit in a diluted form. Robinson (*Ancient Rome*, 111–29) writes of the Roman authorities' "promotion of public health" (111). She makes such statements as, "Public baths were a very suitable way for promoting public health" (116), which leave a strong impression of conscious intent on the part of the Roman authorities in this regard.

53. Note the comment in the speech Dio puts into the mouth of Maecenas that Augustus (by which Dio means any good emperor) should adorn Rome as a matter of course; see Dio 52.30.1. The *Res Gestae* (19–24) and imperial biographers (see, e.g., Suet. *Jul.* 44; *Aug.* 28.3–30.2; *Calig.* 21; *Claud.* 20; *Vesp.* 8.5–9.1) list the various *opera publica* of rulers without comment—contributing to public works was expected imperial behavior, part of what Veyne (542–43, 622, 639) terms "le style monarchique." Indeed, the prologue of the *Res Gestae* describes the document as an account of Augustus' deeds, "by which he brought the world under the rule of the Roman people, and of the expenses he incurred for the state and the Roman people." The personal outlay, much of it spent on buildings, is thus presented as a cardinal benefit of the imperial regime.

54. See Veyne, 689–701.

be enshrined in the urban topography of Rome alongside the likes of Trajan, who ruled in less troubled times and for far longer. But one still wonders why baths in particular were built. A reasonable suggestion is that the emperors were reacting to popular demand, though in general it is hard to prove that construction projects were undertaken specifically to appease the people.[55] It may also have been the case that the emperors' building activities helped generate demand for baths; once lavish baths existed, people would surely require little spur to use them. But why should emperors undertake to build such vast, essentially functional structures unless it was anticipated that they would be used? Perhaps it was a case of positive feedback: popular demand encouraged imperial bath building, which in turn encouraged public demand. But all this is speculation, beyond checking in the ancient evidence. Other factors need to be considered.

One such factor is what we may term "dynastic rivalry." A discernible feature in imperial building (indeed, in all ancient public building) is the competitive impulse to outdo predecessors. The construction of a building by one benefactor could be viewed by a successor as a challenge to do better. For the emperors, the process is reflected in the succession of imperial fora and in the emperors' palaces and villas.[56] But the baths illustrate this phenomenon even more richly. From the Thermae of Agrippa to the Thermae of Diocletian, each new set tended to be bigger and more luxuriously appointed than its predecessor. Only the Thermae of Decius and the Thermae of Constantine are the exceptions to this rule, presumably due to the straitened financial circumstances that prevailed when they were constructed. Imperial propaganda, itself a disputed notion, probably also played a role in generating the large-scale *thermae*.[57] Whether such construction projects were pro-

---

55. That there was a popular demand for baths is a reasonable inference from the evidence reviewed in the previous chapters. Note Suetonius' comment (*Aug.* 29.1) that Augustus' forum was built due to a need for more market space. It is far from clear, however, that the need was brought to the emperor's attention by popular demand and that the construction was in response to that demand.

56. For the forum buildings, see J.C. Anderson, *The Historical Topography of the Imperial Fora* (Brussels, 1984), where each forum is treated in sequence. The imperial palaces and villas are too numerous to document in detail here and have yet to be studied in detail as an architectural type, but note, for instance, how the imperial palaces at Rome grew from the simple house of Augustus on the Palatine to the excess of Nero's *Domus Aurea* and then to the imposing *Domus Augustana* of Domitian; see I.M. Barton, "Palaces," in id., ed., *Roman Domestic Buildings* (Exeter, 1996), 91–120. A related phenomenon is the competition to outdo predecessors in staging spectacles; see, e.g., K.M. Coleman, "Launching into History: Aquatic Displays in the Early Empire," *JRS* 83 (1993): 68–69.

57. M.P. Charlesworth ("The Virtues of a Roman Emperor: The Creation of Belief," *PBA* 23 (1937): 105–33) argued that propaganda, or the creation of goodwill toward the ruler, was essential to the empire's survival and that buildings were among the vehicles for such propa-

pagandistic in purpose, in that they attempted to inculcate a certain perception of the state, or whether they were merely an expression of an already existing perception is not germane to the present inquiry. On either view, the construction of baths by the emperor symbolized at the very least the benevolence of his rule, the permanence and power of the state (as embodied by the emperor), and the ruler's concern for the welfare of his subjects, regardless of whether or not it was genuinely felt.[58] The baths provided an especially apt manifestation of all these concepts. The frequent appearance of Hercules in the decorative sculpture of imperial baths makes manifest the ideological associations of these buildings. From the late second century onward, Hercules was increasingly presented as the chief "imperial" deity, the protector of the emperor's person and house; and he is found in such powerfully imperial settings as the Severan buildings in Lepcis Magna.[59] Therefore, to find, for instance, that four representations of Hercules are known from the Thermae of Caracalla alone helps to bring the imperial ideological associations of these buildings into high relief.[60]

---

ganda (109–10). This view has been called into question by Veyne (661–65) who, without direct reference to Charlesworth, denies the existence of propaganda at all, arguing that there was no desire to *create* a belief in the majesty of the state, only a desire to express it. See also A. Wallace-Hadrill, "The Emperor and His Virtues," *Historia* 30 (1981): 298–323. For a recent defense of the existence of an "imperial propaganda," especially in art and architecture, see N. Hannestad, *Roman Art and Imperial Policy* (Århus, 1988), esp. 9–14.

58. For these functions of imperial euergetism, see Veyne, 621–60, 675–701. It is noteworthy, however, that baths never feature as major coin types, although a wide variety of utilitarian buildings—such as aqueducts, *castella,* roads, fountains, and bridges—were commemorated (and advertised?) in this way; see P.V. Hill, *The Monuments of Ancient Rome as Coin Types* (London, 1989). A possible exception is the identification of the entrance to the Thermae of Titus on a coin issued to commemorate the opening of the Colosseum in 80 (see M.J. Price and B.L. Trell, *Coins and Their Cities* [Detroit, 1977], 60–61). Even if this identification is correct, it is hardly encouraging. The baths are represented only by their entrance, which itself is rendered as a constricted series of columns crushed into the periphery of a field dominated by the Colosseum. Baths are not otherwise attested on coins. The explanation for this omission is unclear. Die casters could undertake representations of such complex structures as the *Domus Flaviorum* (see Hill, op. cit., 102–4 [no. 198]), so it seems unlikely that the buildings were too difficult to render. In any event, symbolic representations were always possible, as with the Via Traiana (see ibid., 96 [no. 186]), and legends could be used to identify individual structures. The matter is worth further investigation.

59. For recent treatments of these buildings and their sculptural decoration, see J.B. Ward-Perkins, *The Severan Buildings of Lepcis Magna: An Architectural Survey* (London, 1993); D.E.E. Kleiner, *Roman Sculpture* (New Haven, 1992), 340–43. On Hercules as a *Kaisergott,* see La Follette, "Baths of Trajan Decius," 76–77; M. Jaczynowska, "Le culte de l'Hercule romain au temps du Haut-Empire," *ANRW* 2.17.2 (1981): 631–61; Manderscheid, *Skulpturenausstattung,* 33–34.

60. Manderscheid, *Skulpturenausstattung,* 74 (nos. 51–54). Figured capitals depicting Hercules and a colossal statue of the demigod as an infant once stood in the Thermae of Decius at Rome (see La Follette, "Baths of Trajan Decius," 67–78). Outside Rome, baths with strong

On a metaphysical level, the baths were a manifestation of the emperor's power over nature. This power was also displayed in the beast hunts *(venationes)* of the Roman games, whereby the Romans were assured of their control over otherwise threatening beasts when they were destroyed as a form of entertainment provided at imperial expense.[61] In a similar way, the baths symbolized the harnessing of the primordial elements of water and fire, thereby reiterating the power of the Romans, and especially of the emperor, over the unpredictable forces of nature.[62] As with the beast hunts, that these otherwise unruly elements were not only tamed but deployed for the pleasure of the Roman people only underlined the point. In addition, the imperial baths, with their immense scale and luxurious fittings, were something of a fantasy world, a contrived environment that was the product of the emperor's power and munificence.[63] When compared to other public buildings erected by emperors, such as temples, basilicas, or arches, the baths can be seen to carry particularly direct messages. An arch may beautify the city, a temple may express the emperor's piety (which was certainly important for the state's welfare), but a bath was primarily a functional structure, allowing the citizens to get clean and relax in surroundings that spoke volumes about the power of Rome and its rulers. Although the emperors did provide other public utilities—markets, aqueducts, roads, and so on—the baths were arguably one of the most direct architectural expressions of imperial concern for the welfare of the masses, which, I must reiterate, was not necessarily genuinely felt. As is true of other utilitarian structures, people would have used

---

imperial connections could also feature Hercules: a statue of him was found in the Antonine Baths at Carthage (see Manderscheid, op. cit., 115 [no. 407]); and of the fourteen statues known from the baths at Lambaesis, the headquarters of the Legion III Augusta, eight represent Hercules (see ibid., 123–24 [nos. 489–97]).

61. See T. Wiedemann, *Emperors and Gladiators* (London, 1992), 55–67.

62. N. Zajac made this point in her paper "The Pursuit of Cleanliness in Rome?" delivered at the First International Conference on Roman Baths, Bath, England, April 1992. A similar manifestation of the emperors' near superhuman control over the natural elements is the nautical displays staged in flooded circuses or arenas: ancient commentators (see, e.g., Mart. *Spect.* 24; Dio 62.15.1) seemed most impressed by the speed with which land became sea and vice versa; see Coleman, "Launching into History," 56–57. By way of comparison, the fountains at Versailles were seen by contemporaries as a "sign of supreme domination over a capricious element"; see G. Vigarello, *Concepts of Cleanliness: Changing Attitudes in France since the Middle Ages* (Cambridge, 1988), 25.

63. See H. Drerup, "Bildraum und Realraum in der römischen Architektur," *RM* 66 (1959): 147–74, on the general concern of Roman architects to control internal and external perspectives and so to create a make-believe world in their buildings. A parallel is provided by baths in modern Japan, where there is a demand for "jungle baths," appointed in such a way as to give the bathers the impression they are in such exotic locations as a South Seas island, a futurescape, or Disneyland (see Grilli and Levy, *Furo,* 156–58).

them regularly, but bathers interacted more directly and intimately with the fabric of a set of baths than people did with, say, an aqueduct or a market. As a result, the baths would have had a greater impact on visitors' perceptions. This point makes the progressively larger dimensions of the imperial baths more understandable: the increase in size physically manifested each successive bath-building emperor's greater concern for the public good, while simultaneously overshadowing the efforts of predecessors. These two points lead to another possibility. Looking at the overall pattern of imperial bath building in the capital, it is noticeable that most of the large-scale *thermae* were put up by emperors or their associates close to the start of a new dynasty, on the occasion of a shift in the nature of the succession, or at the end of a civil war.[64] This timing may be pure coincidence, but it is possible that these emperors were trying to emphasize the stability of the new age and the concern of the new rulers for their people by erecting the very structure that best symbolized peace, stability, and prosperity, as well as power and benevolence.

Private Citizens

Because Rome was primarily the emperor's preserve, extensive public construction in the city by private benefactors or even by other representatives of the imperial authorities was a rarity, except in the cases of emperors' favorites, such as Agrippa, or late Imperial officials, such as urban prefects. Under the Republic, *triumphatores* had traditionally earned the right to build *opera publica* with the spoils of their victories *(manubiae),* but after Augustus, there were no *triumphatores* other than emperors. The last recorded case of "private," nonimperially funded public construction at Rome is the restoration and adornment of the Basilica of Paullus by M. Lepidus in 22.[65] In the case of baths not associated with emperors or their families, almost three

---

64. So Agrippa built his *thermae* for Augustus and the Julio-Claudians, Titus for the Flavians, Trajan and Licinius Sura for the Antonines, Commodus and Cleander for the transition from adoptive to blood dynasty, Septimius Severus and Caracalla for the Severans, Decius for the chaotic third century, Diocletian for the restoration of order, and Constantine after the civil war with Maxentius. The exception to this scheme is the Thermae of Nero, the construction of which may be set against the backdrop of Nero's desire to be popular among the masses; see M.T. Griffin, *Nero: The End of a Dynasty* (New Haven, 1984), 104–5. Note, by way of comparison, that just such occasions as those listed above prompted the Athenians to set up statues of emperors or members of the imperial family; see D.J. Geagan, "Imperial Visits to Athens: The Epigraphical Evidence," in Πρακτικα του Η Διεθνους Συνεδριου Ελλενικης και Λατινικης Επιγραφικης, Αθηνα, *3–9 Οκτωβριου 1982* (Athens, 1984), 69–78.

65. See Tac. *Ann.* 3.72.1. Tacitus comments on this incident (my emphasis), *"at that time, public munificence was still customary" (erat etiam tum in more publica munificentia).*

dozen are known by name from Rome. Presumably all were of modest dimensions and did not approach the scale of even the smaller imperial facilities. The names of some of these privately built baths suggest that they were owned and/or possibly built by high-ranking families and imperial officials. If so, such people appear to have been acting as private citizens, as were others of more obscure station who gave their names to the modest baths they erected (see appendix 2). The main problem is that all of these buildings took their names from the cognomens of their builders or owners, so that several known individuals can be associated with the same facility. Also, it is rarely clear exactly when a specific bath was built or if its name changed to reflect shifts in ownership or the activities of benefactors who carried out repairs or extensions. As a result, it is entirely possible that none of the notables I suggest as builders or owners were at all concerned with the baths that shared their names, although in some cases (e.g., the *Balneum Tigellini* or *Balneum/Thermulae Claudii Etrusci*), the connection appears secure.

In specific cases, additional problems of interpretation arise. For example, the *Notitia* lists a *Balneum Bolani et Mamertini* and a *Balneum Abascanti et Antiochiani* in Regio I of the city (see appendix 2). Do the names denote two buildings or four? If the former, the doubling up of names for each structure may be a consequence of repairs, extensions, or transferals of ownership bearing a later builder or owner's name.[66] Despite the unusual mode of expression used in the *Notitia* (for separate buildings, we should expect "*Balnea Bolani et Mamertini*" etc.),[67] support for the separate-building view can be found in the parallel entry in the *Curiosum,* where only a *Balneum Abascantis et Mamertini* is mentioned, with no mention of a corresponding Bolanus or Antiochianus. As the names are here crossed, it seems likely either that the *Curiosum* has made two omissions, or that the *Balneum Bolani* and *Balneum Antiochiani* had ceased to function (or exist) in the intervening period.[68] On either view, the names probably denote separate buildings.

---

66. Lugli (*FTUR* 3.8.147–50, 3.8.165–66) treats each separately, as does E. de Ruggiero (*Dizionario epigrafico di antichità romane* [Rome, 1895; reprint, 1961], 1.970, s.v. "Balneum"). More recently, D. Palombi (*LTUR* 1.155, s.v. "Balneum Abascanti") maintains that it is impossible to be sure whether the names indicate separate, neighboring structures or single buildings with multiple owners.

67. Compare the *balinea Sergium et Put[inium]* at Altinum (no. 168/69).

68. C. Lega's inverse suggestion (*LTUR* 1.156–57, s.v. "Balneum Bolani")—that the missing names of Bolanus and Antiochianus suggest that their baths were built between the publication of the *Curiosum* and the *Notitia*—requires that, besides the *Balneum Bolani,* the *Balneum Antiochiani* and *Balneum Vespasiani* were erected at this time (both are mentioned in the *Notitia* but not in the *Curiosum*). This concurrence seems unlikely, since the *Balneum Vespa-*

A similar difficulty pertains to the *Balneum Torquati et Vespasiani* (listed only as *Balneum Torquati* in the *Curiosum*). If the arguments just presented are accepted, these would also be separate structures: a *Balneum Torquati* and a *Balneum Vespasiani*.[69] A possible builder for the former is D. Junius Silanus Torquatus, who was consul in 53.[70] The *Balneum Vespasiani* (mentioned only in the *Notitia*) is more interesting. Because the cognomen is not attested for any other individual, it seems that the emperor of that name is the strongest candidate for the Vespasianus concerned and thus possibly for the builder or owner of the bath.[71] Such a facility, however, is not connected with Vespasian in any other source, which is not necessarily conclusive but noteworthy.[72] That it was a *balneum* suggests a modest structure in comparison to the two larger imperial *thermae* then in existence (those of Agrippa and Nero); the construction may therefore have taken place before Vespasian's elevation, when he was still a private citizen.[73] Vespasian suffered a miserly reputation among the masses, so his building of a mere *balneum* as emperor, after Nero had offered his huge *thermae* complex, is most unlikely (see Suet. *Vesp.* 16, 19.2). Finally, we can account for the name of the building by other possibilities that in no way require the involvement of Vespasian in its construction, namely, that the bath was dedicated to the emperor or that it was named after a statue or other decorative feature associated with the emperor. The same possibilities pertain for a *Balneum Caenidianum* attested in an inscription and probably associated with, if not

---

siani, by its name alone, is not likely to date to so late a period, and such prolific construction of baths in late Imperial Rome as Lega's suggestion assumes is not otherwise attested.

69. They are so listed in *FTUR* 3.8.178–79 (*Balneum Torquati*), 3.8.180 (*Balneum Vespasiani*).

70. See *PIR*[2] I 837 (the baths are not mentioned in this article).

71. See *RE* 8A.1711, s.v. "Vespasianus" (Chochole).

72. E.g., Suetonius (*Vesp.* 8.5–9.1) does not mention a bath building in his list of the emperor's *opera publica*. See also L. Homo, *Vespasien, l'empereur du bon sens* (Paris, 1949), 365–81; *RE* 6.2623–95, s.v. "Flavius 206" (Weynand), esp. 2688–90 for his construction activities (with no mention of the bath).

73. He was suffect consul in 51 (see Suet. *Vesp.* 4.2) and had by then been in the imperial service for a long time; see *PIR*[2] F 398. For a summary of Vespasian's preimperial career (where the bath finds no mention), see J. Nicols, *Vespasian and the* Partes Flavianae (Wiesbaden, 1978), 1–12. Vespasian's family was of modest means (see Suet. *Vesp.* 1.2–4), and he himself was not outstandingly rich as a private citizen (see ibid., 4.3). However, he must have at least had a senatorial census at his disposal. As a result, whether or not he could have afforded to build a bathhouse, even a *balneum* run for profit (which would certainly be in accordance with his rumored avarice), before becoming emperor remains a moot point. Yet another possibility is that Vespasian's brother, T. Flavius Sabinus, who was *praefectus urbi* for twelve years (see Tac. *Hist.* 3.75) and apparently more generous with his money (see ibid., 3.65), built the bath and named it after Vespasian.

belonging to, Vespasian's concubine Caenis. This bath was probably private, however, and not open to the public.[74]

The foregoing discussion makes glaringly clear the acute difficulties of identifying the builders of privately owned baths at Rome from the names of the buildings alone. Unfortunately, that is all we have to go on in most cases. Where possible identifications occur, they are often plagued with uncertainties and ambiguities. In only a handful of cases can secure identifications be offered. Therefore, for most nonimperial baths at Rome, it is simply not possible to offer any concrete evidence as to who built or owned them. Nevertheless, the majority of the baths discussed above were most probably run as (family?) business investments. Some may have been built or run—or both—by people of relatively low social standing.[75] But if so, such builders/ owners must have been of sufficient substance to construct or buy an urban bathing complex, an endeavor that would not have been possible for the average shopkeeper or craftsman. It is also conceivable that local neighborhood leaders formed consortia to construct baths that would have been beyond the means of any one of them. There is some evidence in this regard from Ostia, where several bathing facilities, such as the Baths of Buticous, the Baths of the Drivers, and the Baths of the Philosopher, may have belonged to guilds or associations of some sort; and Libanius refers to baths owned by the tribes of late Imperial Antioch.[76] But the names of the individual facilities do not seem to reflect this type of arrangement. By and large, it seems likely that the people who built baths, no matter how low their social status was, must have been economically and socially prominent in at least their area of the city. If even some of the identifications with known senators, *equites*, and imperial freedmen proposed above are correct, these lowly baths represent a continuation of the Republican tradition whereby leading citizens assumed responsibility for providing the city with its baths. It might seem to the modern reader that such places could not hope to compete with the luxury available free of charge in the imperial *thermae*, but certain evi-

---

74. See P.R.C. Weaver and P.I. Wilkins, "A Lost Alumna," *ZPE* 99 (1993): 241–44.

75. Such is the case, in all likelihood, with the *Balnea Abascanti (?), Fortunati, Polycliti, Stephani,* and *Ampelidis* listed in appendix 2, many of these names appear to have had slave origins. For example, of the 221 examples of use of the word *Abascantus,* 78 denote slaves or freedmen (see Solin, 2.847); similarly, of 236 attested "Stephani," 87 are of servile origin (see ibid., 3.1186). I am not suggesting that slaves owned or built these buildings, but successful freedmen may have.

76. See R. Mar, "Santuarios e inversion inmobiliaria en la urbanística ostiense del siglo II," in A.G. Zevi and A. Claridge, *"Roman Ostia" Revisited: Archaeological and Historical Papers in Memory of Russell Meiggs* (London, 1996), 115–64, esp. 127–38, 152–60 (Baths of Buticosus and Baths of the Drivers); Boersma, *Amoenissima Civitas,* 35–47 (Baths of the Philosopher); Lib. *Or.* 11.245 (Antioch).

dence suggests that these more modest establishments could on occasion offer splendor to rival the imperial best, albeit on a lesser scale.[77] In addition, many people are likely to have lived nearer to a local *balneum* than to an imperial *thermae,* so the sheer convenience of the former would have attracted custom. We have seen how Martial, with his preference for the Thermae of Titus, would also meet dinner guests in the nearby Baths of Stephanus. Probably, the smaller (less salubrious) facilities also attracted a regular set of clients. The pubs of the British Isles offer a point of comparison: regular customers willingly pass up more comfortable surroundings in favor of their "local."[78] Whatever the case, the figures in the Regionaries—856 *balnea* to 11 imperial *thermae*—are eloquent testimony to the enduring popularity of the Imperial city's descendants of Republican Rome's modest public bathing establishments.

---

77. Note especially the *Balneum/Thermulae Claudii Etrusci* (for which, see above, chapter 1, p. 19–20). For free admittance to imperial *thermae,* see Fronto *Ep. Grec.* 5.1; Heinz, 23–24; Merten, 6–11; Nielsen, 1.133–34. Note also that *CGL* 3.651.10 includes the (unanswered) question, *ad thermas aut in privato? Privato* probably denotes here a privately owned facility open to the public, so the question may indicate that the *thermae* were free (which presumably would be the chief distinction between the *thermae* and *[balneum] privatum*). The alternative— that *privato* refers to a private bathing suite at home—is less likely: the party is clearly about to go out to bathe. When the scene shifts to the bathhouse, an entrance fee is paid and change received—*da balnitori nummos, accipe reliquum* (ibid., 652.10)—but it is not clear if the setting is the *thermae* or *(balneum) privatum.*

78. For "regulars" at Roman baths, see Hor. *Epist.* 1.1.91–93; Mart. 3.25, 3.36.1–6, 12.83; Amm. Marc. 28.4.10. A graffito from the vestibule of the Forum Baths at Pompeii—"I, Speratus, live (here)" (*CIL* 4.1465: *Speratus habito*)—should probably be interpreted in this light.

Chapter 6

Bath Benefactors 2: Italy and the Provinces

If the presence of the emperor at Rome, his special relationship with the city's populace, and the capital's unique status as the residence of the most powerful and influential individuals in a world empire combined to make Rome a special case, then the pattern of imperial and private munificence there cannot be used as a model for predicting similar activity across the empire. As a result, it is to those responsible for the construction and maintenance of public baths in Italy and the provinces that we must now turn our attention. The main focus of what follows is on the benefactors responsible for constructional activity and on their possible motivation, but nonconstructional benefactions, the social status of the benefactors, and other points of interest are not passed over in silence.

General Remarks

The chief medium for this investigation is inscriptions. The abundant physical remains of the empire's baths have been subjected to close scrutiny in other studies, both empire-wide and regional, but the inscriptions that can accompany these structures have not.[1] This chapter is, in part, an attempt to redress this imbalance and should be read in close conjunction with the epigraphic sample later in the book. That said, this is not a comprehensive

---

1. The major books of Nielsen and Yegül contain regional sections, and Farrington *(Roman Baths of Lycia)* has paved the way for future research into variations in local bathing practices; see my remarks in "Bathing in the Backwaters," *JRA* 10 (1997): 520–23. All of these studies utilize the pertinent epigraphic evidence, but they do so primarily as adjuncts to the physical remains. Nielsen, for instance, assembles inscriptions in prodigious footnotes (e.g., 1.39–41 nn. 25–26, 1.85–86 nn. 9–10) but uses them only as bare illustrations of bath-building activity at various sites. In contrast, Rebuffat ("Vocabulaire thèrmal") offers an analysis of bath terminology as recorded in inscriptions, but his conclusions are disappointingly vague— understandably so, given the difficulty of comprehending many of these terms. Note, however, that recent publications of specific bathhouses often include detailed analysis of related inscriptions: see, e.g., H. Broise and Y. Thébert, *Recherches archéologiques franco-tunisiennes à Bulla Regia,* vol. 2, *Les architectures,* pt. 1, *Les thermes memmiens: Étude architecturale et histoire urbaine* (Rome, 1993); Y. Hirschfeld, *The Roman Baths of Hammat Gader* (Jerusalem, 1997).

study of bath-related inscriptions, as such a task would require a book in itself. It is hoped that the epigraphic sample will act as an aid for future research in this area. In what follows, the focus is on the people who populate the inscriptions—the men and women who built, restored, extended, adorned, and maintained baths—rather than on the remains of the buildings and their relationship to the epigraphic evidence. For this reason, detailed investigation of findspots, analysis of bath terminology, and close correlation of epigraphic claims with surviving remains is undertaken neither here nor in the sample, although I do note where the ruins of particular facilities can be associated with specific inscriptions.

Since constructional inscriptions make up the bulk of the entries in the sample,[2] the following remarks pertain primarily to them. (The nature and distribution of nonconstructional benefactions is discussed in more detail below.) For the most part, Roman construction inscriptions are formulaic documents, in that their wording usually adheres to a set pattern. It is worthwhile first to review that pattern for the benefit of those unfamiliar with it. The two essential elements in a construction inscription are, first, the name of the benefactor(s) and, second, the nature of the work done (the first sentence of no. 1/2 is a good example). In inscriptions set up on the building itself, the name of the benefactor often appears in the nominative case, while in honorary texts voted in gratitude to the benefactor, it is usually in the dative or, in the case of statue bases, the genitive, because it denotes the identity of the statue. As to the work done, a variety of phrases can be found recording it, with the building itself usually mentioned and sometimes named. A noteworthy exception is inscriptions that were originally set up on the edifices they commemorated, in which cases the phrase "this building" can be understood (see, e.g., nos. 1/2, 42, 62, 99). A third, very common, but not obligatory, element is an acknowledgment as to how the project was financed, usually expressed with a vague phrase, such as "at his/her own expense" or "with public money." There are, however, cases where more specific financial information is provided, and they are discussed below (chapter 6, pp. 173–75).

A series of optional elements could be added to these basic components: dedication of the inscription and building to a deity or to the emperor(s); the recording of additional work carried out, especially work of a decorative nature; mention of who benefited from the benefaction; inclusion of the names of people who oversaw the work; and notice as to whether extra liberalities had been presented, either as part of the constructional operation itself or when the building was dedicated. In reconstruction inscriptions,

---

2. Nos. 1–196; see figs. 26A–F for the physical appearance of some bath inscriptions.

there may also be a description of the circumstances of the building's deterioration and details of the benefactor's restorative actions. Sometimes multiple actions that took place over many years are commemorated in a single text, providing a sort of "building history" in capsule form. In inscriptions of the later Empire, there is a tendency to wax lyrical about the complexity and thoroughness of the work done, the disgraceful state of the damaged building in cases of restoration, and the praiseworthy qualities of the benefactor(s). (Examples of all of these elements in various combinations can be gained by skimming the epigraphic sample.)

There are difficulties of interpretation. Specific problems are discussed in this chapter, in the introduction to the epigraphic sample, and in the notes attached to individual entries in the sample, so here I draw attention only to those problematic features that affect the immediate inquiry. The 196 constructional entries in the sample record 194 separate acts of benefaction.[3] Of these, the nature of the work can be securely determined in 180 benefactions: 65 (36.1%) are initial constructions, 85 (47.2%) are restorations, and 73 are extensions and adornments, of which only 30 (16.7%) were undertaken as main benefactions in their own right.[4] In addition, some caution is required in reading these materials. Certainly, as argued forcefully in a recent study of reconstruction inscriptions, epigraphic language is often imprecise or misleading, so, for instance, acts of reconstruction can be denoted with words usually reserved for initial construction (e.g., *aedificare* and *facere* in nos. 43 and 69, respectively). This observation throws some doubt on the reliability of epigraphy as a guide to ancient actions, but the language of constructional inscriptions must nevertheless have borne directly on ancient physical conditions to be believable to those who originally read them; approaching such

---

3. The discrepancy between the total for entries (196) and the total for benefactions (194) is due to the fact that, on two occasions, two entries each refer to single acts of benefaction by different classes of benefactor, at Corfinium (nos. 80 and 174) and at Anagnia (nos. 95 and 179). Here the two acts of benefaction, not the four entries, are counted.

4. The relevant entries are, for initial construction, nos. 1, 4, 6, 15, 22, 23, 47, 56, 58, 62, 64, 65, 67, 70, 72, 78, 81, 82, 86, 88, 89, 92, 93, 98, 99, 101, 102, 106–8, 120, 127, 135, 138, 144, 145–48, 151–55, 158, 159, 161, 162, 164, 165, 168, 170–74, 176, 177, 180, 182, 184, 186, 187, 191, 193; for restorations, nos. 2, 3, 5, 7–9, 11–14, 16–19, 24–26, 28, 31–37, 43, 44, 46, 48–50, 53, 59, 61, 63, 69, 73, 74, 76, 77, 84, 85, 87, 90, 91, 94–96, 103, 109–14, 116, 118, 119, 121–26, 128, 129, 131, 134, 136, 137, 139, 140, 141, 143, 149, 156, 169, 181, 185, 188–90, 192, 194, 195; for extensions/adornments alone, nos. 21, 27, 29, 30, 38, 39, 42, 45, 51, 54, 55, 68, 71, 75, 79, 83, 97, 104, 115, 117, 132, 133, 142, 150, 157, 158, 163, 166, 178, 196. The total of 180 benefactions does not include the forty-three extensions/adornments undertaken as adjuncts to other constructional operations or the fourteen entries in which the nature of the work cannot be determined with absolute certainty: seven possible initial constructions (nos. 10, 40, 57, 105, 167, 175, 183), five possible restorations (nos. 41, 52, 60, 100, 130), and two possible extensions/adornments (nos. 20, 66).

texts with a primarily "ideological interpretation" that minimizes or even rejects the usefulness of inscriptions as indicators of ancient reality is unnecessary.[5] In any event, I am interested here more in the benefactors than in their actions, so the manner in which they wished their actions to be presented to their public is of more importance to the current inquiry than what they might or might not have done in reality. Armed with a healthy skepticism, therefore, there is no reason why we cannot analyze these inscriptions for what they can tell us about bath benefactors, their identities, and their motives, as well as their actions.

The geographical distribution of the data for bath construction deserves attention. Unfortunately, a comprehensive survey of Roman building inscriptions has yet to be undertaken, so there is no conclusive body of data with which to compare my figures. Thomas and Witschel's analysis of reconstruction texts offers, at least, a point of partial comparison with the bath inscriptions in my sample.[6] The two sets of data, however, must be made correlative, which requires some adjustments to the figures in both cases. First, since Thomas and Witschel tabulate volumes of *inscriptions,* as opposed to acts of benefaction, we must do the same. This requirement reduces our base figure from 196 (the number of constructional *entries* in the sample) to 184 (the number of constructional *inscriptions* in the sample), since on four occasions two benefactions recorded in the same inscription are counted once each (see nos. 1/2, 73/74, 148/49, 168/69); nine entries refer to inscriptions cited in full elsewhere in the sample and are thus excluded (nos. 80, 145, 147, 152, 154, 155, 162, 181, 185); and one entry comprises two inscriptions and so is counted twice (no. 150). Second, the two samples diverge in geographical scope. Thomas and Witschel restrict themselves to the Latin West and overlook regions represented in my figures, but they include Britain, which is not represented in my sample. The two sets of figures must therefore be adjusted to take this factor into account, reducing the comparable totals to 634 for restorations and 163 for bath benefactions.[7]

---

5. For the ideological interpretation, see Thomas and Witschel, "Constructing Reconstruction"; see, contra that interpretation, G.G. Fagan, "The Reliability of Roman Rebuilding Inscriptions," *BSR* 64 (1996): 81–93.

6. See Thomas and Witschel, "Constructing Reconstruction," 175 (appendix a), where $n = 672$.

7. Among reconstruction inscriptions, Britain accounts for 38 of 672, so that $n = 634$. Among bath inscriptions, the following regions are excluded: Sicily—1/184 (no. 55); Cyrenaeca—2/184 (nos. 4 and 5); Tripolitania—5/184 (nos. 35, 90, 117, 119, 166); Asia Minor—3/184 (nos. 13, 29, 81); Greece—1/184 (no. 60); the Danubian provinces—9/184 (nos. 25, 26, 92, 109, 120, 161, 167, 180, 189). Thus the total for bath inscriptions excluded on the basis of geographic incompatibility with Thomas and Witschel's sample ("Constructing Reconstruction") is 21/184, so that $n = 163$.

A third and final factor, for which no adjustment can be made, may distort the comparison to some degree. Thomas and Witschel restrict their attention to a certain type of inscription as it applies to a wide variety of structures, whereas my epigraphic sample takes the inverse focus and embraces a wide variety of inscriptions as they apply to a single type of structure. Ideally, we would be able to compare the bath inscriptions with those pertaining to another, specific type of public building, but Thomas and Witschel's figures cannot be broken down in this manner. The net effect of all of these factors and adjustments is to counsel caution in drawing dramatic conclusions from any divergences between the sets of data.

In general, Latin inscriptions do not survive in equal proportions across the empire: Italy and North Africa predominate, with the other western regions variously represented.[8] The figures for both reconstruction and bath inscriptions bear this observation out, with Italy and North Africa combining to account for over 80 percent of the texts in both samples. A chart offers the most convenient means of comparing the two sets of data, which show some divergences, but none so serious that they that cannot be accounted for by the differences in the size, scope, and focus of the samples. If anything, the distribution between the two sets of data is notably consistent (see chart 1).

The chronological distribution of bath-related inscriptions can also be compared to that of reconstruction texts.[9] It is now widely recognized that the survival rate of Latin inscriptions across time is not constant but peaks in the second century and especially in the Severan period, falls off in the third century, and rises again in the fourth.[10] Given that Latin inscriptions survive in great numbers (an estimated 250,000 are known), it seems more likely that the peaks reflect less the vagaries of survival and more the pattern of production. An explanation for this pattern, however, remains elusive. A recent analysis has argued that it was generated, in part, by a desire for status display linked to the spread of citizenship in the second century, which, understandably, declined after the declaration of universal citizenship, the *Constitutio Antoniniana*, of 212. Unfortunately, this argument is restricted to epitaphs, which constitute a special type of inscription that accounts for 68 to 76 percent of all surviving Latin inscriptions; conclusions drawn about

---

8. The proportion of *CIL* volumes devoted to these two regions makes this pattern manifest, as does the Italic and North African focus of such epigraphically based studies as Duncan-Jones' *Economy* or Jouffroy's *Construction publique*.

9. See Thomas and Witschel, "Constructing Reconstruction," 175 (appendix b).

10. See R. MacMullen, "The Epigraphic Habit in the Roman Empire," *AJP* 103 (1982): 233–46; S. Mrozek, "À propos de la répartition chronologique des inscriptions latines dans le Haut-Empire," *Epigraphica* 35 (1973): 113–18 and, under the same title, *Epigraphica* 50 (1988): 61–64.

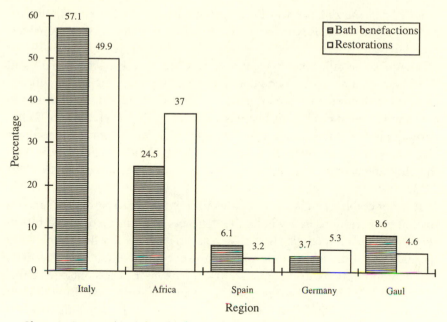

Chart 1. Geographical distribution of construction texts.

Data (by region):

Restorations (*n* = 634): Italy: 316/634 (49.9%); Africa: 235/634 (37%); Spain: 20/634 (3.2%); Germany: 34/634 (5.3%); Gaul: 29/634 (4.6%).

Bath benefactions (*n* = 163): Italy: 93/163 (57.1%); Africa (including Numidia and Mauretania): 40/163 (24.5%); Spain: 10/163 (6.1%); Germany: 6/163 (3.7%); Gaul (including Alpes): 14/163 (8.6%).

References:

Italy: nos. 1/2, 3, 6, 7, 10, 11, 14, 16–20, 22–24, 27, 30–33, 36, 37, 39–41, 43–50, 56, 57, 69, 61–70, 73/74–76, 84, 85, 87, 88, 91, 95, 96, 98, 99, 102, 108, 112, 116, 118, 121, 124–26, 136, 139, 141, 143, 144, 146, 151, 153, 157, 159, 160, 164, 168/69, 171, 173, 174, 176, 177, 179, 184, 188, 190, 191, 193, 195, 196; Africa: nos. 12, 21, 34, 38, 42, 83, 86, 89, 93, 94, 105, 107, 110, 111, 113–15, 123, 127–34, 137, 138, 140, 142, 148/49, 150 (two inscriptions), 156, 182, 183, 186, 187, 192, 194; Spain: nos. 28, 71, 72, 78, 101, 122, 158, 165, 172, 175; Germany: nos. 53, 54, 103, 104, 163, 178; Gaul: nos. 8, 9, 15, 51, 52, 58, 77, 79, 82, 97, 100, 106, 135, 170.

epitaphs cannot be transferred wholesale to construction inscriptions.[11] The overall chronological pattern of epigraphic production must be borne in

---

11. See E.A. Meyer, "Explaining the Epigraphic Habit in the Roman Empire: The Evidence of Epitaphs," *JRS* 80 (1990): 74–96 (spread of citizenship); R.P. Saller and B.D. Shaw, "Tombstones and Roman Family Relations in the Principate: Civilians, Soldiers, and Slaves," *JRS* 74 (1984): 124 n. 1 (proportion of epitaphs). Meyer's conclusions have been challenged, in part, by D. Cherry, "Re-Figuring the Roman Epigraphic Habit," *AHB* 9 (1995): 143–56.

mind when analyzing the distribution of the data, and a strict chronological analysis of inscriptions is a risky endeavor, since so many texts are of uncertain date.

Again, some adjustments to the figures are necessary if Thomas and Witschel's data are to be made comparable to my own. First, a significant proportion of both samples comprises undated texts; second, some entries in my sample cannot be fitted to Thomas and Witschel's periodization, which is here adopted to enable comparison. These considerations reduce the comparable totals to 421 for restorations and 120 for bath benefactions.[12] As with the geographical distribution, the data are best presented in a chart (see chart 2).

It is noticeable that bath inscriptions follow the broad pattern of survival for Latin inscriptions as a whole; there are peaks in the second and fourth centuries (roughly periods III and V, respectively), with a dip in the third (period IV). In the first two periods, the proportions of dated restorations and bath inscriptions are close. In contrast, bath inscriptions outstrip restorations in period III, while in period IV, the inverse is the case. In periods V and VI, the totals once more converge, more so in the latter than in the former. It is tempting to start speculating reasons for the divergences. The archaeologically attested growth in the construction of baths in the second century may explain the discrepancy for period III; and indeed, of the thirty-two bath inscriptions datable to this period, fifteen are initial constructions, and nine are restorations.[13] Likewise, the decline in bath inscriptions in period IV, a time of great unrest and uncertainty in the Roman empire, might be explained by a tendency to favor more practical buildings over "luxury" structures, such as baths; however, the differences in the samples, above all the low overall figures involved in both cases, make such speculation hazardous and inadvisable. For the moment, the differences can be noted, perhaps to await a more complete study of Latin building inscriptions. Nev-

---

12. The starting samples are, for restorations, $n = 634$ and, for bath inscriptions, $n = 163$, since the geographical exclusions explained above (chapter 6, n. 7) are still in effect. The respective totals for texts excluded on the basis of dating uncertainties are 213/634 (33.6%) for undatable restorations, and 43/163 (26.4%) for bath inscriptions, which includes both undatable texts and those that cannot be fitted into Thomas and Witschel's periods ("Constructing Reconstruction"). The references for undated texts are nos. 20, 46–54, 56–59, 143, 144, 146, 148/49, 150 (two inscriptions), 151, 153, 156. The references for nonfitters are nos. 164, 165 (first or second century); 95, 96, 179 (late second century and so in either periods III or IV); 104, 182, 183 (second or third century); 114, 115, 190 (late third century and so in either periods IV or V); 28, 43–45, 139 (fourth or fifth century); 136, 137 (late fourth century and so in either periods V or VI); 195, 196 (late Imperial and so in either periods V or VI).

13. Initial constructions: nos. 6, 22, 78, 82, 86, 98, 99, 101, 170–74, 176, 177. Restorations: nos. 3, 7–9, 84, 85, 87, 90, 91.

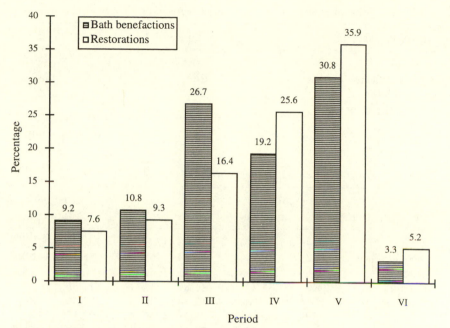

Chart 2. Chronological distribution of construction texts.
Key to periods:
Period I: Late second century B.C. to 14; period II: 14–98; period III: 98–192;
  period IV: 192–284; period V: 284–392; period VI: 392–500.
Data (by period):
Restorations (*n* = 421): I: 32/421 (7.6%); II: 39/421 (9.3%); III: 69/421
  (16.4%); IV: 108/421 (25.6%); V: 151/421 (35.9%); VI: 22/421 (5.2%).
Bath benefactions (*n* = 120): I: 11/120 (9.2%); II: 13/120 (10.8%); III: 32/120
  (26.7%); IV: 23/120 (19.2%); V: 37/120 (30.8%); VI: 4/120 (3.3%).
References: I: nos. 21, 61–68, 157, 158; II: nos. 1, 69–77, 159, 160, 163; III:
  nos. 3, 6–10, 22, 78, 79, 82–87, 89–91, 97–101, 170–78; IV: nos. 11, 12,
  23, 24, 27, 93, 94, 102, 103, 105–8, 110–12, 116, 118, 184, 186–88, 191;
  V: nos. 14–19, 30–34, 36, 37–42, 113, 121–35, 192–94; VI: nos. 138, 140–
  42.

ertheless, the figures for bath construction alone corroborate the archaeological record in marking the second century as central in the history of
Roman bathing culture.

Such is the character of the construction inscriptions. In the analysis that
follows, the chief topics of investigation are how the benefactions are
distributed among the various types of benefactor, what social status the
benefactors enjoyed, and what motives, if any, can be discerned or postu-

TABLE 2.   Distribution of Entries by Type of Benefactor

Type of Benefactor	No. of Entries	% of Total
Emperors	19	9.7
Imperial officials	26	13.3
Local authorities	97	49.5
Private benefactors	54	27.5
Total	196	100

TABLE 3.   Distribution of Bath Benefactions by Type of Benefactor

Type of Benefactor	Initial Construction	Restoration	Extension/ Adornment
Emperors	4/18 [22.3%]	14/18 [77.7%]	—
Imperial officials	2/23 [8.7%]	13/23 [56.5%]	8/23 [34.8%]
Subtotal	6/41 [14.6%]	27/41 [65.9%]	8/41 [19.5%]
Local authorities	28/89 [31.5%]	46/89 [51.7%]	15/89 [16.8%]
Private benefactors	31/50 [62%]	12/50 [24%]	7/50 [14%]
Subtotal	59/139 [42.5%]	58/139 [41.7%]	22/139 [15.8%]
Total	65/180 [36.1%]	85/180 [47.2%]	30/180 [16.7%]

lated for their acts of benefaction. Among the construction inscriptions, a simple and obvious prediction can be made before the evidence is approached. Baths were expensive commodities.[14] As a result, only those who could afford them are represented in the texts. We cannot expect to and do not find slaves or shopkeepers building baths, although some ex-slaves did.[15] Since the focus of the investigation is on the benefactors, the analysis proceeds accordingly, with the benefactions considered under the rubric of type of benefactor. The breakdown of benefactors is presented in table 2. The distribution of the different types of constructional benefaction within these categories of benefactor is presented in table 3.[16]

14. On the costs of baths, see below, chapter 6, pp. 173–75.

15. It is possible, as suggested in the previous chapter, that consortia of humbler Romans (collegia, etc.) built baths, but such projects do not seem to have been commemorated with formal inscriptions.

16. The total for clearly discernible constructional benefactions is 180 (see above, chapter 6, n. 4), hence the apparent discrepancy between the number of entries for benefactors, as laid out in table 2, and the totals for benefactions, as presented in table 3.

Emperors and Imperial Officials (nos. 1–45; see also nos. 288–91)

Emperors are attested as constructional benefactors in only nineteen entries in the epigraphic sample (nos. 1–19; compare nos. 288–90). That bath benefactions by emperors derive mostly from Italy (12/19 [63%]) is in broad accord with the general pattern of survival of such inscriptions and cannot therefore be put down to special treatment of Italian communities due to their proximity to Rome. Chronologically, the greatest intensity of imperial action is displayed in the second (8/19) and fourth (6/19) centuries, which is again in keeping with the overall chronological distribution of Latin inscriptions.[17] Noteworthy is the almost even split of imperial benefactions between the periods of Italy's "privileged" and "provincial" status. Emperors appear to have continued to benefit the peninsula, regardless of its "official" status.[18] The benefactions to non-Italian communities cover North Africa (nos. 4, 5, 12), Gaul and the Alps (nos. 8, 9, 15), and Asia Minor (no. 13; see also nos. 288–90).

In some cases, the emperor enjoyed a special connection with the favored community. Diocletian, for instance, took up residence among the Nicomedians (no. 13), while Gordian III repaired a bath that was attached to imperial property at Volubilis (no. 12). Other reasons for imperial action seem standard, such as offering relief after a revolt (no. 5) or local disasters (nos. 8, 9); in such cases, there must be a suspicion that the emperor's actions were in response to embassies sent from the stricken communities. But most of the commemorations of imperial bath benefactions contain no hints as to why the emperor acted as he did, beyond a vague and obsequious statement concerning the emperor's "customary generosity" (no. 15). In these cases, as in most, the emperor's reasons for action can be put down to what has been termed "le style monarchique," that is, the ruler's role as the empire's preeminent patron and benefactor.[19] It is possible that the actions of some emperors flowed from a special relationship with the locals, hinted at by the appearance of such phrases as "for his town/people," although the phrase need be little more than epigraphic rhetoric and can be found in nonimperial inscrip-

---

17. Italy: nos. 1–3, 6, 7, 10, 11, 14, 16–19. Second century: nos. 3–10. Fourth century: nos. 14–19.

18. The "provincialization" of Italy was a gradual process, with roots even in the Augustan period; see W. Simshäuser, "Untersuchungen zur Entstehung der Provinzialverfassung Italiens," *ANRW* 2.13 (1980): 401–52.

19. See above, chapter 5, n. 53.

tions as well.[20] Whatever the case, the evidence is clear that emperors did not go about the empire building baths for local populations as a matter of course. The small overall total of benefactions from emperors, even in Italy (19/194 [9.8%]), makes this point still stronger.

Of the nineteen entries for emperors, the nature of the work in eighteen cases can be securely identified. Of these, restorations (14/18 [77.7%]) are far more common than initial constructions (4/18 [22.3%]); the single uncertain entry (no. 10) was probably an initial construction.[21] In several cases, emperors are praised as the benefactors of a building either promised and/or worked on by a predecessor (nos. 2, 5, 6, 13, 17, 19) or standing on imperial property (no. 12). In other words, many emperors are again seen to enjoy some special connection with the buildings they benefit. That certain baths bore emperors' names is insufficient grounds for deducing an original imperial benefactor, since in one case (no. 81) a bath is reported as built and paid for by the local authorities but dedicated to and named after Hadrian; the same is likely true of most of the other baths named after emperors (see below, chapter 8, p. 171). Members of the imperial family or others linked with emperors could also act as benefactors (nos. 179, 188, 315 [?]), but they are best interpreted as doing so in the guise of rich, private individuals rather than as direct representatives of the state or the imperial majesty. This is particularly clear in the case of Marcia Aurelia at Anagnia (no. 179), who despite being the concubine of Commodus and hence a *stolata femina,* chose to commemorate her actions in conjunction with her father (no. 95) and makes no mention of her imperial connections.

In several bath benefactions credited to the emperor, his representatives are said to have supervised the implementation of imperial munificence (nos. 4, 12, 17–19). Twenty-six inscriptions credit construction work on baths to the officials themselves; that is, whereas in the former instances these men acted as agents of the emperor's *liberalitas,* in the latter they themselves are presented as the chief benefactors (nos. 20–45; see also no. 291). It remains possible in such cases that the officials were perceived as representatives of the central authorities and hence of the emperor, but even if so, they are nonetheless commemorated on the stone as independent and autonomous agents.

A closer look at these texts reveals some interesting features. As with the emperors, Italy predominates (17/26 [65.4%]) as the focus of imperial offi-

---

20. Nos. 13–15, 18 ("his people"). For rhetorical uses of similar phrases, especially in later texts, see, e.g., nos. 90, 104, 125, 141, 165. Note also that Hadrian, who had promised the Neptune Baths to Ostia, had held the duovirate there; see Meiggs, 175–76.

21. Restorations: nos. 2, 3, 5, 7–9, 11–14, 16–19. Initial constructions: nos. 1, 4, 6, 15.

cials' attention, with North Africa coming in a distant second (5/26 [19.2%]).[22] The other regions represented are Dalmatia (nos. 25, 26), Spain (no. 28), and Asia Minor (no. 29). Nine of the Italian instances date to the fourth century, the period that, overall, dominates this benefactor category with fourteen entries (nos. 29–42); the third century, with five entries (nos. 23–27), is second in overall frequency. The absence of any benefactions from the first century is also noteworthy. Again, Italy's gradual shift to the status of a province does not seem to have affected the degree of benefaction by the emperor's representatives—if anything, it increased it. Also comparable to the actions of emperors is the distribution of the benefactions themselves. In three instances, the exact nature of the work is uncertain (nos. 20, 40, 41). Among definitely identifiable benefactions, the majority are of the restorative kind (13/23 [56.5%]). In addition, imperial officials, more than any other benefactor type, show the highest proportion of extensions/adornments carried out as benefactions in their own right (8/23 [34.8%]).[23] This latter figure, just over double the percentage for extensions/adornments in the general pattern of distribution, may suggest that when the central officials intervened, they were apt to do so in the manner of a "quick fix," dealing more often than other benefactors with the surface of a building rather than embarking on larger, more time-consuming projects. Indeed, in only two cases are imperial officials definitely credited with the initial construction of a bath (nos. 22, 23).

The highest imperial office recorded is a *praefectus praetorio* acting at Ostia (no. 22). Governors *(praesides, proconsules)* are well represented (nos. 28, 29, 35, 38, 42), but all of them are late-Imperial appointments, made at a time when the provincial administration had grown and the size of individual jurisdictions had contracted. From the Principate, there is a procurator (no. 26), a *legatus Augusti pro praetore* (no. 25), and three imperially appointed *curatores rei publicae* (nos. 23, 24, 27). This latter office, primarily concerned with the financial welfare of a community, was originally an imperial appointment, but in the course of the later third century and especially in the fourth, it was transformed into a local magistracy.[24] *Curatores rei publicae,*

---

22. Italy: nos. 20, 22–24, 27, 30–33, 36, 37, 39–41, 43–45. N. Africa: nos. 21, 34, 35, 38, 42.

23. Restorations: nos. 24–26, 28, 31–37, 43, 44. Adornments/extensions: nos. 21, 27, 29, 30, 38, 39, 42, 45.

24. *Curatores rei publicae* have received much scholarly attention in recent years, but the details of the office's functions remain obscure, and the date of its transformation into a local magistracy is also disputed: see G. P. Burton, "The Curator Rei Publicae: Towards a Reappraisal," *Chiron* 9 (1979): 465–87; G. Camodeca, "Ricerche sui *curatores rei publicae,*" *ANRW* 2.13 (1980): 453–534; R. Duthoy, "Curatores rei publicae en Occident durant le

even in their imperially appointed guise, are therefore something of a special case, with their duties restricted to specific communities. Indeed, localized officials predominate in the later Empire, and by and large, the officials represented in the sample are the less prestigious officials in the Dominate's extensive bureaucratic hierarchy: *correctores* (nos. 30, 45), *rectores* (nos. 31–33, 40), *consulares* (nos. 34, 36, 39, 43, 44), and *proconsules* (nos. 37, 42).[25]

The motivation for constructional intervention by imperial officials remains particularly obscure. There seems little reason for such men, stationed in a region for a fixed period of time and usually lacking extensive local connections, to spend their money in attending to bathhouses. The habitual euergetistic desires for prestige, prominence, and social recognition, to be explored more fully below, may have played their part, but in the cases of imperial officials, one suspects that these aspirations were largely met by the status such men already enjoyed by virtue of their high birth and proximity to the seat of power. A possibly compelling motive may have been the desire to earn imperial favor. Part of a governor's mandate was to ensure that the physical appearance of communities under his jurisdiction did not dilapidate unduly.[26] As in the case of Pliny the Younger in Bithynia, however, it was usually the locals who footed the bill for any recommended repairs or improvements. At Olisipo in Lusitania, for instance, the local authorities are reported to have been "following the order of Numerius Albanus, . . . gover-

---

Principat," *AncSoc* 10 (1979): 171–238; W. Eck, *Die staatliche Organisation Italiens in der hohen Kaiserzeit* (Munich, 1979), 190–246, esp. 198–205; F. Jacques, *Les curateurs des cités dans l'Occident romain de Trajan à Gallien: Études prosopographiques* (Paris, 1983); id., *Le privilège de liberté: Politique impériale et autonomie municipale dans les cités de l'Occident romain (161–244)* (Rome, 1984), 282–300. In the epigraphic sample, it is clear from such entries as nos. 125–27, among others, that late Imperial *curatores rei publicae* were local officials. The latest possible centrally appointed curator in the sample is Sattius Crescens in the second half of the third century (see no. 27); his senatorial status suggests, but does not prove, an imperial assignment.

25. There is as yet no succinct account of late-Imperial provincial administration, so the best method for assessing the relative status of these officials is through the relevant entries in *RE*. See also A.H.M. Jones, *The Later Roman Empire, 284–602: A Social, Economic, and Administrative Survey* (Oxford, 1964; reprint, Baltimore, 1986), esp. 1.366–83.

26. See *Dig.* 1.16.7.1, 1.18.7. See also the *senatus consultum* of Claudius prohibiting the demolition of buildings for profit (*CIL* 10.1401 = *ILS* 6043); it was modified under Nero to exempt certain individuals but made the point that the destruction of a single edifice was a blot on the entire Roman empire. This latter sentiment fits well with Vitruvius' contention (1 *praef.* 2) that the state is manifest in its public buildings. Note also Hadrian's edict to Stratonicea (*SIG*[3] 837 = *IGRR* 4.1156a) expressing concern that the house of a certain Ti. Claudius Socrates in the city maintain a proper appearance. The imperial lead was followed by local authorities. The *lex municipii Malacitani* (of Flavian date; *CIL* 2.1964 = *ILS* 6089, §62) stipulates that no building may be destroyed without being restored within a year.

nor of the province," when they restored a bathhouse.[27] For an official on
the spot to take the extra step of undertaking the work himself may have
been a way of demonstrating enthusiasm for his job and a commitment to the
imperial ideology in this regard. (A cynic might suggest that such deeds may
also have served to divert suspicion of fiscal mischief away from the official.)
Benefactions to local communities may therefore have been used by some
imperial officials as stepping stones in their political careers. The alternative
possibility that these men were altruists cannot be ruled out entirely, especially when dealing with the likes of Fabius Maximus, who, as *rector* of
Samnium, is remembered in fifteen building inscriptions from the region,
three of them involving baths.[28] Finally, D. Laelius Balbus, the only provincial official of Republican date represented in the epigraphic sample, is a
special case. As *quaestor pro praetore* of Africa Vetus under Q. Cornificius in
43–42 B.C., he lived in unstable times and, indeed, was to fight and die
attempting to resist the triumvirs' appointee to the governorship, T. Sextius
(see no. 21 and note there). As a result, he had a particular interest in currying
local favor.

The central authorities, whether represented by emperors or by their officials, display a particular pattern of bath benefaction. The distribution of
their actions and its comparison with the general pattern of bath benefactions are presented above in table 3 (chapter 6, p. 136). It can be seen from
these figures that the central authorities tended to restore, extend, and adorn
baths rather than build them in the first place. This pattern broadly matches
the general distribution of benefactions, but the total percentage for their
initial constructions (6/41 [14.6%]) is less than half that of the general
pattern (65/180 [36.1%]), while that for their restorations and extensions/
adornments (35/41 [85.4%]) is higher by more than 20 percent (115/180
[63.9%]). While the small totals involved counsel caution in using these
divergences to draw far-reaching conclusions, the figures as presented may
suggest that the central authorities tended more to the superficial and restorative role than to the provisionary one. Such a tendency would be entirely appropriate, given that most of the emperor's business got done on a
reactionary basis, in response to embassies or other specific requests, and
that imperial officials had no inherent motive for building expensive baths

27. No. 122. See also Pliny *Ep.* 10.23, 10.24 (Prusa). On Pliny's position in Bithynia, see
R.J.A. Talbert, "Pliny the Younger as Governor of Bithynia-Pontus," in C. Deroux, ed., *Studies
in Latin Literature and Roman History,* vol. 2 (Brussels, 1980), 423–24.

28. Nos. 31–33. Duncan-Jones ("The Procurator as Civic Benefactor," *JRS* 64 [1974]: 79–
85), when faced with the massive benefactions of Q. Torius Culleo at Castulo in Spain (no. 249),
concludes that altruism cannot be ruled out as a motive for his actions.

for communities over which they were temporarily stationed. In both cases, therefore, the outcome of a benefaction from such an authority was more likely to be the restoration, extension, or adornment of an existing bath than the construction of an entirely new facility.

As a whole, the central authorities account for only 23.2 percent (45/194) of the constructional benefactions listed in the sample. This situation is consistent with the "remote" model of the imperial authorities in the daily life of the empire, whereby the emperor and his agents were concerned with security and taxation and impinged but little on the everyday existence of the populace.[29] It is worth noting that in Pliny's Bithynian correspondence with Trajan, the emperor's interest in local conditions is minimal, at least in the case of those circumstances that did not bear directly on the smooth administration of the region. Similarly, imperial concern with bath-related matters in the laws assembled in the *Digest* is superficial; for the most part, baths appear as part of illustrations of broader legal principles, such as transfer of property and ownership, criminality, and personal litigation.[30] The laws are not concerned with dictating who is to be responsible for bath construction or to regulate how baths should be built or under what circumstances. Evidently, the provision and maintenance of public baths was, in the eyes of the central authorities, not their responsibility. The possibility that public baths somehow reflected imperial concern for the health and welfare of the general populace becomes yet more remote.

Local Authorities and Private Benefactors (nos. 46–196; see also nos. 292–328)

The vast majority of constructional bath benefactions listed in the epigraphic sample were undertaken by locals, in the guise of either local authorities or private benefactors. Overall, benefactions undertaken by locals outnumber

---

29. This position is most fully laid out in Millar, *Emperor in the Roman World*. Note also P. Garnsey and R. Saller, *The Roman Empire: Economy, Society, and Culture* (Berkeley, 1987), 20–40; MacMullen, *Roman Social Relations*, 1–27; F. Millar, "The World of the *Golden Ass*," *JRS* 71 (1981): 66–69; id., *The Roman Empire and Its Neighbours*[2] (London, 1981), 52–80 (at 52 Millar states baldly, "The Roman Empire had no Government").

30. See *Dig.* 7.1.13.8, 7.1.15.1, 7.4.12, 8.5.8.7, 9.2.50, 13.6.5.15, 30.41.8, 32.55.3, 32.91.4, 33.7.13.1, 33.7.17.2, 34.2.40.1, 35.2.80.1 (property and ownership); 1.15.3.5, 2.4.20, 3.2.4.2, 47.17, 48.5.10(9).1 (criminal activity); 16.3.1.8, 17.1.16, 19.2.30.1, 19.2.58.2, 20.4.9, 43.21.3.7, 47.10.13.7 (personal litigation). (I am indebted to R.J.A. Talbert for these references.)

those offered by the central benefactors by a ratio of 3.3:1 (149:45).[31] The chief means of distinguishing local authorities from private benefactors in the inscriptions is the presence or absence of offices or honorary titles. Local authorities are represented by a community's municipal council and its magistrates, by its priests and *patroni,* while private benefactors record only their names. Given the Roman elite's obsession with status, and given the inherent link between rank and public appearance, for a person with an extensive local career to be silent about it in such a major monument as a building inscription appears all but inconceivable. That some benefactors emphasize their *honores* while others do not is therefore more than a matter of personal choice—in all likelihood the officeless benefactors had no offices to boast of.

It must be stressed at the outset that the distinction between local authorities and private benefactors should not be drawn too strictly. In reality, funding for the public buildings of a Roman community tended to come from the same pockets, whether the inscriptions vaunt the actions of municipal councilors acting in concert, individual magistrates, or wealthy private citizens.[32] A good illustration of the fluidity between privately and publicly funded munificence is an inscription from Corfinium (no. 174) reporting that a private benefactor began work on a bathhouse but then died. The *possessores* of his estate contributed 100,000 sesterces toward the work, and the local council completed the project at a further cost of 152,000 (or, possibly, 103,000) sesterces. In the sample, the actions of these agents are assigned to different categories of benefactor (compare no. 80), but it is questionable to what extent contemporaries would have drawn this distinction, if at all. Similar is a case from Paestum (no. 108) in which a man who was a *duovir* and *patronus* built a bathhouse that was later rebuilt by his son. The actions of the *duovir* and the son are assigned to separate categories of benefactor in the sample (compare no. 185), but once more it is unlikely that in ancient times such a distinction would have been drawn. Both men stemmed from the same local family, and the son may well have been destined for a civic career (he is not credited with any local offices in the text). Finally, note that a generous Republican benefactor at Aletrium (no. 157) appears to have been

---

31. This general pattern is, of course, consistent with all public construction in the Roman world, as suggested by the preliminary investigations of H. Jouffroy in "Le financement des constructions publiques en Italie: Initiative municipale, initiative impériale, évergétisme privé," *Ktema* 2 (1977): 329–37, which is expanded on in the relevant sections of id., *Construction publique;* see also Duncan-Jones, *Structure,* 174–84.

32. See R. Duncan-Jones, "Who Paid for Public Buildings in Roman Cities?" in F. Grew and B. Hobley, eds., *Roman Urban Topography in Britain and the Western Empire* (London, 1985), 28–33; id., *Structure,* 184. On the social status and wealth of decurions in Spain, which is probably representative of the Latin West, see Curchin, 71–84, 103–14.

a private citizen until major constructional operations, including work on the local baths, earned him the municipal censorship—a good illustration of the thin line between private benefaction and office holding. In short, local authorities and private benefactors were, on one level, one and the same people.

There are, however, two important respects in which these categories of benefactor diverge, justifying their distinction both in the epigraphic sample and in the analysis that follows. A commemorative inscription, whether set up on the building by the benefactor(s) or voted in gratitude by the beneficiaries, was a permanent monument to a euergete's generosity and social prestige. For those who took part in local politics, it was also a political tool; as a testament to the local family's public service, it could be used by future generations of candidates to gain popular favor (as I suspect was the case at Paestum; no. 108). Therefore, the purpose of these inscriptions, and the motivation for undertaking the benefaction in the first place, would differ somewhat between local authorities and private benefactors.

The other divergence lies in the nature and distribution of the benefactions, which raise several interesting, if unresolvable, possibilities. By and large, private benefactors tend to cluster in the second century and before and are responsible more often for initial construction than for restoration. Local authorities, in contrast, show an inverse distribution: they are more frequent in the third century and later and are associated more often with restorations than with initial constructions. By the fifth century, no private benefactors are represented at all.[33] Given the smallness of the sample for local benefactors (151 entries), this pattern may be put down to pure coincidence. Alternatively, it could reflect a historical process, such as a declining sense of civic responsibility on the part of private citizens, who were unwilling to act without either the social payback of municipal office or the expectation of munificence that came with it. Or, in the face of reluctance, it could be that local authorities took to pushing their magistracies on wealthy private citizens, to spur them to benefaction (note the exhortation in this respect in the closing lines of no. 117). There is so little evidence of enforced office holding, however, and so few bath benefactions are expressly said to be funded by "payments for office" *(summae honorariae)*, that this possibility is largely unsupported by the evidence. The proposed ideological nature of

---

33. Among inscriptions mentioning private benefactors, nos. 157–79 date to the second century or before. Of these entries, 14/23 (53.8%) record initial constructions; see nos. 158, 159, 161, 162, 164, 165, 168, 170–74, 176, 177. Among inscriptions mentioning local authorities, nos. 105–42 date to the third century or later. Of these, 24/38 (63.2%) record restorations; see nos. 109–14, 116, 118, 119, 121–26, 128, 129, 131, 134, 136, 137, 139–41.

epigraphic language raises another possibility: that the distribution pattern merely reflects a change in the way language was used in inscriptions, with a greater emphasis placed on reconstruction at a time when the concept of *restitutio* was especially important to an empire under threat. Again, the weaknesses of this argument in the face of ancient conditions render it unconvincing in itself as an explanation for the divergent distribution. Whatever the case, the evidence assembled in the epigraphic sample suggests that there was a chronological and qualitative difference between the activities of private benefactors and those of local authorities, justifying the distinction drawn between them in the following analysis, despite the underlying coincidence of the socioeconomic identities of the two groups.

In light of these points, I first present an overview of the distribution of benefactions for both types of local benefactor taken together. In all, 149 separate acts of benefaction are recorded in 151 entries.[34] As with the activities of the central authorities, those for locals stem mainly from Italy (72/149 [48.3%]), with Africa second in frequency (39/149 [26.2%]).[35] Gaul (including the Alpine provinces) and Spain are exactly equal, with eleven benefactions each (for a combined proportion of 14.8%); and the Danubian provinces contribute seven (4.7%). Other regions are variously represented, but all in small proportion.[36] The chronological distribution has just been alluded to, with the concentration of activity in the second and fourth centuries corresponding well to the overall pattern for bath-related texts, although the figures are not evenly distributed across the two benefactor categories. Of the 149 benefactions, 139 are securely determinable; and among these 139, initial constructions (59/139 [42.5%]) and restorations (58/139 [41.7%]) are all but equally represented, while extensions and adornments account for only a fraction (22/139 [15.8%]).

Of the two categories of benefactor—and I am now including the ten projects of uncertain nature—local authorities (96/149 [64.4%]) greatly out-

---

34. As before, four entries are counted for a total of two (see above, chapter 6, n. 3), thus generating the total of 149 for the number of separate benefactions.

35. Italy: nos. 46–50, 56, 57, 59, 61–70, 73–76, 80 (+174, not counted), 84, 85, 87, 88, 91, 95 (+179, not counted) 96, 98, 99, 102, 108, 112, 116, 118, 121, 124–26, 136, 139, 141, 143–46, 151–53, 155, 157, 159, 160, 162, 164, 168/69, 171, 173, 176, 177, 181, 184, 185, 188, 190, 191, 193, 195, 196. N. Africa: nos. 83, 86, 89, 90, 93, 94, 105, 107, 110, 111, 113–15, 117, 119, 123, 127–34, 137, 138, 140, 142, 148/49, 150, 156, 166, 182, 183, 186, 187, 192, 194.

36. Gaul: nos. 51, 52, 58, 77, 79, 82, 97, 100, 106, 135, 170. Spain: nos. 71, 72, 78, 101, 122, 147, 154, 158, 165, 172, 175. Danubian provinces: nos. 92, 109, 120, 161, 167, 180, 189. The other regions are Germany—6/149 (nos. 53, 54, 103, 104, 163, 178); Sicily—1/149 (no. 55); Greece—1/149 (no. 60); and Bithynia et Pontus—1/149 (no. 81).

weigh private benefactors (53/149 [35.6%]).[37] The former, therefore, offer an initial focus for closer investigation. In terms of geographic distribution, the pattern is the predictable one of Italy (43/96 [44.8%]) and North Africa (28/96 [29.2%] dominating, with other regions represented in far smaller proportion.[38] The chronological distribution of the benefactions by local authorities is also consistent with the overall pattern of survival of bath-related inscriptions, with the greatest proportion representing the second (nos. 78–101) and fourth (nos. 121–37) centuries. In addition, the local authorities are the most active of the benefactor types represented in the Republic (nos. 61–67), in the first century (nos. 68–77), and in the third (nos. 105–19). Naturally, they are also responsible for the lion's share of the securely determinable benefactions (89/139 [64%]), the breakdown of which is presented above in table 3.[39] As I have noted (above, chapter 6, pp. 144–45), local authorities were more often restorers than builders of baths, especially in the third century and later. What is the identity of the local benefactors? What types of local authority are represented in the inscriptions?

The municipal government of the Roman West came in a wide variety of forms.[40] In most municipalities, the two chief wings of administration were a council of landed gentry and the local magistrates, who acted as the executive officers of the council. In inscriptions, each of the two wings is denoted by titles and terms that usually vary by community, since the institutions sometimes adhered to local, even pre-Roman traditions (e.g., the presence of *sufetes* in North Africa). The Romans, with their hierarchy of community status and their inclination toward regularization, imposed a certain uniformity on these institutions, especially in regions that had lacked an urban

---

37. Of the dual-entry single benefactions, one (nos. 80 and 174) was primarily the work of private benefactors; the other (nos. 95 and 179) was primarily the work of a local official, if we assume that the father took precedence over his daughter, even if she enjoyed imperial connections. The ten entries of uncertain nature are nos. 52, 57, 60, 66, 100, 105, 130, 167, 175, 183.

38. See above, chapter 6, nn. 35, 36, for the references, where all the entries falling between nos. 46 and 142 are assigned to the local authorities. (Excluded from the count for Italy here is no. 80; see above, chapter 6, n. 3.)

39. The references are, for initial constructions, nos. 47, 56, 58, 62, 64, 65, 67, 70, 72, 78, 81, 82, 86, 88, 89, 92, 93, 98, 99, 101, 102, 106–8, 120, 127, 135, 138; for restorations, nos. 46, 48, 49, 50, 53, 59, 61, 63, 69, 73/74, 76, 77, 84, 85, 87, 90, 91, 94–96, 103, 109–14, 116, 118, 119, 121–26, 128, 129, 131, 134, 136, 137, 139–41; for extensions/adornments, nos. 51, 54, 55, 68, 71, 75, 79, 83, 97, 104, 115, 117, 132, 133, 142.

40. For accounts of municipal administration, on which the following discussion relies, see F.F. Abbot and A.E. Johnson, *Municipal Administration in the Roman Empire* (Princeton, 1926); Curchin, esp. 1–70; Jacques, *Liberté,* esp. 321–503; A. Lintott, Imperium Romanum: *Politics and Administration* (London, 1993), esp. 129–53; H. Rudolph, *Stadt und Staat im römischen Italien* (Leipzig, 1935; reprint, Göttingen, 1965); A.N. Sherwin-White, *The Roman Citizenship*[2] (Oxford, 1973). (Rudolph and Lintott deal mostly with the Republic.)

tradition before their arrival, but nevertheless a wide variety of offices and titles are represented in the epigraphic example. Given the permutations of local variation, comparison of the relative importance of magistrates across communities, not to mention across regions, is largely fruitless. Therefore, we must concentrate on the similarities.

The local landed gentry were usually grouped into an *ordo* and termed *decuriones* or *curiales*. The normal vehicle for decurional administration was a municipal council that met, discussed, and voted on issues of local importance. Qualifications for membership of the decurional *ordo* varied from place to place, but a minimum property census and age limit, combined with election to a local magistracy, were habitual requirements. Decurions sitting in session had the power to issue decrees *(decreta)* that publicized their decisions, the enactment of which was then entrusted to the local magistrates, who were usually elected annually by popular vote. The titles, duties, and jurisdictions of these magistrates varied more widely than those of the councils and depended in part on the status of the community. Colonies of Roman citizens, for instance, tended to be headed by dual magistrates, called *duoviri* or *duumviri*, with two aediles below them, and sometimes with quaestors below the aediles. A censorial *duovir* could be elected every five years and was hence marked by the title *quinquennalis*. (Over time, *municipia* and noncitizen communities adopted these administrative forms of *quinquennales, duoviri*, and aediles.) The office of *quattuorvir* also appears in the epigraphic record. Its precise significance, especially its distinctiveness, if any, from the duovirate, is most unclear. The confusion is well illustrated by an inscription from Brixia that commemorates a man who was both *quattuorvir* and *duovir* of the town (no. 66). Like *duoviri*, censorial *quattuorviri* were termed *quinquennales*. A habitual epithet attached in inscriptions to the titles *duovir* and *quattuorvir* is *iure dicundo* (meaning "for administering the law"), which reveals something of these officials' chief duties: to hear and rule on local disputes. For our immediate purposes, it is noteworthy that the *lex Ursonensis,* a municipal charter of Triumviral date, adds to the mandate of the local magistrates, especially aediles, responsibility for the maintenance of the physical fabric of the town.[41] There is little point in reviewing here the numerous other offices mentioned in the epigraphic sample—they usually mimic the duties, if not the titles, of *duoviri* and *quattuorviri,* and many are discussed below—but their variety is itself an illustration of the vitality and variation of local political life under the empire.

Parallel to the civic *cursus* stood the religious offices, in the form of

---

41. *CIL* 2.5439 = *ILS* 6087, §98.

priesthoods devoted to cults of both local and wider significance. Chief among the latter was the flaminate of the imperial cult. Other *flamines* are also attested in the sample, but their cultic affiliation goes unstated. In such cases, they can be assumed to have been priests either of the imperial cult or of some other deity with special relevance to the community. *Sacerdos,* another priestly term found in the texts, can also, but does not necessarily, apply to the imperial cult. Also mentioned in the sample are augurs and *seviri Augustales,* the latter again attached to the imperial cult, although, as freedmen, barred from other civic offices.[42] Finally, there were municipal patrons. Originally, these men were not local officials at all but influential outsiders adopted by a community. Insofar as such men, having been formally selected by the decurions, enjoyed a degree of public recognition within a client community, I include them among the local authorities. Like the *curator rei publicae,* the municipal patronate shifted over time from the adoption of a prominent outsider to the appointment of a local magnate, and this shift is reflected in our inscriptions: at Verona, an ex-consul was curator and patron of the town in the early third century (no. 23), but many late Imperial *patroni* were evidently men of local stock (e.g., nos. 125, 126).[43]

Just as the Roman system of local government in the West varied by region, it also changed over time. Such changes, however, are hard to detect, due to the generally sparse and uneven survival of the evidence. Italy and North Africa, particularly well endowed with epigraphic material, are somewhat exceptional in this regard, and broad trends are, to a degree, traceable. One observable phenomenon is that of towns adding new magistracies to their municipal *cursus.* A notable from late-second-century Corfinium, for instance, boasted that he was "the first ever quaestor at Corfinium" (no. 88), and the existence of a man who was both *quattuorvir* and *duovir* at Brixia (no. 66) possibly reflects an adjustment to the local *cursus.* The slate of magistrates at a given community should not therefore be considered as fixed; it could and did change over time. Besides adding new offices or adjusting existing ones, certain offices or combinations thereof could rise to prominence in the course of a town or region's history. It seems from the sample, for instance, that from the late third century onward, the curatorship *rei publicae,* often in combination with a lifetime flaminate, had become the leading municipal post in Africa and Numidia; the inscriptions credit many

---

42. *Flamines:* nos. 52, 84, 88, 97 (imperial cult); 83, 90, 91, 100, 114, 127, 130, 132, 137 (unaffiliated). *Sacerdotes:* no. 77 (imperial cult); 71, 126 (unaffiliated). Augurs: nos. 47, 90, 99, 106, 130. *Seviri:* nos. 57, 58, 59, 72.

43. For this change as attested among North African patrons, see B.H. Warmington, "The Municipal Patrons of Roman North Africa," *BSR* 22 (1954): 46, 52–53.

holders of these offices with carrying out bath benefactions (nos. 114, 123, 127, 129–34, 137, 140, 142). Earlier bath benefactions in these same areas had been recorded as undertaken primarily by local councils (nos. 86, 89, 94, 107, 111, 113). In North Africa, then, there seems to have been a shift in responsibility for constructional bath benefactions, from local council to magistrates, or at least a change in the way such benefactions were described in the commemorative inscriptions.[44] In Italy, the local *curator rei publicae* is also attested in the late Empire (nos. 125, 126, 139), but unlike North African bath benefactions, Italian bath benefactions had long been pro- claimed in inscriptions as the work of local magistrates, rather than of the decurions acting together (e.g., nos. 46, 55, 59, 61, 66). Here, then, the curator is little more than a variation on a preexisting theme. The possibility of such regional and chronological variations as these must be borne in mind as we survey the evidence, although there is not enough material from the different regions of the West to write regional "histories" of responsibility for bath construction and maintenance. We have little choice but to examine the material as a whole, always wary of the possibility that the impression we gain may be distorted by regional and chronological variation.

By far the most active arm of the local authorities in carrying out bath benefactions was the local council. There are several ways to detect the actions of the decurions in their formal role. They could identify themselves by an institutional title, such as *senatus* (no. 102) or, in the case of smaller places, *vicani* (nos. 53, 120); but more often than not they simply employed the name of the town or designated their actions as those of the *respublica* and as ordered by a *decretum decurionum* (nos. 73/74, 80, 81, 86, 89, 93, 94, 105, 111, 112, 115, 116). In other cases, the work is expressly said to be financed "with public money" *(pecunia publica)*, thereby revealing the hand of the council (nos. 48, 49, 62, 64, 68, 96, 128, 129). In Republican and early Imperial Italy, the work was often reported as carried out by local magis- trates, but when a formula appears, such as "X saw to the work in accor- dance with a decree of the decurions, and Y approved it," it denotes the ultimate responsibility of the decurions, with the magistrates acting as their agents.[45] It is probable, though not certain, that the mysterious *curatores refectionis* of the Hadrianic Baths at Lepcis Magna were acting under the council's orders (no. 119). Less certain are those instances when the work is

---

44. Some late Imperial inscriptions, however, record the work of local councils; see, e.g., nos. 128, 129. In addition, some texts apparently commemorating the work of curators actually reflect the combined actions of the local authorities; see below, chapter 6, p. 150.

45. Nos. 61, 63, 65, 66 (?), 67, 76, 85. The formula could also be employed by private benefactors (see, e.g., no. 188), perhaps emulating its "official" tone.

reported simply in the passive voice (nos. 107, 113, 122). Here the local authorities are by far the most likely agent, especially in cases like that from Olisipo in Spain, where the work was done on the order of the governor (no. 122). On another occasion, the passive voice is employed with *pecunia publica* to make the agency of the council clear (no. 48), although the actions of a *patronus* might also be described in this way (no. 56 [?]). Taking all of these forms of inscription together, municipal councils are attested as responsible for constructional bath benefactions in the largest proportion of any single benefactor type among the local authorities (38/96 [39.6%]).[46]

When we turn to the magistrates themselves, it would be useful to categorize and tabulate the officers responsible for constructional activity. There are, however, considerable difficulties in determining responsibility for the work in some of these inscriptions. The ambiguous role of some *curatores rei publicae* in late Imperial African benefactions is a case in point. In several inscriptions, the work is reported as carried out by the *curator rei publicae* "along with the decurions/*ordo*" (nos. 123, 127, 131, 142), making ultimate responsibility for the work difficult to deduce. Likewise, although a *curator rei publicae* is credited with extending and restoring baths at Abbir Maius, the project is reported as funded by "contributions from the most eminent *ordo*," belying the curator's responsibility for the project (no. 133); and in an inscription from Madaurus, a curator is presented as the main benefactor but is said to have acted "with public money" *(pecunia publica)*, which thus lays responsibility squarely at the council's feet (no. 129). A text from Thibursicum Bure in Africa (no. 115) reveals a possible role for the curators in these confusing inscriptions. The inscription notes that when the local council moved some statues into the baths, the work was done "through the foresight and insistence" of the *curator rei publicae*, suggesting that he proposed the transferal in the first place. In another instance from Italy, a curator *(rei publicae?)* is reported as supervising the work (no. 112), which offers another possible explanation for the curatorial role in the unclear North African examples. In such cases, then, the benefaction is best considered the work of the council, with the curator acting as its agent or in some supervisory capacity.

Even when local officials are clearly the responsible party, the task of assigning specific acts of benefaction to specific types of magistrate quickly becomes difficult. In some cases, determination is straightforward, since the inscriptions mention only single offices: for example, quaestor (no. 136),

---

46. Nos. 48, 49, 53, 61–68, 74, 76, 80, 81, 85, 86, 89, 93, 94, 96, 102, 105, 107, 111–13, 115, 116, 120, 122, 123, 127–29, 131, 133, 142.

aedile (nos. 54, 91), *duovir* (nos. 55, 117), *quinquennalis* (nos. 60, 73), or *flamen* (nos. 52, 84, 91, 97, 100). But most individuals held multiple civic and religious offices, often in conjunction, so that it is impossible to say which office was the more prominent in order to assign the benefaction to the appropriate "guise" of the benefactor and thereby tabulate the data (e.g., nos. 87, 88, 90, 99, 126). As with the broader distinction between local authorities and private benefactors, the ancients probably did not recognize such differences at all but rather read the assemblage of offices and honors together and took it to mean "important person." Nevertheless, that some sort of ranking among *honores* took place is indeed hinted at by the evidence. At Ocriculum, for instance, a bath benefactor's daughter was honored by the town with an inscription in which her father is named as a *patronus municipi;* but in another inscription from the same town, the father is revealed to have had an extensive local career, of which the patronate was only one element (no. 98). For the patronate, and that alone, to be mentioned in his daughter's inscription strongly suggests that it was the pick of all the titles to which the father could lay claim. It is also clear that in the municipal "run of office" *(cursus honorum)*, gradation of office applied, just as in the senatorial *cursus* at Rome. Thus the quinquennalate, elected only every five years, was more prestigious than the annual duovirate or quattuorvirate, and the aedileship was more important than the quaestorship. Such offices were usually held in sequence of seniority, although, as I have noted, not every town had a complete slate. Thus, when a benefactor declared himself a *duovir* and an aedile (e.g., no. 87), he was undoubtedly commemorating his actions as a holder of the former office. But ranking importance of title is not so clear for a man who was a flamen of the imperial cult, *patronus* of the town, and *quattuorvir quinquennalis* (no. 88).[47] Due to these considerations, it is not practical to arrive at firm figures for the actions of each type of magistrate, which would require inordinate guesswork and arbitrary drawing of distinctions. Instead, therefore, I undertake a broad survey of the evidence.

On the whole, it is noticeable that men who advanced to the higher local offices and priesthoods are represented in the epigraphic sample far more frequently than those who held only the more lowly ones. Thus *duoviri, quattuorviri,* and *quinquennales* are the most frequently represented magistrates, even if they are often noted as having held the lower offices earlier in their careers (nos. 47, 55, 60, 70, 73/74, 75, 78, 87, 92, 97, 99, 101, 117). Similarly, men credited with having completed "all the offices and duties" of

47. The order of citation is of little use in determining the relative seniority of positions listed, since in some cases the order moves from highest to lowest (see, e.g., no. 47), while in others it is vice versa (see, e.g., nos. 46, 70, 87, 92).

a town are well represented (nos. 104, 106, 118, 124, 141), as are *flamines* (nos. 52, 83, 84, 91, 97, 100) and *patroni* (nos. 50, 56, 69, 95, 98, 110, 121, 138). In the later Empire and especially in Africa, as we have seen, *curatores rei publicae* of local origin rise to prominence, often as concurrent *flamines perpetui.* Some individuals cite a combination of important posts, including many of those just mentioned, thus highlighting their sustained social and political importance in a number of capacities (nos. 88, 90, 108, 125, 126, 139). Worth noting are three other offices that were evidently in the upper echelons of the *cursus* in their respective communities: a dictator (no. 46), two *praefecti civitatis* (nos. 51, 79), and a *magistratus* (?; no. 135). Among the *sacerdotes* is a woman, described as "the leading lady in the town of Cartima" (no. 71). (The role of women in bath benefactions is examined in more detail below.) The frequent mention of senior *honores* can be contrasted to the infrequency of humbler offices cited as the highest posts earned by the benefactor: aedile (no. 54, 91), *curator refectionis* (no. 119), *decurio* (nos. 103, 109), *praefectus fabrum* (no. 82), and quaestor (no. 136). This pattern of representation is hardly surprising. Lowly offices were not likely to act as an incentive for expensive benefactions of the sort baths demanded. In contrast, men who had reached the pinnacles of the municipal *cursus,* who stood as the leading lights of their communities, might wish to crown their success or propel themselves still farther into the stratospheres of esteem by deploying their wealth on a structure that was regularly and heavily frequented by all the people of their town. Thus *quinquennales, patroni, curatores,* and *omnibus honoribus functi* predominate among the local officials.

Private individuals make up a significant proportion of local bath benefactors (53/149 [35.6%]). They are responsible for fifty clearly determinable benefactions, more often initial constructions than restorations (see table 3). The geographic and chronological distribution of their actions fit the overall patterns so far reviewed and have already been alluded to above.[48] The outstanding examples in this category come from the Greek East, where Opromoas and a contemporary anonymous benefactor were responsible for staggering outlays to benefit dozens of communities in Asia Minor and Greece, many of which were applied to baths (nos. 311, 313, 314). In the

---

48. Among private benefactors, as in all the benefactor categories, Italy (29/53 [54.7%]) and North Africa (11/53 [20.8%]) dominate the geographic distribution. Italy: nos. 143–46, 151–53, 155, 157, 159, 160, 162, 164, 168, 169, 171, 173, 174, 176, 177, 181, 184, 185, 188, 190, 191, 193, 195, 196. N. Africa: nos. 148–50, 156, 166, 182, 183, 186, 187, 192, 194. The other regions represented are: Spain—6/53 (11.3%; nos. 147, 154, 158, 165, 172, 175); Danubian provinces—4/53 (7.5%; nos. 161, 167, 180, 189); Germany—2/53 (3.8%; nos. 163, 178); Gaul—1/53 (1.9%; no. 170). For the chronological spread, see above, chapter 6, n. 33.

West, most of the private benefactors are otherwise unknown locals, but not invariably so. One discernible type is the native son who did well in the central administration and either returned home as a rich man, enjoying the esteem of his compatriots, or cast a backward eye at his roots as he moved further up the imperial ladder. Thus a *praefectus Aegypti* built a bath for his native Volsinii (no. 159), a *primipilaris* and *tribunus* did likewise at Fanum Fortunae (no. 162), and the ex-consul Pliny the Younger left money in his will for the construction and decoration of baths at his native Comum (no. 171).[49] In some of these cases, however, it is also possible that we are dealing not with men of local stock but with affluent outsiders who owned property in the territory of the communities they benefited. Of particular interest are women who were connected to the imperial house and who acted as private benefactors either to their native towns or to places they stayed in or visited. Marcia Aurelia, a concubine of Commodus who took part in his assassination, helped restore a bathhouse at Anagnia along with her father, an imperial freedman (no. 179; compare no. 95); Vibia Galla, possibly the daughter of the ill-fated emperor Trebonian, saw to the restoration of baths at Alba Fucens (no. 188); and Faustina, the wife of Antoninus Pius, may have erected baths at Miletus when she was touring the East (no. 315).

Mention of Miletus prompts a brief assessment of the bath benefactors of the Greek East. As stressed in the introduction to the epigraphic sample, the Greek inscriptions cannot be taken as representative, since they have been collected under rather arbitrary and restricted criteria. Therefore, no quantitative analysis of them is undertaken here. Nevertheless, they bear some interesting testimony. As with the Latin texts, both local authorities (nos. 292–301) and private benefactors (nos. 302–28) are represented. Some of the magistrates and titles are analogous to those in the West: for example, the names of towns and councils (nos. 293 and 298); an ἀγοράνομος, or aedile (no. 299); and λογιστεύσαντες, the Greek equivalent of *curatores rei publicae* (no. 300). Most, however, are not. The most notable example is the gymnasiarch, a Greek official with duties specific to places of exercise and under whose aegis the baths naturally fell (nos. 292, 297); but there are also appearances of other peculiarly Greek officials, such as the "general" (στρατηγός, no. 295), the "secretary" (γραμματεύς, no. 296), or the "ruler" (ἄρχων, no. 299).[50] The last named, in particular, had a heritage stretching back to the Geometric period of Greek history. Despite the divergences from

---

49. Other examples are nos. 172 (two men with extensive imperial careers), 173–74 (three ex-consuls), 176 (ex-consul), 184 (two ex-consuls), and 189 *(ducenarius)*.

50. See H.J. Mason, *Greek Terms for Roman Institutions: A Lexicon and Analysis* (Toronto, 1974), esp. 1–16.

the offices and titles of the Latin West, and excepting the unusual position of the gymnasiarch, the underlying pattern appears similar: men who held the higher, rather than lower, offices in their communities acted as bath benefactors. Among private benefactors, the exceptional cases of Opromoas and the anonymous benefactor in Lycia have already been mentioned. Other notable examples include the putative benefactions of Faustina at Miletus, followed by a repair and renaming of the building by the locals Makarios and Eucharia (no. 315/16); the bath at the very edge of the empire at Palmyra, which may have been temple property (no. 317); the construction activity of consular woman Curtia Julia Valentilla (no. 321); and the benefactions that a leading lady of Julia Gordos in Asia Minor carried out in a nearby village (no. 324). As was the case in the Latin West, these private citizens must have been among the leading people in their localities.

The activities of local bath benefactors, whether municipal authorities or private individuals, therefore offer a clear window onto the operation of urban euergetism in the Roman world. The actions of municipal authorities illustrate the importance of local government in providing public amenities for the majority of the empire's inhabitants. The actions of apparently politically inactive but wealthy local magnates drives home a point essential to understanding the socioeconomic operation of the Roman empire: with wealth and social prominence among the Romans came an expectation of munificence. The pattern of constructional bath benefactions I have examined in this chapter makes it clear that this expectation was yielded to most often not by the emperor or his representatives but by the decurions and notables at hand in the community. The place of local euergetism as a cornerstone of life in the Roman World has been reinforced by these inscriptions—without it, few baths would have existed in the first place.

Social Status

Among imperial officials, the social status of the benefactors is readily identifiable from the offices and titles they held. Of the twenty-six bath benefactions attributable to representatives of the central authorities (excluding emperors, of course), those attributed to senators account for the vast majority (19/26 [73.1%]), in comparison to those credited to *equites* (7/26 [26.9%]).[51] The reason for the disparity cannot be put down solely to relative wealth, since *equites* could match senators in riches. It may lie to some extent in the greater need for prestige and ostentation among senatorial

---

51. Senators: nos. 21, 23–25, 27, 29–34, 36, 37, 39, 40, 42–45. *Equites:* nos. 20, 22, 26, 28, 35, 38, 41.

officials. The senatorial *cursus* was more extensive than the equestrian and so demanded greater effort to complete successfully. In contrast, determining the social status of local benefactors is a difficult task. First, we must exclude from consideration the benefactions of local councils, since theirs are official collective actions, albeit attributable as a whole to the decurional *ordo*. Second, individual and joint benefactions must be distinguished from each other if a true picture of status varieties is to emerge. Third, in many cases, the difficulty of discerning social status has to be admitted. Where benefactors record only their names, their social status remains open to question. Despite these problems, some headway can be made. Of the 151 entries for local benefactors in the epigraphic sample, 38 (25.2%) are attributable to local councils and so to the decurional class acting in its official capacity as the guardians of regional interests.[52] This total includes those cases where the local council acts alongside a *curator rei publicae,* discussed above (chapter 6, p. 150). In other of these cases, the responsibility for the actions is not readily apparent. At Cures Sabini, for instance, a bath construction is credited to the council and five *sevirales* acting in concert (no. 96). Likewise, when the council at Thibursicum Bure in Africa built a bathhouse, several decurions contributed money for the addition of a *musaeum* (no. 111). A bath at Corfinium required the attention of three consulars and the local council to reach completion (nos. 80, 174). Most of these instances are best considered the collective actions of the local authorities and are usually counted as single actions, unless there is reason to consider them separately.[53] Of the remaining 113 entries for locals, 28 (24.8%) are the actions of two or more benefactors acting in conjunction, and 85 (75.2%) are attributable to individuals.[54]

The status of many individual local benefactors can be deduced from the offices they held or, during the second century and later, from the honorific

---

52. Since I am now focusing on the social identity of the benefactors, rather than on the nature of their actions, all 151 entries are counted. For the references to local councils, see above, chapter 6, n. 46.

53. Thus nos. 96 and 111 are counted as single actions funded by two representatives of the same benefactor category; in contrast, nos. 80 and 174 and nos. 95 and 179 are counted as single benefactions funded by different categories of benefactor. For clarification, see the notes to the individual entries.

54. Joint: nos. 55, 57–60, 70, 75, 78, 84, 91, 95, 97, 104, 114, 119, 124, 144, 147, 159, 161, 164, 167, 172, 174, 176, 179, 182, 184. Individual: nos. 46, 47, 50–52, 54, 56, 69, 71–73, 77, 79, 82, 83, 87, 88, 90, 92, 98–101, 103, 106, 108–10, 117, 118, 121, 125, 126, 130, 132, 134–41, 143, 145, 146, 148–58, 160, 162, 163, 165, 166, 168–71, 173, 175, 177, 178, 180, 181, 183, 185–96. (In the joint benefactor category, nos. 95 and 179 are listed and counted separately; see below, chapter 6, n. 61. Similarly, entry no. 80 is excluded as referring to a local council, but no. 174 is counted as a single entry recording a joint action of three ex-consuls.)

titles they bore.[55] Senators and *equites* account for only a handful of the total number of individual local benefactors (10/85 [11.8%]). Only four senators are represented (nos. 110, 171, 173, 180), not including two women from senatorial families (nos. 187, 188) and a youth bearing the title *clarissimus iuvenis* (no. 191). These senators were mostly scions of local families who had either done well in imperial service—an example is Pliny the Younger at Comum (no. 171)—or were acting as local *patroni* (no. 110, 173, 180 [?]). Securely identifiable *equites* are similarly rare, accounting for only six benefactions (7.1%; nos. 73, 79, 109, 162, 170, 189). Half of the six benefactors were "functionary" equestrians, that is, men who were active in the imperial service before returning to their hometowns, often to local magistracies (nos. 79, 162, 189). The other half were "honorary" equestrians, that is, men who enjoyed their status primarily by virtue of their wealth and local standing.[56] This latter circumstance raises the difficulty of distinguishing wealthy decurions from *equites*. The latter was a fluid *ordo,* defined as much as anything else by the status symbols to which its members were entitled.[57] Many members of the decurional class must have qualified for and enjoyed equestrian status. Pliny the Younger, for instance, assisted a man at Comum by giving him the balance of the requisite property qualification, so that he could rise from decurional status to equestrian (see Pliny *Ep.* 1.19). A good illustration of the difficulty of identifying local *equites* is an inscription from Furfo: a decurion with an extensive local career was joined in a bath benefaction by his son, who also enjoyed a local career but reports service as a *tribunus militum* (no. 70). The son was therefore a "functionary" *eques,* and his father was probably an "honorary" one, although this distinction is not made explicit in the surviving portions of the inscription. In the face of such uncertainty, it must be recognized that an unknown proportion of local notables may have belonged to the equestrian *ordo*. Nevertheless, without evidence to the contrary, individuals who held local office are best assigned, tentatively, to the decurional class. On this criterion, decurions comprise the largest proportion of individual bath benefactors (37/85 [43.5%]).[58] This total includes three somewhat unusual cases—a Republican magnate who

---

55. The history of these titles (e.g., *vir clarissimus, egregius, perfectissimus*) can be traced through the relevant entries in *RE*. For an overview, see H.-G. Pflaum, "Titulature et rang social sous le Haut-Empire," in C. Nicolet, ed., *Recherches sur les structures sociales dans l'antiquité classique* (Paris, 1970), 159–85.

56. For this classification of *equites*, see R. Duthoy, "Le profil social des patrons municipaux en Italie sous le Haut-Empire," *AncSoc* 15–17 (1984–86): 123–27.

57. See F. Kolb, "Zur Statussymbolik im antiken Rom," *Chiron* 7 (1977): 239–59.

58. Nos. 46, 47, 51, 52, 54, 77, 82, 83, 87, 88, 90, 92, 98–101, 103, 106, 108, 117, 118, 121, 125, 126, 130, 132, 134–41, 157, 160, 185.

earned the local censorship from his benefactions (no. 157), a member of a known leading Pompeian family (no. 160), and the son of a decurion (no. 185). In contrast, individual freedmen account for only one benefaction, that of a *sevir* at Murgi in Baetica (no. 72).

The remaining individual benefactors (34/85 [40%]) are of indeterminate social status, since their names are missing from the inscriptions, only their names are recorded, or they are women.[59] Three men, identified only as *patroni* (nos. 50, 56, 69), may have been of local stock—compare the evidently decurional *patroni* who benefited Ocriculum (no. 98), Amiternum (no. 121), or Thuburbo Maius (no. 138)—but this identification is not securely determinable, since an inscription at Vreu records the actions of a senatorial *patronus* (no. 110). Of the remaining "indeterminates," the majority are probably to be assigned to the decurional class, while allowing the possibility that an unknown proportion of them might have been equestrians. With two notable exceptions (nos. 187 and 188), lone female benefactors undoubtedly stemmed from influential local families (nos. 143, 146, 151, 165, 196). In the case of a female *sacerdos* (no. 71), decurional status for her family seems assured. (This woman, incidentally, is the only female official represented in the sample.) It is interesting to note that one of the female benefactors provided a bath specifically for other women (no. 151), although the others appear to have opened their baths to the general populace—one, for instance, built the facility "for her city of Tagilis" (no. 165).

Turning now to joint benefactions, a slightly different pattern emerges. Senators and *equites* are again in the minority (6/28 [21.4%]).[60] As with the individual senators, these eminent benefactors probably stemmed from local families or at least owned property in the area. Some benefactions, however, were undertaken in noteworthy circumstances. The consular Cornelius Dolabella Metilianus died when his bath project at Corfinium was still in progress, and two consular executors of his estate contributed money from his will to the work (no. 174). Similarly, when the senatorial benefactor Valerius Bradua Mauricus died as work was in progress, a friend and fellow senator finished the job (no. 184). These cases reflect the strong Roman concern to respect the wishes of the dead more than they reflect any prearranged division of labor or of responsibilities. The two equestrian benefactions were offered by men who had reached high posts in the imperial

---

59. Names only: nos. 145, 148–50, 152–56, 158, 163, 166, 168/69, 177, 178, 181, 183, 185, 190, 192, 193. Women: nos. 71, 143, 146, 151, 165, 196. Missing names: nos. 175, 194, 195.

60. Senators: nos. 172, 174, 176, 184. *Equites:* nos. 84, 159.

service—a procurator of Britain and his wife (no. 84), and an unnamed *praefectus Aegypti* along with several female relatives (no. 159). In addition, the joint actions of a decurion and his equestrian son should again be noted here (no. 70). One marked divergence from the status distribution for individual benefactors is the greater representation among joint benefactions of freedmen *(liberti)*. I found only one freedman among individual benefactors (no. 72), but among joint benefactors, freedmen almost match senators and *equites* in frequency (5/28 [17.9%]).[61] These men were either *seviri* (nos. 57–59) or imperial freedmen (nos. 95, 164; see also no. 306) and so hailed from the upper echelons of the freed population. Interestingly, in the majority of these cases, wives and daughters are mentioned alongside husbands and fathers (nos. 57, 58, 95 and 179, 164; see also no. 306). The particular desire of freedmen to advertise their social status, both for themselves and their families, probably explains the frequency of the appearance of women in these inscriptions. It is also possible that some of the wives were freeborn and thus lent further weight to establishing their husbands' status.[62] In only one instance do *seviri* act together (no. 59), excepting the bath restoration at Cures Sabini carried out by the local council and five *sevirales* in conjunction (no. 96).

As with individual benefactors, decurions represent the majority in this category (11/28 [39.3%]). (Bear in mind that the thirty-eight entries for local councils can also be considered joint actions of the decurional class.) A significant segment of this category comprises father-and-son benefactions, mostly commemorating the successful acquisition of office in successive generations (nos. 55, 70, 91, 97). In one case, the mention of the son appears entirely gratuitous, serving only as an advertisement for his existence (no. 114). The other cases are the actions of colleagues in office (nos. 60, 75, 119)—on two occasions related by blood (nos. 104, 124)—and one instance

---

61. Nos. 57–59, 95 (compare no. 179), 164. Nos. 95 and 179 represent an unusual situation that requires elucidation. These two inscriptions record a single joint benefaction by two classes of benefactor, therefore each earns a separate entry in the epigraphic sample (compare nos. 80 and 174). Unlike other joint benefactions by members of the same family, which are often recorded on one stone (e.g., see the entries listed at the head of this note), the benefactors here were felt to be sufficiently important and distinct to warrant separate stones. Furthermore, the daughter enjoyed connections to the imperial house, as a concubine of Commodus. Her social status is therefore unclear. In light of this distinction, each entry is counted separately, no. 95 as commemorating a freedman and no. 179 as commemorating a woman of indeterminate status.

62. Some of the wives' names seem securely names of ex-slaves; see, e.g., nos. 57 and 164, where the nomenclature of the husband and wife suggests freedpeople from the same household, probably former slave *contubernales*. In other cases, the issue is not so clear-cut. Clodia Agathe, the wife of the *sevir* Chrysanthus (see no. 58), may have been freeborn.

of a *duovir* acting with his daughter (no. 78). Benefactors of uncertain status are not represented as frequently among joint benefactors as they are among individual benefactors (6/28 [21.4%]). Family relations continue to dominate here, with two father-and-son combinations (nos. 144 and 182), one father-and-daughter pair (no. 179; compare no. 95), one husband-and-wife couple (no. 161), and one indeterminate relationship (no. 147). The form of the names in the husband-and-wife benefaction (no. 161) suggests that the benefactors might have been imperial freedpeople, but this fact is not stated in the inscription. A unique benefaction in this category is the action of an unspecified number of Roman citizens settled at a place called "Sixty Boats" in Moesia, who assert that they built the baths there, at the very frontier of the empire (no. 167). It is possible that they acted for their own exclusive benefit, but it is more probable, given what we shall see in chapter 8, that they were providing a typically Roman comfort both for themselves and for their fellow townspeople.

Before moving on to the issues of nonconstructional benefactions and motivation, it is useful to pause and look at the women represented in the sample. Given the hierarchical nature of Roman society and the snobbery displayed by the privileged toward those below them, it is a dubious method to treat the women separately from the male members of their social class; indeed, most of these women have already been discussed in the appropriate sections above. It is noteworthy that, as if to emphasize their status, many of the women represented in the sample appear in conjunction with their husbands or fathers (nos. 57, 58, 78, 84, 95 and 179, 159, 161, 164). Their exact roles are not usually described, so their appearance seems little more than a general promotion of the family. An exception is a woman of senatorial status who bequeathed two hundred thousand sesterces toward the restoration of a bath initiated by her husband (no. 84). In a large number of commemorations, however, the women did indeed stand alone and acted as the main benefactors (nos. 71, 143, 146, 151, 165, 187, 188, 196), making it likely that they belonged to the prominent families of their communities. In one of these cases, the woman took the lead and used her benefaction to advertise her husband and son (no. 146). On another occasion, the daughter of an imperial freedman was honored at Anagnia with her own inscription, even though she had acted in conjunction with her father. The daughter, however, was a concubine of Commodus and so probably enjoyed a special status above her peers; interestingly, no mention is made of her imperial connections in the inscription (no. 179). These lone female benefactors, then, appear to have been people of considerable substance and significant social standing in their communities. A good example is Julia Lucilia at Ocriculum, who was honored by the authorities with a monument for no other stated reason than that her father was *patronus* and had built a bathhouse (no. 98). To merit such special attention, winning Julia's favor was evidently a matter of some importance to the local authorities. In the Greek East, several of the individual benefactors are females (nos. 304, 307, 315 [?], 317, 321, 324, 325), although others appear in association with their menfolk (nos. 306, 309, 310, 316, 320, 327). The phenomenon of such powerful local women is, among ancient Mediterranean societies, specific to the Roman empire.[63]

Nonconstructional Benefactions (nos. 197–252; see also nos. 329–39)

Before examining the motivation of bath benefactors, it is worthwhile to pause and look at the nonconstructional largesse attested in the inscriptions. Baths, by their functional nature, offered a variety of alternatives for benefaction, beyond merely constructional actions. Several such benefactions are collected in part B of the epigraphic sample, even if in many cases they were offered in association with constructional activity (e.g., nos. 200, 202, 240–48). Nonconstructional benefactions fall into two broad categories: those directed at the bathers and those directed at the baths. It is noteworthy that all but one of these benefactions are the work of locals, and the single "central" entry is only a possibility (no. 236). Nonconstructional benefactions to communities other than Rome were manifestly not an imperial concern. A good illustration of this fact comes from Bononia, where a bathhouse was built by Augustus and repaired by Gaius. Some time following the repair, a local notable, T. Aviasius Servandus, provided in his will that a foundation be established for men and minors of both sexes to bathe in these baths for free (no. 202).

An offer of free bathing is one of the most obvious and frequently attested benefactions offered in connection with a bathhouse.[64] It raises the question

---

63. See R. MacMullen, "Woman in Public in the Roman Empire," *Historia* 29 (1980): 208–18 (= id., *Changes in the Roman Empire: Essays in the Ordinary* [Princeton, 1990], 162–68); J. Nicols, "*Patrona Civitatis*: Gender and Civic Patronage," in C. Deroux, ed., *Studies in Latin Literature and Roman History*, vol. 5 (Brussels, 1989), 134–36.

64. Nos. 197–213. Naturally, emperors and those close to them provided such benefactions at Rome (see Dio 49.43.2, 54.25.4; Pliny *HN* 36.121). Most noteworthy is Agrippa's provision of estates to allow the *populus* to use his *thermae* for free, following the transfer of the building to public ownership (see Dio 54.29.4). There is also literary evidence for analogous actions by less elevated individuals at the local level, such as the man at Tibur who left a bathhouse to the people so they could use it for free (see *Dig.* 32.35.3), but the most voluminous testimony comes from epigraphy. The whole issue of free bathing has been most thoroughly treated by

of entrance fees for baths *(balneatica),* but there is no need to delve deeply into that issue here, since it has been more fully investigated in prior studies.[65] An offer of free bathing could be expressly restricted to a single bathhouse, as at Bononia, or, in most cases, it can be assumed to have applied only to the building on which the inscription stood. It could be offered for a restricted period (nos. 197, 203, 210, 213) or continuously and forever *(in perpetuum)* by means of a foundation (nos. 200–202, 204–7, 209). The privilege could also be extended to an entire town or to certain groups within it. Thus there are benefactions that are given *populo* (no. 197, 210) or to a community's various members, listed in descending order of status—*colonis, municipibus,* and so on (nos. 198, 199, 201, 204–6). Other inscriptions restrict the privilege to women (nos. 203, 209 [?], 213), men and minors of both sexes (no. 202), or people of a particular status (no. 208). In one unique instance, the right of free bathing was voted by the local council to a veteran upon his honorable discharge from service (no. 207). This text in particular raises serious problems for the notion that all publicly owned baths were free of charge, since here the town's main facility was undoubtedly the building in question, and yet the veteran is deemed exempt from the *balneaticum.*[66] The situation offers yet another warning about using specific evidence to draw broad conclusions about how bathing culture operated across the empire. In those cases where the beneficiaries are not specified, it must be assumed that the privilege extended to all comers (nos. 200, 211, 212). A notable case is that of Caesia Sabina, who invited the women of Veii to partake of an oil distribution and free bathing while the men attended the games and a banquet offered by her husband (no. 213). In the Greek East, a gymnasiarch is attested as offering free baths (no. 329), as are the managers of an association of wool sellers (no. 330).

F. Cenerini, "Evergetismo ed epigrafia: *Lavationem in perpetuom,*" *RivStorAnt* 17–18 (1987–88): 199–220.

65. See Heinz, 23–25, 149–50; Merten, 3–6; Nielsen, 1.131–35. The evidence is scattered and patchy, so determination of empire-wide norms for the cost of a bath is impossible. Little noted in the works just cited, however, is the ruling in the Mishnah (*m. Meil.* 5:4) whereby the man who uses consecrated money to pay for a bath is judged to have committed sacrilege, even if he does not actually enter the building. He is so judged because, the man having paid his entrance fee, the bath-keeper says to him, "Lo, the bath is open to you. Go in and take a bath." This ruling offers a rare glimpse of a transaction that must have occurred countless times a day in the Roman world; compare *CGL* 3.652.10 *(colloquia Monecensia):* "Pay the bathman his fee; take the change" *(da balnitori nummos; accipe reliquum).*

66. All of the authors cited in the preceding note argue for free publicly owned baths. In all likelihood many other offers of free bathing applied to such facilities; see esp. nos. 202 (a bath built for the community by Augustus) and 211 (a village bath).

An interesting problem with these inscriptions is envisioning how the benefaction was administered. In cases where free bathing was offered for a specific period, an obvious method would have been to hire out the bath for the duration of the benefaction and then throw open the doors.[67] Alternatively, the bath-owner could have been paid a fixed sum to cover his costs, regardless of the number of bathers involved. In cases where there were restrictions on who was entitled to the privilege, some screening at the door would have been necessary. On these occasions, the most logical method of implementing the benefaction was to give the beneficiaries bath chips *(tesserae)*, which could then be redeemed at the entrance.[68] A recent proposal that the benefactor provided wood sufficient for each beneficiary to use the baths gratis appears unduly cumbersome and impractical.[69]

Since oil was such an integral part of the bathing process, its provision provided another opportunity for displays of liberality to bathers. This benefaction had a long heritage in the Greek East, where it had been associated for centuries with gymnasia and their supervising magistrates, gymnasiarchs.[70] The tradition continued into the Roman period and extended to Roman-style baths, with the oil often distributed to individuals in small vials from larger vessels (nos. 331–36). In the West, however, the gymnasiarchy was unknown, so it fell to others to undertake the task. These others were usually local officials, although no specific office in the West appears to have carried with it the expectation of oil provision (nos. 214–21). The method seems to have been to set up in the favored building vessels from which the bathers could then take their oil, as is reflected in the formula "X put oil in the baths" (e.g., nos. 216, 219). Only once is there mention of the smaller vials so common in the East, termed *conchae* in Latin (no. 214). Like offers of free bathing, the oil could be made available for set periods (nos. 215, 216, 218). In most cases where a period is unspecified, it was probably a onetime occasion that applied only to a specific building (e.g., nos. 214, 217, 219–21). An exception is the bequest of a *quattuorvir aedilicia potestate* at

---

67. A municipal aedile is reported as doing just that in the *Digest* (19.2.30.1). A legal question was raised, however, when the bath burned down after three months: was the owner of the bath entitled to recompense from the aedile for the period of the bath's inoperation? (He was.)

68. Some such *tesserae* have been found. They are usually made of lead and are occasionally inscribed with the name of the bath to which they applied and with appropriate images, such as strigils or deities (e.g., Fortuna or Neptune); see *Syll.* 111–13 (nos. 886–904). See also appendix 2; Nielsen, 1.134.

69. See P. Le Roux, "Cité et culture municipale en Bétique sous Trajan," *Ktema* 12 (1987): 275–76.

70. See the notes to no. 292.

Comum that specified that the oil be given "in all the *thermae* and *balineae* that are in Comum" (no. 215).

Aside from free bathing and oil, there is the possibility that an African benefactor of uncertain identity provided cash handouts *(sportulae)* to the bathers of Bisica (no. 252). Distribution of *sportulae* to clients at the baths of Rome is known from Martial's *Epigrams* (e.g., 10.70.13–14), but the wording and interpretation of this text from Bisica remain unclear. An inscription from Narbo records the construction of baths and the distribution of *sportulae* at their dedication (no. 58). It is possible that here, as perhaps with the baths in Bisica, the *sportulae* were given out in the building itself, albeit on a special occasion.

Among the benefactions directed at the baths rather than at the bathers, the most common type was the provision or improvement of the water supply (nos. 222–38). It is true that this benefaction was often constructional, insofar as it involved the provision or maintenance of aqueducts or other means of water conveyance. Its special nature, however, is suggested by the separate mention it often garners in constructional inscriptions, distinguishing it from the main benefaction (nos. 222–25, 227–30, 232–36). In some cases, the addition of an aqueduct for the baths is a benefaction in and of itself (nos. 231, 237, 238). Interesting variations are also recorded. An astute and generous *duovir* at Forum Novum, having provided for public use water from his own property, extended the supply to the town's bathhouse, since there was no guarantee of a good supply to that facility (no. 226). At Vicus Albinnensis in Gaul, a *praefectus fabrum* who had built a bath and other buildings also provided a water supply, possibly from springs, along with the right to channel it in pipes (no. 230). In late Imperial Africa, a benefactor whose name is lost saw to it that the hot tub of the summer baths was supplied with water from a purer source (no. 233), and at Calama in Numidia, a *flamen* and *curator rei publicae* repaired a *piscina* so that its water supply was improved from a trickle to a torrent (no. 234). Finally, at Tarentum, a freedman improved the water supply to the *lavacra* of an existing bathhouse, "for their better use" (no. 238).

In addition to water, the baths needed heat: as a mosaic inscription from Miletus poetically puts it, the baths operated when "the fire-wedded nymphs" were summoned (no. 315/16). The provision of heat could be effected in a number of ways.[71] The most obvious was the establishment of a foundation to pay for wood (no. 240). Another possibility was the agree-

---

71. See nos. 239–41; compare no. 338. That this benefaction was burdensome is suggested by its becoming an unpopular liturgy by the third century; see Robinson, "Baths," 1077–78.

ment that woodland on the benefactor's property could be used by the baths (no. 241). The most intriguing method attested in the sample is that of the *duovir quinquennalis* at Misenum who arranged for four hundred wagon-loads of wood to be given to heat the baths and stipulated that the town's magistrates pass this arrangement on to their successors from year to year (no. 239).

A Roman bath was a complex structure. The combination of heat, humidity, and frequent use must have taken a heavy toll on the building's fabric. The establishment of funds for the maintenance of baths was therefore another way a benefactor could advertise his or her generosity.[72] The size and nature of the foundations vary from place to place, but usually a set sum is given, the proceeds from which could then be used to pay for the maintenance. It is noteworthy that all the funds were established as part of larger acts of benefaction, so that none is presented as a benefaction in itself. Regular maintenance, then, appears to have been an ancillary concern for benefactors. But it is also an unusual benefaction in that, of the actions we have seen so far, it is forward-looking. When the benefactors looked ahead and made provision for the future welfare of the building, they were breaking with the habitual ancient pattern of reacting to expedience. One wonders, in fact, whether they preferred buildings to fall into disrepair, so that their acts of restoration—higher profile by their very nature—would appear all the more dramatic and gratifying.

Finally, there are miscellaneous benefactions pertaining to the baths. A female *sacerdos* at Cartima gave ground for baths (no. 248), as did the generous Q. Torius Culleo at Castulo (no. 249). At Teanum Sidicinum, the local council bought a privately owned bathhouse with money collected from six *Augustales* and made it public property.[73] Finally, a benefactor at Nemus Dianae gave a quantity of lead to the "old bath," probably for the repair and maintenance of various working parts (no. 251).

The foregoing evidence illustrates the great range of possibilities that the baths offered the potential benefactor. Indeed, it is possible that the variety of euergetistic options made baths especially attractive to the benefactor looking for a way to spend money in return for social prestige. This suggestion brings us to the issue of motivation for bath benefactors.

---

72. See nos. 242–47. Note also a passage in the *Digest* (19.2.58.2) where a man furnishes baths and where one hundred coins *(nummi)* are needed specifically to repair the furnaces and pipes.

73. No. 250. Note also P. Oxy. 44.3173, 44.3176, where the baths of Arrius Apolinarius come into public ownership; see A.K. Bowman, "Public Buildings in Roman Egypt," *JRA* 5 (1992): 497 n. 10.

The Motivation of Local Benefactors

The motivation of local benefactors has been touched on at various junctures above, but the whole topic deserves fuller consideration in its own right. Very few inscriptions give clues as to why baths were built, restored, or adorned. Consonant with what we have seen about the association of bathing with healthfulness, the villagers of a Moesian community declared that they built their baths "for the sake of their bodily health" (no. 120). Popular demand for baths may be reflected in the opening lines of an inscription from Narona in Dalmatia recording that a benefactor acted "when the people asked" (no. 189); however, the reading is uncertain, since the text is fragmentary at this point. A late Imperial inscription from Interamna Lirenas is clearer when it states that "his people came to him [i.e., the benefactor] on account his kindness" (no. 141) and stimulated him to action, while another from Baetica reports that honors were paid to a benefactor "since the people demanded it" (no. 203). Popular agitation, therefore, appears to have played a role in these euergetistic transactions, but such popular requests very rarely appear in the inscriptions. When a *curator rei publicae* began, completed, and dedicated some extensions to the baths at Abbir Maius, he is said to have done so "with the enthusiasm of the people"; had they demanded he act in the first place?[74] It is possible that the silence of the inscriptions in this regard is purposeful. Benefactors would want to portray their actions more as the result of spontaneous, unsought generosity than as reactions to pressing demands. As a result, it is not possible to gauge with confidence the extent to which local magnates regularly built and maintained baths in response to popular demand, although it is certainly a plausible suggestion; if, after all, provincial communities habitually petitioned the emperor for favors by means of embassies, it is not a stretch to envision similar behavior taking place on a more local level. The only other motive for action specified in the inscriptions is the fulfillment of a religious vow. The people who pay their vows with constructional activity vary from priests (no. 77), to municipal officials (nos. 92, 103, 119), to private citizens (nos. 166, 180). There is no discernible pattern among them.

Thus general explanations must be sought for the phenomenon of bath benefaction. One factor is the symbolic role of architecture as a manifesta-

---

74. No. 133. The phrase *cum amore populi* might also mean "out of love for the people." If so, the benefactor is nonetheless said to have acted on the people's perceived needs. Note also no. 95, where a local benefactor is reported to have acted "on account of his affection for his hometown and its citizens." By way of comparison, Pliny notes (*Ep.* 6.34.2) that his friend Maximus put on a *munus* at Verona, because the people demanded he do so.

tion of the Roman state. From the second century onward, when cities all across the empire were equipping themselves with elaborate public buildings, the construction of baths was entirely natural, almost *de rigeur,* for any community with pretensions of importance.[75] When petitioning Constantine for a grant of city status, the people of Orcistus in Phrygia pointed to their baths and other public buildings as evidence of their community's worth.[76] Some inscriptions reflect the specific value of baths in this regard. Julia Memmia's impressive bath establishment at Bulla Regia is said to beautify the town, as do the baths at Oxyrhynchos.[77] The summer baths at Madaurus are reported, if the text is restored correctly, to have been "once the most splendid ornament" of that colony (no. 129). A restored bath at Antium became "a better emblem of the city" (no. 37), while the transferal of statues into the Severan *thermae* at Liternum was "for the fame of the baths" (no. 39). When a benefactor at Serdjilla in Syria built baths, he was praised for "glorifying his hometown" (no. 327). When an imperial official at Kenchela in Numidia repaired a bathhouse, he did so "for the splendor of the city and of the province" (no. 34). Conversely, the dilapidated appearance of rundown baths was a mar on the face of the city; for instance, the decrepit aqueduct that fed the baths at Thignica was "shrouded in a horrible and ugly mist and in no respect pleasing to the eye" (no. 237). It is clear from such references that baths enhanced the dignity of a city, making it almost natural that local councils and magistrates would see to their provision and maintenance.

A related motive is intercity rivalry. Neighboring communities often competed with one another in the size and splendor of their public buildings, in the honors they sought from the central authorities, and, particularly in the Greek East, in the grandiloquence of the titles they bore.[78] The construction of ever larger and more elaborate baths was quite possibly stimulated by these local rivalries. Both Pliny the Younger's description of the vast baths at

---

75. See Vitr. 1 *praef.* 1 (symbolic value of buildings). On the importance of buildings in establishing the dignity of a town, see Pliny *Ep.* 10.23.2; Dio Chrys. *Or.* 40.10. W. L. MacDonald (*The Architecture of the Roman Empire,* vol. 2 [New Haven, 1986], 253–78) has stressed the underlying uniformity of urban elements in provincial towns across the empire.

76. No. 287. In the Mishnah, bathhouses are considered one of the defining fixed features of a town (*m. B. Bat.* 4:7). Pride in a city, especially as embodied in its baths, is also reflected in such passages as Apul. *Met.* 2.19; Ael. Arist. 13.189, 15.232.

77. No. 187 (Julia Memmia); *P. Oxy.* 43.3088 (Oxyrhynchos).

78. See Ael. Arist. 23, 27.44; Dio 52.37.9–10; Dio Chrys. *Or.* 34.47–48; *Dig.* 50.10.3. See also S.R.F. Price, *Rituals and Power: The Roman Imperial Cult in Asia Minor* (Cambridge, 1984), 126–32; L. Robert, "La titulature de Nicée et de Nicomédie: La gloire et la haine," *HSCP* 81 (1977): 1–39 (= id., *Opera Minora Selecta* 6.211–49); R. Syme, "Rival Cities, Notably Tarraco and Barcino," *Ktema* 6 (1981): 271–85.

Claudiopolis and the desire of the Prusans and the Lanuvians to replace their old-fashioned baths with bigger and better facilities ought to be viewed against this background.[79] A glimpse into the motivational power of these rivalries is revealed in an inscription stipulating various benefactions to Barcino in Spain (no. 218). A local magnate left a foundation of 7,500 denarii for games and free oil in the baths, on the condition that his freedmen not be burdened with the obligations of the sevirate. He ended his bequest with a telling threat: "But if any of them [i.e., the freedmen] should be called to the duties of office, then I order that the 7,500 denarii be transferred to Tarraco [i.e., the neighboring rival community], subject to the staging of games at Tarraco of the same type as described above."

Rivalry may also have played its part in motivating local magistrates within a given community. Tenure of local offices *(honores)* carried with it an expectation of expenditure for the community from the official's personal funds *(munera)*.[80] Only a handful of our inscriptions record acts of benefaction expressly associated with office holding (*ob honorem, pro honore,* or *summae honorariae*).[81] Silence in this regard is not, of course, conclusive. Many magistrates may have acted *ob honorem* but chose not to say so in their inscriptions. Where five *sevirales* at Cures Sabini each contributed three thousand sesterces to the construction of a bathhouse, there is a valid suspicion that the figure represents a *summa honoraria,* which was a common and compulsory fee for holding local office (no. 96). Similarly, when six Augustales contributed sixty thousand sesterces to the purchase of a bathhouse at Teanum Sidicinum, the sum was probably comprised of *summae honorariae* (no. 250). In such cases, the payments were tantamount to a tax. Magistrates or their relatives could, of course, add more money beyond that required and so parade their exceptional generosity before their peers (e.g., no. 84). Such political rivalry can be considered as accounting for many bath benefactions by local officials.

On another level, the agonistic ethic among the Roman elite as a whole appears to have played its role in stimulating bath benefactions. The construction or repair of a bathhouse would have added to the prestige and prominence of an official's family in the community and would have acted as

---

79. See Pliny *Ep.* 10.23, 10.24, 10.70, 10.71 (Prusa); ibid., 10.39.5–6, 10.40.3 (Claudiopolis); no. 102 (Lanuvium).

80. The seminal work on this subject remains that of Veyne. See also, Curchin, 106–12; Duncan-Jones, *Structure,* 159–63; Jacques, *Liberté,* 687–765.

81. Nos. 55, 59, 91, 97, 102. Note also nos. 61 (money earmarked for games or building used in a bath reconstruction) and 90 (money promised for games *ob honorem quinquennalitatis* and diverted to restoring an *apodyterium*).

a manifestation of past service if and when future generations stood for local office.[82] Several joint benefactions appear to reflect this situation directly. At Burgvillos in Spain, a man who was twice *duovir* built a bathhouse, and his son, a *duovir designatus,* "gave it to the town at his own expense," which presumably means he opened the building to the locals for free (nos. 101, 212). At Furfo, a *quinquennalis* and his son and namesake, also a *quinquennalis,* built baths at their own expense (no. 70). Two texts from Intermna Lirenas are suggestive. In one, summer baths were restored, extended, and adorned by M. Sentius Crispinus, *omnibus honoribus functus,* at some indeterminate date but possibly as early as the third century (no. 118). Crispinus was apparently deceased when the council set up a statue honoring him, since it was erected "to amplify his memory." Such amplification can be imagined as having been a boon to any family members with local political aspirations who survived him, and indeed, in the early fifth century, we see another Sentius, also *omnibus honoribus functus,* restoring the building once again; a statue erected in Sentius' honor by the local authorities was expressly "for his everlasting fame" (no. 141). Both men appear to have stemmed from the same local family; it may be surmised that an earlier Sentius had built the facility in the first place. Such was the case at Paestum, where a *duovir* and *patronus coloniae* built a set of baths that his son rebuilt after a fire (nos. 108, 185). It is not unreasonable to suppose that in all these cases, the bath benefactions in earlier generations could only have helped the family's subsequent attainment of high *honores.* Illustrative is the blatant advertisement of an upcoming family member attached to a bath benefaction at Turca in Africa. A *flamen perpetuus* and *curator rei publicae* is said to have added an *apodyterium* and carried out various restorations and adornments "along with his son Magnilianus, a most distinguished and fine young man" (no. 114). Magnilianus is not credited with contributing anything to the actual work, and his inclusion in the inscription bears all the appearances of a "plug," aimed perhaps at injecting life into Magnilianus' local political career. But politics did not stand behind such mentions of family members in every case: officials also mention wives, mothers, and daughters, none of whom could hold local office, except for priesthoods (nos. 57, 58, 78, 84). In the case of wives, it is likely that they are included because they added

---

82. If one generation overspent, it could condemn descendants to relative obscurity for years to come; see Plut. *Mor.* 821F–22 (risk of overspending); Duncan-Jones, *Structure,* 170–71 (generational difficulties). This factor and the scattered survival rate of inscriptions make tracking the fortunes of prominent families in specific localities very difficult. Notable exceptions are the Lucilii Gamalae at Ostia (see Meiggs, 493–502) or the Sallii at Amiternum (see Dyson, *Community,* 231–32).

something to the prestige of their husbands, perhaps because they were members of other prominent families. If so, their appearance in the inscriptions acted as a testimonial to local political alliances.

The rhetorical tone of late Imperial epigraphy provides detailed descriptions of damage to buildings and sometimes of the work done to remedy that damage. As a result, some overtly bombastic texts that highlighted the immensity of the benefactor's efforts on the public's behalf survive. These texts echo the sort of prestige and esteem that benefactors were fishing for when they undertook bath benefactions. A *flamen* and *curator rei publicae* at Thuburbo Maius, for instance, restored baths "within the seventh month [of his year in office?], after eight whole years" (no. 127). Another *flamen* and *curator rei publicae* at Thugga repaired the atrium of the Licinian Baths, "which had been started by the ancients with the demolition of cisterns at the site"; the inscription claims that originally "the work was substandard and the foundations unsound" (no. 132). At Ocriculum two *omnibus honoribus functi* restored the winter baths "in accordance with their civic-mindedness" (no. 124). At Abbir Maius, a *principalis* and *curator rei publicae* added a pool to the baths and repaired the *soliaris,* and "he decorated the new entrances, brought to the point of perfection and beauty with statues set up alongside" (no. 133). A patron of Carthage acting at Thuburbo Maius "raised the roof of the winter baths, from the lowest levels of the foundations to the pediments."[83] The purpose of such boasts is to emphasize the outstanding civic-mindedness of the pertinent officials, no doubt in contrast to their idler rivals.

Whereas a desire to enhance the *dignitas* of the community, rivalry between neighboring towns and among leading families within towns, and the demands of local politics help explain why local authorities acted as they did, the motivation of private benefactors remains more obscure. The texts commemorating private benefactors are silent as to motivation. To be sure, some of the motives advanced above for local officials—the desires to beautify the community and to enhance the family's prestige and so heighten its profile in the community—applied here too. The construction of baths could take a long time (see no. 127), and perhaps temporary signs at the site announced the benefactor's identity while work was in progress.[84] If so, the benefactor did not have to wait for the completion of a project to enjoy the kudos of the

---

83. No. 138. By way of a parallel, note that Dunbabin (*"Baiarum Grata Voluptas,"* 33–34) cites mosaic inscriptions aimed at those who doubted that construction work on various baths could be completed.

84. See J. DeLaine, "Baths and Benefactors in Roman Italy," in Johnston and DeLaine, *Roman Baths and Bathing.*

community. Other motives could include a desire to be remembered after death and a concern to outstrip predecessors.[85] The habit of naming baths after their original builders was an excellent way of achieving both these goals (see below).

On the whole, the activities of private bath benefactors and those of most of the local officials are best explained by the concept of voluntary euergetism (as opposed to euergetism *ob honorem*). This phenomenon derived partly from an ideology of magnificence among upper classes (the benefactors) and partly from an expectation of munificence among the lower classes (the beneficiaries).[86] The system amounted to a widely held social contract, so that it appeared strange and contemptible for a wealthy family to refuse completely to benefit a community (see Plut. *Mor.* 822A). Aside from the social and euergetistic elements in motivation, more prosaic, functional stimuli may have played their part. Given the inefficient tax system and the generally poor budgetary state of most Roman communities, there was often no other source of funding for public buildings except from the pockets of the affluent. For the benefactors, public donations and acts of munificence may have been one of the few outlets open to them for disposing of surplus cash, since investment for profit on the modern model was almost unheard of.[87] The question of motivation is therefore moot but is best elucidated by the socioeconomic system of euergetism that generated so many of the empire's public buildings. Rich locals were induced to part with their money for the public good by a desire for prestige and all-important status, by local and regional rivalries, and by demands placed on them if they opted to stand for municipal office. One particularly clear sign that magistrates and local notables earned kudos from association with baths is the presence there of inscriptions and statues dedicated to them.[88]

---

85. Note again the statues erected "to amplify the memory" of one benefactor (no. 118) or for the "everlasting fame" of another (no. 141). Cicero (*Off.* 2.55) disparages games, banquets, and distributions of money and food as leaving little memory, whereas buildings leave something for posterity. See also Plut. *Mor.* 821F; Wesch-Klein, 41–46; Veyne, 272–76. Note no. 28, where a benefaction by a governor in Spain puts him "above all the other governors" *(super omnes reliquos praesides)*.

86. See Veyne, esp. 20–43. See also Duncan-Jones, *Structure,* 159–62. Apuleius (*Apol.* 87) reports that he got married some distance from town, to avoid the mobs who would show up expecting cash handouts.

87. See R. Duncan-Jones, "Wealth and Munificence in Roman Africa," *BSR* 31 (1963): 161–62.

88. The Varius Baths at Ephesos yielded dozens of inscriptional dedications to local magnates (see the relevant entries in *IK* 12 [Ephesos 2] and 13 [Ephesos 3]), as did the Forum Baths at Ostia (see P. Cicerchia and A. Marinucci, *Scavi di Ostia,* vol. 11, *Le Terme del Foro o di Gavio Massimo* [Rome, 1992], 165–228). Magistrates are identifiable among the statuary of

Ancillary Information: Named Baths and Financial Details

To close our consideration of the inscriptions, it is worthwhile to survey the ancillary information contained in the epigraphic sample. Some of the baths mentioned in the sample are given names. A common source of inspiration was the emperor himself, which does not mean that the emperor was responsible for the original construction of the facility but rather reflects the unwavering devotion of the locals to his person.[89] The people of Siga in Mauretania expressed as much when they dedicated their new baths and recorded that "the town of Siga, faithful to his [Caracalla's] spirit and majesty, [built *and/or* dedicated] the Antonine Baths" (no. 105). Likewise, a *Balineum Hadrianum* was built and dedicated to the emperor by the local council at Apamea (no. 81), while the authorities of the village of Zorava dedicated the baths they built to Severus Alexander (no. 323). Many other inscriptions in the sample implicitly link the emperor and the building by including a preamble dedicated to the ruler (e.g., nos. 83, 86, 89, 90, 92, 93, etc.). I am not arguing that emperors did not build baths and name them accordingly: the imperial baths of Rome comply with this pattern, as do the *Thermae Commodianae* at Beneventum (no. 195), which appear to have been constructed by that emperor (compare no. 10). Septimius Severus is also reported to have built the *Thermae Severianae* at Antioch (see Hieron. *Chron. sub anno* 200 [p. 212 Helm]). Rather, it is safe to conclude, first, that baths named after emperors cannot be assumed to have been the work of those emperors and, second, that communities saw their baths as buildings worthy of dedication to the imperial majesty.[90] This latter factor speaks volumes as to the prestige status of a community's bath building.

In contrast, when baths are named after private benefactors, that some actual work on the building was done by the named individual(s) seems the

---

several establishments; see, e.g., Manderscheid, *Skulpturenausstattung*, 97–98 (nos. 238–39), 108 (no. 328), 131 (no. 560). Many of the anonymous male portraits and statues found in baths probably also depict local magnates, but they do not necessarily depict people connected to the baths; see ibid., 34–35.

89. See *Balineum Hadrianum* (no. 81), *Thermae Commodianae* (no. 195), *Thermae Severianae* (no. 39), *Thermae Antoninianae* (nos. 13, 105), *Thermae Gallienianae* (no. 111), *Thermae Licinianae* (no. 132), *Balneum Aurelianum* (no. 112), *Thermae Constantianae* (nos. 29, 126), *Thermae Gratianae* (no. 135). See also the Σεβαστὸν βαλανεῖον (no. 304); Διοκλητιανὸν βαλάνιον (*AE* 1932.79 [Palmyra]), τὸ βαλανεῖον τοῦ / τῶν Σεβαστου / ῶν (*IGRR* 4.1519 [Sardis]; *SEG* 27 [1977] 746 [Ephesos]). Note also that in at least two cases, statues of emperors are reported to have been erected in baths; see nos. 86 and 132.

90. Imperial visits appear to have occasioned dedications of local facilities to emperors; see Farrington, *Roman Baths of Lycia*, 27, 54–56.

most likely explanation.[91] In these instances, the original builder is the most probable source of the name, as when an Avelius donated to Corfinium a women's bath aptly named the *Balneum Avelianum* (no. 88) or when a Pacatus at Cirta constructed the *Balineum Pacatianum* (no. 186). Joint benefactions could also be enshrined in a facility's name, as in the case of the *Thermae Cassiorum* at Olisipo in Spain (no. 122). For the most part, the social status of the eponymous benefactors is unknowable, with the notable exceptions of the praetorian prefect M. Gavius Maximus (no. 22) or Corfinium's local patron Avelius (no. 88). The erection of a building that would bear the family's name must have been a particularly appealing incentive for the prestige-minded local benefactor to construct baths.

Gods also provided names for baths, possibly stemming from decorative features peculiar to the structure, or possibly deriving from some special association of the building with the deity. Several baths in Rome follow this pattern (see appendix 2), and a further three that can be added from the sample are the *Thermae Herculis* at Allifae (no. 32), the *Thermae Silvani* at Saepinum (no. 33), and the *Balneum Veneris* at Liternum (no. 43). We have seen already that Hercules and Venus are two of the deities most commonly associated with baths in general (above, chapter 4, p. 89 [Venus], chapter 5, p. 121 [Hercules]), making the naming of an entire establishment after them particularly apt. Similarly, the healthful and imperial associations of Apollo and Serapis may have prompted the naming of a bathhouse at Smyrna (no. 302).

There are also baths named for some other reason, such as the *Thermae Maritimae* at Ostia (no. 19), the *Balneae Novae* at Paestum (no. 108), the *Balneum Novum* at Baetulo (no. 267), or the *Thermae Iuventianae* at Verona (no. 23). The last name may indicate that the baths were designed for use by the youth *(iuventus)* of the city, as was common for baths and gymnasia in the Greek East (e.g., no. 292), but this conclusion is a tenuous one to draw from a name alone. The name could just as easily have been designed to make the facility more attractive by advertising the freshness and vitality of the baths and/or by laying claim to a certain set of customers. It is interesting that, in contrast to these "Baths for the Young," there is no corresponding mention in the Latin texts of "Baths for the Old," such as is found in the Greek East (e.g., those implicit in no. 297). A more solid reflection of Greek influence is found in the title of the *Thermae Pentascinenses* at Tarentum (no.

---

91. *Thermae Gav(i) Maximi* (no. 22), *Thermae Montanae* (no. 28), *Thermae Sabinianae* (no. 31), *Balneum Avelianum* (no. 88), *Thermae Cassiorum* (no. 122), *Thermae Noviani* (no. 125), *Thermae Tusciani* (no. 139), *Balneum Terenti Donati* (no. 148/49), *Balinea Sergium et Putinium* (no. 168/69), *Balneum Pacatianum* (no. 186). Note also a *Thermae Urbanae* at Patavium (no. 284), although here it is not clear that the baths were named after a person.

238). These "Baths of the Five Stages *or* Five Drawings" were apparently named after some decorative feature of the building.[92]

Finally, we turn to the financial information included in some inscriptions. The subject of bath costs has been treated in other studies,[93] so there is no need to review it in detail here. It has already been noted that most financial information in the inscriptions is vaguely expressed in such formulae as "at his own expense," "with public money," and so on. Occasionally, however, more details are provided that give some idea of the expense of constructing and maintaining baths. For instance, Hadrian promised 2,000,000 sesterces to Ostia for the construction of the Baths of Neptune, and Antoninus Pius completed the task, "having added all the extra money required" (no. 6). The final cost of the baths was therefore more than the original 2,000,000 sesterces.[94] The emperor's involvement makes this case special, and it cannot be taken as typical for bath costs. Nevertheless, the extraordinary expense of this building provides a caliber against which the astronomical cost of the much larger imperial *thermae* can be gauged.[95] The next highest specified outlay in the epigraphic sample is the huge donation by an anonymous

----

92. The text is not skillfully carved and caution is required in interpreting it. Nevertheless, the name of the building appears derived from a Latinized compound of πεντάς (meaning "five") and a root drawn from σκηνή (equivalent to the Lain *scaena*) or σκιά (in the sense of "drawing"). If the former, the reference may be to a columnar display, of the sort commonly found in Greco-Roman cities and not unknown in baths (although more usually those located in the Greek East): see MacDonald, *Architecture of the Roman Empire*, 2.183–220; Yegül, 422–23. If the epithet means "Five Drawings/Etchings" a possible parallel is provided by the vestibule of the Baths of the Seven Sages in Ostia, which is adorned with depictions of famous Greek philosophers dispensing advice on bowel movements: see G. Calza, "Die Taverne der Sieben Weisen in Ostia," *Die Antike* 15 (1939): 99–115; Meiggs, 417–19, 429; Nielsen, 2.5 (C.22); Pavolini, *Ostia*, 135. However, neither of these suggestions can be confirmed, since the remains of the *Thermae Pentascinenses* are not particularly informative; see E. Lippolis, "Le Thermae Pentascinenses di Taranto," *Taras* 4 (1984): 119–53.

93. The fullest study is Meusel, *Verwaltung und Finanzierung*. For more general assessments, see Nielsen, 1.122–25; Yegül, 43–46.

94. In Duncan-Jones' list of Italian prices (*Economy*, 156–237), this final cost is the single most expensive construction cost (see ibid., 124–26). Indeed, it is noteworthy that of the fourteen building costs assignable to a specific type of structure, baths account for six; see ibid., 157 (nos. 439–51). Perhaps, being so large, the outlays for baths were thought especially worthy of specific mention.

95. Janet DeLaine investigates the construction costs associated with the Thermae of Caracalla in some detail in her study of the building; see DeLaine, *Baths of Caracalla*, 207–24. According to her estimates, which are admittedly speculative and are expressed in *kastrenses modii* of wheat, the *thermae* cost twelve million *kastrenses modii* (for the central block alone) or fourteen million *kastrenses modii* (with the precinct included). Since she implies (220–23) that one *kastrensis modius* is equivalent to about 10 sesterces, the cost of the central block alone can be estimated at 120 million sesterces, which is ca. 60 times the stated cost of the Baths of Neptune. (My thanks to Dr. DeLaine for sending me a prepublication copy of the relevant text.)

benefactor to the baths at Altinum, totaling 1,400,000 sesterces (no. 168/69). This amount was given to the town for expenditure on two bathing facilities, in specified amounts for various tasks: 800,000 for repair, 400,000 for heating, and 200,000 for upkeep.

It is all but certain that Pliny's bequest to Comum included a sum for the construction of baths, but the precise figure is lost on the stone (no. 171). By way of comparison, a consular benefactor bequeathed 330,000 sesterces for the construction of baths at Tarquinii (no. 176), and an estimate for a bath to be built by Fronto totaled 300,000 sesterces (see Gell. *NA* 19.10.1–4). These must have been modest establishments, since Pliny the Younger spent 300,000 alone in decorating the baths at Comum (no. 171). Without knowledge of the relative size and grandeur of these facilities, it is impossible to estimate Pliny's construction cost, but the large bequest for the decoration suggests it was not inconsiderable. A benefactor at Epamanduodurum in Germany left the same amount for marbling the baths there (no. 178), suggesting that decoration accounted for one of the chief expenses in providing baths.[96] This possibility seems confirmed by the high cost of a *labrum* alone at Pompeii (no. 68) and by the financially detailed inscription from Corfinium in which a bath that had been built and roofed at an unspecified cost required a further 252,000 (or 103,000) sesterces to bring it to completion (no. 174). Given that the building was structurally complete, the extra expenditure must have been applied primarily to its decoration. A bath restoration by a senator at Novaria consumed two years and an unspecified amount of money but required a further 200,000 sesterces bequeathed in his wife's will before reaching completion (no. 84). Another type of attested expenditure is the contribution of funds toward the expense of a bath project, but in quantities insufficient to cover the entire cost. At Lanuvium, two local officials contributed 15,000 sesterces toward the restoration of a bath (no. 91), five *sevirales* spent 3,000 sesterces each on a bath restoration at Cures Sabini (no. 96), and a benefactor at Tifernum Tiberinum left 150,000 sesterces in his will for the construction of a bath (no. 177). The latter may be a complete bath cost, if the facility was modest in size and appointment. Also, an unspecified number of decurions contributed 41,200 sesterces for the addition

---

96. A decorative element—sculpture—has been proposed as among the most costly element in the construction of baths; see Marvin, "Freestanding Sculptures," 380–81. Janet DeLaine describes the decoration of the Thermae of Caracalla and estimates its cost, see *Baths of Caracalla*, 24–37, 69–84 (description), 217–18 (cost). She concludes that the greatest costs in the erection of the building lay in materials and transport. Decoration, in her estimate, accounted for some 29 percent of the total cost of the structure, which is still a significant proportion.

of a *musaeum* to the baths at Thibursicum Bure in Africa (no. 111). Again, this may be a complete cost for this room.

This review of bath benefactions and their agents has shown the dominance of local sources of euergetism in providing baths, as well as other amenities, for the use of the common people of the Roman empire. The central authorities played a minor role in this regard and tended to remain largely aloof and removed from the experience of the average inhabitant of the empire. Occasionally, the emperor or his representative might benefit a community, but by and large the local authorities and private magnates built and maintained the empire's baths. The importance of the cities in defining the empire's civilization is thereby reinforced insofar as the decurions and local luminaries, as landowners and so theoretically agriculturists, often spent their money in beautifying the towns and cities in whose locale they lived. Baths, a defining feature of urban living (see nos. 182 [?], 254, 256, 259), were among the most prominent and heavily frequented structures in those towns and so were well worthy of the local benefactor's attention. It remains a moot point to what extent the widespread popularity and essentially functional nature of baths proved especially attractive for the potential benefactor; certainly, when benefiting a community's bathhouse, the euergete had available a greater variety of possibilities than was the case with many public buildings. The building or the bathers could be the target of liberality. In either case, the outcome was usually the same—the erection by the grateful beneficiaries of an inscription honoring the benefactor. Surviving examples of such inscriptions have proven a valuable source of evidence for the operation of local euergetism and for the vitality of public bathing culture in the myriad towns and communities of Italy and the provinces.

Chapter 7

The Physical Environment: Splendor and Squalor

Visiting the baths could be a pleasurable experience, and much ancient testimony attests to this fact. Literary descriptions of baths focus on their splendor and magnificence. The Baths of Hippias, according to Lucian, were a paradigm of comfort, brightly lit throughout, adorned with marbles from Phrygia and Numidia, and inscribed with citations from Pindar (*Hipp.* 4–8). The opulence of the Thermulae (or Balneum) of Etruscus at Rome, commented on by Martial and Statius, has already been alluded to on several occasions.[1] Statius, in fact, provides the more glowing description of the two, placing his emphasis on the sumptuous decoration, including various marbles of foreign origin, bronze and silver fittings, and fine mosaics (*Silv.* 1.5). Similarly, Pliny's descriptions of the fine baths at his Laurentine and Tuscan villas reinforce further the general impression of bath-related grandeur and indicate what an upper-class Roman expected of a bathing establishment.[2] Late Imperial epigrams often praise the physical beauty and luxury of the baths, and appreciation of such beauty appears to have been one of the principal joys of bathing at its best.[3] Such pleasures find further corroboration in the negative reaction to them voiced by certain authors, such as Seneca or Pliny the Elder, as they deplore the luxury that they claim contemporary bathers expected of the baths (see above, chapter 2, pp. 51–52). Literary sources also describe the bathing excesses of certain emperors (usually those emperors characterized as "bad"), and these descriptions, whether historically accurate or not, contribute to the overall impression of bathing

---

1. See above, chapter 1, pp. 16–17, 19–20.

2. Pliny *Ep.* 2.17.11 (Laurentine Villa), 5.6.25–27 (Tuscan villa). It is interesting to compare the pleasure Pliny takes in his fine baths to that of the fifth-century bishop Sidonius Apollinaris, who, out of a Christian modesty entirely lacking in Pliny, is keen to stress the simplicity and lack of ostentation in his establishment, but who, just like Pliny, wishes nevertheless to vaunt the pleasures that await its users; see Sid. Apoll. *Ep.* 2.2.4–10.

3. See Dunbabin, *"Baiarum Grata Voluptas,"* 8–10, 12–32.

luxury.[4] The private Baths of Pompeianus attached to a villa near Cuicul in Numidia provide a good example of the refinement and sophistication often associated with Roman bathing establishments, in both their architecture and their decoration. One heated room features mosaics of gardens, buildings, and two human figures and carries the inscription "The place of the philosopher."[5] In this label may lie an echo of the worthwhile and high-class *otium* that was passed by Pompeianus and his guests, if not in this specific room, then at least in the establishment.

Inscriptions also bear witness to the fine physical environment found at the baths. Mention of baths or parts of baths built or restored "with every refinement" *(omni cultu)* are frequent, and occasionally more specific details of grand adornment with marbles and other decorative features are provided.[6] Some inscriptions advertise the fine facilities and comfort of certain bathhouses, such as the well-known *Balneum Venerium et Nongentum* of Julia Felix at Pompeii. Typical is the claim *Lavatur more urbico,* meaning that one can bathe at a particular location in comfort like that in the city; on occasion a supplementary claim is found, such as *Omnia commoda praestantur,* which advertised the full range of conveniences offered in the facility.[7] There are also inscriptions that expressly say that baths served the public

4. To take just some examples: Caligula is said to have perfumed his bath water (see Suet. *Calig.* 37.1), a practice that Pliny the Elder (*HN* 13.22) reports was imitated by people of private station. Poppaea Sabina, the wife of Nero, is reported to have bathed in ass' milk (see Pliny *HN* 11.238). The bathing excesses of Heliogabalus are a frequent feature of his biography in the *Historia Augusta:* see, e.g., HA *Heliogab.* 8.6, 19.8, 21.6, 23.7, 25.6, 30.5, 30.7, 31.7; but note the reservations of Merten (114–31, esp. 117–20) about the veracity of these and other imperial bath-excess stories in the *Historia Augusta.*

5. *CIL* 8.10890: *filosofi lolocus (sic).* MacMullen (*Roman Social Relations,* 80) is surely mistaken in asserting that this inscription shows that the room was reserved for a philosophers' club, since the mosaic also makes mention of "the place of the cow-herd" *(pecuari locus)* and the "hunting enclosure" *(septum venationis).* These inscriptions, then, act as labels for elements in the mosaic and are not likely to mean that the room was also reserved for cattle-herders and hunters. For the remains of this fine building, see Yegül, 249.

6. See, e.g., nos. 10, 14, 18, 20, 29, 83, 97, 100, 110, 111, 116, 118 121, 127–29, 159, 163 (*omni cultu, cum ornamentis,* and variants). For more detailed decorative elements, see nos. 27, 39, 115 (statues moved into baths for their splendor); 34 (baths as a splendor of the city and the province); 51, 58, 79, 143, 196 (marbles); 59 (various decorative elements added); 71 (portico, pool, and statue of Cupid); 86 (statue of the emperor and Numidian marble); 90 (marbles, columns, statues); 114 (marble statues, paintings, and columns); 117 (Numidian marble and mosaics); 121 (beauty of baths restored with porticoes and statues); 124 (baths restored to a higher degree of beauty); 131 (colored marbles and mosaics); 132 (statue of the emperor); 133 (beauty effected by statuary); 142 (statues); 151 (colored stone, bronze *labrum,* and seats); 294 (columns). Note also *CIL* 6.1130 = *ILS* 646 (*thermas . . . omni cultu perfectas*).

7. See no. 258 *(Balneum Venerium)*; 182(?), 254, 256, 259 *(more urbico).* Note also *CIL* 8.20579, where a *balneum Cy[—] | more prep[—]* is mentioned, the phrase probably advertising the comfort of the facilities. A bath at Patavium was called *Thermae Urbanae* (no. 284). The

good or comfort.[8] One inscription mentions a museum attached to a set of baths, where works of art could be displayed, and where discussions and lectures would take place.[9]

Finally, the physical remains of the baths themselves offer corroboration for the picture of magnificence gained from the written material. This is especially the case with the imperial establishments at Rome, lavish not only in scale but in decoration.[10] The huge shells of the imperial *thermae* still standing in Rome effectively convey their enormous size, but little remains of the decorative skin that once enhanced these buildings. Finds from the Thermae of Caracalla, for instance, reveal that in ancient times the interior was adorned with such opulence as to be virtually unimaginable to the modern visitor confronted only with the exposed brick-and-concrete core. In its original state, the building contained dozens of columns in varying sizes, fashioned from marble and other stones imported from all over the empire. The floors and walls were covered with stone and marble paneling in at least ten different colors, and some floors were decorated with mosaics, both polychrome and black-and-white. There is evidence for brightly painted stucco, and on the vaulting of the roof glittered glass mosaics made from *tesserae* in seven striking colors and some clear *tesserae,* which presumably were painted or gilded. Over one hundred niches for statues have been identified in the building, and there were additional freestanding pieces situated throughout the complex. Many of the statues were colossi, including such famous pieces as the Farnese Bull and the Weary Hercules. In their original state, all the statues would have been brightly painted, and some would have been gilded. Indeed, it is possible that many of the carved elements in the building—column capitals, statues, and friezes—were gilded. The establishment would also have been fitted with numerous bronze and copper elements, including the remarkable lattice singled out for mention in the *Historia Augusta* (*M. Ant.* 9.4–5). The exterior, especially the north facade, where the main entrances were located, was similarly impressive, with niches for fountains and statues and with doorways framed by granite columns and carved entablatures. At the south end, the whole upper portion

---

adjective *urbicus* probably refers specifically to *the* city, i.e., Rome; see *OLD, s.v.*

8. E.g., nos. 120, 159, 187, 226. The public good is also implied in such texts as nos. 37, 133, 135, and 189.

9. No. 111. See *RE* 16.797–821, s.v. "Museion" (Müller-Graupa).

10. See Dunbabin, *"Baiarum Grata Voluptas,"* for the ideal of the pleasurable bath and its manifestation in bath decoration. Sculpture was a particularly luxurious (and expensive) element of bath decoration: see Manderscheid, *Skulpturenausstattung;* Marvin, "Freestanding Sculptures."

of the facade was covered with glass mosaic.[11] The Thermae of Caracalla, then, must have been a stunning sight, both inside and out. Admittedly, these baths were exceptionally luxurious, since they were the work of the emperor and his practically limitless resources. But excavations of baths all over the empire habitually turn up evidence of marble paneling, mosaics, painted stucco, and statuary. Public baths appear to have been places where a high degree of decorative opulence was expected. It is not surprising that many modern commentators, inspired by such evidence as this, have presented the baths as palaces of hygiene, towering testaments to the Roman appreciation of beauty, cleanliness, and good order.[12]

Another side to the bathing experience is traceable through the written and archaeological evidence and is somewhat less salubrious. We have seen that Rome featured baths that were not so pleasant to visit, for example, those of Gryllus and Lupus denigrated by Martial or the simple *balneum* that has been excavated near the Palatine Hill.[13] Many of the empire's *balnea*, on the model of these buildings, were no doubt far from magnificent (see, e.g., Ath. 8.351c). A small corner-bath depicted on a fragment of the *Forma Urbis* near the Horrea Lolliana may well be representative.[14] It is hemmed in on all sides by streets, a laneway, and shops, and its rooms are many but small. It has an odd-shaped exercise ground with a cramped-looking peristyle tucked away at one end. Pompeii offers some surviving examples for comparison. Besides the main showcase facilities (the Stabian Baths, the Forum Baths, and especially the up-to-date Central Baths), there were the splendid baths in the Premises of Julia Felix, privately owned and finely appointed. These facilities may be of a sort similar to the Baths of Etruscus at Rome. The Sarno Baths at Pompeii, however, no matter what their planned final appearance, were approached directly from the street via a long and dingy corridor (see fig. 21A). The Palaestra Baths were somewhat larger than the Sarno complex and were in use when the city's volcanic disaster struck, but they were modestly

---

11. On the physical remains of the Thermae of Caracalla, see DeLaine, *Baths of Caracalla,* 69–84; Marvin "Freestanding Sculptures." See above, chapter 5 n. 36, for a fuller bibliography.

12. See Lord Amulree, "Hygienic Conditions in Ancient Rome and Modern London," *Medical History* 17 (1973): 244–55; Carcopino, *Daily Life,* 277; Scarborough, 78–80; Yegül, 31–32.

13. See above, chapter 1, pp. 20–21 (Martial); chapter 2, n. 4 (Palatine bath).

14. See *FUR* fr. 25. For the identification of the complex as a bathhouse, see R.A. Staccioli, "Terme minori e balnea nella documentazione della 'Forma Urbis,'" *ArchClass* 13 (1961): 92–102. The utilitarian nature of the surrounding buildings has been used to suggest that this facility served mainly workers; see Yegül, 66. On the difficulty of deducing clientele from siting alone, see above chapter 5, n. 50.

decorated with a wooden colonnade on a stone stylobate—hardly a paradigm of magnificence.

These baths are all of a type. If Roman communities featured less inviting baths alongside their finer ones, could not the discerning bather simply avoid the latter and bathe amid the splendor of the more refined establishments? In this regard, the sources present hints of physical conditions, apparently fairly common, that the modern bather would find unacceptably unpleasant but that the Romans appear to have tolerated as a matter of course. Unfortunately, the very nonchalance of the sources about these conditions has had the effect of reducing the volume of pertinent references to them, so that what is available is largely allusive and indirect in nature; but the clues are there to be found, nonetheless.

Some inscriptions record that baths were repaired after they had fallen into a state of rather advanced decay. When the council at Lanuvium built a set of *thermae* to replace the older *balneae,* they did so because the latter "through old age had ceased to be used"; and at Antium the baths had deteriorated into such a hazardous condition that the people were afraid to use them.[15] In these cases, it seems that either inutility or outright danger was required to deter bathers and stimulate repair. Most inscriptions, however, do not mention the virtual abandonment of the baths but simply record the various states of decline that preceded restoration.[16] Even if we factor in the formulaic nature of epigraphic language, it seems that baths, initially of splendid appearance, could present a far from magnificent aspect after some years of operation. This deterioration is only natural. The daily use of these buildings by an eager public, their habitually elaborate decoration, and their sustained exposure to combined heat and humidity must have ensured that dilapidation crept in quickly. An obvious conclusion is that bath maintenance was not always the best; but a converse, and reasonable, inference is that Roman baths must regularly have been operating under less-than-perfect conditions. Indeed, many of the facilities recorded as having been renovated seem to have been frequented right up to the moment of restoration. Several inscriptions comment that the baths had been in a poor condition for some time before the repair work was carried out; presumably they were still in use over this period. Other texts celebrate the return of the bathhouse to its "original appearance" (*ad pristinam faciem* and variants),

---

15. Nos. 102 (Lanuvium), 37 (Antium). For other cases where baths or elements thereof had become unusable, see nos. 35, 113, 125, 135, 140, 237.

16. There are many such inscriptions employing various phrases to describe the dilapidated condition of the baths, *vetustate conlapsae/corruptae* (and variants) being the most frequent; see e.g., nos. 7, 11, 33, 50, 53, 77, 95, 116, 118, 123, 126, 129, 131–33, 141, 189, 192.

which suggests that the public had grown accustomed to its rundown aspect.[17] In such cases as these, then, the baths would have presented to the everyday user an appearance far short of dazzling beauty, even if they had been an impressive sight on completion of their initial construction (see no. 129). The converse was also possible. A bath at Corfinium appears to have been built, opened, and dedicated despite requiring considerably more work to complete (nos. 173, 174). Naturally, the evidence precludes quantification of how many baths in a given community would have presented a rundown appearance and how many were in the full bloom of their splendor. But given the considerations of use and circumstance mentioned above, many baths across the empire must have been at least in an undesirable state for much of their operative lives, if not actually "collapsed with old age" (*vetustate conlapsae*). In fact, it is noticeable that the literary eulogies of baths tend to focus much of their attention on the fineness of the decorative elements in the building. Perhaps they do so precisely because so many baths operated in a substandard condition and because the authors are, in effect, highlighting the well-maintained quality of the facilities they are praising, as a contrast to the more widely encountered circumstance of rundown or substandard operating conditions.

There are hints in the sources, however, that general conditions even in well-maintained and finely appointed buildings may well have fallen far short of modern hygienic expectations. The water quality, for instance, seems to have left a lot to be desired. While Seneca claims that the bathers of his day were very fussy about water purity, Frontinus reports that in the Republican period the baths of Rome used runoff water from public troughs.[18] Elsewhere Frontinus says that until the reign of Nerva, the city endured muddy water after heavy rains, and that when he became *curator aquarum* in 97, he found that many watermen *(aquarii)* were mixing the waters of the different aqueducts, producing a substandard quality for all—although this probably affected drinking water more than that used for bathing.[19] A fragmentary inscription from Africa apparently records the improvement of the water supply to the *solium* (a heated communal pool) in a set of summer baths, by drawing it from a pure source; the implication is that previously the water

---

17. Long period of disrepair: nos. 14, 17, 43, 95, 127, 179. *Ad pristinam faciem:* nos. 11, 17, 26, 43, 136, 143, 179. Presumably, baths damaged or destroyed by fire (see nos. 8, 16, 74, 87, 185), earthquake (see nos. 13[?], 18, 32, 69), flooding (see nos. 9[?], 110), or other forms of violence were not in use when they were repaired; see also nos. 5 and 195 (war), 106 (bad foundations), 156 (overgrown with thornbushes), 325 (structural instability).

18. Sen. *Ep.* 86.9; Frontin. *Aq.* 94.3–4.

19. Frontin. *Aq.* 89.3 (muddy water), 91.3–5 *(aquarii).* See also Ath. 8.351e.

had not been entirely clean.[20] Whatever the quality of the water was as it entered the bathhouse, the Roman habit of immersion in communal pools—one of the defining features of their bathing practices—should cause some concern as to water quality in these pools. Celsus, for instance, warns that one of the worst things to do for a fresh wound that has not been fully cleaned is go to the baths, "for this renders the wound both wet and dirty, which normally results in gangrene"[21]—a piece of advice that adopts a suspicious attitude toward the water quality in the baths. Martial provides evidence that, similar to so many of the details he offers about life at the baths, makes no bones about the dangers of life in the communal *solium*.

Zoile, quod solium subluto podice perdis,
　　spurcius ut fiat, Zoile, merge caput.

(2.42)

[Zoilus, you spoil the *solium* washing your arse. To make it filthier, Zoilus, stick your head in it. (trans. adapted)]

Non vis in solio prius lavari
quemquam, Cotile: causa quae, nisi haec est,
undis ne fovearis irrumatis?
primus te licet abluas, necesse est
ante hic mentula quam caput lavetur.

(2.70)

[You don't like anyone to wash in the *solium* before yourself, Cotilus. What is the reason except that you would rather not be laved by irrumated water? But though you are the first in the bath, it needs must be that your cock is washed here before your head. (trans. adapted)]

Iratus tamquam populo, Charideme, lavaris:
　　inguina sic toto subluis in solio.
nec caput hic vellem sic te, Charideme, lavare.
　　et caput ecce lavas: inguina malo laves.

(6.81)

---

20. No. 233. See also nos. 230 and 238 for records of a poor water supply. On the *solium*, see A. Maiuri, "Significato e natura del *solium* nelle terme romane," *PP* 5 (1950): 223–27; Nielsen, 1.157, s.v. "solium."

21. Celsus 5.26.28d: *balneum quoque, dum parum vulnus purum est, inter res infestissimas est: nam id et umidum et sordidum reddit, ex quibus cancrum transitus esse consuevit.*

[You bathe as though you were angry with the public, Charidemus, washing your groin all over the *solium*. I wouldn't have you wash your head here like that, Charidemus. There now, you're washing your head. I'd sooner you washed your groin. (trans. adapted)]

All of these passages take it for granted that the water in the *solium* will be dirty or at least that it is previously used by other bathers—the jokes are on what part of the bathers' anatomy is the filthiest. When Martial refers to bathers entering the tubs caked in ointments or mud,[22] the state of the water in many baths becomes even more dubious. Bear in mind that the Romans had no chemicals to maintain water cleanliness, and we have no idea how often the water in the baths was changed.[23] That it was one of the duties of aediles to inspect the public baths and enforce cleanliness shows that the ancients expected corners to be cut in this regard by the baths' owners and managers.[24] To be sure, many pools enjoyed a constant supply of running water that generated an overflow onto the bathroom floor. Such overflow could have restricted the reproductive opportunities for some microbes and, over time, would also have replaced the water in the pools. Short of torrential currents, however, the water in communal pools could not have been re-

---

22. Mart. 3.3, 6.93, 11.47 (caked bathers). Note that in the schoolbooks, the bathing children are anointed before entering the *solium* and only strigiled after the immersion in water is over: see *CGL* 3.652.10 *(colloquia Monacensia)*, 3.657.16 *(colloquium Montepessulanum);* Dionisotti, "From Ausonius's Schooldays?" 102–3 (§§56–61).

23. There is no ancient evidence. Farrington *(Roman Baths of Lycia,* 108) tentatively estimates the frequency of water changes in the cistern-fed baths at Rhodiapolis at once every week or twice every three weeks, if the baths operated year-round. But he doubts his own conclusions, on the basis that such conditions would have been unacceptable to bathers "used to such high standards of cleanliness." In truth, however, we do not have to suppose that Lycian (or Roman) standards of cleanliness were particularly high. Today, disinfection is regarded as vital to the maintenance of public swimming pools, especially given the variety and virulence of the microorganisms that thrive in untreated bodies of standing water; see F.V. Kroeber, *Public Swimming Pools: A Manual of Operation* (New York, 1976), 82–118 (disinfection), 153–80 (viruses and bacteria). In the Japanese public bath and the Tunisian *hammam,* washing is done from buckets of water drawn from the communal heated pool, thus maintaining water cleanliness in the pool itself (see Grilli and Levy, *Furo,* 100), but there is no evidence for analogous practices among the Romans.

24. See Sen. *Ep.* 86.10 and *Dial.* 7.7.3. Seneca portrays inspection as the job of "the most noble aediles" of the past—the context mentions Cato, Fabius Maximus, and the Cornelii—but there is no reason to suppose that the duty did not continue into the Principate. Indeed, some inscriptions from the provinces—e.g., the *lex Irnitana (AE* 1986.333.XIX; see also J. Gonzalez, "The *Lex Irnitana:* A New Copy of the Flavian Municipal Law," *JRS* 76 [1986]: 147–243)— show that aediles in local municipalities were still in charge of conditions at the baths in the Flavian period, while Plutarch suggests the continuance of this duty into the second century (see below, chapter 7, n. 29). See also Curchin, 61–63. Note that the actual work of cleaning baths appears to have been carried out by criminals used as public servants; see Pliny *Ep.* 10.32.2.

placed sufficiently quickly to preclude the accumulation of grime from the circulating visitors, especially at peak hours of use—hence the comments in the sources about not-so-clean water in bathtubs used by multiple bathers.

The sources blithely accept a situation that perhaps raises the most unpleasant implications for water quality in Roman baths: the bathing together of the ill and the healthy. This practice could only have contributed further to poor water quality in communal pools. We have seen already the major role that baths played in Roman preventive and remedial medicine (see chapter 4). When a medical writer like Celsus recommends a bath for treating an illness, as he does frequently, where was the patient to go? For the majority of ailing Romans, the only option would have been a trip to the nearest public facility. The wealthier patient might indeed enjoy the privilege of treatment in his own bathing suite, but in the absence of hospitals and separate bathing establishments for the sick, we must assume that public baths would have been the resort of the majority.[25]

There is positive testimony to this effect. Martial comments how Laetinus' fever accompanied him everywhere he went, including to the baths (12.17.1– 3). Fabianus, another character in the *Epigrams,* used to deride the ruptured, until he looked at himself in the Thermae of Nero (12.83). Both quips seem to assume that the sight of ill people at the baths was not uncommon. The impressive litany of Heliogabalus' perversions as documented by the *Historia Augusta* includes a proclivity for bathing with hernia victims in the palace baths, having first picked out his guests from the city's public establishments (*Heliogab.* 25.6). Perhaps the most famous evidence for the sick bathing with the healthy is the report, also in the *Historia Augusta,* that Hadrian reserved certain hours in the public baths for the use of the ill (*Hadr.* 22.7). If we assume that the report is not an invention of the author, it suggests that prior to Hadrian's ruling, the sick and healthy had bathed simultaneously as a matter of course. Several features of the notice merit comment. First, it is not clear how far-reaching the measure was, but if it was applied in the provinces, we find no sign of it there. Examples do survive of inscriptions, one of Hadrianic date, assigning specific bathing hours for men and women, but no texts mention a similar segregation of the sick and the healthy.[26] Second,

---

25. This aspect of the bathing experience is emphasized by Scobie in "Slums, Sanitation, and Mortality," 425–27. A sixth-century inscription from Scythopolis in Palestine records the benefaction by a local bishop, Theodorus, of a special bath for lepers; see M. Avi-Yonah, "The Bath of the Lepers at Scythopolis," *IEJ* 13 (1963): 325–26. Lepers, however, were something of a special case; other Byzantine sources make it clear that most ailments would be treated at public baths: see Magoulias, "Bathhouse, Inn, Tavern," 234–35.

26. The Hadrianic text is the *lex Metalli Vipascensis* (no. 282); see also *SEG* 26 (1976/77) 1043/44 (first century, at the earliest).

even if the regulation was restricted to Rome, it is unclear whether it applied equally to all the baths in the city, which would have presented considerable difficulties of enforcement. It is more likely that only the imperially controlled *thermae* were affected, since they were the emperor's administrative concern. Third, there is no way of knowing what motivated Hadrian to take this measure. We cannot assume that it was for reasons of public health. No Roman medical writer, either before or after Hadrian, expressly warns against bathing with the ill.[27] Perhaps Hadrian was motivated by a desire to keep people with often unsightly illnesses out of the public eye or to prevent them from sullying the golden image of the imperial baths. Alternatively, he may have wished to close the baths to the able-bodied but lazy, who should have been at work until the seventh or eighth hour (which was about midday).[28] Finally, we do not know how effective the measure was. Did the sick and healthy really not bathe together in post-Hadrianic Rome? The notice in the *Historia Augusta* about ruptured people in the public baths of Heliogabalus' Rome suggests that they did.

It seems from the available evidence, as well as from general considerations, that it would have been normal to find people with all kinds of illnesses frequenting the public baths of a Roman community. Exhortations in medical treatises to use baths as remedies for illness would only have added to their numbers. Typical, and especially repulsive, are the assumptions behind Scribonius Largus' observations on the qualities of different plasters.

Emplastrum coloris incerti facit ad omnia mediocria vulnera, quadrupedum morsus, contusa vel incisa articulamenta, ut fit, cum ad dentem pervenit pugnus. eadem ad furunculos mire facit et strumas omnemque duritiem discutit, si quis perseveranter eam imponat. eadem cicatricem ducit diutini ulceris et in totum ad omnia levia in quotidianos usus mirifica est: tumorem non patitur fieri neque pus;

27. Contrast, for instance, the injunctions of medieval writers to avoid public baths for fear of contracting the plague. For example, G. Bunel writes (1513), "Steam-baths and bath-houses, I beg you, flee them or you will die" (cited in Vigarello, *Concepts of Cleanliness,* 8). It is probable that the Romans, unaware of the existence of germs, conceptualized the microbiological hazards of bathing in divine terms, as demons, the evil eye, and so on (see Dunbabin, *"Baiarum Grata Voluptas,"* 35–37). It still remains the case, however, that no source expressly makes a connection between public bathing and falling ill (except where people abuse the baths, by drinking in them, eating too much before or after bathing, etc.: see, e.g., Juv. 1.140–46; Pliny *HN* 7.183; Plut. *Mor.* 124C).

28. For Roman working hours, see above, chapter 1, p. 22; see below, chapter 8, pp. 210–11.

haeret, ut fascia non sit opus; in balineo non excidet. (Scribonius Largus 214)

[A plaster of indistinct color is useful for all moderate wounds, animal bites, and contusions or cuts on joints, as when teeth are punched in. Likewise it is remarkably helpful for boils and swellings of the lymphatic glands, completely dissipating hardness as long as it is used for some time. It also draws fluids off long-term ulcer scars and is generally wonderfully good for all sorts of light tasks in daily usage: it doesn't allow tumors or pus to develop; it sticks, so that bandages are unnecessary; and it will not fall off in the bath.]

Noteworthy in the passage is the remarkably casual manner in which Largus comments on the plaster's ability to stay on in a bath; presumably other plasters did fall off under these conditions. When this passage is combined with the equally casual comments of Martial on water quality, the picture of life in a communal *solium* becomes still less pleasant.

Whereas the water in Roman baths could leave much to be desired, a further unpleasantness derived from the other essential component of the facilities' operation—the furnaces. It seems that it was possible for gases and odors from the fires to reach and, on occasion, inconvenience the bathers. Plutarch reports that conscientious aediles would not allow people who ran baths to put darnel (a weedy grass) into the furnaces, "since the resultant fumes induce headaches and dizziness in the bathers."[29] Pliny the Elder confirms this effect, commenting that he has heard that *balneatores* in Greece and Asia would put darnel seed onto hot coals to clear out unwanted crowds.[30] Fronto, writing to M. Aurelius in 143, says he prefers the natural grottos of Baiae to the furnaces of other baths, which are lit "with expense and smoke" (*M. Aur. Caes.* 1.3.4). Considering Fronto's elevated social standing, this comment is revealing: if the sorts of baths he regularly visited could be smoky, what was the situation like in the more lowly establishments? Finally, the *Historia Augusta* provides a typically colorful anecdote, the veracity of which is not as important as the assumptions that lie behind it.

---

29. Plut. *Mor.* 658E: οἱ, χαρίεντες ἀγορανόμοι τοὺς ἐργολαβοῦντας οὐκ ἐῶσιν . . . αἴρας ἐμβαλεῖν εἰς τὴν ὑπόκαυσιν, αἱ γὰρ ἀπὸ τούτων ἀναθυμιάσεις καρηβαρίας καὶ σκοτώματα τοῖς λουομένοις ἐμποιοῦσιν.

30. Pliny *HN* 18.156. Direct access from the hypocaust to the bathroom has been archaeologically proven only in the case of Bath IV at Olympia and the men's *caldarium* in the Stabian Baths: see E. Kunze and H. Schleif, *IV. Bericht über die Ausgrabungen in Olympia* (Berlin, 1944), 52–53; Nielsen, 1.20.

The young Commodus, dissatisfied with the heat of his bath, ordered that the *balneator* be thrown into the furnace as punishment. The slave ordered to carry out the deed threw a sheepskin onto the fire instead, thus fooling the prince, by the resulting smell, into believing his cruel order had been carried out (*Comm.* 1.9).

There is no way of knowing how common it was for gases from the heating system to reach the bathers, but if fumes and odors from the like of darnel seed or sheepskins could reach them, as the evidence cited above indicates, it is not impossible that fumes or even smoke from regular furnace fuel did also. Considering the great amount of fuel burned to maintain the heat in large baths, the general occurrence of this circumstance seems a strong likelihood. Indeed, such conditions may even have been so accepted and unremarkable a feature of a visit to the baths that only the occasional indirect reference (of the sort just surveyed) survives. It must be admitted, however, that these notices give little indication as to the intensity of the fumes or as to where in the bathhouse the bathers were likely to encounter them. It is surely unrealistic to envision bathing rooms habitually filled with smoke—rather, I am suggesting that smoke and odors from the furnaces may have filtered into the buildings, possibly affecting the heated rooms to a greater degree than elsewhere. The use of darnel to clear out facilities in Asia Minor appears to assume that all or most of the building would be sufficiently affected.

The operation of strigiling—scraping off with a tool called a strigil—appears to have taken place indoors, in *destrictaria* or possibly in the *tepidarium*.[31] If so, the combined oil, sweat, and dirt (onomatopoeically termed γλοιός in Greek) was doubtless splashed onto the floor and the walls. The medical writer Aetius Amidenus, who used this substance as a binding agent in his medicaments, certainly had no trouble collecting it "from the bathhouse or from the hot water,"[32] which reflects badly not only on the water quality but also on the state of the baths' interior. Conditions such as these probably prompted Trajan to characterize the task of cleaning the

---

31. Strigiling was part of the massage process and so probably took place indoors: see Celsus 1.4.2 (strigiling in the *tepidarium*); Galen *Hipp. acut. morb.* 47 (15.715 Kühn; strigiling in a sweat bath). It must be admitted that *destrictaria* (see nos. 21 and 61) may have been open areas off the palaestra, and strigiling could also have taken place in the palaestra itself. It seems clear from various sources, however, that the *tepidarium* was often the room where anointing took place, so oil spillage must have been a common occurrence in this room, if not elsewhere: see, e.g., Luc. *Hipp.* 6; Celsus loc cit.

32. Aet. Amid. 1.P84 (γλοιός ἀπὸ βαλανείου), 2.3 (γλοιὸν τὸν ἀπὸ τοῦ βαλανείου ἢ ἀπὸ τοῦ θερμοῦ ὕδατος μίξας τῇ πλυθείσῃ μελαίνῃ χρῶ . . .).

baths as "tantamount to punishment."[33] Two final notices deserve comment: Pliny the Elder notes that baths were favorite breeding grounds for cockroaches, and as Petronius' heroes are at one stage required to leave a bath in haste, they do so via "a dark and dirty exit."[34]

The cumulative effect of the evidence presented here is to suggest that whereas some baths were paradigms of refinement and splendor, others were not. This is an obvious inference to draw, but the evidence also suggests strongly that many of the empire's baths operated in a condition far below even ancient expectations, as suggested by restoration inscriptions. Once fine baths, after continuous use, must have been less pleasing to the eye and must have offered a bathing experience far removed from the idealized picture presented in poetry and laudatory epigrams. The most far-reaching conclusion, however, is that general sanitary conditions, even at the finer and well-maintained establishments, left a lot to be desired. That said, it is nonetheless true that the Romans usually associated a visit to the baths with hygiene, getting clean (or at least cleaner), and having a good time, rather than with wallowing in filth and having a repulsive experience. But the Roman threshold for what constituted acceptable hygienic conditions undoubtedly fell well below its modern counterpart. Thus, despite the evidence for luxurious decoration and other splendors, the physical environment at Roman baths should not be unduly idealized. It seems that certain conditions—such as the simultaneous bathing of the sick and the healthy, the everyday reality of preused and dirty water, and the presence in some rooms of smells or even smoke from the furnaces—may have been far more common features of a visit to the baths than many today might suspect. The last word should perhaps go to the saturnine Marcus Aurelius, who asks, "What is bathing when you think about it—oil, sweat, filth, greasy water, everything loathsome."[35]

---

33. Pliny *Ep.* 10.32.2 *(non longe a poena)*. Trajan, in making this judgment, may also have had in mind the dreadful job of cleaning the hypocaust. Since most hypocaust cavities are one meter high, the task must have been horrendous for those who had to do it. Note that the *Tosefta* makes mention of "the hook of the scrapers of the bathhouses" that "is made only for use in connection with the ground" (*t. Kelim B. Bat* 2:12). Given their expressed function, these scrapers are not likely strigils but rather implements for cleaning the fabric of the building.

34. Pliny *HN* 11.99 (see Sen. *Ep.* 86.8); Petron. *Sat.* 91.

35. M. Aur. *Med.* 8.24: ὁποῖόν σοι φαίνεται τὸ λούεσθαι· ἔλαιον, ἱδρώς, ῥύπος, ὕδωρ γλοιῶδες, πάντα σικχαντά.

Chapter 8

The Bathers

The most important element of the bathing experience was the people who went through it. The baths have long been recognized as social centers in the Roman world,[1] but the social identities of the bathers and the degree of interclass mixing that prevailed among them have never been closely investigated. At first glance, the hierarchical nature of Roman society would seem to preclude that all classes used the baths together—it appears inconceivable that snobbish senators and lowly slaves could rub shoulders in any social context.[2] Yet the evidence seems clear that they did just that in the baths. A common response to this situation has been to suggest that the baths represented an anomaly, a remarkably egalitarian feature of Roman daily life, a place where social distinctions broke down. The baths were, in short, social levelers.[3] In the following pages, I present an effort to identify who used the baths, from emperors to slaves. From this effort emerges evidence that all the social groups, in varying degrees, can be located there. Also investigated are the issues that stem from this circumstance: the extent to which the different classes mixed and mingled at the baths, and the overall significance of bathing as a social process. The resultant picture of the baths' broad social function is rather different from their proposed role as mechanisms of equalization.

---

1. This point is made in most studies of Roman daily life and urbanism. For some recent examples in English, see L. Adkins and R.A. Adkins, *Handbook to Life in Ancient Rome* (New York, 1994), 350, s.v. "baths"; Balsdon, *Life and Leisure,* 27; J.E. Stambaugh, *The Ancient Roman City* (Baltimore, 1988), 201–6; R. Tomlinson, *From Mycenae to Constantinople: The Evolution of the Ancient City* (London, 1992), 161; Toner, 53–54; P. Veyne, ed., *A History of Private Life,* vol. 1, *From Pagan Rome to Byzantium* (Cambridge, MA, 1987), 198.

2. On the contempt of the elite for the lower orders as reflected in the pejorative vocabulary used by the upper classes in reference to the lower, see R. MacMullen's "The Lexicon of Snobbery," in his *Roman Social Relations,* 138–41.

3. See, e.g., Dyson, *Community,* 174; Sherwin-White, *Letters of Pliny,* 247; Stambaugh, *Roman City,* 205; Toner, 57; Yegül, 32; id., "Thermo-Mineral Complex," 161.

The Emperor

A famous story in the *Historia Augusta* locates Hadrian in the baths with the general public, an occurrence said to have been frequent. On one of these occasions, so the story goes, Hadrian encountered an army veteran rubbing his back against a wall and asked the man what he was doing. The veteran replied that he was too poor to have a slave rub his back for him. The emperor promptly donated some slaves to him, along with funds for their upkeep. When visiting the baths on a later occasion, Hadrian was confronted by a crowd of old men rubbing their backs against the walls, in the hope of exciting his generosity. Not to be fooled, the emperor advised that the old men rub each other's backs instead (*Hadr.* 17.5–7). This passage and a handful of others have been used to justify the claim that "many a Roman emperor visited the public baths and enjoyed bathing in the company of his subjects."[4] But closer analysis of the evidence reveals that the issue is not as clear-cut as this assertion implies.

Aside from the question of the veracity of this anecdote, was Hadrian's alleged behavior typical for emperors? That is the crux of the issue. There seems, at first, to be some support for an affirmative response. In addition to the story about Hadrian, the *Historia Augusta* reports that Caracalla bathed with the populace when his *thermae* were dedicated at Rome (in 215), and it is also claimed that Severus Alexander bathed with the people frequently. Similarly, Suetonius reports that Titus used the baths in Rome that bore his name.[5] But certain features of these notices need to be stressed. Suetonius, for instance, reports that Titus bathed publicly only "sometimes" *(nonnumquam),* and he states that the emperor visited the baths "so as not to pass up any opportunity of courting popular favor" *(ne quid popularitatis praetermitteret).* In other words, by bathing in public, Titus was exercising his well-documented instinct for public relations. If this is so, his behavior is hardly applicable to emperors as a group, especially those less sensitive to public opinion, such as his father. Also, Suetonius says that "the plebs were admit-

---

4. Yegül, 32. The other passages cited by Yegül—in Suetonius and the *Historia Augusta*—are discussed below.

5. HA *Heliogab.* 17.9 (Caracalla), *Alex. Sev.* 42.1 (Severus Alexander); Suet. *Tit.* 8.2 (Titus). Other evidence in the *Historia Augusta* is ambiguous. For instance, it reports that Antoninus Pius opened a bath, "which he had previously used himself, to the people free of charge" *(Ant. Pius* 7.6: *balneum, quo usus fuisset, sine mercede populo exhibuit),* but it is unclear whether or not the bath was a private or public one, whether the people had been excluded when Pius had used it and were now merely admitted free, and whether he continued to use it after it was opened to the people.

ted" *(admissa plebe)* on these occasions, which suggests that on other occasions they were not, or which at least implies that some distance existed between the bathing emperor and the watching plebs. All of these observations tend to vitiate the claim that Titus bathed with the populace frequently or as a matter of course. As to the alleged public bathing of Caracalla and Severus Alexander reported in the *Historia Augusta,* these notices are, at best, dubious. The report about Caracalla appears to be entirely fictional. In 214 the emperor left for the East, where he was assassinated three years later; there is no report of him ever returning to Rome in the interim (see Dio 77[78].16.7–78[79].10.3). This discrepancy reflects the general unreliability of the *Historia Augusta* as a source, and a recent study of the bath-related passages in it argues that the anecdotes about Hadrian and Severus Alexander may derive directly from Suetonius' *Life of Titus,* since mixing with the populace is the sort of thing a "good" emperor was likely to do, and Titus had long been fossilized as a paradigmatic "good" ruler.[6]

However, with the exception of the story about Caracalla, there is no reason to believe that all the vignettes of emperors at public baths are complete fiction. They may contain a kernel of truth, in which particular circumstances played a role. The extensive provincial tours of Hadrian, for instance, probably required him to use local public facilities as a matter of necessity.[7] More stationary emperors did not face the same need, or else they had other options open to them: a procurator of Egypt is said to have been banished for using baths built specifically for a planned visit by Nero (see Suet. *Ner.* 35.5). Whose bathing inclinations were typical for itinerant emperors, Hadrian's or Nero's? On a broader view, most literary sources that portray emperors in their baths give no hint of a public setting, so most imperial bathing should be seen as taking place in palaces and imperial villas, which archaeology

---

6. See Merten, 130–31. The similarities of wording in both the *Historia Augusta*'s notice about Caracalla (*Heliogab.* 17.9: *et lavacrum quidem Antoninus Caracallus dedicaverat et lavando et populum admittendo*) and Suetonius' about Titus (*Tit.* 8.2: *admissa plebe*) tend to support the proposal that some borrowing has taken place; at the very least, similar staged events ought to be envisioned. In general, the motif of "ruler at the public baths" goes back at least to Hellenistic times: similar stories are told of Antiochus Epiphanes (see Polyb. 26.1.12–14) and Herod the Great (see Joseph. *BJ* 1.340–41). Note that the depraved Heliogabalus is said to have done the opposite: he made his private baths in the palace public, so that he could gather around him especially well-endowed men (see HA *Heliogab.* 8.6). This story is just one of many such "bath-excess" stories told about this and other "bad" emperors; see Merten, 132–33.

7. The visits of Hadrian to Asia Minor in 129 have been plausibly proposed as the stimulus for the renovation of baths and other public buildings in the various cities of the region; see above, chapter 6, n. 90.

reveals were habitually equipped with the requisite facilities.[8] In addition, inscriptions record the existence of slaves whose function was to attend to the emperor's bathing needs, and in one case the slave is said to have been attached to the private bathing suite of the palace.[9] In short, the evidence for emperors at public baths is open to question, and it tends not to support the notion that it was commonplace for ruler and people to share bathing facilities. If such sharing took place at all, the occasion was more likely a rarity, possibly limited to emperors on the road or staged as a special event designed to foster public goodwill. The notice about Titus using his baths along with the public should be read in this light. Likewise, although Nero, the senate, and the entire equestrian order were present in Nero's baths on the day of the building's dedication (see Phil. *VA* 4.42), there is no need to believe that the emperor's presence was thereafter habitual.

Beyond the question of their individual historicity, however, the reports of emperors bathing with the public carry a different weight as evidence. As a group, they reveal something of a broader social attitude toward the public bathhouse and its clientele. The stories, and presumably their audience, do not consider it at all implausible to portray bathing in a public bath as a situation in which people of the most elevated social station could be found alongside the most lowly. If emperors are an extreme case, other evidence is quite clear that Romans of varying status used public baths and often did so simultaneously.

Senators, *Equites,* and the Elite

The presence of the elite at public baths is attested in numerous sources. In contrast to the stories of emperors bathing in public, none of these sources in any way implies that it was unusual or remarkable for the upper class to be seen at the baths. On the contrary, to the Roman tastes of Valerius Maximus, it was indicative of their *insolentia* that the rulers of Carthage bathed separately from the populace (see Val. Max. 9.5 ext. 4; compare HA *Gallien.* 17.8). Senators could use public baths, as Pliny the Younger makes clear

8. For emperors bathing, see, e.g., Suet. *Aug.* 76.2, 82.2, 85.2, *Calig.* 37.1–2, *Ner.* 20.2, 27.2, 31.2. In some cases, private baths appear more certain: see Suet. *Galb.* 10.5, *Vesp.* 21; Fronto *M. Aur. Caes.* 2.13, 4.6.2, *M. Ant. Imp.* 1.5.4; Plut. *Mor.* 124C; HA *Comm.* 5.4. Domestic baths are known from such palaces as the *Domus Augustana* on the Palatine or the imperial villas, among others, at Tibur (see W.L. MacDonald and J. A. Pinto, *Hadrian's Villa and Its Legacy* [New Haven, 1995]) and Capri (see De Caro and Greco, *Campania,* 111–14).

9. See, e.g., a *praepositus balneariorum domus Aug(usti)* (CIL 6.8642), and *mag(ister) a balneis Aug(usti)* (CIL 6.8512). Such servants were clearly part of the emperor's private staff, comparable to the *praepositus vestis albae triumphalis* (CIL 6.8546 = ILS 1763) and others concerned with the imperial wardrobe; see *ILS* 1755–66.

when, in describing the amenities of his Laurentine villa, he adds that if his private bathing suite was unavailable, the nearby *vicus* contained three *balnea meritoria* (i.e., privately owned but publicly accessible facilities).[10] Pliny expresses a preference for his private baths but has no qualms about using local public establishments if necessary. Others appear less fastidious. Pliny's anecdote about Larcius Macedo suffering a blow at the hands of an angry *eques* is set in a public bath at Rome (*Ep.* 3.14.6–8); the raw fact of Macedo's presence at the public baths draws no comment whatsoever from Pliny. Likewise, Seneca's story about the violence done to Cato the Elder in a bath (*Dial.* 4.32.2), whether true or not, reveals something of the matter-of-fact attitude among these writers—themselves privileged—toward the use of public baths by members of their class.

There is other specific evidence. Aulus Gellius records the story of a consul and his wife using public baths while traveling in Italy—with disastrous results for the locals (*NA* 10.3.1–3; see below, chapter 8, p. 212, for a fuller discussion of this passage). We have already seen how Cicero's ridiculing of the plot to poison Clodia portrays *amici* of both Clodia and Caelius, among them the *prudens adulescens et bonus* Licinius, meeting at public baths in Rome. Despite the overall sarcastic tone of the passage, nowhere does Cicero suggest that the presence of men of such evident good breeding was in itself unusual or noteworthy for a public bathhouse (*Cael.* 61–67). The character Ulpianus in Athenaeus' *Deipnosophistae* (1.1d–e) is most probably the famous jurist Domitius Ulpianus of Tyre, and he is portrayed as regularly visiting public baths. Governors appear to have used local public facilities while in the provinces, as would be consistent with what I postulated about traveling emperors doing so. The *Historia Augusta* claims to reproduce a letter from Valerian to an otherwise unknown and probably fictitious procurator of Syria, in which it is recommended that if the governor's personal firewood is lacking, he should use public baths.[11] Despite the doubtlessly spurious nature of the letter and its possibly sarcastic tone, that its contents are not pure fantasy is implied by a passage in the *Digest*. In describing the conditions under which a magistrate can sanction a manumission, the jurist Gaius writes, "slaves are very commonly manumitted when [the magistrate

---

10. Pliny *Ep.* 2.17.26. On *balnea meritoria*, see Heinz, 23–26; Merten, 3–6; Meusel, *Verwaltung und Finanzierung*, 23–27; Nielsen, 1.119–20, 122–25.

11. HA *Claud.* 14.12–13. Note also that the governor Julius Priscus held court at the Baths of Hadrian at Antioch, though in this case he is not present to bathe; see D. Feissel and J. Gascou, "Documents d'archives romains inédits au Moyen Euphrate (IIIe siècle après J.-C.)," *CRAI*, 1989, 545–57. A similar story is told of Aurelian sitting in state in the baths at Byzantium; see HA *Aurel.* 10.3, 13.1.

is] moving about, when [for instance] the praetor or proconsul or legate of Caesar has come out to bathe, or drive, or attend the games."[12] The point is that the magistrate can be called on to witness a manumission when in public at times other than when he appears formally on the tribunal, and one of those instances—indeed the first one cited—is when he is on his way to the public baths, an apparently common occurrence for governors or other magistrates.

Aside from this material pertaining to senators and *equites,* there are general indications that the elite, whether "imperial" or local, used public baths as a matter of course. We have seen how inscriptions place responsibility for bath construction and maintenance firmly on the shoulders of local notables, either individually or collectively. For them to have invested in these buildings but not to have used them would be surprising, to say the least. The *Digest* defines a man's *domicilium* not as the place where he cultivates farmland but as that place where he conducts his business *(negotia);* visits the forum, baths, and theater; and celebrates festivals (*Dig.* 50.1.27.1). Since the individual is said to live either in a *colonia* or a *municipium* and to own property at more than one location, a person of at least modest wealth and social standing is inferred. The logic behind the ruling is clear: wherever a man participates in a community's public activities, there lies his legal *domicilium.*[13] That visiting the baths is included as a defining communal activity is revealing and suggests that it was not only normal but expected behavior for people of substance to be found in the local bathhouse. It is probably in this connection that we should read Lucian's description of the Baths of Hippias, which includes a reception room for the rich (*Hipp.* 5). Isolating examples of such reception halls in surviving physical remains has proven virtually impossible, although the *atrium* or *basilica thermarum* mentioned in written sources is certainly a good candidate.[14] Such poets as Martial and Juvenal, usually men of modest wealth and social status who associated with the rich and powerful of the city, regularly used the public baths of Rome; indeed, Martial complains that he was expected to accompany one of his patrons to the Thermae of Agrippa, evidently that man's

---

12. *Dig.* 40.2.7 (trans. P.A. Brunt): *plerumque in transitu servi manumitti solent, cum aut lavandi aut gestandi aut ludorum gratia prodierit praetor aut proconsul legatusve Caesaris.* See also Gaius *Inst.* 1.20.

13. Note that among the restrictions imposed on Christians during the second-century persecutions was exclusion from houses, baths, and markets, i.e., from communal life; see Euseb. *Hist. eccl.* 5.1.5.

14. See appendix 3 for a list of parts of baths found in the epigraphic sample. See also Nielsen, 1.162–63, s.vv. "basilica thermarum," "vestibulum, atrium."

favorite establishment.[15] Ammianus Marcellinus describes aristocrats of the fourth century A.D. going to the public baths and adds the detail that it was polite to ask a stranger what baths he used (Amm. Marc. 28.4.8–10).

Iconographic evidence for the elite at the baths—and indeed for people of any status there—is extremely slim. The Romans appear to have preferred decoration evoking the metaphorical joys of bathing over direct representation of bathers actually utilizing the facilities. There are exceptions, however. From the private baths at the late-Imperial villa at Piazza Armerina in Sicily come several particularly good depictions of privileged bathers in action. In one, from the vestibule of the baths, a procession makes its way into the establishment led by a servant carrying a box of bathing gear, the Roman equivalent of a toilet bag, with another servant holding up the rear and carrying a chest of towels and clothes (see fig. 27). From the *frigidarium* come representations of particularly self-satisfied bathers, their needs attended to by slaves. In one case, a slave moves to dry a seated female figure with a towel, while another presents her with fresh clothes (or more towels; see fig. 28). In another vignette, one slave offers a dressing bather a fresh cloak while another attends to his footwear (see fig. 29). Although the context is that of a private establishment, there is no reason to doubt that similar scenes were not enacted daily in public establishments across the empire.

Few inscriptions give indications as to who used baths, let alone specify the presence of the elite among the clientele. An unusual text from Rome is an exception. It purports to be a commemoration of one Ursus who claims mastery of the "glass ball" game to the delight of crowds in the Thermae of Agrippa, Nero, Titus, and Trajan (no. 283). If taken at face value, the inscription appears to be little more than a quaint commemoration of a quainter old man, but a recent interpretation argues that it is, in fact, a subtle allegory for participation in imperial politics, represented by the slippery and fragile "glass ball." The protagonists are the consular rivals of Hadrianic date, L. Julius Ursus Servianus (twice consul, in 91 and 102) and M. Annius Verus (three times consul, in 98, 121, and 126).[16] It might seem that acceptance of

---

15. Mart. 3.36.5–6. For Martial's wealth and social status, see Sullivan, 26–30. Juvenal owned a house in Rome (11.171, 11.190) and perhaps a farm at Tibur (11.65).

16. For this view, see E. Champlin, "The Glass Ball Game," *ZPE* 60 (1985): 159–63. The proposal is that Verus' third consulship, among other things, heralded the death of Ursus' political career; this explains the references to revering Ursus' statue as if paying homage to a dead man, despite his being "alive and willing." E. Courtney (*ML*, p. 331) dismisses Champlin's views as "a fantastic and untenable interpretation." Such a harsh judgment, however, cannot be accepted without detailed argumentation, and Courtney refrains from presenting any. Courtney provides no alternative explanation, for instance, for the otherwise unattested glass ball game and passes over in silence those odd features of this text that Champlin seeks to explain.

this ingenious interpretation of the inscription requires that it be thrown out as evidence for the upper classes at the baths. But this assumption is far from true. For the allegory to be successful, it is essential that a senator's/ex-consul's participation in a ball game at the baths was a plausible scenario for the ancient reader.[17]

Plebs, Commoners, and Others of Low Station

The presence of the general populace in the baths is rarely attested directly in the sources but is clearly implied in several of the passages already discussed: they are the poor veterans who accost Hadrian, the crowd that obstructs Larcius Macedo, those excluded from Lucian's reception hall for the rich, and the spectators cheering at the ball games of Ursus in the great baths of Rome. When Martial contemplates what life would be like if he did not move among the elevated circles at Rome, he muses:

> Nec nos atria nec domos potentum
> nec litis tetricas forumque triste
> nossemus nec imagines superbas;
> sed gestatio, fabulae, libelli,
> campus, porticus, umbra, Virgo, thermae,
> haec essent loca semper, hi labores.
>
> (5.20.5–10)

> [We should know nothing of the halls and mansions of the mighty, nor sour lawsuits and the gloomy Forum, nor haughty death masks: but riding, chatting, books, the Field, the colonnade, the shade, the Virgin, the baths—these should be our daily haunts, these our labors.]

Despite its overtly romanticized view of the "simple life," the poem assumes that those unacquainted with wealth and power loitered around the public buildings of the city. Since the living conditions of the city's less well-off would have been deplorable, their frequenting the more opulent public structures seems entirely understandable. Large public baths, with their heated elements and often finely appointed surroundings, must have been among the most attractive destinations for the hard-pressed or the indigent, especially in colder weather.

---

17. Ball games were very popular pastimes at the baths, as attested by specific areas or rooms given over to them *(sphaeristeria)*: see Pliny *Ep.* 2.17.11, 5.6.27; appendix 3, s.v. "sphaeristerium." For ball games, see Mart. 7.32; no. 83; Balsdon, *Life and Leisure,* 163–67; Blümner, *Privataltertümer,* 439–41.

There is more explicit evidence for the presence of commoners at the baths than this, however. The most direct is the graffiti from the towns buried by Vesuvius. The Forum Baths and Sarno Baths at Pompeii and the Suburban Baths at Herculaneum have yielded the scribblings of visitors, usually little more than their names.[18] Such graffiti writers were, then as now, most likely of common station. In a more formal context, epitaphs of humble Romans mention visits to the baths, and an inscription from Claudiopolis in Bithynia records the unexpected death of a dancer "while bathing in the hot baths."[19] Occasionally, *instrumenta balnei* are inscribed with their owners names (see, e.g., *CIL* 15.7084–95), but these people were at least wealthy enough to be able to afford such paraphernalia. Other inscriptions suggest that families would go to the baths together. Two epitaphs—one from Ostia, the other from Lugdunum—commemorate deceased wives who used to bathe with their husbands (nos. 263 and 264). In the text from Lugdunum, the grieving husband, Pompeius Catussa, describes himself as a "Sequanian citizen, a plasterer." The bereaved Ostian husband was a Roman citizen but gives no hint as to his profession or his status; his silence in this regard may suggest a person of little social consequence, like Catussa. When husbands and wives visited the baths together, they seem to have brought their children along. In an inscription from Rome, two freedpeople mourn the loss of their eight-year-old son who drowned in the *piscina* of the Baths of Mars.[20] A drawing of stick-men on the wall of the ramp leading to the Sarno Baths has been interpreted as the work of a waiting child.[21] Of the five teeth found in the baths at Caerleon, three were from children, and the descriptions of the bathing process in ancient schoolbooks are by their very nature aimed at children.[22] All these fragments of evidence seem to suggest that families and children would have been a regular part of the Roman bathing scene, although they were perhaps not found in every establishment.[23]

Further evidence for commoners at the baths derives from benefactions that expressly mention the beneficiaries. Thus an inscription from Nemausus

---

18. See nos. 278–81. See also *CIL* 4.1462–69 (Forum), 4.10674–83 (Suburban); Koloski-Ostrow, 54–59 (Sarno).

19. See nos. 261–64 (epitaphs); *SEG* 36 (1986) 1139 (dancer).

20. No. 260. Compare a similar text from Teate Marrucinorum (*CIL* 9.6318): *ipse pa[ter infelicissimus]* | *sculpsi puero* | *qui miser in piscina p[eriit];* | *vixit annis III mens VI.* Here, however, it is not made explicit that the *piscina* was part of a bathhouse.

21. See Koloski-Ostrow, 59.

22. See above, chapter 4, n. 30 (teeth); chapter 1, p. 12 (schoolbooks). Note HA *Clod. Alb.* 5.6 where it is implied that baths were considered good for children.

23. Aelius Aristides (40.511) refers to women and children at the baths chanting slanderous verses from comedy; nothing suggests that their presence was remarkable or atypical.

records that a benefactor opened a bath more speedily for the use of the plebs (no. 170). The text has been read, unnecessarily, as indicating that these baths were reserved for the exclusive use of the plebs (see below, n. 53 in this chapter), but at the very least their presence in this establishment is made explicit. Other texts record work carried out for the benefit and with the support of the *populus*—once, as we have seen, in response to its demands.[24] Among the clearest testimony in this regard are the inscriptions recording the provision of free bathing to named categories of beneficiaries. Bathing, as we have seen, can be given simply "to the people," a designation that probably denotes the entire citizen body of a community, even if, strictly speaking, the designation excludes decurions and Augustales.[25] Other texts are more specific. Free bathing can be stipulated for all or some of the citizens of the community *(municipes* or *coloni); noncitizen residents (incolae);* guests of the community *(hospites);* visitors, probably from neighboring villages and towns *(adventores);* and foreigners, either resident aliens or the rough equivalents of visitors *(peregrini).*[26] Again, it is far from certain that use of the baths was restricted only to the groups named; rather, the texts mention those to whom the benefaction applied, and it must be assumed that other classes of people could attend the baths but had to pay. In all of these cases, however, the commoners are discernibly present.

Finally, in many communities, especially larger colonies and *municipia,* the urban baths must also have served the *territorium* of the city. It is unlikely that farmers and other rustics would have had the time or opportunity to visit the baths every day, but presumably market days, festivals, local elections, assizes, spectacles, and other special occasions offered these people a golden opportunity to "bathe in the manner of the city," as bath advertisements regularly put it.[27] On these days, the baths of a Roman community, whether

24. For benefactions expressly aimed at the *populus,* see, e.g., nos. 13, 20, 37, 161, 303, 329–36. For popular demand and baths, see above, chapter 6, p. 165.

25. See nos. 197 *(populus),* 211 *(pagani),* 329 (ὁ δῆμος), 330 (οἱ κατοίκοι). Note also oil distributions, which are often given *populo:* see nos. 215, 218, 219 *(populus);* 331 (πολὶς), 332 (ὁ δῆμος). On the meaning of *populus,* see Duncan-Jones, *Economy,* 141–43; Mrozek, *Distributions,* 94–102. Note that in one text (no. 210) "all the people" *(populus universus)* are distinguished from the "inhabitants" *(incolae),* presumably of the surrounding countryside. Even here, though, the term *populus* denotes persons of differing social status.

26. For the references, see above, chapter 6, pp. 160–61. Note also no. 334, where oil is provided "for the councillors and all the citizens."

27. For *lavatio more urbico,* see above, chapter 7, n. 7. For the living conditions of the peasantry, see J.K. Evans, "*Plebs Rustica:* The Peasantry of Classical Italy," part 2, "The Peasant Economy," *AJAH* 5 (1980): 134–73. For market days as social occasions, see L. de Ligt and P.W. de Neeve, "Ancient Periodic Markets: Festivals and Fairs," *Athenaeum* 66 (1988): 391–416; J.M. Frayn, *Markets and Fairs in Roman Italy* (Oxford, 1993), esp. 133–44; R. MacMullen, "Market-Days in the Roman Empire," *Phoenix* 24 (1970): 333–41.

in a village or city, must have been especially full of visitors, many of them lowly *rustici* come to town for a taste of high living.[28]

Slaves as Attendants and Customers

Perhaps the most remarkable possibility for social variety among the bathers is the presence of slaves as customers.[29] At the very least, their presence as attendants, in an "official" capacity, is amply attested in the sources. A mosaic from Piazza Armerina depicts slaves carrying buckets and names them in the vocative—"Tite!" "Cassi!"—as if they are being summoned (see fig. 30).[30] In the surviving schoolbooks, many of the bathing scenes are expressed as orders issued to silent slaves.[31] When Trimalchio first appears in the *Satyricon,* he is at the baths with three wine-drinking masseurs.[32] They are presumably members of Trimalchio's retinue, since bringing slave attendants to the baths was not unusual for those who could afford it. Juvenal makes great sport of the woman who bathes at night, has all her bath equipment transported to the baths (presumably by slaves), and is accompanied by a masseur *(aliptes).*[33] The satirist also pokes fun at one Tongilius who "usually bathes with a huge oil-flask made from rhinoceros horn and

28. See, e.g., Macrob. *Sat.* 1.16.34 (farmers shave and bathe on market days); Amm. Marc. 14.3.3 (town of Batnae near the Euphrates filled every September during a great market in exotic goods); *CIL* 9.2689 = *ILS* 7478 (a comic conversation between a hotelier and a *rusticus* who has visited town and racked up expenses on wine, food, women, and hay for his mule—"That mule will ruin me!" exclaims the customer).

29. The following discussion is an extended reworking of the second part of my article "Interpreting the Evidence," in Johnston and DeLaine, *Roman Baths and Bathing.*

30. Note also Amm. Marc. 28.4.16, where a slave receives three hundred lashes for not bringing hot water quickly enough. The baths offer an apt context for this notice, but a dining context is also possible, since the Romans habitually mixed their wine with hot water; see K.M.D. Dunbabin, "Wine and Water at the Roman *Convivium,*" *JRA* 6 (1993): 116–41.

31. See Dionisotti, "From Ausonius's Schooldays?" 102 (§55) and 103 (§61): *deferte res ad balneum mutatoria* and *da strigilem, destringe me.* Compare similar wording in *CGL* 3.651–52.10, 3.657–58.14–16.

32. Petron. *Sat.* 28. For a selection of bath personnel, see nos. 265, 266, 268, 269, 271–73. On the mostly servile status of such bath personnel as masseurs, see Ch. Bruun, "Lotores: Roman Bath-Attendants," *ZPE* 98 (1993): 222–28; Nielsen, 1.125–31; Wissemann, "Personal"; Yegül, 47. Note also Youtie, "Records of a Roman Bath," where the names recorded in the archive of a first- or second-century military bathhouse at Apollinopolis Magna (Edfu) show the slave status of the staff. An inscription (no. 284) mentions a *familia thermensis Thermarum Urbana[r(um)],* i.e., the slave workers at the baths. On masseurs *(iatraliptae)* in particular, see Wissemann (op. cit., 88) who concludes that they were mostly freedmen but could also be part of an upper-class Roman's slave household (see, e.g., Pliny *Ep.* 10.5.1–2, 10.6.1). This latter situation appears to be the case with Trimalchio's attendants, as there is no hint in the *Satyricon* that his masseurs were attached to the bathhouse, as Wisseman suggests.

33. Juv. 6.418–47. On the opening hours of baths, see Heinz, 145–46; Merten, 59–78; Nielsen, 1.135–38. There appears to have been no strict regulation of opening hours.

disrupts the baths with a mob of dirty retainers."[34] The reality behind this quip is reflected in Ammianus Marcellinus' description of retinues of up to fifty servants accompanying late Imperial aristocrats to the baths at Rome, and Plutarch, with typical moderation, counts it among the virtues of the good man (χρηστός) that he does not have an immoderate number of servants at the baths.[35] But the size of the retinue need not have been especially large—a retinue of one or two was also possible.[36] It seems probable that one of the functions of the benches found outside public baths—as are visible outside the entrance to the *Balneum Venerium et Nongentum* at Pompeii (see fig. 19)—was to accommodate slaves waiting for their masters, as well as other bathers waiting for access when the establishments were busy. Lucian also mentions a room in the Baths of Hippias that was specifically for servants and attendants (*Hipp.* 5). Slave staff could also guard clothes or serve baser functions.

So slaves could be found at the baths—that much is certain. But could they use the baths as customers? It might seem highly unlikely for this to be so, but there is strong evidence that they could. In addressing this issue, however, circumspection is required, since the question of the typicality of the evidence is particularly acute. In general, what was "normal" practice for one bathhouse might not have been for another. Also, one of the many consequences of servitude was the limitation placed on freedom of movement, since slaves were, by their nature, at the behest of their owners. Trimalchio placed a sign on the door of his house that read, "Any slave who goes outside without the master's order will receive one hundred lashes."[37] Such an injunction, however, would have affected the members of a slave *familia* to different degrees. The trusted slave, such as, to name but a few, the *paedagogus,* the personal valet, or the servant put in charge of a workshop or retail outlet (sometimes overseas), would surely have been able to move about more freely than the menial laborers tied to a specific location, such as the kitchen staff, house cleaners, farmhands, and so on. Nevertheless, for

---

34. Juv. 7.130–31: *magno cum rhinocerote lavari / qui solet et vexat lutulenta balnea turba.* See Sen. *Dial.* 10.12.7, where the pampered bather is lifted by his slaves out of the bath and into his litter.

35. Amm. Marc. 28.4.8–9 (fifty-strong retinue); Plut. *Mor.* 823B (χρηστός).

36. See Mart. 11.75; Petron. *Sat.* 91, 97 (single slave attendants); Juv. 6.374–76 (a single eunuch attendant?); Mart. 12.70 (one slave to carry towels and one to watch clothes); Pliny *Ep.* 3.14.7–8 (slave to make way for Larcius Macedo, although the ex-praetor may have had more unmentioned slaves in his retinue); Anon. *Life of Aesop* 32 (handsome slave attends mistress at [a private?] bath), 38 and 66 (Aesop, the only slave in his master's townhouse, attends to his master at the public baths).

37. Petron. *Sat.* 28: *quisquis servus sine dominico iussu foras exierit, accipiet plagas centum.* See further Bradley, *Slavery and Society,* 81–106, esp. 84–87.

many slaves, the restriction on mobility would have interfered directly with their ability to use public baths. This concern is vitiated somewhat for the slave members of a bathing retinue, if the distinction between slave attendants and customers is not drawn too firmly. It is quite possible that some slave attendants "on duty" at the baths also took the opportunity to bathe while performing their tasks. If so, these slaves could have visited the baths to bathe, presumably simultaneously with their owners—a remarkable occurrence in itself. Not all attendants, however, would have been given this opportunity, since their duties required vigilance (e.g., as clothes guards) or precluded entrance to the baths in the first place (e.g., as litter carriers). In contrast, the likes of *perfusores* (water pourers; see fig. 30), masseurs, anointers, strigilers, dryers, and others who attended their owners while they bathed may well have had a chance to use the facilities.[38] In this way limitation of movement would have affected individuals differently, even within a particular slave retinue. Altogether, the possibility that at least some slaves could work and bathe at the same time ought to be allowed.

The direct evidence for slaves at the baths specifically as customers is scant. Graffiti can locate a slave or *libertus* at the baths, but they usually give no indication as to whether the person was using the facilities, attending an owner, or merely loitering during a quiet moment.[39] There are exceptions. From the Suburban Baths at Herculaneum, two graffiti tell us that Apelles Mus, who calls himself a "chamberlain of the emperor" *(cubicularius Caesaris),* ate and enjoyed sex at the baths along with his "brother" Dexter; clearly they were customers.[40] Assuming that the claim to membership of the imperial *familia* is not spurious (it is certainly plausible, given that a number of imperial villas were located in the vicinity of the town) and that the "brotherhood" between Apelles and Dexter lies in social status and not in blood, here were two slaves enjoying the pleasures of Herculaneum's newest facility. That they were imperial slaves may be significant—perhaps only such high-ranking servants as chamberlains, who had direct access to mem-

---

38. For instance, Caelia enjoys the attentions of a slave while in the pool (see Mart. 11.75), but it is not made explicit that the slave also washes, although it would make sense for him to do so.

39. Typical is the notice *[F]usci Cilix* (CIL 4.10681; the Suburban Baths, Herculaneum). See also no. 280 for the possible slave Hermeros at the baths.

40. For the texts, see nos. 278 and 279. Imperial *cubicularii* were usually slaves: see G. Boulvert, *Esclaves et affranchis impériaux sous le Haut-Empire romain: Rôle politique et administratif* (Naples, 1970), 241–47; *RE* 4.1734–37, s.v. "a cubiculo, cubicularius" (Rostovtzeff), esp. 1734. There are two chief indications that Apelles was a slave, not a *libertus*: (1) he uses only one nomen (although, admittedly, the text is a graffito); and (2) the possessive *Caesaris* was generally used by slaves, while freedmen preferred *Augusti*. See P.R.C. Weaver, Familia Caesaris: *A Social Study of the Emperor's Freedmen and Slaves* (Cambridge, 1972), 48–54.

bers of the imperial house, enjoyed the degree of freedom sufficient to spend a day in town.

More formal inscriptions also provide useful testimony. In two benefactions of free bathing to specified classes of beneficiary, the offer is expressly extended "to their slaves" *(servisqu[e] eorum)* and "to their slaves and their maids" *(serveis ancilleisque eor(um))*.[41] It is conceivable that these servants were members of a retinue, that is, that they were "on duty." But if so, they were nonetheless granted the right of *lavatio gratuita,* "free bathing," and so they must have used the facilities as customers. This point raises the question of whether a bather arriving at the baths with slaves in tow was expected to pay an entrance fee for each attendant or whether slaves counted among the *instrumenta balnei* (like towels or strigils) and were automatically exempt. A passage in the *Digest* states that in legacies involving bathhouses, the property was to include, as *instrumenta balnei,* the bathmen *(balneatores)* and furnace attendants *(fornacatores),* both of which were slave positions.[42] If this principle was applied generally to slave bath attendants—and we do not know for certain that it was—it would be no benefaction at all to extend an offer of free bathing to slaves, unless they were included among the groups of customers listed. Whatever the case, the two inscriptions recording extensions of free bathing to slaves and maids provide concrete evidence that slaves could use the baths as customers, at least at the places where the texts were found. A negative inference in support of this proposition can also be drawn. That the slaves are mentioned in these inscriptions and absent from the majority of such benefactions implies that they usually would not be beneficiaries of *lavatio gratuita.*[43] The wording, in fact, shows not that slaves were excluded from the baths per se but rather that they could use the baths but had to pay.

In this connection, the *lex Metalli Vipascensis* is pertinent. In this instance, however, the issue of typicality comes to the fore, since the place was an imperial mining facility; regulations governing the usage of the baths there

---

41. Nos. 204 *(servi),* 206 *(ancillae);* see also no. 198 where mention of the bathers' *familia* no doubt includes slaves. The implications for slave bathers in such texts are taken at face value by Cenerini ("Evergetismo ed epigrafia," 212) and Mrozek *(Distributions,* 101 n. 48).

42. *Dig.* 33.7.13.1, 33.7.17.2 *(balneator);* 33.7.14.1 *(fornacator).* The ruling is justified on the basis that these staff were essential to the running of the facility. It is therefore conceivable that perhaps only essential staff were considered *instrumenta balnei.* This approach, however, appears unduly legalistic; Velleius Paterculus (2.114.2) implies that the term applied to whatever was necessary for bathing. See also Nielsen, 1.142–44.

43. Such is the conclusion of Mrozek *(Distributions,* 100–102), who proposes the habitual exclusion of slaves from money and food distributions in Italian towns. However, at Sen. *Dial.* 7.24.3, it is claimed that slaves could, in principle, be beneficiaries of liberality. See also Cenerini, "Evergetismo ed epigrafia," 212.

might be entirely inapplicable to the everyday "civic" facilities that are the chief focus of this study. Despite this issue, in the case of slaves using baths—attested, as we have just seen, in some urban centers—the *lex* stipulates that slaves and freedmen who were in the employ of the procurator in charge of the mine or who enjoyed other privileges could use the baths free of charge (no. 282, lines 23–24). As with free-bathing inscriptions from more ordinary contexts, the wording can be read to imply that slaves not in the employ of the imperial service would be charged, which in turn implies that slaves of any kind, such as the personal chattels of local people serving the mining community, had access to this bath as customers. Another inscription, also from the emperor's estates (this time in Coela, Thrace), records the building of baths for "the people and the *familia* of our Caesar," that is, for the local inhabitants and the emperor's slaves who served his estates in the region (no. 161). It would seem from these inscriptions that imperial slaves on certain of the emperor's properties could use public baths and that in the latter case at least, they shared them with the locals. That the inscriptions come from opposite ends of the empire and are separated chronologically by almost a century suggests that the practice may have been commonplace on imperial property; however, two inscriptions do not establish a general practice, and neither text proves that imperial slaves could use public facilities elsewhere, although Apelles and Dexter's action-packed visits to the Suburban Baths at Herculaneum ought to be borne in mind here (nos. 278 and 279).

The rules of the Lanuvian burial club are also instructive. It seems clear that the collegium had slave members, who appear to have been treated on an equal footing with the others.[44] When free oil was prescribed for the collegium at the public baths prior to their annual banquets, the slave members presumably benefited as well; certainly, they are not explicitly excluded in the regulations (no. 216). The rules of the club therefore indicate that collegium members, of varying social status and including slaves, bathed together on these occasions. An inscription from Puteoli prohibits the slaves who removed corpses in the town from using the baths before the first hour of night,[45] a time restriction probably imposed for religious reasons—but they *could* use the baths. In this latter case, as with the slaves using the baths at imperial mines in Metallum Vipascense, a purely practical consideration must be factored into the discussion. Mining and handling corpses are partic-

44. See *CIL* 14.2112 = *ILS* 7212.I.20–II.10, where the burial rights of the slave and freed members are outlined (esp. II.3–10 for slave members); see also Mrozek (*Distributions*, 101–2) on slave members in collegia.

45. *AE* 1971.88.II.3–4.

ularly dirty jobs, and it is entirely possible that slaves involved in such work were permitted baths whereas others generally were not. These slaves, therefore, may be special cases.

Literary sources, however, offer testimony that counters this possibility by portraying slaves at the baths in a matter-of-fact way. In Petronius' *Satyricon* (30), the heroes meet a slave who is about to be punished for losing the clothes of a *dispensator* while at the baths. A *dispensator* resembled an accountant in charge of financial and other domestic affairs in a household. Though on occasion a freedman, he was commonly a slave who enjoyed high status in the domestic slave hierarchy.[46] If Trimalchio's *dispensator* was a slave—the man claims to have had clients, which argues against slave status, unless the comment is intended as a jab at his inflated sense of self-importance—he is seen here using the baths as a customer, with another, less-elevated slave as a robe guard. Juvenal offers more secure evidence, when he comments that one of his two simple serving slaves "does not carry his pubescent testicles noisily into the baths, nor offer his armpits for depilation, nor timidly cover his stout groin with a flask held in front."[47] Presumably other slaves did, and the reference to depilation demonstrates that Juvenal was thinking of these slaves as going to the baths to bathe, not to serve. Pliny the Elder complains of gold-adorned *paedagogi*, also household slaves, who had transformed the appearance of the baths,[48] but in this case it is not clear if the *paedagogi* are part of a retinue accompanying a minor or are visiting the baths independently as customers. A dinner guest who arrives early at Martial's house finds the place practically deserted, because the servants are all at the baths (8.67). It is noteworthy that in all of these instances, the slaves in question either stand high in the slave hierarchy or enjoy close proximity to their owners; there is no evidence that menials would have had the same opportunities as these fortunates. An apparent exception are the slave brothers who harbor the transformed Lucius in Apuleius' *Metamorphoses* (10.13–17). The brothers work as skilled cooks for a rich master and are

---

46. In the *Digest, dispensatores* are habitually presented as slaves; see *Dig.* 11.3.16, 14.3.12, 34.2.1.1, 40.4.24, 40.5.35, 40.7.21, 46.3.51 and 62, 47.10.15.44, 50.16.166 and 203. For the status and duties of a *dispensator,* see *RE* 5.1189–98, s.v. (Liebenam); S.M. Treggiari, "Domestic Staff at Rome in the Julio-Claudian Period, 27 B.C. to A.D. 68," *Histoire Sociale/Social History* 6 (1973): 241–55. Imperial *dispensatores* were normally slaves of the highest rank: in the emperor's *familia,* they are the group most frequently attested as slaves who owned slaves (termed *servi vicarii*). See *CIL* 6.5197 = *ILS* 1514; Weaver, *Familia Caesaris,* 200–206. Note that Trimalchio, himself a freedman, had once held this position in his former owner's household (see Petron. *Sat.* 29).

47. Juv. 11.156–58: *nec pupillares defert in balnea raucus / testiculos, nec vellendas iam praebuit alas, / crassa nec opposito pavidus tegit inguina guto.*

48. Pliny *HN* 33.40; see Juv. 6.374–76.

presented as taking baths on a daily basis but only in the evening, after they
had come back from preparing the evening meal. Even in this case, however,
the slaves are portrayed as enjoying an amiable relationship with their
master.

It must also be stressed that the above discussion applies to public baths in
an urban context. In the countryside, conditions may have dictated separate
bathing for master and slave. It would be unrealistic to expect that a villa's
private bath suite would be available to farmhands, though baths shared by
workers and owners have been postulated for some early country villas in
southeast England.[49] A villa excavated at Ashstead in Surrey has a small bath
built into it and a larger, detached bath building located fifty meters down the
road approaching the house. The most logical explanation for this arrangement is that the detached bathhouse was for the use of the workers, with the
villa's bath suite reserved for the owners of the estate.[50] Most villas, though,
do not feature such detached bath buildings, so presumably the workers had
to fend for themselves when it came to getting clean; perhaps they used the
public facilities in nearby villages. Columella recommends allowing farm
slaves to bathe only on festival days, so they seem to have enjoyed a full
Roman-style bath only on these special occasions. Otherwise they would
have to improvise. But it remains unclear how typical and widely applied
Columella's prescriptions were. Altogether, access to public bathing among
the inhabitants of the countryside is a topic in need of further investigation.[51]

The evidence so far reviewed, when assessed cumulatively, makes strong
the possibility that slaves were allowed to use urban public baths as customers. It is probable that the practice varied from district to district and
from bath to bath within a town or region. Had it been a common practice, it
might be expected that some evidence would survive, no matter how indirect, either of the reservation of a bathhouse for the use of slaves alone or of
their exclusion from other baths. None does. The sort of lowly establishment
likely frequented by slaves would hardly have been graced with grandiose

---

49. See E.W. Black, *The Roman Villas of South-East England* (Oxford, 1987), 51–55.

50. See Black, *Roman Villas*, 105–16. Similar arrangements are found at Angmering in
Sussex and at Darenth and Hartlip in Kent (see ibid., 87–89, 52–53, and 124–25, respectively).

51. See Columella 1.6.19–20. Pliny (*Ep.* 8.16) deplores such a cold-blooded attitude toward the treatment of slaves and outlines his own, more benign approach. Pliny's comments,
unsurprisingly, apply to his domestic chattels and cannot be shown to have extended to the
laborers on his agricultural estates. Rural public baths have received scant attention, see Pasquinucci, 95–96 (by S. Menchelli). Farrington (*Roman Baths of Lycia*, 119) notes that all the
baths of Lycia are urban facilities and that there is "no indication that bathing was popular in
the countryside." This lack of evidence, however, may be due to the concentration of scholarly
attention on the urbanized sites of the province.

inscriptions, but it is noteworthy that there is a complete absence of any compelling evidence (even graffiti or literary asides) that slaves were not welcome in some public facilities for the mere fact of their being slaves. The volume and diversity of the evidence for Roman bathing culture makes this argument from silence somewhat more persuasive than is usually the case with this weakest form of deduction. If we assume that slaves had to get clean just as much as anyone else, their presence as customers at certain public facilities would seem logical enough. It is probable, however, that only privileged classes of slaves, such as high-ranking servants—imperial *servi,* household *dispensatores,* and personal attendants and favorites—or slaves employed in especially dirty work, enjoyed the freedom of movement and/or permission to visit baths on anything like a regular basis.[52]

Social Mixing: The Baths as Social Levelers?

Because various classes of Roman can be located at the baths, it is natural to ask what degree of social interaction prevailed among them as they bathed. I have just noted that no evidence exists for the formal exclusion of slaves from baths. In fact, the same is true for any formal social segregation among baths, in whole or in part.[53] It would certainly have been possible for the Romans to

---

52. In the *Life of Aesop,* for instance, Aesop is never depicted as going to the baths except as an attendant to his master. Aesop is clearly an all-purpose chattel and perhaps lacked the necessary status to use public baths independently of his master.

53. Formal segregation should be differentiated from de facto exclusivity: certainly "rich" and "poor" baths existed, but by and large bathing facilities were open to all. For this reason, the evidence marshaled by Nielsen (1.146 n. 2) to argue for socially segregated baths is unconvincing. For instance, when she uses Val. Max. 9.5 ext. 4 to show that "the classes were separated in Carthage and Campania, with respect to fora and baths," she misrepresents the passage: as we have seen above (chapter 8, p. 192), Valerius states that the Carthaginian oligarchs (not the Campanians) bathed separately from the plebs, and he uses this habit to illustrate their *insolentia.* It was not behavior Valerius condoned. Likewise, while it is true that Lucian (*Hipp.* 5) mentions a "room for the reception of the rich," that is only half the story: the room served only the *arrival* of the affluent—everywhere else in the facility, they would have mingled with the other bathers. The inscriptions Nielsen cites are similarly dubious: *CIL* 4.1136 (= no. 258; not *CIL* 9.1136, as printed in Nielsen) is of disputed interpretation and does not prove that the *Balneum Venerium et Nongentum* was "for the better-off," as she claims, while *CIL* 12.3165b (= no. 170) merely states that the baths were open for the use of the plebs, which is not the same as being reserved for their exclusive use. This, incidentally, is also true of inscriptions that mention baths built by or for the Roman citizens of a community (see nos. 131 and 167): it is not at all clear that such baths were reserved for the use of this group alone. In a highly stratified society, exclusivity was doubtless an attractive claim for an establishment (it remains so today in our supposedly egalitarian society), so advertisements stressing exclusivity—such as *Anth. Pal.* 9.624—can hardly be taken at face value. There is other evidence, not addressed by Nielsen, that might seem to support the notion of social segregation,

impose such segregation—it was possible in the case of men and women—but there is no sign of a desire on their part to do so.[54] Typically illustrative of the open access to public baths is the benefaction at Comum whereby oil was given "to the people in the Campus and in all the *thermae* and *balineae* that are in Comum" (no. 215; compare nos. 333 and 336). There is no hint here of socially differentiated bathhouses, but rather there appear to have been a variety of communal facilities, all used by the *populus*. Baths operated by collegia are exceptions, to be sure, since they were not open to the general public; in any case, individual collegia could have a socially diverse membership, so that even within these organizations, different classes could attend the same bathhouse.[55] It is noteworthy also that Jewish sources do not consider it improper for Jews and gentiles to share the bathhouses of their communities, which constitutes strong testimony as to the social promiscuity of Roman bathing culture.[56]

Archaeology contributes clues. The physical distribution of bath buildings within specific urban contexts (the study of which has yet to be undertaken in any systematic manner) suggests that, for the most part, particular establishments were not intentionally aimed at particular classes of clientele. I am not

but all of it is questionable. The report in the *Historia Augusta* (*Gord.* 32.5) concerning certain *balnea* built and fitted out "for private persons" is too obscure to merit serious consideration, while a notice in Malalas (306.22–307.2) that fifth-century Antioch featured a "Senate Bath" might be taken to suggest that the bath was reserved for the use of senators (so argues Yegül, 324 and 461 n. 82). But it seems rather tenuous to argue restricted entry on the basis of a mere name, when other possibilities have to be admitted (for instance, that it was built by, dedicated to, or featured decorative statues of senators or that it stood near the senate house). Anderson's suggestion ("Date of the *Thermae Traiani*," 501) that the Thermae of Titus served "women or the lower classes" has no basis in ancient testimony.

54. Social segregation could have been enforced without too much difficulty, even if only on a very broad basis (e.g., separate bathing times for each *ordo* or separate facilities for freeborn and freed/slaves). Contrast, for instance, the socially restricted use of baths in Umayyad Syria (see Yegül, 339–49); the fourteenth-century rulings at Digne, Dijon, and Rouen stipulating alternate days at public baths for men, women, Jews, and actors (see Vigarello, *Concepts*, 29); and the restricted clientele of seventeenth-century public baths in Paris (see ibid., 22–23). In the medieval Islamic world, Jews and Christians were allowed to share public baths with Muslims but were often required to wear bells, crosses, seals, or similar identifying markers; see Grotzfeld, *Bad im arabsich-islamish Mittelalter,* 123–28. There is no evidence for any comparable restrictions or requirements in Roman baths.

55. See Lib. *Or.* 11.245 (bathhouses run by tribes in Antioch). For socially diverse collegia membership, see above, chapter 8, pp. 203–4.

56. See, for instance, *m. Maks.* 2:5; *t. Miqw.* 6:4; *b. Sabb.* 33b. There are some restrictions, however, on the recommended degree of interaction and the activities permitted within the bathhouse: see *t. Abod. Zar.* 3:4; *t. Ber.* 2:20. On Jewish attitudes toward Roman baths, see Goodman, *State and Society in Roman Galilee,* 81–84. On the interaction of Jews and gentiles in the ancient urban context, see D. Sperber, *The City in Roman Palestine* (Oxford, 1998), 58–72 (baths).

claiming that individual bathhouses did not have their regular patrons, perhaps often drawn from relatively homogenous social groups, but I do wish to
emphasize that nothing in the location of specific public facilities suggests a
purposeful exclusion of any group.[57] The large *thermae* of Rome, for instance, are so sited as to afford access from any region of the city, and
although their specific locations are rarely known, the humbler *balnea* appear
similarly distributed (see appendix 2). A recent study of Pompeii argues that
zoning on the modern model did not exist in the Roman city, so residences,
shops, taverns, and baths were spread evenly throughout the urban landscape.[58] Such an arrangement does not facilitate the limiting of bath access
to certain classes. Further, study of the streets on which the Pompeian baths
stand shows that in all cases, the main facilities (Stabian, Forum, Republican,
and Central) front onto streets of particularly high activity.[59] It is fair to
conclude that the siting of these baths was aimed at attracting the widest
possible customer base, not at restricting admission to members of particular
social groups. Of course, means other than location could be employed to
restrict access, such as higher entrance fees,[60] more expensive services,
screening of "undesirables" at the door, and so on, so exclusive bathhouses
doubtless existed at Pompeii (the Sarno Baths?) and elsewhere (the Baths of
Claudius Etruscus at Rome?). But as a rule, the location of the main bath-

---

57. This situation can be contrasted to the siting of public baths in nineteenth-century and
early twentieth-century American cities, which were often situated in slum neighborhoods and
designed to serve the working classes or particular immigrant groups; see Williams, *Washing
"The Great Unwashed,"* 61–64, 91–94. For "regulars" at Roman baths, see above, chapter 5,
n. 78.

58. See Laurence, esp. 12–19, 122–32. He reiterates these arguments in "The Organization
of Space in Pompeii," in Cornell and Lomas, *Urban Society,* 63–78. Certainly, the baths of
Pompeii, especially in the last years, amply served the residential areas (see map 2). A similar
situation pertains to the baths of Timgad; see Nielsen, 2.75 (fig. 39).

59. See Laurence, 104–21, esp. 105–7 (on the Forum and Central Baths). The Stabian Baths
stand on the corner of two of the city's main thoroughfares (the Via dell'Abbondanza and the
Strada Stabiana), as do the Forum Baths (on the Via del Foro and Via di Nola) and the Central
Baths (on the Strada Stabiana and Via di Nola). The defunct Republican Baths were located at
the corner of the Strada Stabiana and the Via dei Teatri, immediately outside the entrance to the
Triangular Forum (see fig. 14), and the *Balneum Venerium et Nongentum* was advantageously
located near the amphitheater.

60. Entrance fees, even at privately run public establishments, appear to have been generally
small, though variation must be expected: see Heinz, 149–50; Nielsen, 1.131–35. The maximum price for a bath stipulated in Diocletian's price edict (no. 286) is two denarii. In modern
Turkish baths, the cost of admission is usually a fraction of the cumulative costs of the various
personal services on offer, which are often mandatory. Note, by way of contrast, that in 1849–
50, the commercially run public baths in Philadelphia and Boston were too expensive for the
poor; see Williams, *Washing "The Great Unwashed,"* 14, 15.

houses of a Roman community—often at gates or near the forum—seems to suggest that they stood available for all comers.[61]

In an ideal world, it would be possible not only to study bathing facilities within their broad urban context but also to assess a particular bath's operation by comparing its remains with a known clientele. Unfortunately, this assessment is usually impossible. A unique exception is the bathhouse of the Arval Brethren, located at Magliana, outside Rome.[62] We know that there were twelve brethren, yet the pools of the bathhouse have twice that capacity. Since the facility was employed on formal occasions, it is unlikely that anyone other than officials attached to the college would have used it.[63] So the best explanation for the large capacity is that the brethren and their personal footmen *(calatores)* used the baths together, one *calator* per Arval brother. It is fortunate that, by way of contrast, we also know the seating arrangements for the Arval college at the Colosseum. Here seats were assigned in three grades, and the measurements for each grade suggest that the twelve brethren and their families occupied the best grade, officials of the college (scribes, *ministri,* and *calatores*) occupied the second, and slaves sat at the back in the wooden bleachers.[64] Similar arrangements are attested in municipal charters,

---

61. For the siting of baths near gates, see above, chapter 2, n. 69. For baths near fora, see Nielsen's geographical index (1.184–91), where the following places have "Agora," "Forum," or "Central" Baths (listed in alphabetical order, with Nielsen's catalogue entries or page numbers in parentheses where applicable): Augusta Raurica (C.157), Cales (C.35), Cumae (1.29), Ephesos (C.299), Forum Trajani (C.131), Herculaneum (C.38), Lugdunum Convenarum (C.75), Lutetia (C.92), Ostia (C.27), Paestum (1.49 n. 91), Pompeii (C.42, 47), Side (C.373), Thubursicum Numidarum (C.251), Timgad (C.241), Turris Libysonis (C.135). Additions from Manderscheid (with page numbers in parentheses) are Avenches/Aventicum (70), Cherchel/Iol Caesarea (97), Gigthis (117), Lausanne-Vidy/Lousonna (135), Lisieux/Noviomagus Lexoviorum (139), Lucus Feroniae (141), Nocera Superiore/Nuceria Alfaterna (155), Nora (155), Sabratha (189), Saepinum (191), Side (Selimiye; 198), Vaison-la-Romaine/Vasio Vocontiorum (218), Volubilis (226). This list, of course, is far from complete. The designations "Agora," "Forum," and "Central" are modern ones, so other baths can also be located near fora but are not so named: examples are the baths of M. Tullius Venneianus at Paestum (see no. 108) and the so-called Baths of Seius Strabo at Volsinii (see no. 159), both of which were adjacent to the forum.

62. See H. Broise and J. Scheid, *Recherches archéologiques à la Magliana: Le balneum des frères Arvales* (Rome, 1987). See also J. DeLaine, "The *Balneum* of the Arval Brethren," *JRA* 3 (1990): 321–24.

63. See the entry for the year 218 (*CIL* 6.2104.10 [pp. 568–69, s.v. "a. 218"] = Henzen, *Acta,* 203): *item post meridiem a balneo cathedris considerunt.* And see that for 241 (*CIL* 6.2114.14–18 [pp. 580–81, s.v. "a. 241"] = Henzen, *Acta,* 225): *[item post meri]die⟨m⟩ mag⟨ister⟩ lo[t]us cenatorio albo ac pue[ri praetextati patri]mi et matr[i]mi senatorum filii Bo[. . .] conseder(unt) et epulati sunt.* Unfortunately, these laconic notices are our only two witnesses to the Arval Brethren at their bath.

64. See *CIL* 6.2059.25–34 = Henzen, *Acta,* 106–7; J. Kolendo, "La répartition des places aux spectacles et la stratification sociale dans l'empire romaine," *Ktema* 6 (1981): 304–5.

where specific blocks of seats at the theater are assigned to *coloni, incolae, hospites,* and *adventores,* but in free-bathing benefactions in which the very same groups are named as beneficiaries, there is no hint of separate use of the facilities.[65] Although this point of difference cannot be pushed too far— since segregation at shows and spectacles, where members of a community were assembled formally, is only to be expected—the situations evidenced by the charters and benefactions nicely illustrate social mixing at the baths, by providing an explicit contrast whereby the same groups are strictly separated in one context but not in the other.[66]

If, in principle, baths were open to and used by all, there might nonethe-less have been a broad de facto social segregation that separated the bathers by class, as suggested in a recent study of Pompeii. Considering the shape of the Roman day, Ray Laurence argues that only the elite would have had the free time to use the baths at the optimum time (between the sixth and eighth hours), while the lower classes—such as the owners of snack bars (*popinae*) or laborers *(mercennarii)*—visited the facilities only later. He even goes so far as to suggest that perhaps the commoners rarely enjoyed a hot bath.[67] This interesting suggestion is flawed for two reasons. First, even within the pa-rameters of his reconstruction, Laurence's conclusion is unwarranted. Ac-cording to the data he supplies, *mercennarii* and other manual laborers enjoyed a break at the sixth hour, during which time they could have visited the baths, where a light lunch might also be taken. Second, his scheme appears too rigid to offer a realistic reflection of the full gamut of Roman conditions. Owners of *popinae,* for instance, would be busiest at night, so a trip to the baths during the afternoon would not have been beyond them.

---

65. Compare, e.g., *CIL* 2.5439 = *ILS* 6087, §§125, 126 *(lex Ursonensis)* with the benefac-tions at nos. 198, 199, 201, and 204–6. E. Rawson *("Discrimina Ordinum:* The *Lex Julia Theatralis," BSR* 55 [1987]: 93 n. 63) is unsure whether or not the bath provisions were separate for each group. Given the logistics of implementation, separate benefactions seem unlikely.

66. Again, the nature of the evidence requires restating the caveat that we are dealing with different places and different times. The separation of classes at spectacles, however, was made empire-wide by Augustus (see Suet. *Aug.* 44.1) and can be traced in seating inscriptions from all over the empire (see Kolendo, "La répartition"; C. Roueché, *Performers and Partisans at Aphrodisias in the Roman and Late Roman Periods* [London, 1993], 83–128). The formulaic nature of the listed beneficiaries of free baths (specified in descending order as *coloneis/ municipibus, incolis, hospitibus,* etc.) mirrors that of legal regulations and so suggests a formal and widespread application of the practice (at least in the Latin West).

67. Laurence, 122–32, esp. 128–29. In a similar vein, Yegül (429 n. 18), on the basis of Mart. 8.67, suggests that slaves used public baths between the hours reserved women and men. Apparently supportive of this case is the anonymous epigram "The immortals bathe when the bath is first opened, the demi-gods at the fifth hour, and later all the rubbish" *(Anth. Pal.* 9.640: ἀθάνατοι λούονται ἀνοιγομένου βαλανείου, / πέμπτῃ δ' ἡμίθεοι, μετέπειτα δὲ πήματα πάντα).

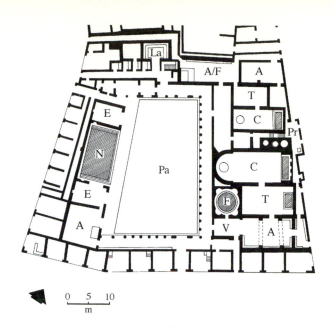

Key to Plans of Baths

A = Apodyterium
C = Caldarium
Ca = Calida Piscina
E = Exedra
F = Frigidarium
N = Natatio
La = Latrine
Lc = Laconicum
Pa = Palaestra
Pr = Praefurnium
T = Tepidarium
V = Vestibule

Fig. 1. Stabian Baths, Pompeii. Groundplan. (G. Fagan after original supplied by F. Yegül; with permission.)

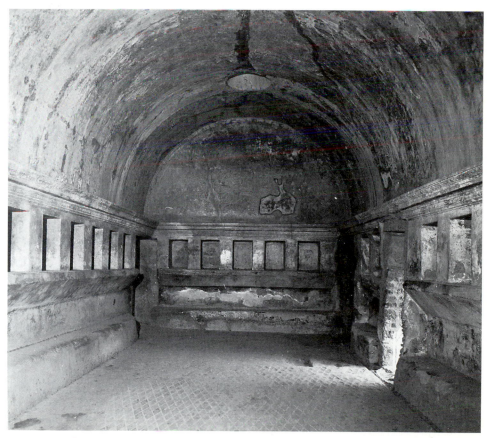

Fig. 2. Stabian Baths, Pompeii. Interior of women's *apodyterium,* looking northeast. (Photo: DAI, Rome.)

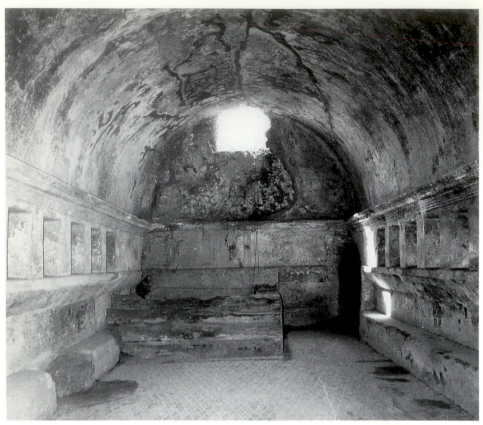

Fig. 3. Stabian Baths, Pompeii. Interior of women's *apodyterium*, looking southwest. (Photo: DAI, Rome.)

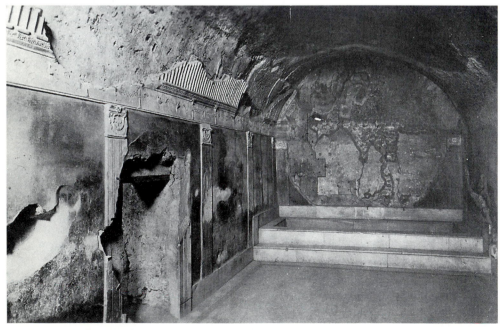

Fig. 4. Stabian Baths, Pompeii. Interior of the women's *caldarium*, looking north. (Photo: DAI, Rome.)

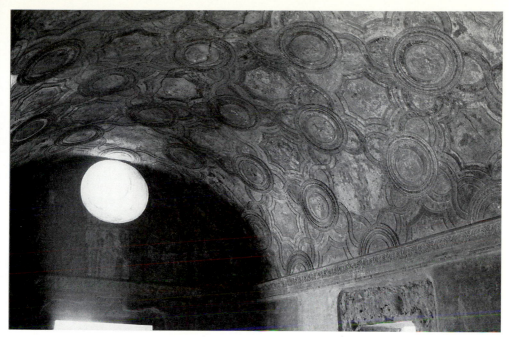

Fig. 5. Stabian Baths, Pompeii. Stucco decoration on vault of men's vestibule.
(Photo: G. Fagan.)

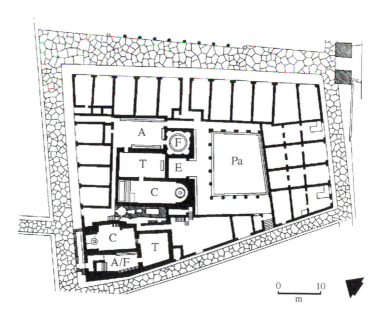

Fig. 6. Forum Baths, Pompeii. Groundplan. (G. Fagan
after E. la Rocca, M. De Vos, and A. De Vos, *Guida
archeoligica di Pompei* [Verona, 1976], 131.)

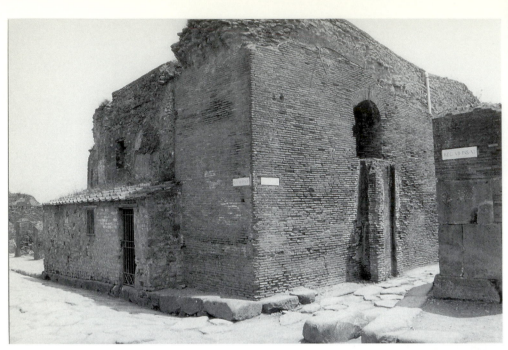

Fig. 7. Forum Baths,
Pompeii. Exterior of the
women's section, which can
be seen to encroach onto
the original pavement.
(Photo: G. Fagan.)

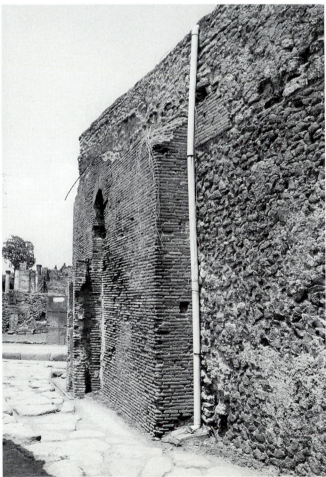

Fig. 8. Forum Baths,
Pompeii. Difference in
construction technique
between the women's
section, in brick on the left,
and the original walling.
(Photo: G. Fagan.)

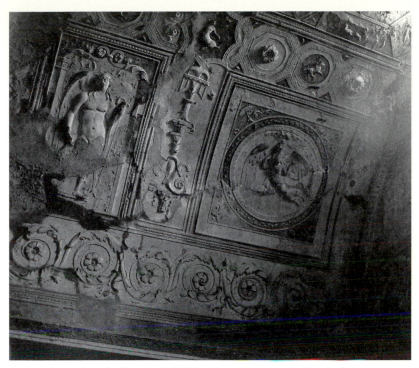

Fig. 9. Forum Baths, Pompeii. Stucco decoration on the roof of the men's *tepidarium*. (Photo: G. Fagan.)

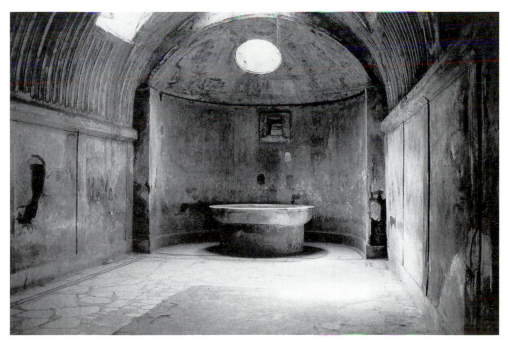

Fig. 10. Forum Baths, Pompeii. Interior of the men's *caldarium*. (Photo: G. Fagan.)

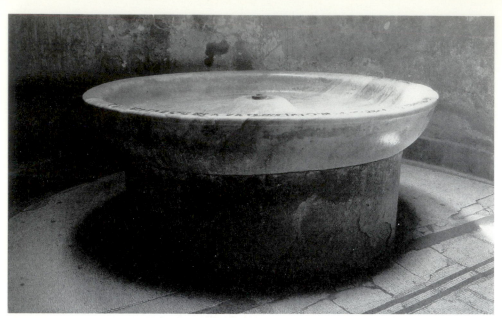

Fig. 11. Forum Baths, Pompeii. Detail of the *labrum* in the men's *caldarium*. (Photo: G. Fagan.)

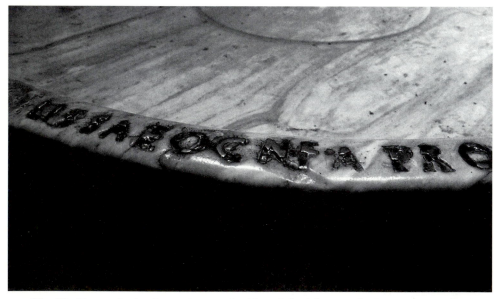

Fig. 12. Forum Baths, Pompeii. Inscribed lip of the *labrum*. The letters M]ELISSAEO CN F. APRO are visible. For full text, see no. 68. (Photo: G. Fagan.)

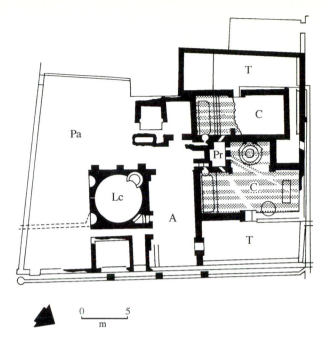

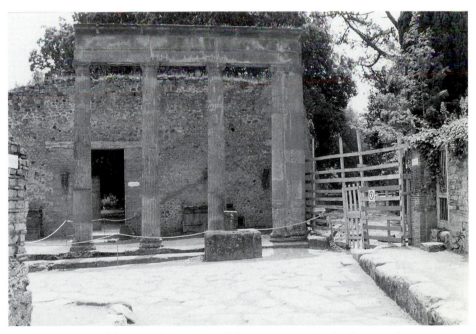

Fig. 13. Republican Baths, Pompeii. Groundplan. (G. Fagan after Nielsen, 2.99 [fig. 77]; with permission.)

Fig. 14. Republican Baths, Pompeii. The entrance to the baths, at right, was located near the monumental entrance to the Triangular Forum and the theater beyond. (Photo: G. Fagan.)

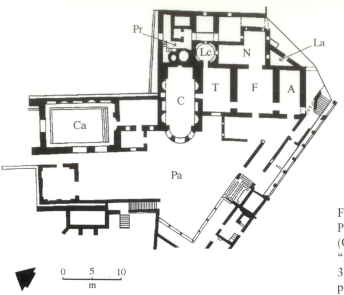

Fig. 15. Suburban Baths,
Pompeii. Groundplan.
(G. Fagan after Jacobelli,
"Suburbanen Thermen,"
328 [fig. 1]; with
permission.)

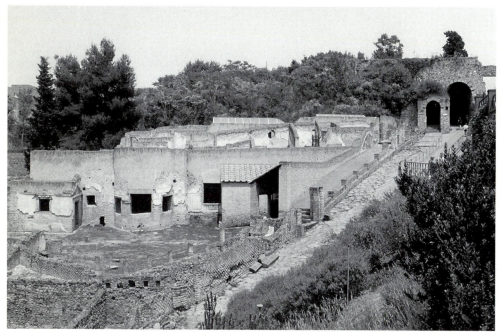

Fig. 16. Suburban Baths, Pompeii. The baths, at left, are located a few meters
outside the Porta Marina, at right. (Photo: G. Fagan.)

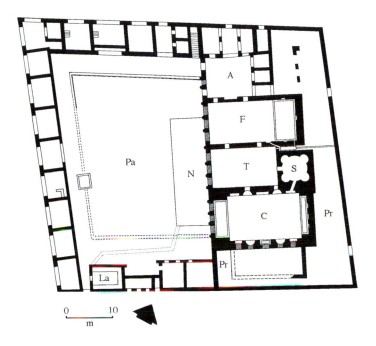

Fig. 17. Central Baths, Pompeii. Groundplan.
(G. Fagan after Nielsen, 2.100 [fig. 79]; with
permission.)

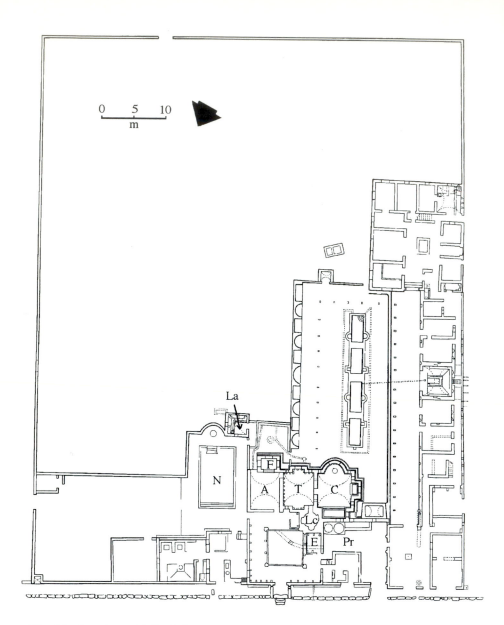

Fig. 18. Premises of Julia Felix, Pompeii. Groundplan indicating the rooms of the *Balneum Venerium et Nongentum*. (G. Fagan after original supplied by C.C. Parslow; with permission.)

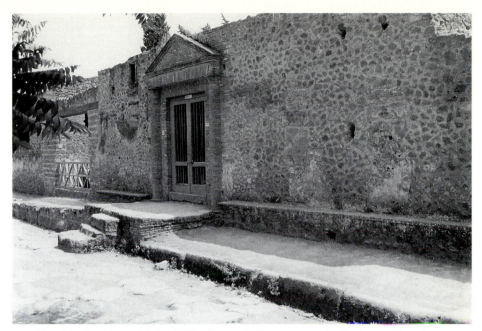

Fig. 19. Premises of Julia Felix, Pompeii. Entrance to the *Balneum Venerium et Nongentum*, with flanking benches. (Photo: G. Fagan.)

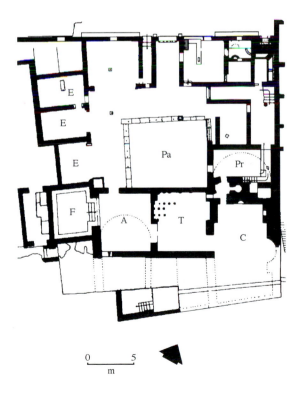

Fig. 20. Palaestra Baths, Pompeii. Groundplan. (G. Fagan after F. Noack and K. Lehmann-Hartleben, *Baugeschichtliche Untersuchungen am Stadtrand von Pompeji* [Berlin, 1936], pl. 13.)

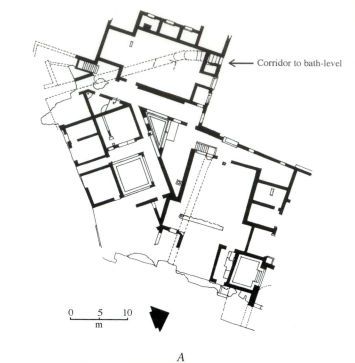

Corridor to bath-level

Fig. 21. Sarno Baths, Pompeii. *(A)* Groundplan of the facilities on level one, that is, street level. *(B)* Groundplan of the baths on level four, that is, on the lowest terrace. (G. Fagan after originals supplied by A.O. Koloski-Ostrow; with permission.)

0   5   10
m

A

B

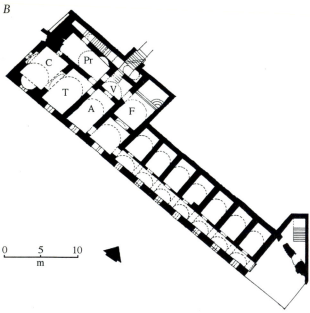

0   5   10
m

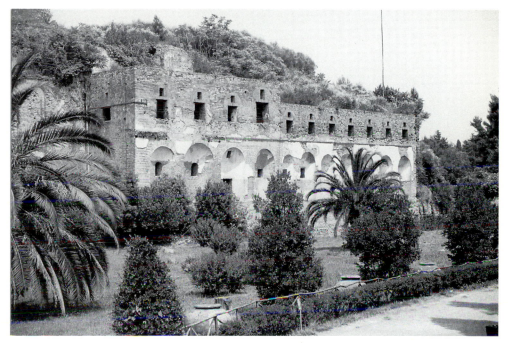

Fig. 22. Sarno Baths, Pompeii. Exterior of the building, showing the bathing suite, at left, with the corridor of seven cells, at right. (Photo: G. Fagan.)

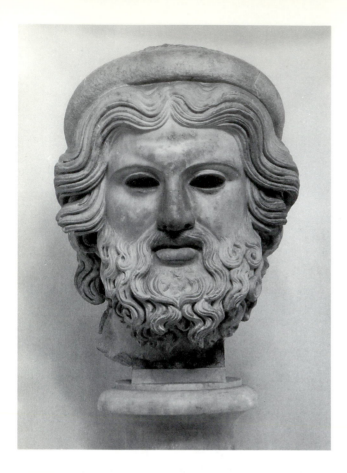

Fig. 23. Baths of Caracalla, Rome. Colossal head of Asclepius. (Photo: DAI, Rome.)

Fig. 24. Baths of Caracalla, Rome. Model. (Photo: DAI, Rome.)

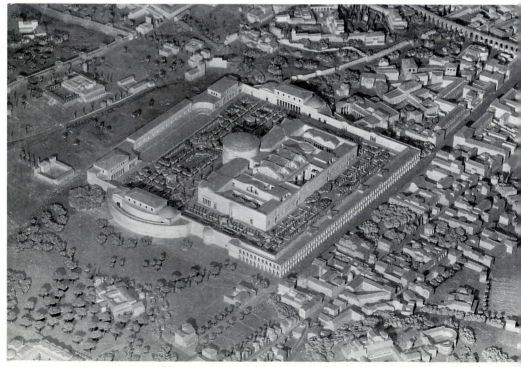

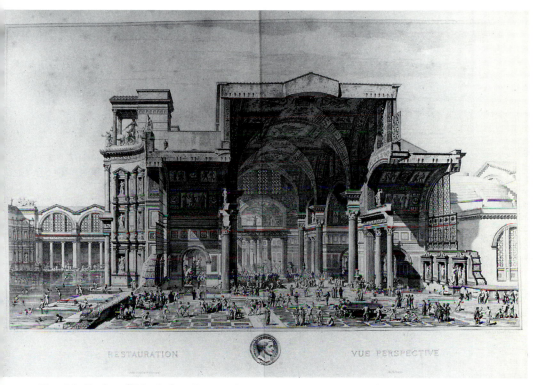

RESTAURATION   VUE PERSPECTIVE

Fig. 25. Baths of Diocletian, Rome. Cutaway reconstruction. (Photo: DAI, Rome.)

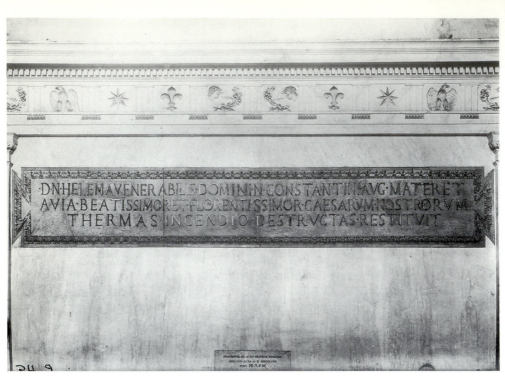

A   Fig. 26. Selected bath inscriptions. *(A)* The Thermae Helenae, Rome.
(B) Dedication to Q. Avelius Priscus; see no. 88. *(C)* Dedication to Euhodus; see
no. 95. *(D)* Commemoration of Q. Volusius Victor's benefactions; see no. 136.
(E) Commemoration of benefactor's actions; see no. 168/69. *(F)* Commemoration of an offer of free bathing; see no. 205. (Photos: DAI, Rome.)

B

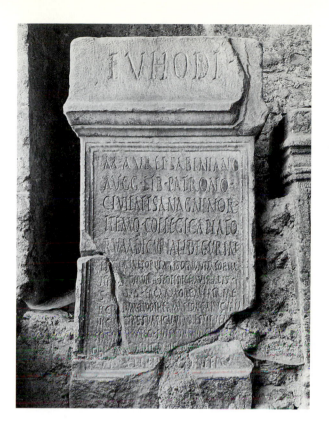

C

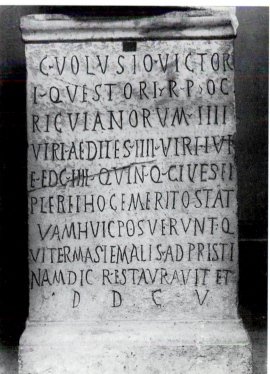

D

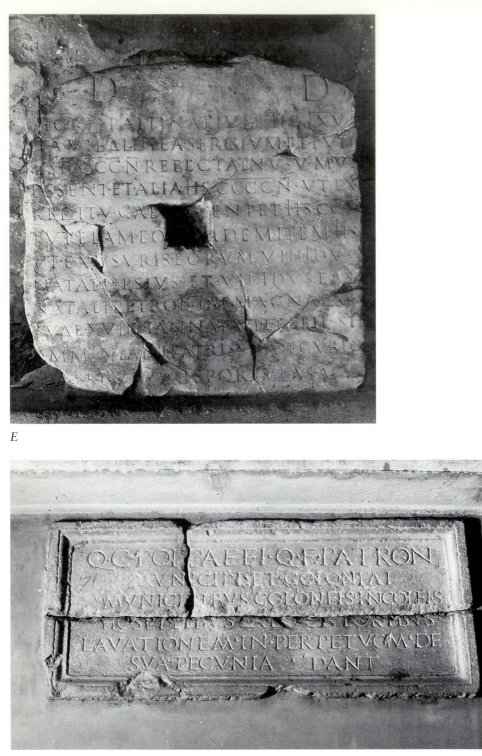

E

F

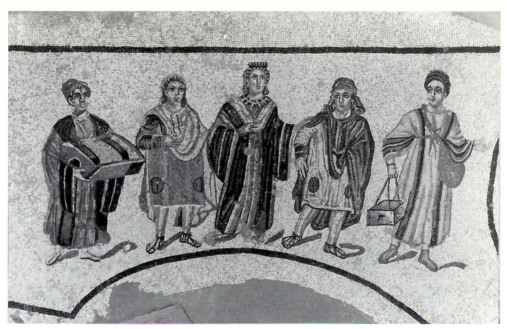

Fig. 27. Piazza Armerina, Sicily. Mosaic of a group of bathers entering the baths. (Photo: DAI, Rome.)

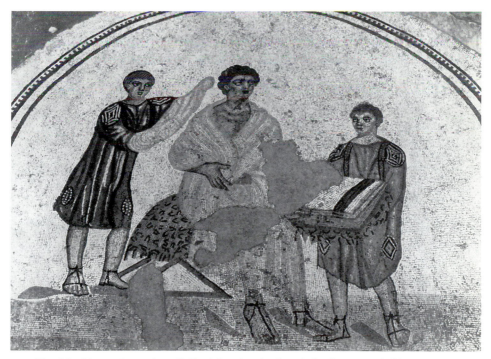

Fig. 28. Piazza Armerina, Sicily. Mosaic of a female bather attended by servants. (Photo: G.V. Gentili, *La villa erculia di Piazza Armerina: I mosaici figurati* [Milan, 1959]; pl. VI; with permission.)

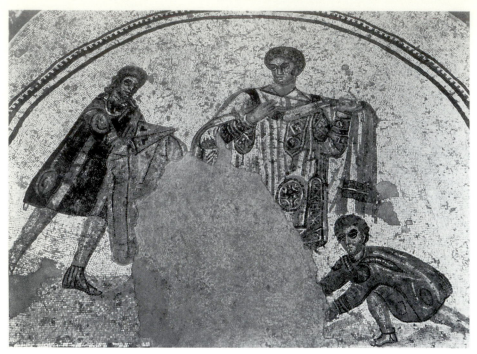

Fig. 29. Piazza Armerina, Sicily. Mosaic of a bather attended by servants, one of whom offers him fresh clothes, while another attends to his footwear. (Photo: Gentili, *Villa erculia*, pl. V; with permission.)

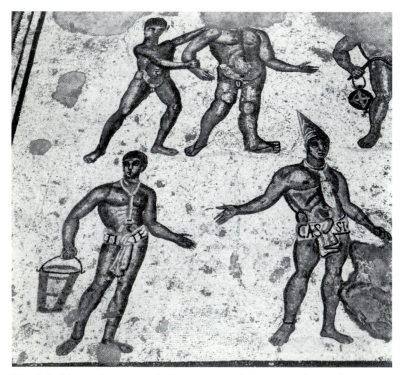

Fig. 30. Piazza Armerina, Sicily. Mosaic of slave attendants; their names are printed on the waistbands of their loincloths. (Photo: Gentili, *Villa erculia*, pl. IV; with permission.)

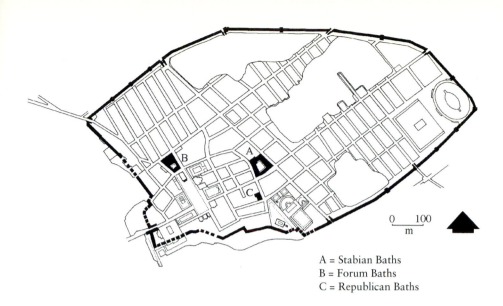

A = Stabian Baths
B = Forum Baths
C = Republican Baths

Map 1. The Public Baths of Pompeii in the Republican Era. (G. Fagan after Eschebach, *Stabianer Thermen*, pl. 1a.)

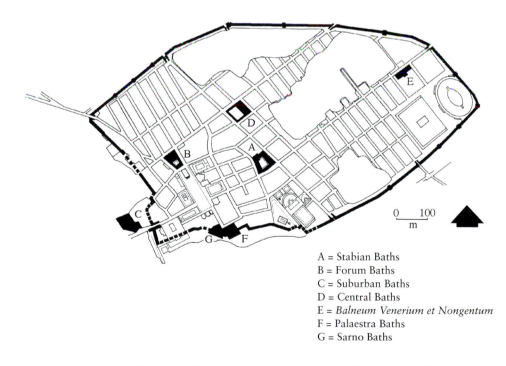

A = Stabian Baths
B = Forum Baths
C = Suburban Baths
D = Central Baths
E = *Balneum Venerium et Nongentum*
F = Palaestra Baths
G = Sarno Baths

Map 2. The Public Baths of Pompeii in the Julio-Claudian and Flavian Eras. (G. Fagan after Eschebach, *Stabianer Thermen*, pl. 1a.)

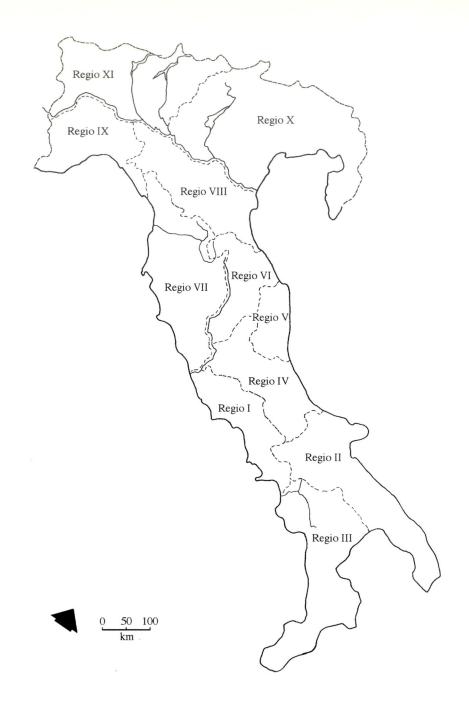

Regio XI

Regio IX

Regio X

Regio VIII

Regio VII

Regio VI

Regio V

Regio IV

Regio I

Regio II

Regio III

0   50   100
km

Map 3. The Regiones of Italy. (G. Fagan after Jouffroy, *Construction publique*; with permission.)

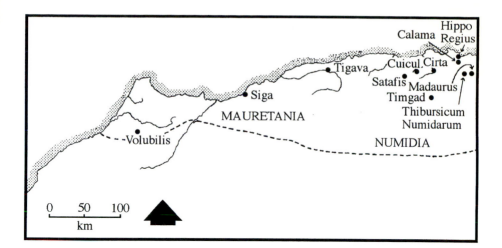

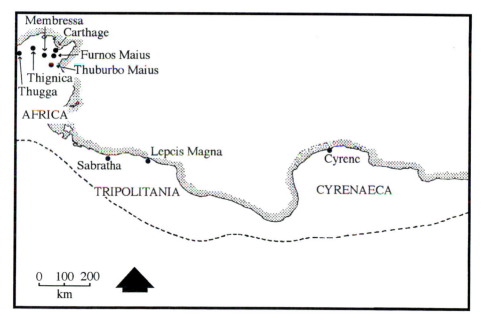

Map 4. The North African Provinces with the Major Sites Mentioned in the
Epigraphic Sample Marked. (G. Fagan after B.H. Warmington in *Atlas of Classical
History*, ed. R.J.A. Talbert [London, 1985], 128; with permission.)

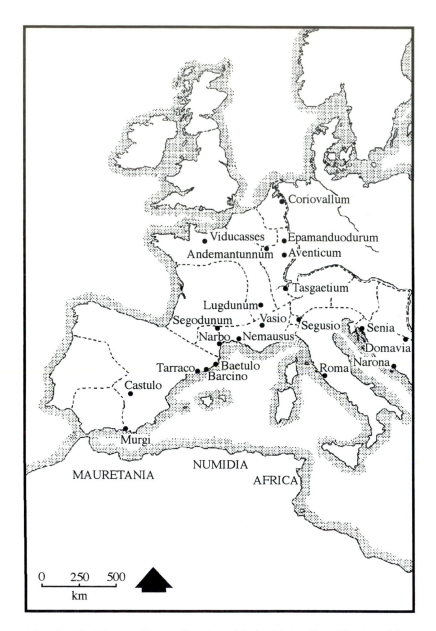

Map 5. The Western Roman Empire with the Major Sites Mentioned in the Epigraphic Sample Marked. (G. Fagan after R.J.A. Talbert in Talbert, *Atlas of Classical History,* 150; with permission.)

The same is true of other shopkeepers who, even if they ran their shops personally throughout the entire day, could leave family members or slaves in charge while they went out for a quick bath in the afternoon. Others conducted their businesses through slave agents *(institores)* and so would have had the opportunity to visit the baths at the optimal hours; and the same is probably true of the *institores* themselves, who appear to have enjoyed considerable freedom of movement.[68] A strict sequence of bathers by class, then, is not a likely scenario.

In any event, the written evidence consistently portrays a social mélange at the public baths and militates against social segregation there, even segregation of a circumstantial nature. Many passages already considered do so, both expressly and implicitly. It would be tedious to go back and draw out the inferences of social mixing from each notice, so some emblematic examples will suffice. The vignettes concerning Larcius Macedo and Hadrian place members of the elite, commoners, and slaves (albeit "on duty") together in the baths simultaneously. In a similar vein, Cicero's refutation of the alleged plot to poison Clodia places well-bred Roman youths in the Senian Baths alongside slaves of Clodia masquerading as conspirators. Cicero's scenario requires a high degree of interaction between the slaves and the noble young men; the baths appear to have been chosen for the transfer of the poison precisely because such open mingling between privileged youths and slaves could occur without drawing unwelcome attention. It is worth noting here that Plutarch, writing centuries after Cicero, offers corroboration of this situation from a different perspective. Pondering the origin of the *bulla,* an amulet worn by freeborn aristocratic youths, he wonders whether it was designed to distinguish them from slaves, so that whenever older men "happened upon them nude" (γυμνοῖς ἐντυχόντες), they could tell the difference and so avoid debauching a boy of free birth.[69] The likeliest context for such

---

68. See Laurence 125 (fig. 8.2; break at sixth hour) and 81–84 (*popinae* busiest at night). On *mercennarii* and shop owners, see S.M. Treggiari, "Urban Labour in Rome: *Mercennarii* and *Tabernarii,*" in P. Garnsey, ed., *Non-Slave Labour in the Greco-Roman World* (Cambridge, 1980), 48–64. On *institores,* see J.-J. Aubert, *Business Managers in Ancient Rome: A Social and Economic Study of* Institores 200 B.C.–A.D. 250 (Leiden, 1994), esp. 22–24 (on *institores* moving about and seducing wives in their homes). Even the jocular epigram cited in previous note (n. 67) need not be taken too literally: it is odd that the bathers attend the baths so early (the eighth hour appears to have been normal, at least in Rome), and the text may reflect the relative densities of the different classes rather than any strictly adhered-to bathing order.

69. Plut. *Mor.* 288A; see further P.G. Warden, "Bullae, Roman Custom, and Italic Tradition," *OpRom* 14 (1983): 69–75. Compare Petron. *Sat.* 92, where an *eques,* a slave, a youth, and the amateur poet Eumolpus are placed together, if not in a bathhouse, then in its immediate vicinity (the young man is naked, implying perhaps that he was still at least within the confines of the bathing complex).

naked encounters among Romans is at the baths. More generally, it seems unlikely that when Pliny visited the public baths in the village near his Laurentine villa, he had the locals thrown out so he could enjoy some privacy. Rather, he would have joined them. To be sure, an infamous story of unpalatable upper-class arrogance at the baths is on record. Gaius Gracchus, in an anecdote cited by Aulus Gellius, reports how a traveling consul's wife cleared the men's baths at Teanum Sidicinum so she could use them—and then had the local magistrate flogged in the forum for not complying quickly enough. Interestingly, a nearby town reacted by issuing a decree banning the locals from their bathhouse if a Roman magistrate was in town; otherwise, presumably, they would have continued to use it along with visiting magistrates.[70] Most interesting about these events is the indignation with which they are recorded. Evidently such occurrences were exceptions to the rule. For the Romans, a town's public baths seem to have been places where everyone could and did go, and anyone who insisted otherwise was transgressing an unwritten social code.

The question remains open as to how free the interclass mingling was in the baths. At first glance, there seems little hope of detecting such mingling. Explicit evidence for it is lacking, and the general shape of Roman society would seem to militate against it. Among the Romans, wealth, status, and privilege were paramount concerns, especially for those who enjoyed them.[71] Divisions between the wealthy upper classes (broadly designated *honestiores* from the second century onward) and everyone else (termed *humiliores* or *tenuiores*) were visible and enshrined in the laws.[72] Citizens were organized

---

70. Gell. *NA* 10.3.1–3. The consul's wife wanted to use the men's baths, which were presumably bigger and better appointed than the implied women's facility, and so the local people were not removed solely out of class snobbery, though it was certainly a factor. The same passage reports that a Roman praetor had the local quaestors at Ferentinum flogged for not clearing the baths for his use, presumably out of pure social arrogance.

71. This point is made repeatedly in modern studies of the Roman social order: see, e.g., G.E.M. de Ste. Croix, *The Class Struggle in the Ancient Greek World* (London, 1981), 327–408, 425; Duncan-Jones, *Economy,* 12; Garnsey and Saller, *Roman Empire,* 107–25; MacMullen, *Roman Social Relations,* 88–120; id., *Corruption and the Decline of Rome* (New Haven, 1988), 60–84; M. Reinhold, "Usurpation of Status and Status Symbols in the Roman Empire," *Historia* 20 (1971): 275. The hierarchy is further crystallized in such studies as J. Gagé, *Les classes sociales dans l'empire romaine* (Paris, 1964), where each class is treated separately, with little or no attention paid to interclass relations. An excellent overview is provided by G. Alföldy, *The Social History of Rome*[3] (Baltimore, 1988), esp. 106–15.

72. The divisions were most palpable in the different punishments meted out to the different groups: for *honestiores,* fines, loss of property, and exile; for *humiliores,* flogging, torture, condemnation to the arena, and crucifixion. See P. Garnsey, *Social Status and Legal Privilege in the Roman Empire* (Oxford, 1970), 103–52 (differentiated punishments); 222–23, 260–80 (*honestior/humilior* division). See also K.M. Coleman, "Fatal Charades: Roman Executions Staged as Mythological Enactments," *JRS* 80 (1990): 54–57.

into officially regulated "orders" *(ordines),* of which the senators, *equites,* and decurions constituted the elite. Each order carried property qualifications for admission, legal distinctions were assigned according to rank, and legally regulated status symbols identified members. In fact, status symbols— such as particular articles of clothing, rings, or reserved seats at spectacles— were essential for maintaining and displaying the *dignitas* of the upper classes as they moved about in public. The strict laws against usurpation of such symbols constitute strong testimony to the seriousness with which public appearance was treated by those formulating the legal codes, namely, the upper classes.[73] Further complications were added to this system in the form of distinctions between citizen and noncitizen (until 212), slave and free, and freeborn and freed, as well as by the complex social contract of *clientela.* Within the privileged *ordines* themselves, added status accrued to people who enjoyed proximity to sources of power and influence, that is, to the emperor or his family, officials in the central administration, or prominent local aristocrats.[74] The nature of the whole towering edifice is summed up by Pliny when he advises a fellow senator in the provincial service to preserve the distinction of the orders in legal hearings, since "nothing is more unequal than equality itself" (*Ep.* 9.5.3: *nihil est ipsa aequalitate inaequalius*).

In such a social environment, it seems inconceivable that the upper classes would have exposed themselves to (and at) public baths: surely their *dignitas* would have been compromised by doing so. Yet the evidence reviewed above suggests that the mingling of rich and poor, *honestior* and *humilior,* and slave and free was a daily occurrence at the baths. This circumstance has prompted some scholars to conclude that the baths acted as social levelers. Indeed, a recent study of Roman leisure includes a sustained analysis of the baths as places of social tension where the elite's social identity was threatened and moral ambiguity abounded: J.P. Toner argues, "The baths represented a hole in the ozone layer of the social hierarchy."[75]

---

73. The *lex Ursonensis* stipulates fines of five thousand sesterces for transgression of reserved seating arrangements, suggesting that the measure was aimed more at the socially ambitious decurion or *eques* than at the lowly *humilior* (*CIL* 2.5439 = *ILS* 6087, §§126–27). Note the shocked reaction in the sources to usurpation of status symbols: see Cic. *Phil.* 2.44; Pliny *HN* 33.32; Suet. *Aug.* 40, *Calig.* 26.4, *Dom.* 8.3; Mart. 5.8, 5.14, 5.23, 5.35, 5.38. See further Kolb, "Statussymbolik im antiken Rom."; Reinhold, "Usurpation."

74. See Alföldy, *Social History,* 115–33; R. MacMullen, "Personal Power in the Roman Empire," *AJP* 107 (1986): 512–24 (= id., *Changes in the Roman Empire,* 190–97); id., *Corruption,* 96–104.

75. See esp. Toner, 53–64 (quote at 57); see also above, chapter 8, n. 3. This conclusion is certainly defensible. By way of comparison, note that public baths in Japan of the Edo era, itself marked by a rigidly hierarchical social order, were seen to promote a "democracy of nudity" (see

In my view, this conclusion is unconvincing. In the first place, we have seen that members of the elite built and maintained the empire's public baths at great personal expense and visited them as a matter of course. Why would they do so only to face potential humiliation and degradation in front of the common mob? Further, the Romans themselves rarely speak of baths in terms of equalization. Unlike the dinner party *(convivium)*, any ideology of bathing equality that may have existed was not systematically worked out and appears to have been minimally pervasive.[76] Even if such an ideology were present and prevalent, there is no reason to believe that it played itself out in reality.[77] A point of comparison is the common moralistic trope that hot baths were ruinous to military discipline.[78] Despite this widely attested belief among ancient writers, bathhouses fully equipped with heated sections are found attached to Roman military installations of all kinds, from Syria to Scotland. The opinions of certain members of the elite cannot therefore be used to circumscribe mass behavior. In fact, it is arguably the imposition of modern Western attitudes toward public nudity that gives rise to the belief that it was compromising for the upper-class Roman bather to be seen naked at the baths.[79] Roman attitudes toward the body and toward bodily functions were more open than they are today, and we may safely assume that if the elite felt their *dignitas* would be impugned by visiting the baths, they would have stayed away.[80] It seems highly unlikely that members of the elite,

---

Grilli and Levy, *Furo*, 76, 79); and Frans Emil Sillanpää, Finnish Nobel laureate, writes: "The understanding shared by all decent sauna-men transcends distinctions of class and party. Should a sauna bench turn literally into a field of heated contention, it is even then a great unifier" (cited in Bremer and Raevuori, *World of the Sauna*, 173).

76. A comment in Clement of Alexandria (*Paid.* 3.47.3 [Stählin]) is the only place I have encountered an open expression of baths as social equalizers, and Clement's peculiar worldview can hardly be applied to an entire culture that is largely silent on the matter. On the ideal of equality at dinner parties, see J.H. D'Arms, "The Roman *Convivium* and the Idea of Equality," in O. Murray, ed., *Sympotica: A Symposium on the* Symposion (Oxford, 1990), 311–14.

77. At dinner parties, despite the egalitarian ideology, social segregation was regularly implemented; see D'Arms, "Roman *Convivium*," 314–17.

78. See, e.g., Plut. *Alex.* 40.1, *Luc.* 7.5; Dio 27.94.2, 62.6.4; HA *Avid. Cass.* 5.5, *Pesc. Nig.* 3.10.

79. Whether bathers were fully or partially naked does not affect the argument—the Latin word *nudus* implies, at the very least, a person stripped of their proper apparel; see above, chapter 1, pp. 24–25.

80. There have been, as yet, no serious studies of Roman attitudes toward public nudity, although there are such studies of the Greek attitudes, notably L. Bonfante, "Nudity as a Costume in Classical Art," *AJA* 93 (1989): 543–70; J.-P. Thuillier, "La nudité athlétique (Grèce, Etrurie, Rome)," *Nikephoros* 1 (1988): 29–48. Due to the specific cultural context of much Greek nudity (i.e., athletics and the gymnasium), these attitudes cannot be extrapolated wholesale to Roman public baths. For a preliminary consideration of Roman attitudes, see Hallett, "Roman Heroic Portrait," 67–117, esp. 90–99 on public baths. In general, Roman attitudes are

obsessed with their social status and with the public appearance that declared it to the world, checked their *dignitas* at the bath door along with their cloaks.

Far from offering an "equalizing" atmosphere that threatened the social identity of elite bathers, it seems more plausible that the baths functioned very much like any other public venue—as places where the rich went deliberately to flaunt, show off, and thereby reinforce their claim to social superiority. At Pompeii, the spatial relationship of the houses of the rich to the forum and public baths can be interpreted in this light. The buildings are so located as to allow the elite to process in style to the forum in the morning, to the baths in the afternoon, and then back home for dinner in the evening, ever mindful of the public's gaze. Indeed, the entire urban landscape of the Roman city was, in some respects, a product of this social process and others, in which the baths had their role.[81] Even when at the baths, there are indications that signals of status followed the privileged bather past the *balneator* and into the establishment. Chief among these would be the size (and cut) of the slave retinue: we have seen Macedo's path-clearing slave and late Imperial retinues of fifty or more (above, chapter 1, p. 30 [Macedo] and chapter 8, pp. 199–200 [retinue]). The behavior of such bathers and their slaves could further distinguish the important personage from the surrounding nonentities. For instance, Lucian (*Nigr.* 34) complains of people whose slaves carry them around in litters at the baths or go before them crying out warnings of impending obstacles. Such pampered bathers could also bring *instrumenta balnei* of fine metals; be oiled with perfumed unguents; drink expensive wine from ostentatiously fine goblets; be dried with woolen, rather than linen, towels; and have multiple changes of clothes to chose from at the end of it all. Jewelry could also be worn throughout the bathing process, as a constant indicator of rank. Corroboration comes from the drains of baths,

---

relaxed, at least in relation to the baths. Note that Aesop's master feels no compunction about urinating or defecating in front of him—the two even discuss the latter process (Anon. *Life of Aesop* 28, 67). The remarkably open form of the Roman public latrine appears related; see above, chapter 3, pp. 77–78. Relatively open attitudes toward public nakedness may have come to Rome with the Greeks (see Plut. *Cat. Maj.* 20.8), but, interestingly, there were still restrictions on bathing naked with certain family members (see above, chapter 2, n. 28). Instructive is the reaction of A. Selkirk in reviewing M. Henig, *Classical Gems: Ancient and Modern Intaglios and Cameos in the Fitzwilliam Museum in Cambridge* (Cambridge, 1994). Selkirk, a non-specialist, is struck by how many Roman gems depict male nudes (mostly gods)—and aged and corpulent nudes at that. He adds, "It is not at all to our modern tastes: but who is the odd one out—the Romans or us?" (*Current Archaeology* 144 [1995]: 475). Note also the shocked reaction of early European visitors to Japanese public baths: "They wash twice a day and do not worry if their privy parts are seen" (Jorge Alvares, cited in Grilli and Levy, *Furo,* 68).

81. See Laurence, esp. 131–32.

which have proven fertile fields for finds of gems and beads, washed away as their owners soaked.[82] No doubt such status indicators as these allowed Clement of Alexandria to recognize rich women at the baths (*Paid.* 3.31.1–33.3 [Stählin]) and caused the Jewish Mishnah to assume that "a gentile of high estate" would be instantly identifiable there (*m. Maks.* 2:5). When Encolpius and his friends first encounter Trimalchio in the palaestra of a set of public baths before adjourning to dinner, they identify him by his fine clothes and slave attendants (Petron. *Sat.* 27–28). Just as instructive, but more pathetic, are those individuals who attempted to imitate the bathing finesse of their social superiors, to little effect. Martial's Aper, though poor, brings along defective slaves to carry his towels and guard his equally defective clothing and to anoint him with a drop of oil (12.70). Juvenal, in a similar vein, comments that Tongilius risks bankruptcy through maintaining a lavish public front, to which end he brings to the baths a huge flask of oil and droves of (hired?) retainers (7.129–31).

The social environment at the baths, then, was far from "equalizing." Although the various classes bathed together and were not formally segregated, there can be little doubt that everybody knew their place in the social pageant.[83] Slave attendants kept curious plebs at bay and cleared paths through crowds, the finery of bathing accessories announced rank to onlookers, and accent, vocabulary, and demeanor presumably helped to discourage uninvited and unwanted contact.[84] Social deference to the elite must have characterized the atmosphere, for instance, when a governor entered a public bath in the provinces or when the ex-consul Pliny dropped in on one of the facilities in the *vicus* near his Laurentine villa. Pliny also makes

---

82. See *Dig.* 34.2.40.1 (a man has two sets of silver bath ware *[argentum balneare]*, one for use only on festival days, the other presumably for ordinary days); *CIL* 13.5708.II.23–25 (a man orders various of his favorite personal belongings, including his bathing gear *[balnearia]*, to be cremated with him); Juv. 7.129–31 (unguents and retinue); Petron. *Sat.* 28 (unguents, towels, and wine); Amm. Marc. 28.4.19 (fine linens, multiple changes of clothes, and jewelry); Mart. 11.59, Pliny *HN* 33.40, Plut. *Mor.* 288A (jewelry in the baths); Mart. 12.70.9 (fine goblets and pretty slaves). *Bullae* may also be considered jewelry that denoted rank; see above, chapter 8, pp. 211–12. For finds of jewelry in the drains of baths, note the substantial deposits—including gemstones, rings, and glass beads—in the conduit under the *frigidarium* of the Legionary Fortress Baths at Caerleon (see Zienkiewicz, *Legionary Fortress Baths,* 117–56) and the discovery of gemstones in the drain at Bath (see M. Henig, "The Gemstones from the Main Drain," in B. Cunliffe, ed., *Roman Bath* [Oxford, 1969], 71–88).

83. J. DeLaine is surely right when she claims ("Recent Research," 29) that at the *thermae* "the principal characters must have always been the rich, who went to be seen, and the rest, who went to gape as much as to bathe."

84. On demeanor and accent as signposts of class and breeding, see Pliny *Ep.* 1.14.8; Plut. *Mor.* 439F–440A; Quint. *Inst.* 1.1; Sen. *Ep.* 52.12, 94.8. See also Cic. *Orat.* 59 (reprised in Quint. *Inst.* 11.3.122) on the importance of poise and gesture, at least for the orator.

mention of a book of verses he composed, presumably by dictation, while at the baths (*Ep.* 4.14.2; compare Suet. *Aug.* 85.2)—if ever he did so in a public facility, lowly onlookers would have had few illusions as to the class of bather who was gracing their ablutions with his presence. The same can be said of the person who showed up at the baths with clients in tow (see, e.g., Mart. 3.36, 7.76). The party, itself of diverse social standing, may well have progressed through the baths together but surely did so on different and perceptible social planes, insofar as the patron's needs must have consistently taken precedence over those of his clients. Martial hints at this social difference when he reminds himself that no matter how much he socializes with his patrons, including taking baths with them, he should not believe that they actually like him (7.76). The practice of patrons dispensing cash handouts *(sportulae)* at the baths, in full public view, could only have reinforced this impression of clear social divisions between the bathers, even within individual bathing parties (see Mart. 3.7, 10.70).

It remains unclear how often commoners were subjected to arrogant or degrading treatment by their social betters at the baths. We hear of Cato or Macedo getting struck, but how many unnamed plebs suffered the same indignity in silence? Even if the behavior of the consul's wife at Teanum Sidicinum is taken as the extreme, how often were plebs cleared out of rooms or pools when some luminary desired their use, and how many commoners were cuffed about the ears for not deferring appropriately?[85] Presumably, the elite expected an automatic deference at the baths, as they did elsewhere. A graffito from Herculaneum reports that two companions *(sodales)* threw a useless bathing servant out onto the street (no. 281). No doubt the man was a slave, but did other lowly bathers suffer similar treatment? There is no way of knowing with certainty, but it is unrealistic to imagine that a harmonious and "democratic" atmosphere prevailed at the baths, that they were "holes in the ozone layer of the social hierarchy," where the elite were suddenly divested of their snobbish attitudes and behavior. Thus Aesop's master sends him to the baths to reconnoiter the crowds before venturing out himself, and Trimalchio praises the pleasure of washing "without the crowd" *(sine turba)*.[86] A trip to the baths, although pleasurable, could also be aggravating

---

85. For Cato and Macedo, see above, chapter 1, pp. 30–31. Note that the *Historia Augusta,* in a diatribe against Egyptians, says that they were wont to cause trouble on the slightest pretext, such as "not being granted a place in the bathhouse" (*Tyr. Trig.* 22.2: *locum in balneis non concessum*). The precise meaning of this statement is unclear, but it possibly refers to the sort of jostling for position envisaged above.

86. Anon. *Life of Aesop* 65–67; Petron. *Sat.* 73.

for the privileged bather, precisely because of the close contact that could be expected with the commoners.

It would be fascinating to know how much business was conducted in the informal context of the bathhouse—how many petitions were quietly heard, agreements reached, alliances forged, and favors requested and granted. Or were baths considered havens from public business, inappropriate places for such activity? Unfortunately, there is no solid evidence either way.[87] When Pliny complains about being hounded by petitioners on making an appearance at his rural property (*Ep.* 9.15), one may wonder how likely it was that he would have been left alone when he visited the local public bathhouse. But it is noticeable that among historical writers, baths are never presented as places where plots are hatched or discussed (such activity is more often staged in people's houses, either at dinner parties or in back rooms).[88] One would imagine that the baths, especially a private suite, would have offered ideal venues for conspirators. The silence of the sources in this regard may suggest that a "no-business-here" ethic prevailed at the baths, but this suggestion is hardly conclusive. In the end, the question must remain open, but given the degree to which all manner of business was conducted on a personal level in the Roman world, it is easy to conceive of the baths as natural venues for meetings and negotiations of all sorts; comparative material from better-documented public bathing cultures also points in this direction.[89]

The general social function of Roman public baths, therefore, appears to have been as reproducers of the social order in Roman communities. To be sure, they promoted a broad community spirit, insofar as everyone went and mixed at unusually close quarters and in marked informality compared to

---

87. There are hints, such as the report in Suetonius (*Vesp.* 21) that Vespasian was more inclined to grant indulgences after his bath. In a similar vein, P. Plautius Hypsaeus, charged under the *ambitus* laws in 52 B.C., sought help from his friend Cn. Pompeius "when he had left the bath" *(balineo egressus)*, but the suppliant met with a stony reception: see Val. Max. 9.5.3; for Hypsaeus, see *RE* 21.16–18, s.v. "Plautius 23" (Münzer). Both anecdotes, however, are set just after a bath, not actually inside a bath building.

88. See, e.g., Sall. *Cat.* 20.1; Tac. *Ann.* 4.69 (private rooms). On dinner parties, see G.M. Paul, "Symposia and Deipna in Plutarch's Lives and in Other Historical Writings," in W.J. Slater, ed., *Dining in a Classical Context* (Ann Arbor, 1991), 162–64. In contrast, emperors (and others) are sometimes portrayed as being harmed going to, coming from, or actually in their baths: see, e.g., Suet. *Galb.* 10.5; Joseph. *AJ* 19.104–6, *BJ* 1.340–41; HA *Pert.* 12.8, *M. Ant.* 4.4, *Geta* 6.3.

89. Finnish saunas are found attached to banks and businesses (see above, introduction, n. 4), and Japanese hot-spring resorts are popular venues for business meetings (see Grilli and Levy, *Furo,* 150). An acquaintance from China once told me how a local Communist Party secretary would take the opportunity of a visit to the public baths to encourage her to apply for membership of the party, because the secretary felt that the informal mood at the baths relieved the intensity of the political pressure and lent the serious discussion a casual air.

other venues of general assembly (such as at the forum, in the streets, or at the theater). Everyone, rich and poor, slave and free, seems to have taken advantage of their local baths. Nevertheless, it would be a mistake to conclude from this fact alone that the baths acted as agents of equalization and promoted a dilution of the status-driven Roman social order. Examination of the evidence suggests that the privileged made their presence felt at the baths, where, despite the prevailing nakedness (or at least improper attire) and the informality of the context, rank was maintained by a variety of means. An analogous situation pertained at public banquets, where, though everyone ate together and in sight of each other, distinctions of status were expressed by the unrepresentative numbers from each attending class, the location of the tables, the maintenance of a strict order of place on the dining couches, and the differentiated quality of the food and drink served.[90] From this perspective, going to the baths expressed one's membership in a Roman community, but going in style helped claim leadership of it.

---

90. See J.H. D'Arms, "Control, Companionship, and *Clientela*: Some Social Functions of the Roman Communal Meal," *EchCl* 28 (1984): 338–44; id., "The Roman *Convivium*," 308–11.

Conclusion

One of the chief values of studying Roman public bathing culture lies in those inferences that can be drawn from the baths and set on the wider stage of Roman social history. For instance, the growth of the bathing habit in the late Republic and early Empire can be used, to some degree, as a barometer for the increasingly sophisticated urbanization underway in Rome and Italy at this time. The technology required for the construction of baths and the broad popular appeal of the public bathing habit bespeak a growing community spirit in the places where they are attested, as well as an increasing affluence among the local benefactors who saw to the erection of baths. At Rome, the spread of baths was the result of a series of coincidental processes, including rising public patronage, a greater foreign presence among the city's ever more numerous inhabitants, and improved building techniques.

If the hypothesis about the influence of medical thinking on the rise of the bathing habit is correct, the baths indicate the remarkable degree to which medical precepts could shape the behavior, initially, of a city and, ultimately, of a whole culture. However, the medical "function" of the baths appears to have quickly fallen into the background, as public baths established themselves as social centers and informal places of leisure open to all. In addition, the rise in the popularity of baths and their subsequent export around the empire represent, in a tangible way, the spread of the Roman lifestyle throughout the provinces, even if, ironically, within Italy itself the Romans were not initially at the forefront of the custom. More profitable work needs to be done in tracing and examining the introduction and spread of baths in the various provinces, especially in the eastern empire, where the Roman habit came to coexist with or even supplant the older Greek customs centered on the gymnasium and βαλανεῖον.

The baths can also been used as a laboratory in which to test propositions about imperial munificence and municipal euergetism. Close scrutiny of the epigraphy has revealed that the emperor concerned himself primarily with the imperial capital and only occasionally acted to benefit communities elsewhere. The huge baths of Rome represent, on some level, the ideals of imperial benevolence and control over nature. They are the biggest bathhouses known, as they should be, since the empire's preeminent benefactor stood behind them. In the majority of the empire's towns and cities, however, the local magnates presented their communities with baths (on a more modest scale), just as they presented all public amenities. Instances of imperial representatives providing bathing facilities for communities under their care are not unknown, but they have been shown to comprise a small proportion of the total. The demography of bath benefactors, then, greatly reinforces the picture of a remote central administration overseeing an empire comprised of largely self-sufficient communities. There is also a certain parallelism at work here: as the emperor proffered benefactions to Rome, so did local aristocrats to their communities. This fact raises the issue of motives, for which the evidence is generally poor. The motivation of specific municipal bath builders remains largely unknown, but there can be little doubt that their substantial financial outlays were repaid in greater social prominence for themselves and their families—in short, the baths provide excellent examples of local euergetism. Again, there remains more to be done with the inscriptions. Particularly useful would be a systematic correlation of known baths with surviving inscriptions, including a detailed study of how the latter relate to the physical remains.

The baths' social functioning is perhaps the most important element of their existence. The baths act as a microcosm for emphasizing the importance of public appearance in establishing status in the Roman world. A rich person who was not seen to be rich was hardly a rich person at all.[1] The baths fit neatly into this world of status defined by public appearance. They were used by the elite as arenas for displays of status, no less—and perhaps more—than the forum, the street, or the theater. It remains unclear to what extent, if any, the modern concept of "social control" can be applied to the world of the Roman public bath. Certainly, the baths were built and maintained by the privileged and were open for use by the masses, but whether the baths were vehicles used by the elite to manipulate the behavior or attitudes of the masses is really a matter of modern debate and is beyond checking based on the ancient evidence available to us.[2] Roman society was permeated

---

1. Note here Apuleius' miserly Milo (*Met.* 1.21), whose reticence in spending his money is resented by the townspeople of Hypata.

2. "Social control" is, in any case, a difficult concept to nail down, despite its prevalence in modern sociological literature. A typical definition runs as follows: "Attempted social control is overt behavior by a human, the first party, in the belief that (1) the overt behavior increases or decreases the probability of a change in the behavior of another human or humans, the second party in either case; (2) the overt behavior involves a third party but not in the way of sequential control [defined as control involving a minimum of three individuals]; and (3) the increase or decrease is desirable" (J.P. Gibbs, *Control: Sociology's Central Notion* [Urbana, 1989], 58–59).

with notions of hierarchy, obligation, benefaction, and reciprocity. The provision of leisure was seen as part of the establishment's job and extended equally to games, public banquets, cash handouts, and buildings for public use.[3] The notion of "social control" may limit the scope of interpretation by imputing ulterior motives on a wide variety of phenomena that are largely removed from modern experience.

That said, the baths certainly fit neatly into the pattern of elite provision of popular leisure, which raises a further point about the reasons for bath construction at the municipal level. In a sense, local luminaries built baths for themselves, as places where they could be seen and (possibly) dispense favors. Whether this activity is an example of social control or just another manifestation of the sort of hierarchical practice that permeated ancient society remains moot. Whatever the case, there must have been a particular pleasure in entering a bathhouse that bore your name, reading the impressive inscription recording your actions over the door, and going through the bathing process in the company of appreciative and deferential members of your community. In some cases, statues or other commemorations of bene-factors, sometimes honoring more than one generation of the same family, graced the baths themselves, reinforcing the essentially provisionary nature of the benefactor's relationship not only with the immediate building but with the community at large.[4] For this reason, the baths are poor candidates as media of social equalization. On the contrary, they stand as a striking illustration of just how deeply ingrained in Roman society were the divisions imposed by hierarchy and status, while at the same time the wide popularity of the baths and their socially diverse clientele laid emphasis on the essential unity of the community. Romans of different social status must often have moved in different worlds, but they could contribute jointly to the social environment of their town's bathing facility.

This definition, however, is notably vague and is potentially applicable to practically every type of human interaction.

3. See Toner, 22–33. Note especially the statement by Cicero (*Rep.* 1.52) that the elite must see to it that the commoners never feel that their comforts *(commoda)* are being ignored.

4. An illustrative example is the room at the baths at Tarquinii in which were found five commemorative inscriptions (accompanying statues, now lost?) relating to a local family who built the baths and to another man and his wife who restored them; see no. 176. In a similar vein, the Thermae of Decius in Rome yielded many commemorations of prominent people; see LaFollette, "Baths of Trajan Decius," 83–85 (nos. 8–17).

Epigraphic Sample

Introduction to the Epigraphic Sample

For the most part, bath-related inscriptions have gone largely unstudied.[1] There are understandable reasons for this. The volume of material involved is prodigious, since the ubiquity of baths and the pervasiveness of Roman bathing culture ensure that practically all regions and periods of the empire are represented, especially from the second century onward. As a result, merely collecting pertinent texts represents a daunting task. In addition, much of the material appears, on the surface, to be largely uninformative. Most bath-related inscriptions are formulaic records of construction and have attracted little attention, except as part of broader studies that employ epigraphy to throw light on Roman building activity.[2] Inscriptions recording offers of free bathing or those that offer interesting terminological details have occasionally been examined more closely,[3] but no systematic collection and analysis of bath inscriptions has yet been undertaken. In the following pages, I present a sample of several hundred of the most informative bath-related inscriptions, drawn mostly from Italy and the provinces of the Latin West. Although the sample is not comprehensive (the myriad of regional epigraphic collections, the patchy and inadequate publication of some material, and the constant discovery of new material ensure that it cannot be),[4] it represents the result of systematic searches through all of the major collec-

---

1. See, above, chapter 6, n. 1.

2. See, e.g., T.F.C. Blagg, "Architectural Munificence in Britain: The Evidence of Inscriptions," *Britannia* 21 (1990): 13–31; Duncan-Jones, *Economy,* passim; id., *Structure,* esp. 174–84; Jouffroy, *Construction publique.* Thomas and Witschel ("Constructing Reconstruction") subject rebuilding inscriptions to closer scrutiny than most, but in my opinion, they do so somewhat misleadingly; see Fagan, "Reliability."

3. See, e.g., Cenerini, "Evergetismo ed epigrafia"; J. DeLaine, "The 'Cella Solearis' of the Baths of Caracalla: A Reappraisal," *BSR* 55 (1987): 147–56; Rebuffat, "Vocabulaire thermal."

4. A class of text omitted from consideration in what follows is lead-pipe stamps, which have been studied in detail by Ch. Bruun: see Bruun, "Private Munificence in Italy and the Evidence of Lead Pipe Stamps," in H. Solin, O. Salomies, and U.-M. Liertz, eds., *Acta Colloquii Epigraphici Latini Helsingiae 1991 Habiti* (Helsinki, 1995), 41–58; and on baths in particular, see id., "Ownership of Baths in Rome: The Evidence of Lead Pipe Installations," in Johnston and DeLaine, *Roman Baths and Bathing.* On new material, see, e.g., the inscriptions associated with the Hadrianic Baths at Aphrodisias, found reused in paving nearby; see R.R.R. Smith and C. Ratté, "Archaeological Research at Aphrodisias in Caria, 1994," *AJA* 100 (1996): 18–19.

tions of ancient epigraphy, as well as some of the most prominent regional compilations (see below, "Abbreviations for Collections of Inscriptions Consulted"). I hope, therefore, that the present assemblage of inscriptions can prove useful for future studies of Roman baths and bathing culture.

The inscriptions are arranged by theme. In part A are collected the constructional benefactions, in part B the nonconstructional benefactions. Part C comprises a variety of texts that throw light on bathing culture in general, and part D offers some Greek texts as comparanda.[5] Within each section, the texts are listed under subheadings. The constructional items are presented according to benefactor—emperors, imperial officials, local authorities, and private benefactors—and the nonconstructional inscriptions are presented by type of benefaction. Among the constructional inscriptions are recorded a wide variety of different operations—initial construction, repair, extension, and adornment—which are not differentiated formally in the sample, since there is some doubt about the use of epigraphic language as a sure guide to the nature of work done.[6]

Greek Inscriptions

A large number of Greek texts of Roman date throw light on bathing culture in the eastern half of the empire. Many are directly analogous to Latin texts from the West; others are not. For several reasons, it is prudent to focus on the Latin texts, but to ignore the Greek evidence completely seemed inadvisable, since it often contains useful information. Therefore, a collection of Greek texts is offered in part D of the sample, primarily for comparison with the Latin sections.

Several difficulties in dealing with Greek bath inscriptions limit the sorts of text included in part D. In the first place, and as we have seen, the Greek terms meaning "bath" are varied and have their own pre-Roman heritage. The word *gymnasium,* for instance, originally denoted the traditional Greek educational and athletic center, but the term came to be applied to Roman-style bathing establishments. In addition, the terms βαλανεῖον and λουτρόν, which designated specific types of bathing facility in the Greek context, were also applied to Roman-style bathing facilities. That these terms can indeed refer to different types of building in the Roman context is made clear from

---

5. Since Rome is a special case, it is omitted from the constructional sections of the sample; the epigraphic evidence for bath construction and maintenance at the capital can be found in the notes to chapter 5 and in appendix 2.

6. See above, chapter 6, pp. 130–31.

such inscriptions as that recording the actions of an anonymous benefactor at Xanthos, where a βαλανεῖον for women, a gymnasium, and a βαλανεῖον in the gymnasium are all distinguished from each other (no. 313). Most texts, however, draw no such distinctions and employ the terms casually, presumably because their meaning would have been self-evident to the ancient reader who encountered the inscriptions in their original setting.[7] Such terminological uncertainties as these caution against fully exploiting the Greek texts until a more thorough inquiry into Roman bathing in the Greek East has been undertaken.[8] For the present, I have somewhat arbitrarily chosen to include Greek texts that refer to baths by using the terms βαλανεῖα and λουτρά—terms that, at least, can be said specifically to apply to bath buildings—but not texts referring to buildings by the term *gymnasia* alone, due to the uncertain application of this term. Another problem, already examined, is the difficulty of correlating Greek and Latin municipal institutions and offices.[9] Such complications have made it advisable that the Greek texts be listed and treated separately from the Latin.

Criteria for Inclusion in the Sample

The sample includes only those inscriptions that deal with baths and that are sufficiently well preserved to allow the nature of the benefaction and the identity of the benefactor to be deduced or reasonably postulated in each case. (The "identity" of the benefactor need not necessarily be his or her name; some indication of his or her social status is sufficient.) Many fragmentary inscriptions are therefore not included, even though they reveal the existence of baths that might otherwise have gone undetected or provide other useful information, such as names for parts of bathhouses.[10] Despite

---

7. For instance, the Vedius Bath-Gymnasium at Ephesos is termed simply τὸ γυμνάσιον in its dedicatory inscription; see *SEG* 4 (1929) 533 = *AE* 1930.80 = *IK* 12 (Ephesos 2) 438. On the unclear application of the terms *gymnasium* and βαλανεῖον, see Delorme, *Gymnasion,* 241–50; Farrington, *Roman Baths of Lycia,* 135–36.

8. Something of a start has been made in Farrington, *Roman Baths of Lycia;* Yegül, *Bath-Gymnasium;* and the pertinent sections on Eastern baths in Nielsen (1.95–118) and Yegül (250–313). Much more needs to be done, however, especially on the issues of the terminology applied to these buildings and the differing uses, if any, to which they were put.

9. See above, chapter 6, pp. 153–54.

10. An exhaustive list of such fragmentary texts is unnecessary. However, a list of those from *CIL,* referred to here by volume, gives an indication as to their numbers; most are undated, unless otherwise indicated: 3.1806 = 8422 (Narona), 3.1807 (Narona), 3.8816 (Salona), 5.3457 (Verona), 5.8807 (Acelum), 8.803 = 12274 (Avitta Bibba; 204), 8.808 (Avitta Bibba; second century?), 8.962 (Muncipium Aurelia Vina), 8.1285 = 14781 (Colonia Vallis), 8.1295 (Mem-

these restrictions, the sample runs to 339 entries. Inscriptions that do not contain bath-related words but were discovered in bathhouses were harder to locate in the major epigraphic collections, since findspots are not listed in the indexes. Part C, in particular, must therefore be seen as the product more of happenstance than of anything else.

Dating

A major interpretative issue that involves all the inscriptions is that of dating. Most of the texts can be dated on internal evidence (imperial names and titles, mention of datable officials and/or events, etc.), but some are assigned dates on less solid grounds, such as letterform or other paleographic features.[11] Since this book is not a primarily epigraphic publication, and given the volume of the material presented here, it has been possible for me to view only a few of the texts firsthand and only a handful more by means of photographs (see figs. 26A–F). The vast majority of the entries are therefore drawn from the published collections; indeed, no text is published here for the first time. Where the published collections or other modern works provide dates for inscriptions undatable by internal means, I present those dates but not necessarily without reservation. In the notes attached to the individual entries, I discuss particular dating problems and present evidence supporting the assignation of particular dates. Overall, the picture is encouraging, since 88.2 percent (299/339) of the entries can be dated one way or

bressa; second/third century), 8.2578? (Lambaesis), 8.8457? (Satafis; 288), 8.9547 = 20990 (Caesarea; fourth or fifth century), 8.10607 = 14700 (Thuburnica ad Aquas), 8.20579 (Thamalla; fourth century), 8.20757 (Auzia), 8.22853a, b (Thysdrus; 326–31), 8.23293 (Thala), 8.23690 (Henchir-Faroha), 8.24090? (Civitas Siagitana), 8.24582 (Carthage; 316–18), 8.25845 (Schuhud el Batel; 376–77), 8.25864 (Tichilla; 412–14), 8.26634 (Thugga), 8.28065 = *ILAlg* 1.1033 (Thagora; 326–33), 9.1579 (Beneventum; fourth century), 9.1667 (Beneventum), 9.5121 (Interamnia Praetuttiorum), 10.3161 (Puteoli), 10.3916 (Capua), 10.4718 (Forum Popilii), 10.7018 (Catina), 11.1433 (Pisa; post-Hadrianic), 11.3010 (Ager Viterbiensis; first century?), 11.3622 (Caere), 11.6481 (Mons Ferreter; 148), 12.3304 (Nemausus), 12.5967 (Narbo), 13.601 (Burdigala), 13.1132 (Limonum Pictonum), 13.1169 (Ager Limonum; second century?), 13.1329 (Ager Biturigum Cuborum), 13.3186 (Noviodunum), 13.11151 = *ILS* 9361? (Ager Biturigum), 14.4711 (Ostia; late Republic?).

11. Note, for instance, the complexities of the criteria worked out for "rustic" central Spanish inscriptions by R.C. Knapp in *Latin Inscriptions from Central Spain* (Berkeley, 1992): 339–84. For other criteria of dating inscriptions not datable by internal data, see, e.g., *ML*, pp. 19–21 (Republican texts); Duncan-Jones, *Economy*, 362–63 (a variety of internal criteria); S. Joyce and A.E. Gordon, *Contributions to the Palaeography of Latin Inscriptions* (Berkeley, 1957) (letterform dating). Dates deduced from letterform alone are particularly insecure, and all dates offered in the sample exclusively on this basis should be considered very tentative; see further, L. Robert, "Adeimantos et la ligue de Corinthe: Sur une inscription de Delphes," *Hellenica* 2 (1946): 16–17.

another, most of them securely on the basis of internal evidence.[12] Given what we have seen about the chronological distribution of Latin inscriptions (see chapter 2, pp. 53–54; chapter 6, pp. 132–35), most of the undated inscriptions probably hail from the second, third, or fourth centuries of the Imperial period.

Abbreviations for Collections of Inscriptions Consulted

AE	*L'Année épigraphique.* Paris, 1888–.
Bull. ép.	J. Robert and L. Robert. *Bulletin épigraphique.* 9 vols. to date, covering the years 1938–80. Paris, 1972–.
CIG	*Corpus Inscriptionum Graecarum.* Berlin, 1828–77.
CIL	*Corpus Inscriptionum Latinarum.* Berlin, 1863–.
CLE	F. Bücheler et al. *Carmina Latina Epigraphica.* 3 vols. Leipzig, 1895–1926.
EphEp	*Ephemeris Epigraphica.* 9 vols. Berlin, 1872–1913.
IAM	J. Gascou et al. *Inscriptions antiques du Maroc.* Vol. 2, *Inscriptions latines.* Paris, 1982.
ICI	*Inscriptiones Christianae Italiae Septimo Saeculo Antiquiores.* Bari, 1985–.
IGLS	L. Jalabert et al. *Inscriptions grecques et latines de la Syrie.* Paris, 1929–.
IGRR	R. Cagnat and G. Lafaye. *Inscriptiones Graecae ad Res Romanas Pertinentes.* 4 vols., 3 in print. Paris, 1906–27. Reprint, Chicago, 1975.
IK	*Inschriften griechischer Städte aus Klienasien.* Bonn, 1972–.
ILAfr	R. Cagnat, A. Merlin, and L. Chatelian. *Inscriptions latines d'Afrique.* Paris, 1923.
ILAlg	S. Gsell et al. *Inscriptions latines d'Algérie.* Rome, 1922–.
ILCV	E. Diehl. *Inscriptiones Latinae Christianae Veteres.* 4 vols. Berlin, Dublin, and Zurich, 1925–67.
ILER	J. Vives. *Inscripciones latinas de la España romana.* 2 vols. Barcelona, 1971–72.
ILLRP	A. Degrassi. *Inscriptiones Latinae Liberae Rei Publicae.* 2 vols. Florence, 1957–63. Vol. 1², 1965.
ILM	L. Chatelain. *Inscriptions latines du Maroc.* Paris, 1942.
ILPaest	M. Mello and G. Voza. *Le iscrizioni latine di Paestum.* 2 vols. Naples, 1968–69.
ILS	H. Dessau. *Inscriptiones Latinae Selectae.* 3 vols. Berlin, 1892–1916. Reprint, 5 vols., Chicago, 1979.
ILTG	P. Wuilleumier. *Inscriptions latines des Trois Gaules.* Paris, 1963.
ILTun	A. Merlin. *Inscriptions latines de la Tunisie.* Paris, 1944.
InscrIt	*Inscriptiones Italiae.* Rome, 1931–.

---

12. Undated entries: nos. 46–54, 143–50, 197–201, 214, 251, 253–56, 260, 265–67, 274, 275, 302–5, 331, 338.

IRT	J.M. Reynolds and J.B. Ward-Perkins. *The Inscriptions of Roman Tripolitania*. Rome, 1952.
ML	E. Courtney. *Musa Lapidaria: A Selection of Latin Verse Inscriptions*. Atlanta, 1995.
SEG	*Supplementum Epigraphicum Graecum*. Leiden, Alphen, and Amsterdam, 1923–.
SIG	W. Dittenberger. *Sylloge Inscriptionum Graecarum*[3]. 4 vols. Leipzig, 1915–24.
SuppItal	*Supplementa Italica*. New series. Rome, 1981–.
TAM	*Tituli Asiae Minoris*. Vienna, 1901–.

Abbreviations, Translations, and Epigraphic Conventions

It was common in ancient epigraphy to abbreviate frequently used words. It has not been my policy to fill out every one of these abbreviations, especially when they are repeatedly encountered. Names and titles are usually left in their truncated form: for example, "imp. Aug." for "imp(erator) Aug(ustus)"; "cos." for "co(n)s(ul)"; "v. c." for "v(ir) c(larissimus)"; "f." for "f(ilius)"; and so on. Abbreviations for rarer offices, less obvious formulae, or words abbreviated in the "narrative" part of the text have generally been filled out for ease of comprehension.

To translate all of the entries seemed unnecessarily pedantic, since so many are formulaic and say much the same thing in slightly variant language. Therefore, I have translated some of the more straightforward entries early in the sample, as exemplars of how such inscriptions are to be understood. Inscriptions that are especially informative (as are most of the rhetorical late Imperial entries) have been translated or, at least, paraphrased, since direct translation is often close to impossible. Translated inscriptions are marked with a dagger (†) beside the entry number.

It remains regrettable that use of epigraphic conventions to indicate the condition of the text on the stone has yet to be lent a universal standard and often varies from collection to collection. The potential for confusion is therefore high. Since I have not viewed most of the inscriptions myself, I am wholly at the mercy of previous publishers in regard to such matters as missing letters, unintelligible letters or sections of text, lacunae, and so on. This is especially the case when the precise number of missing letters is involved, which can be very important for suggesting restorations. As a result, where there has been any uncertainty as to the number of missing letters, I have opted to indicate an indeterminate number.

The conventions used in the sample are as follows (adapted from *IRT*, p. 7):

(abcd)   Letters not appearing on the stone that complete abbreviations.

(abc)   When the enclosed text is in Latin, it denotes letters or numbers ex-
            pressed as symbols on the stone.
            When the enclosed text is in English, it denotes some pertinent feature of
            the stone, such as fragmentary text, missing lines, lines skipped, and so
            on.

[abcd]   Letters missing that can be restored or reasonably postulated.

[...]   Letters missing that cannot be restored. One, two, or three dots indicate
            one, two, or three missing letters. For longer gaps, a figure flanked by
            two dots in square brackets indicates the approximate number of missing
            letters; for example, "[..8..]" indicates approximately eight missing
            letters.

[—]   Indeterminate number of missing letters.

/ / /   Letters deliberately erased and not restorable.

[abcd]   Letters deliberately erased but restorable.

⟨abcd⟩   Letters mistakenly excluded by stonecutter.

{abcd}   Letters mistakenly included by stonecutter.

ABCD   Letters that can be read but the meaning of which remains uncertain.

. . .   Words or lines in the text that have been omitted. If lines are omitted,
            this is noted in italics in parentheses—for example, *(six lines skipped)*

I (10)   Line number of resumed text after omitted portion.

Other Notes on the Sample

All entries are numbered consecutively from 1 to 339.

The entry numbers identify acts of benefaction, so that single inscriptions recording multiple benefactions have been assigned several entries, sometimes in the same section of the sample, sometimes in different sections, and sometimes in both (e.g., 1/2 and 202, 73/74 and 162).

The constructional texts are subdivided under four benefactor categories— emperors, imperial officials, local authorities, and private benefactors.

Entries with more than one number denote discrete actions by different benefactors of the same category recorded on a single stone (nos. 1/2, 73/74, 148/49, 168/69).

Entries are listed in chronological order within each of the four parts.

Some inscriptions are datable only to vague periods and appear after the appropriate securely datable entries (e.g., a "mid-second-century" inscription follows one datable to ca. 150).

Undated texts are listed at the head of each section, in Italy by Regio number and then alphabetically within the Regio, in the provinces alphabetically by province and then by site within individual provinces.

Entries only putatively datable are listed among the "undated" entries, with the possible date or period indicated in parentheses.

Entries marked with an asterisk (*) include the involvement of a woman or women.

Epigraphic symbols are usually rendered into the appropriate words, provided in italics in parentheses—for example, *(denarios)* for X̅.

For complex figures, the Roman and Greek systems of numeration are rendered as Arabic numerals provided in italics in parentheses—for example, HS *(2,000,000)* for HS | X̅X̅ |.

The notes to the entries provide relevant sources (e.g., for dates), discussion of difficulties of interpretation, and, where applicable, references to studies or publications of the physical remains of the pertinent baths. Where possible, I refer to Nielsen's catalogue of bath sites, Manderscheid's bibliography, or the relevant pages of Yegül for information on the physical remains. For Italian sites, when these useful and up-to-date sources are silent, I have resorted to the Guide archeologiche Laterza, many of which I realize may now be redundant. Unfortunately, the volume of material covered made comprehensiveness in this regard unrealistic.

Part A

Constructional Benefactions

Emperors

Augustus and Gaius. Bononia (Regio VIII). Precise dates uncertain. *CIL* 11.720 = *ILS* 5674. 1/2†

dívus Aúg. parens | dedit; | / / / / / / / / | Aúgustus | Germanicus / / / | refécit. | in huius balinei lavation(em) HS *(400,000)* | nomin(e) C. Aviasi T. f. Senecae f. sui T. Aviasius Servandus | pater testament(o) legavit, ut ex reditu eius summ(ae) | in perpetuum viri et impuberes utriusq(ue) sexsus | gratis laventur.

Trans.: "The deified Augustus, the parent, built (this bath); [C. Caesar] Augustus Germanicus [father of his country?] rebuilt it. Toward bathing in this bath, T. Aviasius Servandus Senior gave in his will four hundred thousand sesterces in the name of his son C. Aviasius Seneca, son of Titus, so that from the proceeds of this sum, men and minors of both sexes might bathe free of charge in perpetuity."

NOTES: Two imperial benefactors are commemorated here. Augustus is the most likely candidate for the first, Gaius Caligula for the second. The latter's name has been erased, but the available spaces could accommodate his name and titles in the form C. *Caesar Augustus Germanicus* followed by either *imp(erator)* (compare, e.g., *CIL* 2.172 = *ILS* 190) or *p(ater) p(atriae)* (compare, e.g., *CIL* 13.1189 = *ILS* 4675). Cenerini ("Evergetismo ed epigrafia," 217) argues for the identification of the second emperor as Nero, who is reported to have given a speech in the senate on behalf of the Bononians in 53, when the city was devastated by fire (see Tac. *Ann.* 12.58.2; Suet. *Ner.* 7.2). But it is difficult to fit Nero's nomenclature for the years 53/54 into the erased section preceding "Augustus," since it habitually includes mention of Divus Claudius. Barrett (*Caligula,* 195 and 297 n. 31) considers the text Caligulan. If any physical remains of this building are known, they have not been fully investigated; see E. Mangani, F. Rebecchi, and M.J. Strazzulla, *Emilia, Venezie* (Bari, 1981), 86–91. The second part of the inscription (lines 6–10), which records an offer of free bathing in this bathhouse, is a later addition and is carved in letters of a different style to the "imperial" section (see no. 202).

Trajan. Ricina (Regio IX). Precise date uncertain. *CIL* 9.5746 = *ILS* 5675. 3

divos Traianus | Augustus | concessa Tuscili *(sic)* | Nominati heredit(ate) | rei publ(icae) Ricinens(ium) | balneum et platias | rep(arari *or* reparare) mandavit.

NOTES: Interpretation of the text depends on how *rep.* is restored. If *rep(arare)* is postulated, then Trajan ordered the state of Ricina to repair its *balneum* and *platiae,* which had been given to the town in the will of Tusculus Nominatus. Presumably, the work would then have been carried out at the expense of the town, as seems to have been Trajan's preference, at least for Bithynian communities; see Pliny *Ep.* 10.24, 10.40, 10.99. This interpretation is hardly conclusive, however, since Ricina was an Italian citizen community and so enjoyed higher status than the remote and foreign towns of Bithynia and Pontus. Three points make it more likely that the penultimate word should be restored as *rep(arari)* (thus also argues Rebuffat, "Vocabulaire thermal," 13), so that Trajan can be seen as the benefactor: (1) Trajan's name is in the nominative case, which normally indicates the agent in texts recording construction; (2) it is most unusual for a city to record in this fashion that an emperor had ordered it to carry out work, when alternatives, such as *iussu divi Traiani Augusti,* were available (compare no. 122); (3) comparable records of imperial munificence are known (see, e.g., no. 5).

4   Trajan. Cyrene, Cyrenaeca. 98/100. *AE* 1960.198.

im[p.] Caesar Nerva divi f. Traianus [Aug,. Germ., pont. max.,] | tri[b. p]otest., p. p., cos. II, balineum et thermas fecit per C. Memmium [..27..].

NOTES: This inscription was found in fragments near the baths at Cyrene; see J. Reynolds, "Four Inscriptions from Roman Cyrene," *JRS* 49 (1959): 95–96 . Note that Trajan is reported to have built both a *balineum* and a *thermae* in the Sanctuary of Apollo at Cyrene: see Manderscheid, 104, s.v. "Cyrenae (Shahat), Trajanische Thermen (Terme della Myrtusa)"; Nielsen, 2.40 (C.327); Yegül, 397. The *balineum* was restored by Hadrian (see next entry). For Memmius, see *PIR*² M 454.

5†   Hadrian. Cyrene, Cyrenaeca. 118 or 119. *AE* 1928.2.

imp. Caes. divi Traiani | Parthici fil., divi Nervae nepos, | Traianus Hadrianus Aug., pontif. | max., trib. potest. III, cos. III, balineum | cum porticibus et sphaeristeris | ceterisque adiacentibus quae | tumultu Iudaico diruta et exusta | erant civitati Cyrenensium restitui | iussit.

Trans.: "Imperator Caesar Trajan Hadrian Augustus, son of the deified Trajan, conqueror of Parthia, grandson of the deified Nerva, chief priest, holder of tribunician power for the third time, consul for the third time, ordered that the bath with its porticoes and ball courts and other adjacent buildings, which had been destroyed and gutted by fire in the Jewish uprising, be restored for the city of Cyrene."

NOTES: Although the text does not expressly say that Hadrian himself bore the cost of the restoration, the appearance of his name in the nominative would strongly suggest that he was responsible for the work. I interpret *civitati Cyrenensium* as a referential dative (of advantage: "for the city of Cyrene"); similar use of the dative to indicate a favored community is found in, e.g., nos. 14–18, 165. The Jewish uprising mentioned in the text took place in Cyrene and Egypt in the latter part of Trajan's reign (see Dio 68.32).

6†   Antoninus Pius. Ostia (Regio I). 138/39. *CIL* 14.98 = *ILS* 334 (see HA *Ant. Pius* 8.3).

imp. Caes. divi Hadriani fil., divi Traiani Parthici nep., divi [Nervae] | pronepos, T. Aelius Hadrianus Antoninus Aug. Pius pontif. max., trib. potes[t. II, cos. II,] thermas, in quarum exstructionem divos pater suus HS *(2,000,000)* polli[citus erat], | adiecta pecunia, quanta amplius desiderabatur, item marmoribus ad omnem o[rnatum perfecit].

Trans.: "Imperator Caesar T. Aelius Hadrianus Antoninus Augustus Pius, son of the deified Hadrian, grandson of the deified Trajan, conqueror of Parthia, great-grandson of the deified Nerva, chief priest, holder of tribunician power for the second time, consul for the second time, completed the baths, toward the construction of which his deified father had promised two million sesterces; having added all the extra money required, he also completed the work with marbling for its total decoration."

NOTES: The findspot of this inscription was not adequately recorded, but it is generally taken to refer to the Baths of Neptune, the construction of which fits this date; see Meiggs, 409. Dessau (*CIL* 14) thought perhaps the Maritime Baths were apposite; see below, no. 19. C. Pietrangeli (*Otricoli: Un lembo dell'Umbria alle porte di Roma* [Rome, 1978], 69) has argued that this text is Hadrianic and should be assigned to Ocriculum, not Ostia. He is tentative about this proposition, on good grounds. First, no remains of imperially funded baths are known at Ocriculum (the city's two main establishments are epigraphically associated with local magnates; see nos. 98, 124, 136); second, the eighteenth-century excavation diaries that Pietrangeli depends on for his argument are so vague and scrappy as to carry no probative value; third, the imperial name in the inscription is clearly that of Antoninus Pius, not Hadrian, as Pietrangeli claims; and finally, there is mention in another Ostian inscription of *thermas quas divus Pius aedificaverat* (no. 87), making the Ostian attribution of the current text more secure. On the remains of the Baths of Neptune, see Manderscheid, 162–63, s.v. "Terme di Nettuno"; Nielsen, 2.5 (C.24); Yegül, 68.

Antoninus Pius. Tarquinii (Regio VII). 139 or later. *CIL* 11.3363.   7†

imp. Caesar T. Aeli[us Hadrianus] | Antoninus Aug. [Pius pont.] | m[a]x., trib. pot., [cos., p. p.,] | bal[in]eum vetus[tate collapsum] | sua pecunia [restituit].

Trans.: "Imperator Caesar T. Aelius Hadrianus Antoninus Augustus Pius, chief priest, holder of tribunician power, consul, father of his country, restored with his own money the bath that had collapsed with old age."

NOTES: If any physical remains of baths are known from this site, they are incompletely published; see M. Torelli, *Etruria*³ (Bari, 1985), 133–37.

Antoninus Pius. Narbo, Gallia Narbonensis. 145 or later. *CIL* 12.4342 = *ILS* 5685.   8

imp. Caes. divi Hadr[iani fil., divi] | Traiani Parthici n[epos, divi Nervae] | pronepos, T. Aelius H[adrianus Antoninus] | Aug. Pius pont. maxim[us, tribun. potest.—], | imp. II, cos. IIII., p. p., ther[mas incendio] | consumptas cum por[ticibus et—] | et basilicis et omni [apparatu impensa] | sua re[stituit].

NOTES: The fire occurred at Narbo in 145 (see HA *Ant. Pius* 9.2; *PECS*, 607–8 [Gayraud and Solier]).

M. Aurelius and L. Verus. Forum Claudii Ceutronum Axima, Alpes Graiae et Poeninae. 163. *CIL* 12.107 = *ILS* 5868.   9

[imp. Caes. M. Aurelius—et] imp. Caes. Lu[cius] | Aurelius Verus Aug., | trib. potest. III, cos. III, | [vi]as per fines Ceutro[n]um vi torrentium | e[v]ersas, exclusis | [fl]um-inibus et in nat[u]ra]lem alveum redu[ctis, | m]olibus pluribu[s locis] | positis item F[oro Cl. | te]mpla et baline[as | pec(unia)] sua restit[uer(unt)].

Commodus. Beneventum (Regio II). Precise date uncertain. *CIL* 9.1665.   10

[Be]nevent[i—|—baline]um sua pec(unia) [—| omni]que cultu exor[navit | Comm]odus, pius, fe[lix, |—ludo gladi?]atorio dedic[avit—].

NOTES: Despite the fragmentary nature of the inscription, the sense is clear enough. Verusius, in his 1710 description of Beneventum's monuments, restored the main word as *[portic]um,* possibly that of the *Thermae Commodianae* attested elsewhere (see no. 195 and perhaps also no. 27); a fragmentary inscription from the town (*CIL* 9.1579) may also have mentioned the *Thermae Commodianae*. Whatever the case, the text records a bath construction or extension carried out by Commodus. An unpublished bathhouse was known at Beneventum, but it is no longer visible and has been poorly investigated; see De Caro and Greco, *Campania,* 188; A. Zazo, "Benevento romana," *Samnium* 58 (1985): 102.

11   Caracalla. Pinna (Regio V). 213. *AE* 1968.157.

[—divi Trajani Parthici] et divi | [Nervae a]dnepos, | [M. Aureli]us Antoninus Aug. | [Pa]rt. max. Germ. m[ax.] | pont. max., trib. pot. XVI, imp. [II], | cos. IIII, p. p., balneum vetus[tate] | corrupt(um) ad pristin(am) faciem r[estituit].

12   Gordian III. Volubilis, Mauretania. Precise date uncertain. *AE* 1922.57 = *ILAfr* 614 = *ILM* 74 = *IAM* 404.

imp. Caes. M. Antonius | Gordianus, pius, felix, invictus | Augustus domum cum balineo | vetustate conlapsam | a solo restituit curante | M. Ulpio Victore, v. e., proc., | prolegato.

NOTES: The inscription comes from the entrance to the so-called Palace of the Governor at Volubilis, located on the *decumanus maximus* north of the Forum Novum. The building, as the residence of an imperial official, was evidently public in nature, but it is unclear whether the baths were open to the public. Nevertheless, they have an entrance that opens onto the street, suggesting some public access. For the remains, see R. Thouvenot, *Volubilis* (Paris, 1949), 43–44. Nielsen cites *ILAfr* 614 as evidence for a Gallienic restoration of the Baths of Gallienus (2.18 [C.129]) and *AE* 1922.57 for a Gordianic restoration of the North Baths at Volubilis (2.18 [C.130]); in fact, both references are to this same text, and it refers to neither of the baths she associates with it.

13†   Diocletian. Nicomedia, Bithynia. Precise date uncertain. *CIL* 3.324 = *ILS* 613.

perpetuo imp. [d. n.] | C. Aur. Val. Diocletiano, | p., f., Aug., cuius pro|videntia etiam | lavacrum ther|marum Antoni|nianarum fundi|tus | eversum sua | pecunia ampli-|fi|catum populo suo | exhiberi iussit.

Trans.: "To the perpetual emperor, our lord C. Aurelius Valerius Diocletianus, *pius, felix,* Augustus, whose foresight ordered that the *lavacrum* of the *Thermae Antoninianae,* which was completely ruined, also be opened for his people, after it had been restored and enlarged at his own expense."

NOTES: The special relationship between Diocletian and the Nicomedians, among whom he took up residence, is reflected in this text. The meaning of *lavacrum* is generally unclear, but here it apparently describes part of a bathhouse, possibly the heated section (see nos. 238 and 239). It is difficult to see how Yegül's definition of the term—"a bath suite that is part of a house; or, generally, a small bath, a *balneum*" (Yegül, 491, s.v.)—fits with the wording of this inscription. The uncertainty is a good illustration of the difficulties inherent in deciphering ancient bath terminology.

14   Constantine and Licinius. Lavinium (Regio I). Precise date uncertain. *AE* 1984.151.

[dd. nn. Flavius Valerius Consta]ntinus Maximus et Valerius Licinianus Licinius, pii, felices, inv[i]cti, semp[er Augusti, | thermas mult?]i temporis deformatas Laurentibus suis addito cultu restituerunt, curante Camilio Aspro, v. c., c[uratore rei p.?—].

NOTES: The text was found among the ruins of baths in 1962 and seems to refer to the reconstruction of the edifice. The baths have not been adequately investigated; see Pavolini, *Ostia,* 251.

15†   Constantine. Remi, Belgica. Precise date uncertain. *CIL* 13.3255 = *ILS* 703.

imp. Caesar Flav. Constantinus Max. | Aug. sempiternus, divi Constanti Aug. pii filius, | toto orbe victoriis suis semper ac feliciter celebrandus, | thermas fisci sui sumptu a fundamentis coeptas ac peractas | civitati suae Remorum pro solita liberalitate largitus est.

Trans.: "Imperator Caesar Flavius Constantinus Maximus, Augustus everlasting, son of the deified Constantius Augustus, *pius*, is to be praised always and happily throughout the entire world for his victories. He bestowed on his city of Remi, in accordance with his customary generosity, the baths, begun and completed from the foundations at the expense of his imperial purse."

Constantius and Julian. Spoletium (Regio VI). 355/60. *CIL* 11.4781 = *ILS* 739.   16†

reparatores orbis adque urbium resti|tutores dd. nn. Fl. Iul. Constantius, p., f,. semper Aug. | et Iulianus nobilissimus ac victoriosissimus Caes. | ad aeternam | divini nominis propagationem | thermas Spoletinis in praeteritum igne consump|tas sua largitate restituerunt.

Trans.: "Repairers of the world and restorers of cities, our lords Flavius Julius Constantius, *pius, felix,* always Augustus, and Julianus, the most noble and victorious Caesar, to make their hallowed name live forever, restored for the Spoletians, with imperial largesse, the baths that had been destroyed by fire some time ago."

NOTES: See the notes to no. 99.

Constans and Constantius. Ostia (Regio I). Precise date uncertain. *CIL* 14.135.   17

[Cons]tantius et Const[ans | therm]as incuria longi temporis destituta[s | adiectione marmorum nov?]orum ad pristinum statum reforman[das | Ostiensibus? s]uis red[d]iderunt | [curante—]o, v. c., praefecto annona[e] cum iure [gl]adii.

NOTES: It is not clear to which of the Ostian baths this inscription refers, since the findspot is not on record. However, it was probably one of the establishments that was an imperial concern, e.g., the Baths of Neptune (no. 6) or the *Thermae Maritimae* (no. 19). The *praefectus annonae* cannot be identified; see *PLRE* 1.1014, s.v. "Anonymus 51."

Valens, Gratian, and Valentinian. Regium Julium (Regio III). 374. *AE* 1913.227 =   18†
SupplItal 5 (1989): 52–53 (no. 6).

imperator Caesar Flavius Valentinianus, pius, felix, victor | ac triumfator, semper Augustus, et Flavius Valens, pius, felix, | victor ac triumfator, semper Augustus, et Flavius Gratianus, | pius, felix, victor ac triumfator, semper Augustus Reginis suis | [t]hermas vetustate et terrae motu conlabsas in meliorem | cultum formamque auspiciis felicioribus reddiderunt; | reddita basilica marmorum quae numquam habuerat | pulcritudine decorata, nova etiam porticu adiecta; curante | Pontio Attico, v. c., correctore Lucaniae et Brittiorum, dedecatas | quartum Kalendarum Iuliarum die. domino nostro Gratiano | Augusto tertio et Flavio Equitio, v. c., consulibus.

Trans.: "Imperator Caesar Flavius Valentinian, *pius, felix,* victor and triumphator, always Augustus, and Flavius Valens *pius, felix,* victor and triumphator, always Augustus, and Flavius Gratian, *pius, felix,* victor and triumphator, always Augustus, returned the baths, which had collapsed through old age and an earthquake, to their own people, the Rhegians; they improved the baths' refinements and appearance with luckier auspices: the basilica was restored, embellished by the beauty of marbles, which it has never had, and a new portico was added as well. Pontius Atticus, of senatorial rank, corrector of Lucania and Bruttium, saw to the work. The baths were dedicated on 28 June when our lord Gratian Augustus was consul for the third time with Flavius Equitius, of senatorial rank *(i.e., 374).*"

NOTES: The editors of *AE* note that the earthquake may have been that of 365 (see Amm. Marc. 26.10.5). If so, because the restored building was not dedicated until 374, the building may have been unusable for up to nine years. Since it is not known how long the repair operations were underway, the period of actual ruin may have been shorter. For Pontius Atticus, see *PLRE* 1.123, s.v. "Atticus 3." *SupplItal* 5 (1989): 53–54 (no. 7) presents a fragmentary text that probably commemorates the same benefaction: *suffragan[tibus ddd. nnn. Valentiniano, Valente et Gratiano]* | *ppp(rincipibus) mmm(aximis). ther[mae vetustate ..20.. et]* | *ruin[a conlapsae—]*. Ruins of baths datable to the Imperial period are known from Regium Julium, but they have not been seriously investigated; see E. Greco, *Magna Grecia²* (Bari, 1981), 77.

19†   Valens, Gratian, and Valentinian. Ostia (Regio I). Ca. 377. *CIL* 14.137 = *ILS* 5694.

thermas maritimas intresecus refectione cellarum, foris soli adiectione, ddd. nnn. Valens Gratianus et Valentinianus victor(es) ac triumf(atores) semper Au[ggg. |—] Proculo Gregorio, v. c., praefecto annon(ae) urbis Romae, curante decorarunt.

Trans.: "Our masters Valens, Gratian, and Valentinian, victors and triumphators, always Augusti, decorated the maritime baths by rebuilding the rooms inside and by increasing the area outside. [?] Proculus Gregorius, of senatorial rank, grain prefect of the city of Rome, saw to the work."

NOTES: Proculus Gregorius was prefect of the grain supply in 377; see *PLRE* 1.404, s.v. "Gregorius 9." The extension of the facility "outside" probably denotes the addition of amenities associated with the precincts of larger baths: gardens, fountains, exedrae, etc. For the remains of these baths, the so-called *Thermae Maritimae* or Terme di Porta Marina, see Manderscheid, 164, s.v. "Terme di Porta Marina (Terme della Marciana; IV.10.1–2)"; Nielsen, 2.5 (C.25); Yegül, 81.

Imperial Officials

20   Incertus, annonae praefec(tus). Ostia (Regio I). Date uncertain (but possibly fifth century). *CIL* 14.5387.

[la]bebatur ut lava[tum?—|—omni splen]dore excultum ad usum pop[uli—|—] annonae praefec(tus).

NOTES: This is an inscription on a reused stone found near the Forum Baths. Meiggs (551 n. 3) tentatively dates it to the fifth century.

21†   D. Laelius Balbus, q(uaestor) propr(aetore). Carpis, Africa. 43/42 B.C. *CIL* 8.24106 = *ILS* 9367 = *ILLRP* 1275.

D. Laelius D. f. | Balbus, q(uaestor) pro | pr(aetore), assa, destrictar(ium) | sólariumque faciundu(m) coerav(it).

Trans.: "D. Laelius Balbus, son of Decimus, quaestor with praetorian power, saw to the construction of the sweat room, the scraping-off room, and the sundial."

NOTES: This appears to be the same D. Laelius who committed suicide following his defeat in the struggle for Africa in 40 B.C.: see Dio 48.21.6; App. *B Civ.* 4.53–56; *MRR* 2.361–62. An *assa* was a heating device in a bathhouse (see Cic. *Q Fr.* 3.1.2 [= SB 21]), a *destrictarium* was a scraping-off room (see no. 61), and a *solarium* was a sundial (one was found in the Stabian Baths; see Eschebach, *Stabianer Thermen,* 17, XIIB, 19 [fig. 5], 21 [fig. 7]), although the latter could also denote a terrace or balcony. Other Republican texts mention *solaria,* but it is not clear that they were located in bathing establishments; see chapter 2, n. 49).

M. Gavius Maximus, praef(ectus) praetorio. Ostia (Regio I). Antoninus Pius. *AE* 1984.150 (see also 1955.287) = Cicerchia and Marinucci, *Scavi di Ostia* 11.216–19 (no. C 106). **22**

vetustatis incuria [—] conf[i]rm[atis— | ther]mis Gav(i) Max[imi—] | dominorum nostro[rum—] aete[r]no[rum prin|cipum—loca proxi]ma fori et ian[uae—] *(the rest is very fragmentary).*

NOTES: Another fragmentary text, part of an architrave, reads: *Maximus has olim therm[as extruxerat] | divinae mentis ductu cum o[rnaret—]* (*CIL* 6.29769 = *ILCV* 1901a = Cicerchia and Marinucci, *Scavi di Ostia* 11.220–21 [no. C 107bis]), and a lead pipe from the building bears Maximus' name in the genitive case (Cicerchia and Marinucci, *Scavi di Ostia* 11.222 [no. C 109α]). The most likely candidate for the Maximus of all these inscriptions is the praetorian prefect M. Gavius Maximus, who served under Antoninus Pius; see *PIR*[2] G 104. The Forum Baths are of Antonine date, as confirmed by brickstamps; see Meiggs, 411–15. See also Manderscheid, 160, s.v. "Terme del Foro (Terme Nuove; I.12,6)"; add also Cicerchia and Marinucci, *Scavi di Ostia* Nielsen, 2.6 (C.27); Yegül, 80–81. Richardson (*Dictionary,* 395, s.v. "Thermae Novati") associates our inscription with the so-called *Thermae Novati* under the church of Santa Pudenziana at Rome (see appendix 2) and identifies Maximus as a late Imperial presbyter; however, the architrave on which the inscription is carved features the same decoration as the architrave from the Forum Baths at Ostia, and another honorary text from the city mentions Gavius Maximus (*CIL* 14.191, 14.4471): see Meiggs, 415; Cicerchia and Marinucci, *Scavi di Ostia* 11.220–21. On the whole, therefore, the association of our inscription with the Forum Baths at Ostia appears the stronger possibility. Who carried out the late Imperial restoration that was the main subject of this entry is no longer recoverable.

M. Nonius Arrius Mucianus, co(n)s(ul), curator et patronus r(ei) p(ublicae). Verona (Regio X). 201/210. *CIL* 5.3342 = *ILS* 1148. **23†**

M. Nonio M. [f.] | Pob. Arrio | Mucian[o], | cos., pr., XV[viro] | sac(ris) f(aciundis), curat[ori] | et patrono r(ei) [p(ublicae)] | Veronens(is) | ob largitionem [eius] | quod at ther[mas] | iuventia[nas] | perficiend(as) H[S—] | rei public(ae) d[ederit] | ordo [ded(icavit)?].

Trans.: "The *ordo* of the city dedicated (?) (this monument) to Marcus Nonius Arrius Mucianus, son of Marcus, of the voting tribe Poblilia, consul, praetor, member of the College of Fifteen Priests, curator and patron of the city of Verona, on account of his generosity because he gave to the city *(amount lost)* sesterces for the completion of the *Thermae Iuventianae.*"

NOTES: M. Nonius Arrius Mucianus was consul in 201 (see *PIR*[2] N 114; Degrassi, 57). Jacques (*Liberté,* 9 [no. 39]) gives the dates of his curatorship as ca. 193–210. See also id., *Curateurs,* 100–103 (no. 39); Camodeca, "Ricerche," 520–21, s.v. "Verona." He may have been a native of Brixia; if so, Verona was not his hometown. The name of the building may suggest it was reserved for an association of youths, making this tantamount to a collegium bath. Youth organizations are well attested all over the Roman empire and appear to have been the Roman equivalent of Greek ephebes; see P. Ginestet, *Les organisations de la jeunesse dans l'Occident romain* (Brussels, 1991). Alternatively, the name may have been intended to evoke associations of vitality and novelty. If any physical remains are known, they have yet to be properly investigated, see Mangani, Rebecchi, and Strazzulla, *Emilia*, 160–80.

24 Q. Petronius Melior, v. co(n)s(ularis), cur(ator) r(ei) p(ublicae). Tarquinii (Regio VII). Post-230. *CIL* 11.3367 = *ILS* 1180.

Q. Petronio Meliori, viro | cos., cur(atori) r(ei) p(ublicae) Tarquiniens(ium) | et Graviscanor(um), praefec|to frum(enti) dandi, legat(o) leg(ionis) | XXX Ulpiae, curat(ori) Pyrgens(ium) | et Ceretanor(um), leg(ato) leg(ionis) VIII Aug., praet., trib. pleb. | kandid(ato), quaest. prov. Nar|bon., quaest., sodali Aug. | Claudiali, sexvir. turm. | pr., trib. laticl. leg. pr. Min., | Xviro stlitib(us) iudicand(is), | ordo et cives Tarqui|niensium patrono op|timo, quod rem p(ublicam) fove|rit et thermas resti|tuerit.

NOTES: Nielsen (1.41 n. 26) dates the text precisely to 240; Camodeca ("Ricerche," 516–17, s.v. "Tarquinii") prefers a date of 242/44. All that is securely datable here is Q. Petronius Melior's position as *sodalis Claudialis,* an honor he received in 230: see *CIL* 6.1984, s.v. "decuria XXVII," lines 46–49; *RE* 19.1219–20, s.v. "Petronius 47" (Groag). The date of his consulship is unclear; see Degrassi, 132. He was therefore a *curator rei publicae* of senatorial rank; see Duthoy, "Profil social," 147 (no. 288). The present inscription reveals that he was or had been the curator of no less than four communities (Tarquinii, Graviscum, Pyrgi, and Ceretanum). This text is one of five found in a single room of these baths, another of which honors Melior's wife, Domitia Melpis. J. Nicols (*"Patrona Civitatis,"* 133) implies that Domitia may also have carried out some constructional work on these baths, but this is not certain. For the other honorands, see the notes to no. 176.

25 L. Do[mitius] Gal[licanus, leg. Aug. pr. pr.?]. Senia, Dalmatia. Mid–third century. *CIL* 3.10054

balneum vet[ustate con]|lapsum p[ecunia sua] | restitut[it] | L. Do[mitius] | Gal[licanus, leg. Aug. pr. pr.?].

NOTES: If the proposed restoration of L. Domitius Gallicanus' name is correct, the inscription can be roughly dated; he held the post of *legatus Augusti pro praetore* in Dalmatia (see *CIL* 2.4115 = *ILER* 1302) and lived during the reigns of Philip the Arab and Gordian I; see *PIR*² D 148.

26 Aur(elius) Verecundus, v. e., pro(curator) Argentariarum. Domavia, Dalmatia. 274. *CIL* 3.12736.

[imp. Caes. L. Domiti]o [Aureli]ano [A]u[g.] | II et Capitolino cos(s). | Aur. Verecundus, v. e., pro(curator) | Argentariarum balneum | vetustate conlapsum | ad pristinam faciem re|formare curavit.

NOTES: For Verecundus, see *PIR*² A 1629; *PLRE* 1.950, s.v. "Verecundus 3." Domavia was an important mining community in the third and fourth centuries A.D. Its baths have been excavated and are "the most elaborate in the province"; see *PECS*, 280–81, s.v. "Domavia" (Werner). These baths, however, do not appear in Manderscheid's bibliographic catalogue and garner only passing notice from Nielsen (1.111 n. 123). Argentaria was an area of Dalmatia near the border with Moesia, administered by a procurator; see *RE* 2.705, s.v. "Argentaria" (Tomaschek).

27 Sattius Crescens, v. c., cur(ator) r(ei) p(ublicae). Beneventum (Regio II). Second half of the third century. *CIL* 9.1588 = *ILS* 5480.

Sattius Crescens, | v. c., cur(ator) r(ei) p(ublicae) B(e)n(eventanae), ex | locis abditis | usui adque splen|dori thermarum dedit | [..5..]oder[. . .]nso[. .]ho[. .].

NOTES: For Crescens, see *PLRE* 1.230, s.v. "Crescens 4"; Camodeca, "Ricerche," 502–3, s.v. "Beneventum 6." Crescens stands at the cusp of the transformation of the *curatura rei publicae* into a local office; however, his senatorial status tends to suggest he was an external appointment, since local *curatores* did not usually carry the title *vir clarissimus;* compare, e.g., nos. 115, 123, 125–27, 130–32, 134, 137, 140, 142. The wording, especially the phrases *splendori thermarum* (indicating an adornment of the baths) and *ex locis abditis* (meaning "from remote locations"), recalls that of nos. 39 and 115, both of which record the movement of statues from lonely spots into a bathhouse for its enhancement. The building is probably that mentioned in no. 10.

M. A(u)r(elius) Vincentius, v. [p.], p(raeses) [p(rovinciae) H(ispaniae)] Tarraconensis.   28†
Tarraco, Hispania Tarraconensis. Late third or early fourth century. *CIL* 2.4112 = *ILER* 1306.

M. Ar. Vincentio, v. [p.], p(raeses) [p(rovinciae) H(ispaniae)] | Tarraconensis ac su[per] | omnes reliqu[os] praesides, ius|tissimo restitutori | thermarum Montanarum | Mes[s]ius Marianus, | cur. r. p. Tarraconensis.

Trans.: "Messius Marianus, curator of the city of Tarraco, to M. Aurelius Vincentius, *vir perfectissimus,* governor of the province of Hispania Tarraconensis and, above all the other governors, the most just restorer of the *Thermae Montanae.*"

NOTES: This inscription is dated in *PLRE* (1.966, s.v. "Vincentius 7") to the late third/early fourth century because all other *praeses* inscriptions from Tarraco are so dated. In addition, the *curator r. p.* is evidently a local official. Thomasson (1.13–20) omits Vincentius from his lists of governors, indicating thereby a preference for the later date.

L. Caelius Montius, v. c., procons(ul) Asiae. Ephesos, Asia. 340/50. *AE* 1898.121 =   29
CIL 3.14195 = *ILS* 5704 = *IK* 14 (Ephesos 4) 1314/15.

d. n. Constanti | max. vict. ac | triumfatori | semper Aug. | L. Cael. Montius | v. c., procons. | Asiae, iudex | sacr(arum) cognit(ionum), | atrio thermarum | Constantianarum | fabricato excul|toque consti|tutit *(sic)* dedica|vitque.

NOTES: For this man, see *PLRE* 1.608, s.v. "Montius." The building in question is the so-called Harbor Bath-Gymnasium, originally constructed in the first or early second century and rebuilt, and renamed, during the reign of Constantine; for the remains, see Manderscheid, 108, s.v. "Ephesos, Hafenthermen (Hafengymnasium)"; Nielsen, 2.36 (C.295); Yegül, 272–73.

Furius Maecius Gracchus, v. c., corrector Flaminiae et Piceni. Tibur (Regio I). Before   30
ca. 350. *CIL* 14.3594 = *ILS* 5717 = *InscrIt* 4.1.15.

Furius Maecius | Gracchus, v. c., | corrector Fla|miniae et Pice|ni, ornatui | thermarum | dedicavit.

NOTES: The side of the stone bears a considerably older inscription dated to 172; this inscription can be dated to the mid–fourth century; see *PLRE* 1.400, s.v. "Gracchus 3." These baths are insufficiently investigated to allow any solid conclusions to be drawn about them, but their substructures appear to be built in *opus reticulatum* of Republican date, indicating a long history of use: see C. Carducci, *Tibur* (Rome, 1940), 61–63; Coarelli, *Lazio*, 95.

Fabius Maximus, v. c., rect(or) prov(inciae). Telesia (Regio II). 352/57. *CIL* 9.2212 =   31
ILS 5690 (see also *AE* 1972.150).

Fabius Maximus, v. c., | rect(or) prov(inciae) thermas | Sabinianas restituit, | curante ordine splendidissimo Telesinorum.

NOTES: Fifteen inscriptions record the benefactions of this man in Samnium and its environs; see *PLRE* 1.587, s.v. "Maximus 35." This inscription and the following two entries record his bath benefactions. The *AE* article presents a fragmentary sister text that adds the detail *[vi terrae mo]ltus e[versas]*. Its omission from the current entry is curious but not critical. The remains have not been thoroughly investigated; see De Caro and Greco, *Campania*, 198.

32   Fabius Maximus, v. c., rector prov(incae). Allifae (Regio II). 352/57. *CIL* 9.2338 = *ILS* 5691.

Fabius Maximus, v. c., rect. prov., | thermas Herculis vi terrae moltus eversas restituit a fundamentis.

NOTES: See previous entry. If any remains of these baths are known, they have not been sufficiently investigated and published; see De Caro and Greco, *Campania*, 243–47.

33   Fabius Maximus, v. c., re[c]tor prov(inciae). Saepinum (Regio IV). 352/57. *CIL* 9.2447.

Fabius Maximus, v. c., | re[c]tor provinciae, | thermas Silvani vestutat(e) | conlabsas restituit | curante Neratio Consta[nte] | patrono sumtu proprio.

NOTES: See previous two entries. The phrase *sumtu proprio* is undoubtedly to be ascribed to Fabius Maximus, the main benefactor named in the nominative, rather than to the local Neratius Constans who supervised the work; the Neratii, by the way, are a local family attested at Saepinum for centuries; see M. Gaggiotti, "Frammenti epigrafici inediti da Saepinum pertinenti alla gens Neratia," *AnnPerugia* 25 (1987/88): 129–40. These baths are known and are located near the forum: see Coarelli and La Regina, *Abruzzo*, 221; Manderscheid, 191, s.v. "Saepinum, Terme del Foro (Thermae Silvani)." Another bathing facility, of Imperial date, is located near the Porta Boiano, but it has only been partially excavated and remains unpublished: see Coarelli and La Regina, *Abruzzo*, 218–19; Manderscheid, 191, s.v. "Saepinum, Terme del Decumano." Much of the intramural space at Saepinum is undeveloped, since the town served as a station for drovers moving herds and flocks along pastoralist routes in Samnium (see *CIL* 9.2438, a lengthy inscription detailing abuses inflicted on the drovers by local officials). As a result, much of the town's area must have been given over to animal pens. If so, the baths of Saepinum probably served an unusually diverse clientele.

34†   P. Ceionius Cecina Albinus, v. c., cons(ularis) Numidiae. Kenchela, Numidia. 364/67. *AE* 1911.217.

aureis ubique temporibus dd. nn. Valentiniani et Valenltis perpetuorum [Au]gg. statum desperata recipiunt, amilssa renovantur, ruinarum deformitatem decor novitlatis excludit, iamdudum igitur thermarum aestivallium fabulam factam depellens faciemque restituens | Publius Ceionius Cecina Albinus, v. c. consularis, | ad splendorem tam patriae quam provinciae restituit | perfecit dedicavit [—] omninis i[—]antis | Aemilio Flaviano Fabio praetextato lav[—] | Innocentio Mario Secundino [—]XCV[—]antio | TLL BB PP.

Trans.: "In the golden age of our lords Valentinian and Valens, perpetual Augusti, which reigns everywhere, that which is desperate earns status; that which is neglected is renewed; and the beauty of restoration shuts out the ugliness of ruins. At long last Publius Ceionius Cecina Albinus, of senatorial rank and an ex-consul, drove away the widespread gossip about the summer baths and restored their appearance. He restored, completed, and dedicated (the baths), for the splendor of the city and of the province . . . *(the last lines are too fragmentary to make their meaning clear; possibly Aemilius Flavianus Fabius and Innocentius Marius Secundinus approved the work)."*

NOTES: This man is attested in eighteen inscriptions from Numidia; see *PLRE* 1.34–35, s.v. "Albinus 8."

Flavius Vivius Benedictus, v. p., praeses prov(inciae) Trip(olitaniae). Sabratha, Tripolitania. 378. *IRT* 103a.   35†

[Fl. Vivi Benedicti v.]p. | totius integritatis, moderaltionis, iustitiae, provisionis, | fidei, benignitatis, fortitudinis | ac beneficentiae viro Fl. Vivio | Benedicto, v. p., praesildi prov. Tripol. | inter cetera beneficia sua quibus | omnem provinciam conpendiis, relmediis et virtutibus fovit, sublelvabit, erexit etiam ob ea quae sibi | specialiter conlata sunt civitas | Sabrathensis exsultans quod polst ruinam et abnegatum thermalrum populo exercitium citra ullius | dispendium ornamentis patriae | revocavit ordo populusque | concinentibus omnibus voltis statuam patrono pr(a)estanltissimo gratanti studio conlocavit.

Trans.: "(Statue) of Flavius Vivius Benedictus, *vir perfectissimus*. To Flavius Vivius Benedictus, *vir perfectissimus*, governor of the province of Tripolitania, a man of complete integrity, moderation, fairness, foresight, loyalty, charity, bravery, and generosity. Amid the rest of his favors by which he fostered, encouraged, and raised up the entire province with his economies, remedial measures, and abilities, and also because of those benefactions that were bestowed by him in particular, the city of Sabratha was rejoicing because, after the ruin and denial of the baths, he restored exercise to the people without cost to any civic officer. The *ordo* and people unanimously voted and set up a statue to their preeminent patron, with grateful enthusiasm."

NOTES: For Flavius Benedictus, see *PLRE* 1.161, s.v. "Benedictus 4." The editors of *IRT* comment that the baths were probably ruined after the incursion of the Austoriani in 363–65 (see Amm. Marc. 28.6.1–15), in which case they went unrestored for over a decade. For the remains, see Manderscheid, 190, s.v. "Terme della Regio VII (Terme dell'Ufficio; Terme Meridionali)"; Nielsen, 2.28 (C.217); Yegül, 238–42. Nielsen (loc. cit.) states that the baths were abandoned in 365 due to an earthquake and attributes this inscription to the early fourth century; but Benedictus' term in Tripolitania is securely dated to 378 (see *IRT* 571) and there is no mention of an earthquake in the text.

[Avianius] Vindicianus, v. c., cons(ularis) Camp(aniae). Tarracina (Regio I). Ca. 378.   36†
CIL 10.6312.

[Avianius] | Vindicianus, | v. c., cons. Camp., | [t]hermas vi | [ignis consumptas restituit].

Trans.: "Avianius Vindicianus, of senatorial rank, governor of Campania, restored the baths that had been consumed by fire."

NOTES: For Vindicianus, see *PLRE* 1.968, s.v. "Vindicianus 4." Although much of the text is restored, the *vi* makes virtually certain a restoration of the baths, even if they were not destroyed specifically by fire; compare the wording of, e.g., nos. 87 and 108. For the remains of this building, see Coarelli, *Lazio,* 322.

37†   Anicius Auchenius Bassus, v. c., pro consule Campaniae. Antium (Regio I). 379/83. *CIL* 10.6656 = *ILS* 5702.

florente imperio ddd. Aaaggg. q. nnn. Grattiani *(sic)* | Valentiniani et Theodosi principum maximorum, | thermarum speciem ruinae deformitatem *(sic)* sordentem | et periculosis ponderibus inminentem, quae labantem | populum metu sollicitudinis deterrebat, exclusa totius | {s}carie vetustatis ad firmam stabilitate(m) usumq. tectorum | Anicius Auchenius Bassus v. c., pro consule Campaniae, | vice sacra iudicans, r[e]paravi in meliorem civitatis effigiem.

Trans.: "In the flourishing empire of our lords and Augusti Gratian, Valentinian, and Theodosius, greatest emperors. Anicius Auchenius Bassus, of senatorial rank, proconsul of Campania, deputy judge of imperial appeals: the appearance of the baths was ruinous, their ugliness was dirty, and dangerously unstable overhanging structures threatened to collapse, which used to keep the bathing populace away out of a fear of being worried. I repaired the building by entirely shutting out the decay of old age, until it was solid, stable, and usable, and made it into a better emblem of the city."

NOTES: For Bassus, see *PLRE* 1.152–54, s.v. "Bassus 11." If any physical remains of these baths are known at the site, they have yet to be fully explored; see Coarelli, *Lazio,* 292–98.

38†   [F]l(avius) Felix Gentilis, v. p., pr(a)es[es prov(inciae), patr]onus. Satafis, Mauretania. 379/83. *CIL* 8.8393 = *CIL* 8.20266.

[p]ro felicitate clementium seculor[um—principum maximorum? | d]dd. nnn. Gratiani Valentiniani atq(ue) Thaeo[dosi aquae?]ductum therma[rum | nup]er lignis putrib(us) constitutum at [nunc] mirabili opere agpera[—| constr]uctum ins[ti]tuit, perfecit, dedicavitq(ue) [F]l. Felix Gentilis v. p. pr(a)es[es prov(inciae), | patr]onus ex sumptib[us suis] . . . *(the rest is very fragmentary).*

Trans.: "By virtue of the happiness of the merciful age of (the greatest emperors?), our lords Gratian, Valentinian, and Theodosius. Flavius Felix Gentilis, *vir perfectissimus,* governor of the province, patron, at (his own?) expense began constructing, completed, and dedicated the (aque?)duct of the baths, formerly made of rotten wood but now built with remarkable workmanship . . . "

NOTES: For Felix, see *PLRE* 1.391, s.v. "Flavius Felix Gentilis." This text is a composite of three fragments. The likely restoration is *[aquae]ductum therma[rum]* rather than *[aquae]ductum therma[sque],* because the rest of the text refers to putrid wooden structures replaced by the benefactor: *thermae* are not likely to have been made of wood (though *balnea* could be; see Mart. 9.75, and see above, chapter 2, p. 56, for the putative wooden baths at Velsen, Holland). There is mention of the *curator rei publicae* at the end, but the text is too fragmentary to clarify his involvement. For other aqueduct benefactions, see nos. 222–38.

39   Audentius Aemilianus, v. c., cons(ularis) Camp(aniae). Liternum (Regio I). Before 383. *CIL* 10.3714 = *ILS* 5478.

signa translata ex abditis | locis ad celebritatem | thermarum Severianarum | Audentius Aemilanus *(sic),* v. c., cons. | Camp., constituit dedicarique precepit *(sic),* | curante Tannonio Chrysantio, v. p.

NOTES: For Aemilianus, see *PLRE* 1.22, s.v. "Aemilianus 4." The wording here recalls that of nos. 27 and 115. Aemilianus was a patron of Puteoli. Nothing is known of these baths; see De Caro and Greco, *Campania,* 90–91.

[—] Quintilianus, [rector S]amniticus, pa[tronus optim]us. Venafrum (Regio I). Mid-   40
to late fourth century. *CIL* 10.4865.

[Quintil]iani | [pro eius me]ritis et obsel[quis colle]gia urbis Venal[fran(orum) ..4..]
Quintiliano, | [rectori S]amnitico, pal[trono optim]o et examinal[tori aequis]simo
statuam | [loco publi]co positam ob | [atq]ue therm[as].

NOTES: The stone is a statue base. For Quintilianus, see *PLRE* 1.759, s.v. "Quintilianus 2." It
is not exactly clear from the text what Quintilianus did with regard to the baths. However, a
simple reading of the odd-sounding phrase *ob [atq]ue therm[as]* would suggest he built them. It
is also possible that the baths were built after the statue was erected: the phrase appears virtually
tacked on as an afterthought. A large structure with an exedra near the theater at Venafrum (the
so-called Terme di Sant'Aniello) may be a bathhouse, but whether or not it is the facility
mentioned here is uncertain; see Coarelli and La Regina, *Abruzzo*, 180. See no. 47 for another
constructional bath benefaction at Venafrum.

Ragonius Vincentius Celsus, praefectus annonae. Ostia (Regio I). Ca. 389. *CIL*   41
14.4717/18 = Cicerchia and Marinucci, *Scavi di Ostia* 11.165–66 (nos. C 1, 1a, b).

curavit Ragonius Vincentius Celsus, v.c., praefectus annonae urbis Romae et civitas
fecit me[morata de propri]o.

NOTES: The stone is part of a statue base, probably from the Forum Baths. It may record work
on the baths by Ragonius, here honored by the town. For his date and career, see *PLRE* 1.195–
96, s.v. "Celsus 9."

[Jun]iorinus Polemius, v. c., proconsule province *(sic)*. Carthage, Africa. 388/90. *AE*   42
1949.28.

[ddd] nnn Valentiniano, [Te]odosio et Arcadio | [Iun]iorinus Polemius, v. c., procon-
sule provincle *(sic)*, dignissimo decora(vit?) | almae Karthagi.

NOTES: This inscription is from the architrave of the Antonine Baths at Carthage. For Polemius, who went on to become *praefectus praetorio Italiae et Illyrici*, see *PLRE* 1.710, s.v.
"Polemius 5." The text is fragmentary, but the proconsul's actions are clear. These baths had
been built by the local authorities; see no. 86.

Domitius Severianus, v. c., cons(ularis) Campaniae. Liternum (Regio I). Fourth or   43†
fifth century. *EphEp* 8.456 = *ILS* 5693.

balneum Veneris lon[gi tempo]lris vetustate corruptum | Domitius Severianus, v. c.,
con[s.] | Campaniae ad pristinam faciem [aedifi]lcavit, curante hac *(sic)* dedican[te] |
Sentio Marso v. c., comite divinor[um], | curatore Capuensium, Literni[norum] |
Cumanorum.

Trans.: "The Baths of Venus, damaged by the aging of a long period of time, Domitius
Severianus, of senatorial rank, governor of Campania, built to its original appear-
ance. Sentius Marsus, of senatorial rank, companion of the divine rulers, curator of
Capua, Liternum, and Cumae, saw to the work and dedicated it."

NOTES: For the benefactor, see *PLRE* 1.829, s.v. "Severianus 8."

Septimius Rusticus, v. c., cons(ularis) Camp(aniae), patronus praestantissimus.   44
Puteoli (?) (Regio I). Fourth or fifth century. *CIL* 10.1707 = *ILS* 5692.

Septimio Rustilco, v. c., cons. Camp., | provisori ordilnis, restauratolri thermarum, | ob insignem amolrem splendildissimus ordo | et honestissilmus populus | patrono praesltantissimo.

NOTES: The provenance of this text is uncertain, but *CIL* includes it among the material from Puteoli (it is now in Naples). For Rusticus, see *PLRE* 1.787, s.v. "Rusticus 3"; for Marsus, see *PLRE* 1.562, s.v. "Marsus 1." For the unusual title *provisor ordinis,* compare *CIL* 10.3860 = *ILS* 1276. Neither of the unpublished Roman baths of Puteoli has been sufficiently well investigated to make possible an identification with the building mentioned here: see De Caro and Greco, *Campania,* 39; Manderscheid, 177, s.v. "Pozzouli/Puteoli, 'Bagno Ortodonico'" and "'Tempio di Nettuno.'"

45   Rullus Festus, v. c., corr(ector) Luc(aniae) et Brit(tiorum). Grumentum (Regio III). Fourth or fifth century. *CIL* 10.212.

Rullus Festus, | v. c., corr(ector) Luc(aniae) et | Brit(tiorum), ad ornatum | thermarum | collocavit.

NOTES: For Festus, see *PLRE* 1.337, s.v. "Festus 13." A more fragmentary inscription (*CIL* 10.213) may record the same benefaction. Remains of the Roman buildings at Grumentum are insufficient to allow these baths to be identified; see Greco, *Magna Grecia,* 165.

Local Authorities

46†   M. Valerius, aed(ilis), dict(ator). Lanuvium (Regio I). Undated. *CIL* 14.2121 = *ILS* 5683.

M. Valerio M. f., | aed., dict., | praef. iuventutis, | municipes compitenses veicorum | quinque, quod specus millia | passus (3) purgavit refecit, | fistulas reposuit, balnea virilia | utraque et muliebre de sua | pecunia refecit, populo viscerati(onem) | gladiatores dedit, lumina ludos | I(unoni) S(ospitae) m(atri) r(eginae) solus fecit.

Trans.: "The townspeople who share the crossroads of five *vici* (dedicated this monument) to M. Valerius, son of Marcus, aedile, dictator, prefect of the youth, because he cleaned out and rebuilt the drains for a distance of three miles, replaced the pipes, restored at his own expense both the men's baths and the women's bath, gave a sacrificial feast and gladiatorial games to the people, and alone made ornament offerings and gave games in honor of Juno Sospita, mother and queen."

NOTES: Municipal dictators are attested at Lanuvium in the Imperial period (*CIL* 14, p. 191), but no precise date can be offered for this text; on this office, see Rudolph, *Stadt und Staat,* 7–24. It is reasonable to infer, but not certain, that the drains and pipes were associated with the baths mentioned in the text. The *vici* were local neighborhoods at Lanuvium, probably with shared boundaries at a specific crossroads (for a recent study of such neighborhoods and the role of crossroads in shaping local identities, see Laurence, 38–50). Aside from the ruins of the sanctuary of Juno Sospita, the Roman remains at Lanuvium are insufficient to allow the identification of the baths; see F. Coarelli, *Dintorni di Roma* (Bari, 1981), 105–10.

47†   P. Lucanius Quadratus, IIvir, augur, q(uaestor) II. Venafrum (Regio I). Undated. *CIL* 10.4884 = *ILS* 5664.

P. Lucanius L. f. Ter. Quadratus, IIvir, augur, q. II, balneum solo, peq(unia) sua dedit. Cassia P. f. uxor et Lucania P. f. Procula.

Trans.: "P. Lucanius Quadratus, son of Lucius, of the voting tribe Teretina, *duovir,* augur, quaestor twice, gave the bath on his own property (*or* from the ground up), at his own expense. Cassia, daughter of Publius, his wife, and Lucania Procula, daughter of Publius, (made this monument)."

NOTES: *Dedit* here most probably denotes a construction, since the baths are "given . . . at his own expense" and "on his own ground" or "from the ground up," depending on how *solo* is read. The wife and daughter do not appear to have played any part in the bath benefaction. For the putative bath remains at Venafrum, none of which are likely to have been this establishment, see no. 40.

Local council. Aquilonia (Regio II). Undated. *CIL* 9.6261.   48

[—] balneum | [—] at hoc | [publi]ce ex d(ecreto) d(ecurionum) | [p(ecunia)] p(ublica) restitutum.

NOTES: The inscription was found near the ruins of baths, according to the entry in *CIL*. The work was probably the responsibility of the local council; at any rate, it appears to have been carried out at public expense (compare the wording in the next entry).

Pars Peltuinatium. Peltuinum (Regio IV). Undated. *CIL* 9.3430 = *ILS* 5668/69.   49†

balineum refectum | dec(urionum) decr(eto) pecun(ia) public(a) | partis Peltuinatium.

Trans.: "The bath was rebuilt by decree of the decurions, at the public expense of Pars Peltuinatium."

NOTES: Remains of baths are not known at this site; see Coarelli and La Regina, *Abruzzo,* 27–30. An aqueduct, the Aqua Augusta, was built for this place under Tiberius (*CIL* 9.4206) and restored and improved by Sex. Vitulasius Nepos, consul in 78 (*ILS* 9368). If this water supply had any connection with the *balineum* mentioned here, which is far from certain, a possible date can be assigned to it. In the absence of any physical remains, however, such details remain speculative.

Incertus, patronus municipi, *et alii* (?). Pitinum Pisaurense (Regio VI). Undated. *CIL*   50
11.6040 = *ILS* 5711.

[—b]alineum fecit; | [—q.?] q. pavimentum tepidari s(ua) p(ecunia) refecit; | [—patro]nus municipi signum Fortunae | [—] idem balneum suspendit, tubu[los . . . la]cus piscinamque fecit | [—]m vetustate corrup|[tum] . . .] sua pecunia refecit.

NOTES: The text, although fragmentary, clearly commemorates a series of constructional actions, including construction, restoration, and adornment. The variety and nature of the actions suggest that this inscription originally commemorated at least three benefactors, acting in succession over an unspecified period of time (compare, e.g., nos. 1/2, 73/74). The first benefactor built the bath; a second benefactor, possibly a quaestor or a *quinquennalis,* repaired the floor of the *tepidarium;* and a third, the *patronus municipi,* repaired and adorned it. It is conceivable that all of these operations were undertaken by one man at different stages of his career; however, the manner in which the actions are cited here suggests separate individuals. Fragmentary remains of these baths are known; see M. Gaggiotti et al., *Umbria, Marche* (Bari, 1980), 202. Another inscription from this site reports that a "water receptacle" was completed by a patroness for her freedman, but it cannot be securely associated with baths: *Lania M. f. Celerin(a)* | *receptaculum* | *aquae inchoatum* | *ab Amarantho lib(erto)* | *suo consummavit* (*CIL* 11.6038 = *ILS* 5736).

P. Annius, praef. Pa[gi—]. Pa[gus—] (modern Le Pègue), Gallia Narbonensis. Un-   51
dated. *CIL* 12.1708.

P. Annius P. f. V[ol—], | praef. Pa[gi—] | suo et P. Anni [—fil. | n]omine marm[oribus? | ex]cultum ba[lneum].

52   Q. T[—], flam[en Romae et Augusti?]. Segodunum, Gallia Narbonensis. Undated. *AE* 1914.196.

Q. T[—] | flam[en Romae et Augusti?] | mac[ellum—et] | ther[mas—a funda]|men[tis—s(ua) p(ecunia) restituit?].

NOTES: Although the name of the man cannot be made out and his benefaction may just as easily have been an initial construction, enough survives of the text to be sure that a local official did some constructional work on a bathhouse. As of 1976, the site of Segodunum remained largely unexplored, but pottery finds suggested a period of habitation from the first to the fourth centuries; see *PECS*, 818, s.v. "Segodunum" (Labrousse).

53   V[ik(ani)] Tasg[aet(ii)]. Tasgaetium, Germania Superior. Undated. *CIL* 13.5257.

balneum vetustat[e] | consumt(um) V[ik(ani)] Tasg[aet(ium)] | a solo resti[t]uer[unt] | cur. Car. Cai[.]at. [IIviro?] | et fl(amine) adiecto qu[i et—] | Aurel. Celso et Cilt[o] | Cilti fil.

NOTES: The inscription was found among the ruins of baths, according to the entry in *CIL*. The ending may be fragmentary, but the main benefaction is clear.

54†   Ti. Claudius Maternus, aedilis. Aventicum, Germania Superior. Undated (but possibly early Imperial). *AE* 1946.239.

Ti. Claudius Ti. fil. | Maternus, aedilis, | sphaeristerium | d(e) s(uo) d(edit).

Trans.: "Ti. Claudius Maternus, son of Tiberius, aedile, gave the ball court from his own funds."

NOTES: A *sphaeristerium* was part of a bathhouse; compare no. 5. A bath of the first and second centuries is known at Aventicum, but it is not clear if it is the structure referred to here: see Manderscheid, 70, s.v. "Avenches/Aventicum, Forumthermen"; Nielsen, 2.21 (C.158). *Dedit* here undoubtedly denotes a construction.

55   [P.] Cornelius Grammeu[s?—]lipax et P. Cornelius Long[inus?], pater et f(ilius), pro honore IIvira[tus]. Centuripae, Sicily. Undated (but possibly second century). *CIL* 10.7004 = *ILS* 5663.

/ / / / / / / / / / / / | [P.] Cornelius P. f. Grammeu[s?—| . .]lipax et P. Cornelius P. f. P. n. Long[inus?], | pater et f., pro honore IIvira[tus | s]phaeristerium fecerunt.

NOTES: Dessau comments that the erased opening line of the text may have contained an emperor's name, no longer recoverable (Mommsen saw the letters CA / / VI in the middle of the first line; see the entry in *CIL*). The benefactors are reported to have carried out the work "in return for the honor of the duovirate," making this an *ob honorem* benefaction. Fragments of a possibly second-century bathhouse are known from Centuripae, but it is unclear if this text pertains to it; see R.J.A. Wilson, *Sicily under the Roman Empire: The Archaeology of a Roman Province, 36 B.C.–A.D. 535* (London, 1990), 94, 152.

56   [Hero]des, [patro]nus?, c. v. Aquileia (Regio X). Undated (but possibly third century). *CIL* 5.880.

[ex testamento Hero]dis [patro?]ni c. v., [thermae factae] lavant(ibus).

NOTES: Though the text is very fragmentary and the words *thermae factae* are restored, the presence of *lavant(ibus)* gives a clear sign that baths were somehow involved: the most obvious benefaction to bathers is to build baths. Alternatively, *lavant.* could be an abbreviation of *lavantes,* meaning "baths" (as in no. 189). In either case, a bath construction seems the most likely benefaction. Large baths of the third century are known at Aquileia, and this text may refer to them: see A. Calderini, *Aquileia romana: Ricerche di storia e di epigrafia* (Milan, 1930; reprint, Rome, 1973), 115; Manderscheid, 63, s.v. "Aquileia, Grandi Terme."

Cn. Terentius Primus, IIIIIIvir et Terentia coniunx. Brebia (Regio XI). Undated (but sometime in the Principate). *CIL* 5.5504.   57*

There are two versions of this text (cited as versions A and B below), the original of which is now lost.

A. Cyriacus of Ancona (ca. 1441): Cn. Terentio Cn. f. I Primo IIIIII viro et I Terentiae coniugi I iucundissimae I qui vican(is) f(ecerunt) I habitantib(us) lavationem.

B. J. Castilloneus (ca. 1541): Cn. Terentio I Primo IIIIvir I Terentiae cIiuccu I qui vicin. I habitantib. I lavationem I balneo / / I optatiss.

NOTES: Of the two readings, that of Cyriacus reads more naturally (which is not conclusive, since he may have filled in the gaps with his imagination). Whatever the correct text, the construction of a bath is clearly the sense of version A, while an offer of free bathing is the benefaction in the more difficult version B. In the case of A, *lavatio* means "bathhouse" or "bathing facilities," a rare use of the word (for a parallel, see Cic. *Fam.* 9.5.3 [= SB 179]). The sevirate appeared under Augustus and flourished until the mid–third century, thereby providing termini for the date of this inscription: see R. Duthoy, "Les Augustales," *ANRW* 2.16.2 (1978): 1254–1309; P. Kneissl, "Entstehung und Bedeutung der Augustalität: Zur Inschrift der ara Narbonensis (*CIL* XII 4333)," *Chiron* 10 (1980): 291–326; S.E. Ostrow, "The Augustales in the Augustan Scheme," in K. Raaflaub and M. Toher, eds., *Between Republic and Empire: Interpretations of Augustus and His Principate* (Berkeley, 1990), 364–79.

[—] Chrysanthus [VIvir Aug.] et Clodia Agathe uxor. Narbo, Gallia Narbonensis. Undated (but sometime in the Principate). *CIL* 12.4388.   58*

[—] Chrysanthus I [VIvir Aug. C(olonia) I(ulia) P(aterna) N(arbone)] M(artio) et Clodia Agathe uxor I [—loco si]bi dato ex decreto IIIIIIvirorum Aug(ustalium) I [balineum—] et marmoribus exstructum et ductu(m) I [aquae?—feceru?]nt et sportulis datis dedicaverunt.

NOTES: The mention of *ductus* and *marmorbius* in the surviving portions of the text makes the presence of a bath in the lacuna a strong likelihood, although a *nymphaeum* cannot be ruled out. Since the stone was not found in situ, it is now impossible to say with certainty which type of building was commemorated.

[—]oratus et [—] Pr[imi]genius, ob [honore]m sexvir[a]tus. Lanuvium (Regio I). Undated but (sometime in the Principate). *CIL* 14.2119 = *ILS* 5707.   59†

[ex auctori]tate Luci Ocrae I [dictatoris *or* aedilis?] municipi I [—]oratus et I [—] Pr[imi]genius, ob I [honore]m sexvir[a]tus, apodyterium I [ope]re tectorio, quod vetustate del[ficie]bat, refecerunt, [it]em piscinam ab nol[v]o fecerunt, labrum [ae]num cum salientibus, I [r]ostris navalibus tr[ibu]s, posuerunt.

Trans.: "On the authority of Lucius Ocra, dictator (?) *or* aedile (?) of the town, [?]oratus and [?] Primigenius, on account of gaining the office of the sevirate, restored with stucco work the *apodyterium,* which was fading away with old age; in addition, they built anew the *piscina* and set up a bronze *labrum* with spouts, three ships' beaks."

NOTES: The detailed report of the work done is interesting and covers much of the bathhouse. The *apodyterium* is the changing room, the *piscina* is of uncertain location—it could be an outdoor or indoor facility (see Nielsen, 1.154, s.v. "piscina")—and a *labrum* was usually located in the *caldarium* (see ibid., 1.158, s.v. "labrum"). The latter was apparently supplied with water from three spouts in the shape of ships' beaks. For another dictator and aedile from Lanuvium, see no. 46.

60   [—] Sermo, Turpilius Vetidius, IIviri quinqu(ennales). Philippi, Macedonia. Undated (but possibly fourth century). *CIL* 3.7342 = *ILS* 5710.

IIviri quinq. Philipp., augu[r.,—]| Sermo, Turpilius Vetidius [—per] | Oppium Front-onem patrem [thermas? refec(tas)] | adiecta cella natatori[a—].

NOTES: The main benefaction translates as "[through] Oppius Fronto, their father, [they decorated (?) the baths that had been rebuilt (?)] with a *natatio* room added." The question is, what does "through their father" mean? Did Fronto put up the money for the work? The fragmentary nature of the text precludes certainty. Mention, however, of a *cella natatoria* clearly signifies a bath benefaction; the *adiecta* records at least an extension, probably carried out in association with a restoration. A bathhouse of mid-third-century date is known at Philippi and was restored in the fourth century, but it cannot be securely associated with this text; see Nielsen, 2.43 (C.355).

61† C. Vulius and P. Aninius, IIv(iri) i(ure) d(icundo). Pompeii (Regio I). Ca. 80 B.C. *CIL* 1².1635 = *CIL* 10.829 = *ILS* 5706 = *ILLRP* 648.

C. Vulius C. f., P. Aninius C. f., IIv(iri) i(ure) d(icundo), | laconicum et destrictarium | faciund(um) et porticus et palaestr(am) | reficiunda locarunt ex d(ecreto) d(ec-urionum) ex | ea pequnia quod eos e lege | in ludos aut in monumento | consumere oportuit; faciun(da) | coerarunt eidemque probaru(nt).

Trans.: "C. Vulius, son of Gaius, and P. Aninius, son of Gaius, *duoviri* for administer-ing the law, by decree of the decurions, let contracts for the construction of a *lacon-icum* and a *destrictarium,* and for the restoration of the porticoes and the palaestra, from that money that, according to the law, they ought to have spent on games or in building. They saw to the work and also approved it."

NOTES: This inscription is from the Stabian Baths in Pompeii. The dating of the inscription to the earliest phase of the colony seems secure; see H. Mouritsen, *Elections, Magistrates, and Municipal Elite: Studies in Pompeian Epigraphy* (Rome, 1988), 78. Mention of the *lex* here is most probably in reference to the (now lost) colonial charter of Pompeii, which, on analogy with surviving municipal charters, would have included provisions for the spending of money by local magistrates, especially aediles (see, e.g., the *lex Ursonensis, CIL* 2.5439 = *ILS* 6087, §§ 70–71). If so, the expenditure here came from the private funds of Vulius and Aninius, albeit as a public duty. The exact nature of the work cannot be securely identified in the surviving remains, despite numerous efforts to do so: see, e.g., Delorme, *Gymnasion,* 224–26; H. Eschebach, " . . . *Laconicum et destrictarium faciund. . . . locarunt . . . :* Untersuchungen in den Stabianer Thermen zu Pompeji," *RM* 80 (1973): 235–42; id., *Stabianer Thermen,* 68–69; Richardson, *Pompeii,* 102–3.

62† Local council. Pompeii (Regio I). Ca. 80 B.C. *CIL* 1².1628 = *CIL* 10.819 = *ILS* 6356 = *ILLRP* 641.

L. Caesius C. f., d(uum)v(ir) i(ure) d(icundo), | C. Occius M. f., | L. Niraemius A. f., IIv(iri), | d(e) d(ecurionum) s(ententia) ex peq(unia) publ(ica) | fac(iundum) curar(unt) prob(arunt)que.

Trans.: "L. Caesius, son of Gaius, *duovir* for administering the law, and C. Occius, son of Marcus, and L. Niraemius, son of Aulus, *duoviri*, saw to the construction (of the baths) from public money in accordance with a decree of the decurions; they also approved the work."

NOTES: This inscription was found in the Forum Baths in 1823. The baths are evidently the object of the text, even though they are not expressly mentioned. C. Occius and L. Niraemius were aediles, sometimes called *duoviri* at Pompeii; see Mouritsen, *Elections*, 28–30. On the dating of this text, see ibid., 77.

Local council. Praeneste (Regio I). Ca. 80 B.C. *CIL* 1².1473 = *CIL* 14.3013 = *ILS*   63†
5667 = *ILLRP* 659.

Q. Vibuleius L. f., | L. Statius Sal(vi) f., | duovir(i), | balneas reficiund(as), | aquam per publicum | ducendum d(e) d(ecurionum) s(ententia) | coeravere.

Trans.: "Q. Vibuleius, son of Lucius, and L. Statius, son of Salvus, *duoviri*, saw to the reconstruction of the baths and the bringing of water through public land in accordance with a decree of the decurions."

NOTES: Praeneste was first devastated and then colonized by Sulla in 82 B.C., and this text appears to date to a period shortly after these events. It was found among the remains of baths near the Church of Madonna dell'Aquila, which stands in the region of the Sullan colony's forum. Another set of (possible) baths is situated near the *propyleia* of the Sanctuary of Fortuna Primigenia, an advantageous location. Both facilities are insufficiently investigated to allow any solid conclusions to be drawn about them; see Coarelli, *Lazio*, 155. In the context of the aqueduct, the phrase *per publicum* is more likely to mean "through public land" (see Livy 5.55.5) than "at public expense," which is more usually expressed by phrases like *de publico, ex publico,* or simply *publico;* see *OLD*, s.v. "publicum" (2).

Local council. Grumentum (Regio III). Sullan. *CIL* 1².1690 = *CIL* 10.221 = *ILS 5665*   64
= *ILLRP* 606.

Q. Pettius Q. f. Tro. Curva, | C. Maecius C. f. Ouf., pr(aetores), | duovir(i), balneum ex | d(ecreto) d(ecurionum) de peq(unia) pob(lica) fac(iundum) cur(averunt), | Q. Pettius Q. f. probavit.

NOTES: This text appears to date to the establishment of the Sullan colony. It is unlikely that this bath is the same as those mentioned in nos. 45 and 190, recording restorations in the late Empire.

Local council. Herdonia (Regio II). Caesarian. *CIL* 1².3188 = *AE* 1967.96.   65

D. Funius D. f. Gall[us?], | C. Rubrius C. f. Tinti[rius?], | IIIIvir(i) quinq(uennales), | balneum ab solo fa[ciundum] | coiraver(unt) ex d(ecreto) d(ecurionum), eide(m) | probavere.

NOTES: The editors of *AE* suggest a Caesarian date for this text, on the basis of the archaic *coiraver(unt)*. Remains of baths are known just north of the forum at Herdonia and are datable to the mid- to late first century B.C.; see J. Mertens, ed., *Herdonia: Scoperta di una città* (Brussels, 1995), 176–79 (by J. Mertens and F. van Wonterghem). M. Silvestrini (in ibid., 240) also assigns the text to the Caesarian period.

66   Local council (?). Brixia (Regio X). 49–ca. 27 B.C. (?). *CIL* 5.4412.

Q. Cornel[ius—], | IIIIvir i(ure) d(icundo) q(uinquennalis?), IIv(ir), | in balneum facl[—].

NOTES: It is a matter of uncertainty whether any significance can be placed on this man's holding of both the quattuorvirate and the duovirate. Mommsen (*CIL* 5, p. 439) suggested that *quattuorviri* were instituted at Brixia following the grant of citizenship in 49 B.C., but *duoviri* replaced them when colonial status followed under Augustus, possibly around 27 B.C. (on the latter, see L. Keppie, *Colonisation and Veteran Settlement in Italy, 47–14 B.C.* (London, 1983), 192–95. The relative significance of the terms *quattuorvir* and *duovir* is not as clear-cut as Mommsen imagined (see Curchin, 33–34), so this suggestion, and consequently the date, must be considered tentative. Despite the fragmentary text, the appearance of the phrase *in balneum fac[—]* strongly suggests a constructional benefaction of some sort, possibly an extension or a monetary contribution toward an initial construction, expressed in the formula *in balneum fac[iundum . . .]*. Cornelius may also have been a quaestor, if *q.* is restored as *q(uaestor)* rather than as *q(uinquennalis)*.

67†   Local council. Croton (Regio III). Late Republic. *CIL* 1².2542 = *ILLRP* 575.

[—] Lucilius A. f. Macer, T. Annaeus Sex. f. Trhaso *(sic)* [I]Ivirei | q[uin]q[ue]nnales exs s(enatus) c(onsulto) balneum aedeificandum courav⟨e⟩ru(nt).

Trans.: "[—] Lucilius Macer, son of Aulus, and T. Annaeus Thraso, son of Sextus, *duoviri* with censorial powers, saw to the building of the bath in accordance with a decree of the senate."

NOTES: This text is on a mosaic floor in one of the rooms of a small bath associated with the Sanctuary of Hera at Croton and is dated by Degrassi *(ILLRP)* to the end of the Republic. The remains of these poorly preserved baths have not been properly investigated and are no longer visible; the excavator was unsure if the bath was open to the public, as suggested by the involvement of municipal officials, or restricted to priests and custodians of the sanctuary, as suggested by its location: see P. Orsi, "Prima campagna di scavi al santuario di Hera Lacinia," *NSc* Suppl. (1911): 89–91; note also Greco, *Magna Grecia*, 109–10. In general, there is little reason to suspect that sanctuary baths operated on a basis of strictly restricted access.

68   Local council. Pompeii (Regio I). 3–4. *CIL* 10.817 = *ILS* 5726.

Cn. Melissaeo Cn. f. Apro, M. Staio M. f. Rufo IIvir(i) iter(um) i(ure) d(icundo), labrum ex d(ecreto) d(ecurionum) ex p(ecunia) p(ublica) f(aciundum) c(urarunt). constat HS *(5,250)*.

NOTES: This text is from the lip of the *labrum* in the men's *caldarium* in the Forum Baths at Pompeii (see figs. 10–12). It is dated by the *duoviri* Cn. Melissaeus Aper and M. Staius Rufus, who held office in 3 or 4; see P. Castrén, Ordo Populusque Pompeianus: *Polity and Society in Roman Pompeii* (Rome, 1975), 190 (no. 246.7) for Melissaeus and 224 (no. 388.4) for Staius. Because the work was carried out at public expense, it was clearly the responsibilty of the local council. For similar *labrum* dedications, see below, nos. 75 and 166.

69†   Incertus, patronus. Ligures Baebiani (Regio II). Post-62 (?). *CIL* 9.1466.

(there are an uncertain number of missing lines) | patrono qui [con]llapsum terr[a]e mo[tu] | balineum ref[ici] | curavit ac sua [pe]lcunia fecit ob mulnificentiam eius | ordo et populus | [Ligu]rum Baebian[olr]um posuerunt.

Trans.: "On account of his generosity, the *ordo* and people of Ligures Baebiani put up (this monument) to [?], the patron, who saw to it that the bath that had collapsed in the earthquake was rebuilt and did so at his own expense."

NOTES: Mention of an earthquake in the text prompts Nielsen (1.40–41 n. 26) to date this benefaction to the period immediately after the Campanian earthquake of 62; the date is therefore not secure.

L. Caesienus Firm[us?], quaest(or), praef(ectus) i(ure) d(icundo), q(uinquennalis) and   70
L. Caesienus Firm[us?] [—], quaest(or), quinq(uennalis), trib(unus) milit(um) II.
Furfo (Regio IV). Julio-Claudian (?). *CIL* 9.3522.

[L. Caesienus Firm[us—], | quaest(or), praef(ectus) i(ure) d(icundo),
q[uinq(uennalis)—] | L. Caesienus Firm[us, L. f.,—] | L. pron,. quaest(or),
quinq[uennalis—] | trib. mil. II, flam. Aug., q. [—] | [bal]neum d(e) s(ua) p(ecunia)
fec[erunt—].

NOTES: Nielsen (1.40 n. 25) dates this text to the Julio-Claudian period without explanation. The two benefactors appear to be father and son; if so, the father stayed at the municipal level, while the son, an *eques,* received a posting as a military tribune before returning to his *patria* for the quinquennial quaestorship. Such career profiles are not unusual; see Duthoy, "Profil social," 123–27.

Junia Rustica, sacerdos perpetua, et prima in municipio Cartimitan[o]. Cartima,   71†*
Baetica. Flavian (?). *CIL* 2.1956 = *ILS* 5512 = *ILER* 2054.

Iunia D. f. Rustica, sacerdos | perpetua et prima in municipio Cartimitan[o], | porticus
public(as) vetustate corruptas refecit, solum | balinei dedit, vectigalia publica vin-
dicavit, signum | aereum Martis in foro posuit, porticus ad balineum | solo suo cum
piscina et signo Cupidinis epulo dato | et spectaculis editis d(e) p(ecunia) s(ua) d(ono)
d(edit), statuas sibi et C. Fabio | Iuniano f(ilio) suo ab ordine Cartimitanorum
decret[as | remis]sa impensa, item statuam C. Fabio Fabiano viro suo d(e) p(ecunia)
s(ua) f(ecit) d(edicavitque).

Trans.: "Junia Rustica, daughter of Decius, priestess for life and the leading lady in the town of Cartima, rebuilt the public porticoes that were ruined with old age, gave the lot of land for the bath, paid the public taxes of the town, and set up a bronze statue of Mars in the forum. After giving a public banquet and a spectacle, she gave as a gift at her own expense the porticoes at the bath on her own property, along with the pool and a statue of Cupid. After remitting the cost, she made at her own expense and dedicated the statues decreed to her and her son, C. Fabius Junianus, by the *ordo* of Cartima, and she did likewise for a statue to her husband, C. Fabius Fabianus."

NOTES: The extensive list of benefactions from this obviously prominent woman demonstrates that she was in possession of considerable financial power and was not averse to wielding it for the public good; see MacMullen, "Woman in Public"; Nicols, *"Patrona Civitatis,"* 134–36. The *porticus ad balinetum* appear to have been a part of the bathing complex; compare such formulae as *signa . . . ad theatrum posuit* (no. 249).

L. Aemilius Daphnus, sevir. Murgi, Baetica. Flavian (?). *CIL* 2.5489 = *ILER* 2045.   72†

L. Aemilius Daphnus, sevir, thermas | sua omni impensa municipibus Murg(itanis) |
dedit et quodie *(sic)* eas dedicavit *(denarios)* sinl[g]ulos civibus et incolis epulum
dedit. | [q]amdiu vixisset eodem die daturum | [se] *(denarios)* singulos eisdem promisit

et in | [tute]lam earundem thermarum quam|diu ipse vixisset annuos *(denarios) (150)* |
pollicitus est.

Trans.: "L. Aemilius Daphnus, *sevir,* gave the *thermae* to the people of Murgi entirely
at his own expense and, on the day he dedicated them, gave a single denarius to each
citizen and a banquet to the residents. He promised that for as long as he lived, he
would give 1 denarius to each citizen on that same day, and he promised to give 150
denarii a year for the upkeep of the same *thermae,* for as long as he lived."

NOTES: The text is dated tentatively by letterform. *Dedit* here evidently means "built." The
term *incolae* was applied to a wide variety of people but, as a rule, denoted those who resided in
or around a municipality without holding citizenship of that place; see *RE* 9.1249–56, s.v.
"incola" (Groag).

73/74†   T. Varius Rufinus Geganius Facundus Vibius Marcellinus, equo publ(ico), quinquen-
nalic(ius) and Respublica. Fanum Fortunae (Regio VI). First century (and earlier?).
CIL 11.6225 = *ILS* 5679.

T. Várius T. f. Pol. Rúfinus | Gegánius Fácundus Víbius Márcellinus, | equo publ(ico),
quinquennalic(ius), nomine suo et | T. Vári Longi filii sui | balineum á L. Rufellio
Severo p(rimo)p(ilari), tr(ibuno), factum, | quod rés publica á novo refecerat, incendio
ex maxima parte | consúmptum operibus ampliátis pec(unia) sua restituit.

Trans.: "T. Varius Rufinus Geganius Facundus Vibius Marcellinus, son of Titus, of the
voting tribe Pollia, with the public horse [i.e., a knight], former *quinquennalis,* restored, in his own name and that of his son, T. Varius Longus, at his own expense with
larger structures, the bath that had been largely destroyed by fire. The bath had
originally been built by L. Rufellius Severus, chief centurion and tribune, and the city
had rebuilt it anew."

NOTES: This very instructive concise history of the building records three benefactions by two
classes of agent spread over an indeterminate period of time: (1) the restoration by the local
official T. Vibius Marcellinus, which is the main benefaction commemorated here, (2) a prior
restoration by the local council, and (3) the original construction by the private benefactor L.
Rufellius Severus (= no. 162). Presumably, earlier texts comemmorating these actions had been
damaged or destroyed in the fire, necessitating their replacement with this summary. Nielsen
(1.41 n. 26) dates the main benefaction to the first century, although without explanation. If that
date is accepted, the previous building activity may extend back into the Republic. Scattered
ancient remains are known at Fanum, but none can securely be identified as baths; see Gaggiotti
et al., *Umbria,* 207–10.

75   P. Paquius Priamus, Q. Annius Pom[.]n[—] IIIIvir(i). Copia Thurii (Regio III). First
century. *AE* 1976.175.

IV. P. Paquius P. f. Priamus, Q. Annius Q. f. Pom[.]n[—] IIIIvir(i).

NOTES: This inscription appears on the lip of a *labrum* discovered in 1975. It records only the
names of the magistrates, so it is not clear if the work was carried out by the *quattuorviri*
themselves or by the local council with the magistrates acting as agents. The significance of the
"IV" at the start of the text is unclear. Remains of first-century baths are known at the site, near
the theater; see Greco, *Magna Grecia,* 125. For similar dedications of *labra,* see nos. 68 and 166.

76   Local council. Interamnia Praetuttiorum (Regio V). First century (?). *CIL* 9.5067 =
ILS 5666.

L. Agusius Cn. f. L. n. Mussus, | C. Arrenus T. f. Rufus, | octoviri iterum, | balneas refic(iendas) d(e) c(onscriptorum) s(ententia) c(urarunt).

NOTES: Nielsen (1.41 n. 26) dates this inscription as "presumably first century," without elaboration. As with the previous entry, it is not clear who funded the work. For *octoviri,* see E. Manni, *Per la storia dei municipii fino alla guerra sociale* (Rome, 1947), 141–48; Rudolph, *Stadt und Staat,* 66–87. Putative ruins of baths are known at Interamnia, but it is not clear if they pertain to the building referred to here; see Coarelli and La Regina, *Abruzzo,* 41.

M. Pompeius Libo, sacerdos Arensis. Vesunna Petrucoriorum, Aquitania. First cen-   77†
tury (?). *CIL* 13.939 = *ILS* 4638.

[—?] et deo Apollini | Cobledulitavo | M. Pompeius, C. Pomp. | Sancti sacerdot(is) | Arensis fil., Quir. Libo | sacerdos Arensis, | qui templum deae | Tutelae et therma[s] public(as) utraq(ue) ol[im] vetustate collab[sa] | sua pecunia rest(ituit), v(otum) s(olvit) l(ibens) m(erito).

Trans.: "[—?] and to the god Apollo Cobledulitavus. M. Pompeius Libo, priest of the Altar, son of C. Pompeius Sanctus, priest of the Altar, of the voting tribe Quirina, fulfilled his vow willingly and deservedly. He restored at his own expense the temple of the goddess Tutela and the public baths, each of which had collapsed long ago with old age. He fulfilled his vow willingly and deservedly."

NOTES: The unusual opening of the inscription prompted Dessau *(ILS)* to postulate a missing upper portion (perhaps on another block, now lost). The priesthood mentioned is that of the Altar of Augustus and Rome at Lugdunum. Another inscription (*CIL* 13.1704) honoring Libo and Sanctus, as well as Libo's son M. Pompeius Sanctus, is dated by letterform to the first century, thereby suggesting the date of the current text.

C. Sempronius Sempronianus, IIvir bis, pontufex *(sic)* perpet(uus) and Sempronia   78†*
Fusca Fibia Anicilla, filia. Aurgi, Hispania Tarraconensis. Trajan (?). *CIL* 2.3361 =
ILER 2040.

C. Sempronius C. f. Gal. Sempronianus IIvir bis, | pontufex *(sic)* perpet(uus), | Sempronia Fusca Vibia Anicilla | filia, thermas aqua perducta cum silvis agnuar(um) | trecentarum pecunia impensaque sua omni d(ederunt) d(edicaverunt).

Trans.: "C. Sempronius Sempronianus, son of Gaius, of the voting tribe Galeria, *duovir* twice, chief priest for life, and Sempronia Fusca Vibia Anicilla, his daughter, gave and dedicated entirely at their own expense the baths with their water supply, along with three hundred *agnuae* of woodland."

NOTES: This inscription is cited as securely Trajanic by Nielsen (1.123 n. 5), presumably following *CIL* 2.3361, where the date is by letterform only.

C. Sappius Flavus, praefect(us) Iuliensium, tribun(us) militum. Vasio, Gallia Nar-   79†
bonensis. Not later than the early second century. *CIL* 12.1357 = *ILS* 2709.

Vasiens(ibus) Voc(ontiis). | C. Sappió C. filió Volt. | Flávó, | praefect. Iuliénsium, tribún. | mílitum leg. XXI Rapácis, praef. | álae Thrácum Hérculániae, praef. | rípáe flúminis Euphrátis, | quí HS *(1,200,000)* rei publicáe Iuliénsium | quod ad HS *(4,000,000)* ússúris perdúlcerétur, testámentó relíquit, idem | HS *(50,000)* ad por-ticum ante thermás | marmoribus órnandum légávit.

Trans.: "(Dedicated) by the Vocontii of Vasio. To Sappius Flavus, son of Gaius, of the voting tribe Voltinia, prefect of the town of the Julienses, military tribune of Legion XXI Rapax, prefect of the Herculean horse of Thracians, prefect of the bank of the Euphrates River, who left to the town of the Julienses in his will 1,200,000 sesterces, which was increased to 4,000,000 by interest; the same man bequeathed 50,000 sesterces for the decoration with marbles of the portico in front of the baths."

NOTES: The Vocontii were the Gallic tribe who lived in this area. This man had a predominantly military career, although as *praefect(us) Iuliensium* (the town of Vasio styled itself *Respublica Iuliensium*) he also held local office, perhaps following his return after military service. The date is established by mention of Sappius' posting to Legion XXI Rapax, which was raised under Augustus and was probably destroyed fighting the Sarmatians in 92, though perhaps a little later; see *RE* 12.1781–91, s.v. "Legion XXI Rapax" (Ritterling); G.R. Watson, *The Roman Soldier* (Ithaca, 1969), 23 and 164 n. 43. G. Webster (*The Roman Imperial Army*[3] [Totowa, 1985], 107 n. 32) suggests that the erasure of this legion's name from two tombstones—*CIL* 13.5201 and 13.11514—"may indicate that it seriously disgraced itself." If this suggestion is accepted, then Sappius Flavus apparently served before the disgrace (he shows no reluctance to declare his service in XXI Rapax), and so the inscription may date to the first century. It is not clear from the text that the portico was part of the bathhouse, although this can be assumed. The building in question may be the North Baths at Vasio; see Nielsen, 2.14–15 (C.101).

80   Res p(ublica) et populus. Corfinium (Regio IV). Post-122. *CIL* 9.3152 = *ILS* 5676.

The full text is cited at no. 174. Here note the portion that reads:

. . . balineum . . . res p(ublica) et populus Corfiniensis datis HS CLII (i.e., *152,000*) n(ummum) consummavit . . .

81   Col(onia) Iul(ia) Conc(ordia) Apamea. Apamea, Bithynia et Pontus. 129. *CIL* 3.6992 = *ILS* 314.

numini domus Augustor[um] | et imp. Caesari divi Traiani Parthic[i fil.] | divi Nervae nepoti Traiano Hadriano Au[g.] | pont. max., trib. pot. XIII, cos. III, p. p., Sabinae Au[g.], | senatui populoq(ue) Rom(ae), Col(onia) Iul(ia) Conc(ordia) Apamea | balineum Hadrianum ex p(ecunia) public(a) dedicavit.

NOTES: That the baths were built by the local council is certain due to their dedication to Hadrian and the imperial household from public money; had a party other than the colony been responsible for constructing the baths, mention of it could be expected to appear in the text (unless it was on another, now lost, inscription). The dedication may have been occasioned by Hadrian's visit to Asia Minor in 129; see Farrington, *Roman Baths of Lycia,* 54–56.

82†   C. Sennius Sabinus, praef(ectus) fabr(um). Vicus Albinnensis, Gallia Narbonensis. Hadrian/Antoninus Pius. *CIL* 12.2494 = *ILS* 5768.

C. Sennius C. f. Vol. Sabinus, praef(ectus) fabr(um), | balineum, campum, porticus, aquás iúsque | eárum aquarum tubo ducendarum, ita ut récte | perfluere possint, vicanis Albinnensibus d(e) s(uo) d(edit).

Trans.: "Gaius Sennius Sabinus, son of Gaius, of the voting tribe Voltinia, *praefectus fabrum,* gave at his own expense to the villagers of Vicus Albinnensis the bath, playing field, porticoes, and water, along with the right to channel it in pipes, so that water can flow through properly."

NOTES: Sennius was an Italian (he belonged to the voting tribe Voltinia) and lived during the reigns of Hadrian and Antoninus Pius (see *Dig.* 48.18.1, 5; *RE* 2A.1467–68, s.v. "Sennius 1" [Riba]). Here *dedit* most probably means "built"—the presence of *d(e) s(uo)* tends to suggest so. *Praefecti fabrum* were military aides-de-camp under the Republic but became low-level municipal officials under Augustus (see *RE* 6.1918–24, s.v. "fabri V" [Korneman]). *Aquas* is a common term for aqueducts, but it could also denote a water source (from springs?).

L. Annaeus Hermes, flam(en) et trib(unus?). Aubuzza, Africa. Antoninus Pius. *CIL*   83
8.16368.

genio | imp. Caes. Anto|nini Hadriani | Aug. | L. Annaeus Hermes, flam. | et trib(unus) IAR gentis AI[.]IA | (centuria?) Eron(is) paganicu[m] et portic(um) | et caldar(ium) et c(o)horte(m) cum om|nibus ornamentis a solo | s(ua) p(ecunia) fec(it) idq(ue) ded(ica-vit) | curatore Severo Sil|vani Vindicis, flam(ine) p(er)p(etuo).

NOTES: The reading is not entirely clear, especially in lines 5–6, where the local affiliations—*trib. IAR gentis AI[.]AI (centuria?) Eron(is)*—cannot be restored with any certainty, but the main benefaction(s) and the agent can be readily identified. This text is interesting if for no other reason than it names various parts of a bathhouse (see also appendix 3). A *paganicum* would appear to have been an area or room for playing the ball game *pila paganica,* which utilized a down-stuffed ball (see Mart. 7.32.7; Rebuffat, "Vocabulaire thermal," 14, 33–34). An undated, fragmentary inscription from the site (*CIL* 8.16367 = *ILS* 6783) records that the *paganicum* was later restored *([resti]tuer[unt])* by a group, which can no longer be identified; see Wesch-Klein, 64–65 (no. 1). *Porticus* and *caldar(ium)* require no elucidation. A *cohors* was an enclosed area; what specific function such an area served and how it differed from a palaestra, if at all, are unclear.

C. Valerius Claudius Pansa, flamen divorum Vespasiani, Traiani, Hadrian(i) p(er)(pe-   84†*
tuus), proc(urator) Aug(usti) provinc(iae) Britanniae et Albucia Candida, uxor.
Novaria (Regio XI). Antoninus Pius (?). *CIL* 5.6513.

C. Valerius C. f. Claud. Pansa, flamen | divorum Vespasiani Traiani Hadrian(i) p(er)p(etuus) bis, | trib. coh. VIIII pr., proc. Aug. provinc. Britanniae, | [balneum quod vi] consumptum fuerat ampliatis solo | [et operibus intra bie]nnium pecunia sua restituit et dedicavit, | [in quod opus legata] quoque rei p(ublicae) testamento Al-buciae Candidae | [uxoris suae HS *(200, 000)*] consensu ordinis amplius erogavit.

Trans.: "C. Valerius Pansa, son of Gaius, twice priest for life of the deified Vespasian, Trajan, and Hadrian, tribune of the ninth Praetorian cohort, imperial procurator of the province of Britain, within two years restored and dedicated at his own expense, on a larger lot and with larger structures, the bath that had been destroyed by violence. Toward this work, and with the agreement of the *ordo,* he paid out a further two hundred thousand sesterces that had been left to the city in the will of his wife, Albucia Candida."

NOTES: This text is instructive, albeit fragmentary. Valerius Pansa may have been procurator of Britain under Antoninus Pius (see Duthoy, "Profil social," 151 [no. 379]; S. Frere, *Britannia: A History of Roman Britain*[3] [London, 1987], 187). He is here clearly acting in the guise of a local *flamen perpetuus,* an office to which he was elected twice, although his career was mostly in the imperial, rather than the municipal, service. In such cases, it is usual to assume that the benefactor either stemmed from local stock or owned estates in the region. A bath is the most likely object of the benefaction, although no ruins survive at the modern site to test this supposition; see G. Cavalieri Manasse, G. Massari, and M.P. Rossignani, *Piemonte, Valle d'Aosta, Liguria, Lombardia* (Bari, 1982), 80–82. The building appears to have been destroyed by force, possibly a fire. What fraction of the final cost Albucia's two hundred thousand sesterces represents is impossible to say, but it must have been a major project to occupy two years of work and cost so much money to complete.

85   Local council. Aesernia (Regio IV). Mid-second century (?). *CIL* 9.2660.

Q. Fufius Q. f. Bal., | C. Antracius C. f., | IIIIvir(i) q., | d(e) s(enatus) s(ententia) balneum ref(iciundum) cur(averunt), | C. Antracius C. f. probavit.

NOTES: *Quattuorviri* only appear in Aesernia in the Imperial period, and the terse wording points to an earlier, rather than later, date, perhaps no later than the mid–second century. No remains of these baths are known, so a more precise date cannot be offered; see Coarelli and La Regina, *Abruzzo,* 183–89.

86   Col(onia) Con(cordia) Jul(ia) Karthag[o]. Carthage, Africa. 161/62. *AE* 1949.27.

pro salute imp. Caes. M. A[ureli Antonini Aug, pont. max., trib potest. XVI, cos. III et imp. Caes. L. Aureli Veri Aug., trib.] potest. II, cos. II, | divi Antonini filiorum, d[ivi Hadriani nepotum, divi Nerv]ae a[dnepotum totius]que domus eorum. | Col(onia) Con(cordia) Iul(ia) Karthag[o—cum statua—A]ugus[ti—et columnis?] Numidic(is) donavit. Q. Vocon[ius Saxa Fidus, v. c., procos. prov. Africae dedicavit—]o.

NOTES: This inscription from the architrave of the Antonine Baths is in three fragments (no. 42 was carved below it); the text presented here is that restored in *AE.* The inscription records the local council's construction of baths, along with all their finery (hence the reference to Numidian marble, possibly for columns). For Voconius, see *RE* Suppl. 9.1834–35, s.v. "Voconius 14" (Hanslik); Thomasson, 1.382 (no. 92). The final *o* of the text may have belonged to such a phrase as *epulo dato,* indicating some extra benefaction made to comemmorate these enormous baths, the biggest outside Rome itself: see A. Lézine, *Les thermes d'Antonin à Carthage* (Tunis, 1969); Manderscheid, 94–95, s.v. "Carthago (Carthage), Thermes d'Antonin"; Nielsen, 2.27 (C.209); Yegül, 192–96. The same benefaction may be commemorated in a more fragmentary inscription (no. 231), which, if correctly restored, mentions construction *[e]x permissu* of the emperor and "water that will be of great use to the baths" *([aquam magno u]sui futuram thermis).*

87   P. Lucilius Gamala, aed(ilis), decurio, IIvir. Ostia (Regio I). M. Aurelius (?). *CIL* 14.376.

A lengthy text, thirty lines long, honors Lucilius Gamala. Only the opening and bath-related lines are pertinent.

P. Lucilio P. [f.] | P. n. P. pro n. Gamala[e] | aed., sacr. Volcáni, | eiusdem pr. tert., dec.| adléctó d. d. infanti, | IIvir(o), praéfectó L. Caesar. | Aug. f., cens. q. a., pontif. | tabulár. et librorum, | curátori primo constitu[t.| . . . *(eight lines skipped)* | (18) idem thermas quas divus Pius aedif[i]|caverat vi ignis consumptas refecit | porticum reparavit . . .

NOTES: Nielsen appears confused about the attribution of this text and cites it in connection with both the Forum Baths and the Neptune Baths; see Nielsen, 2.5 (C.24) and 2.6 (C.27). The Forum Baths, however, appear to have been the work of M. Gavius Maximus, praetorian prefect under Antoninus Pius (see no. 22). The Lucilii Gamalae played a leading role in Ostia's public life for six generations; all bear the praenomen *Publius* (see Meiggs, 493–502). The family's prominence is clearly reflected in the enrollment of Gamala among the decurions while still an infant (lines 4–5). Although the findspot is not adequately recorded, the Baths of Neptune at Ostia are in all likelihood the facility in question: their main rooms and portico feature repair work dated by brickstamps to the reign of M. Aurelius; see also no. 6 and notes.

Q. Avelius Priscus Severius Severus Annavus Rufus, flamen divi Aug(usti), patronus   88†
municipi, IIIIvir quinq(uennalis). Corfinium (Regio IV). 180 or later. *AE* 1961.109 =
SuppItal 3 (1987): 144–45 (no. 8).

Q. Avelio Q. f. Serg(ia) Prisco | Severio Severo Annavo Rufo, flamini divi | Augusti,
patrono municipii, | primo omnium Corfiniensium quaestori reipublicae, | IIIIvir.
aedili, IIIIvir. i. d., IIIIvir quinq., pontif. Laurenti(um) Lavinati(um); | hic ob honorem
quinq(uennalitatis) munus gladiatorium edidit, et ob | honorem IIIIvir(atus) ludos
scaenicos dedit, et ob honor(em) aedilitat(is) ludos deae Vetidinae | fecit, et in sub-
sidium annonae frument(ariae) HS L m(ilia) n(ummum) reip(ublicae) Corfiniens(ium)
et balineum Avelianum | muliebre cum HS XXX m(ilia) n(ummum) donavit, frequen-
terque epulationes et divisiones nummar(ias) | universis civibus ex suo distribuit, et
onera rei p(ublicae) gratuita pecunia saepius iuvit. Corfinienses publice ob insignem |
eius erga rem publicam adfectum. | Avelius Priscus honore usus inpens(am) remisit.

Trans.: "To Q. Avelius Priscus Severius Severus Annavus Rufus, son of Quintus, of the
voting tribe Sergia, priest of the deified Augustus, patron of the town, the first ever
quaestor at Corfinium, *quattuorvir* aedile, *quattuorvir* for administering the law,
quattuorvir with censorial powers, *pontifex* of Laurentum and Lavinium. This man,
on account of the honor of the quinquennalate, gave gladiatorial games; and on
account of the honor of the quattuorvirate, he gave theatrical games; and on account
of the honor of the aedileship, he gave games for the goddess Vetidina; and toward the
subsidizing of the grain dole, he gave fifty thousand sesterces to the town of Corfinium; he also gave the women's Avelian Bath, along with thirty thousand sesterces.
At his own expense he frequently gave public banquets and distributed cash handouts
to the entire citizen body of Corfinium, and he very often helped the public expenses
with donations. The people of Corfinium (made this monument) at public expense on
account of his outstanding affection toward the town. Avelius Priscus, while in office,
remitted the expense (of this monument)."

NOTES: For a photograph of the stone, see fig. 26B. The precise nature of the bath benefaction
is not immediately clear, but it probably records the construction of a bath; both *SuppItal* (3
[1987]: 145) and Nielsen (1.40 n. 25) opt for the constructional imputation of *donavit* here. The
sense, however, could just as easily be that Avelius gave an existing structure over to public
ownership. The name of the bath is not particularly helpful in deciding which benefaction is
more likely, since an existing structure that became public property would retain the benefactor's name after the transaction. The accompanying gift of money was no doubt to fund
maintenance and upkeep; see nos. 242–47.

Respublica [C]uicu[litan(orum)]. Cuicul, Numidia. 183/84. *AE* 1920.16 = *AE*   89
1935.45.

[imp. Caes. M. Aur]elio [Commodo | Antonino Augusto Pio S]arm(atico), Ger-
man(ico) M[axi]mo, ponif(ici) max(imo), | [trib. pot. VIII *or* IX, imp. VI *or* VII], cos.
IIII, p(atri) p(atriae), divi M. Antonini Pii Germ(anici) | [Sarm. f]il(io), div[i P]ii nep.,
divi Hadriani pronep(os), divi Traiani | [Part]hici abnep., divi Nervae adnep. re-
spublica | [C]uicu[litan(orum) the]rmas a solo fecit dedicante | [M. Valerio Max-
imi]ano, leg. Aug. pr. pr.

NOTES: The text cited is that of *AE* 1935, restored with reference to a different version of the
same inscription (*AE* 1920). The latter version also adds the detail that Valerius Maximianus
was *patronus col(oniae)*. For Valerius, see *RE* 8A.86–90, s.v. "Valerius 236" (von Lunzer);

Thomasson, 1.401 (no. 49). For the remains, see Manderscheid, 103, s.v. "Cuicul, Grands thermes du Sud"; Nielsen, 2.29 (C.229); Yegül, 201–2.

90   [—] Rusonianus, fl[amen], augur, IIvir q(uin)q(uennalis). Lepcis Magna, Tripolitania. Commodus. *IRT* 396 (see *AE* 1991.1619).

[—imp. Caes. L. Septimi S]eve[ri Pii Pertinacis Aug., Arabici, A]diaben[ici, Par]thici maximi, [pontificis max]imi, [tribunici]ae potes[tati]s X[. .], imp[eratoris?, cos.?, p.] p., et i[mp.] | [Caes. M. Aurelii Antonini [—] et I]uliae [Augu]stae, [matris Augusti et cas]tror[um, totiusque] divinae domus | [—] Rusonianus fl[am.,] augur, IIvir q(uin)q(uennalis), cellam f[rigi]darii et [c]ryl[ptam?] *or* [apodyte]r⟨i⟩[um?] rui[na con]labsas [e]x pollicitatione m[un]eris gladiato[ri o]b honorem | [quinquennalita]tis p[..7..] permissu sacratiss[imi pr]incipis divi M. Antonin[i f.] a fundamentis | [—] marmoribus et co[l]umnis exornavit, stat[u]am Aesculapii novam | [—res]tituit, ceter[as] refe[c]it, ex [multi]is aliis [m]une[ribu]s rei p(ublicae) suae conlatis et | *(the last line is very fragmentary).*

NOTES: This inscription was found in the *frigidarium* of the Hadrianic Baths. Another dedication to Severus from this same room is also known; see *AE* 1925.104 = *IRT* 393. The text is dated by the imperial nomenclature and titles in lines 1–2. These lines, however, originally contained the names and titles of Commodus, to whom a reference survives in line 5. The main body of the text (lines 3–8) is carved in a finer style than the recarved opening lines, which are in the rustic style. All this indicates that the benefaction here commemorated originally took place in the second century; the inscription was then "updated" to make it politically current—which is understandable, since Severus was a native son of Lepcis. On the basis of the imperial titles, Wesch-Klein (121–23 [no. 18]) suggests that the baths were imperially owned, but the titles alone do not offer a firm basis for such a conclusion (compare, e.g., no. 86). Note that Rusonianus had promised games for the quinquennalate but diverted the funds to the bath restoration instead. For recent discussions of the inscriptions of this building and their relationship to the physical remains, see J.C. Fant, "*IRT* 794b and the Building History of the Hadrianic Baths at Lepcis Magna," *ZPE* 75 (1988): 291–94; Thomas and Witschel, "Constructing Reconstruction," 162–63; G. di Vita-Évrard, "Lepcis Magna: Contribution à la terminologie des thermes," in *Thermes*, 35–42. For another inscription from these baths, and their physical remains, see no. 119; see no. 19 and notes.

91   [. .] Dastidius Celer, pro honore ae[d(ilitatis)], [C.] Dastidius Apollonaris, pater, pro honor[e] flamoni. Lanuvium (Regio I). Antonine (?). *CIL* 14.2115 = *ILS* 6198.

[. .] Dastidius C. f. Celer, pro honore ae[d.], | [C.] Dastidius Sp. f. Apollonaris, pater, pro honor[e] | flamoni, HS *(15,000)* | in refectionem balinei intulerunt.

NOTES: The date given for the inscription is that assigned by Nielsen (1.41 n. 26); Duncan-Jones (*Economy,* 161 [no. 479]) dates it to pre-200.

92   Ti. Gavillius Claud(ius) Lambicus, aed(ilis), IIvir. Albona, Dalmatia. 193 (?). *CIL* 3.3047.

Nimphis | Aug. sacr. | ex voto sus|cepto pro sa|lute municip(i) | balineo effect(o) | Ti. Gavillius C. f. | Claud(ius) Lambicus, | aed(ilis), IIvir posuit.

NOTES: The inscription is dated by Nielsen (1.97 n. 12) to 193 without explanation. It is clear that Gavillius completed the bath as part of his vow.

93   Municipium Aelii Chobae. Choba, Mauretania. 196. *CIL* 8.8375 = *ILS* 6876.

imp. Caes. L. Septimio Severo Pio | Pertinace Aug. balneae municipum | municipii Aelii Chobae p(ecunia) p(ublica) factae, | dedicantibus L. Aiedio M. fil. Quir. | Victore, M. Aemili[o . .] Arn. Hono|rato IIviris, a. [pr.] CLVII.

NOTES: Since the findspot of this text was not well recorded, it cannot be tied to the known ruins of baths at Choba, for which see Manderscheid, 98–99, s.v. "Choba (Ziama)."

[C]oloni[a] Augusta Hippo Regius. Hippo Regius, Africa. 198/99. *AE* 1958.141 and   94
1958.142.

141: [C]oloni[a] | Augusta | Hippo | Regius | restituit | felic(iter).

142: L. Septimii [Sev]eri Pii Pertinacis Aug. | [fel]icissimo principi iuventutis splendidis[sima]|m anno procos L. Cossoni [Eg]gi Marulli, c. v., | [O]rfito, c. v., leg. et filio eius *(the rest is missing)*.

NOTES: These two stones were found in the South Baths at Hippo Regius, so the word *thermae* is to be understood. The editors of *AE* link the two entries, which provides a date of 198 for the restoration. For the proconsul L. Cossonius Eggius Marullus, consul in 184, see *PIR*² E 10; Thomasson, 1.385 (no. 115). For the remains, see Manderscheid, 56 s.v. "Annaba, Thermes du Sud"; Nielsen, 2.29 (C.231).

M. Aurelius Sabinianus Euhodus, Augg(ustorum) lib(ertus), patronus civitatis,   95†
decurialis decuriae lictoriae popularis denuntiatorum, decemviralis. Anagnia (Regio I). Late second century. *CIL* 10.5917 = *ILS* 1909.

Euhodi. | M. Aurel. Sabiniano, | Augg(ustorum) lib(erto), patrono | civitatis Anagninor(um) | itemq(ue) collegi cap(u)lato|rum, decuriali decuriae | lictoriae popularis denuntiatorum | itemq(ue) gerulor(um), sed et decemviralis, | s(enatus) p(opulus)q(ue) A(nagninorum) erga amorem patriae | et civium, quod thermas longa incuria | neglectas sua pecunia restituerit, | statuam ex leg(atis) suis ponend(am) censuer(unt); | ob cuius dedic(ationem) dedit decur(ionibus) *(denarios)* V, sexv(iris) | *(denarios)* II, pop(ulo) *(denarios)* I, et epul(um) suffic(iens).

Trans.: "(Statue) of Euhodus. To M. Aurelius Sabinianus, freedman of the emperors, patron of the town of Anagnia and also of the college of *capulatores,* member of the club of *lictores populares* of announcers and likewise of porters, and also *decemvir* (for judging lawsuits). On account of his affection for his hometown and its citizens, because he restored at his own expense the baths that had been neglected through prolonged indifference, the senate and people of Anagnia decreed that a statue be set up to him in accordance with (the advice of?) his *legati.* On the occasion of the statue's dedication, he gave five denarii to each of the decurions, two to each of the *seviri,* and one to each of the people, and a public banquet sufficient for all."

NOTES: For a photograph of this stone, see fig. 26C. The date is suggested by the form of Euhodus' name: he was an imperial freedman who had been manumitted by emperors with the name *Aurelius,* one in particular with the praenomen *Marcus.* The names given point to a manumission under M. Aurelius and L. Verus, a date accepted by Nielsen (1.41 n. 26) and Duthoy ("Profil social," 139 [no. 61]). The involvement of his daughter Marcia with Commodus confirms this interpretation (see no. 179). For *decuriae* of *apparitores,* see N. Purcell, "The *Apparitores:* A Study in Social Mobility," *BSR* 51 (1983): 128–31; *RE* 4.2316–18, s.v. "decuria" (Kübler); ibid., 4.2318–19, s.v. "decurialis" (Schulten). *Legati* were mediators in the cooptation of a *patronus;* see J. Nicols, "*Tabulae Patronatus:* A Study of the Agreement between

Patron and Client-Community," *ANRW* 2.13 (1980): 545–47. Remains of these baths were once known at Anagnia, but they have since completely disappeared; see Coarelli, *Lazio*, 180.

96† Local council and sevirales. Cures Sabini (Regio IV). Late second century (?). *CIL* 9.4978 = *ILS* 5670.

decreto centumvir[um | b]alneum refectum cu[ra | . .] Valeri Cerialis, IIIIvir., pe[c(unia) | pu]blica et ex HS ternis milli[bus | q]uae contulerunt sevirales ii quo[rum | no]mina infra scripta sunt: | *(five fragmentary names follow).*

Trans.: "By decree of the *centumviri* the bath was restored under the care of [?] Valerius Cerialis, *quattuorvir,* with public money and from the contributions of three thousand sesterces from each of those *sevirales* whose names are written below . . . "

NOTES: Nielsen (1.41 n. 26) includes this text among her second-century material. Duncan-Jones (*Economy,* 152; see 161 [no. 478]), who dates the inscription to "pre-200," suggests that the contributions may have been *summae honorariae,* because each *sevir* gave three thousand sesterces. If so, this text commemorates a single official action of the local authorities, funded from different sources. Remains of baths, dated to the Hadrianic period, are known at Cures and may be identified with the building mentioned here: see Coarelli, *Lazio,* 33; Manderscheid, 103, s.v. "Cures Sabini."

97 L. Ju[lius] Equester, IIvir, flam(en) Rom(ae) et Aug(usti), et Lucii Julii Equestris filii Cimber et Equester, flam(ines) Rom(ae) et Aug(usti). Aquae Neri, Aquitania. Second century. *CIL* 13.1376 and 1377.

Two fragmentary texts commemorate the same benefaction. I present here the re-stored composite suggested in *CIL.*

[nu]uminib(us) Aug. et Nerio deo usibusq. r(ei) p(ublicae) B[it(urigum) Cub(orum) et Vic(anorum) Ner(iomagensium)? | L. Iulius Equestr?]is fil. Equester, IIvir II, flam(en) Rom(ae) et Aug(usti) itemque flamen p[rovinc(iae) Aqu(itanicae?) | et] Lucii Iulii Equestris filii Cimber et Equester, flamin[es Rom(ae) et Aug(usti), | diribitoria, t]ab-ernas, porticus, quibus fontes Nerii et thermae p[ublicae? cinguntur, | cu]m omnibus suis ornamentis ob hono[r(em)] flam[o]ni c[onsummaverunt] *or* o[btulerunt].

NOTES: A third fragment from the baths (*CIL* 13.1378) also mentions Equester, but it is too brief to be comprehensible. The town of Aquae Neri had, as its name suggests, springs sacred to the god Nerius. However, assuming that *thermae p[—]* is correctly restored as *thermae p[ublicae],* the wording clearly differentiates the springs from the public baths. The sense of the inscription would seem to demand that as porticoes surround both the baths and springs, the two were separate parts of a single complex, a phenomenon known from other thermal sites (see above, chapter 2, n. 75). The remains of these baths, the Thermes Sud, were unearthed in 1819 but unfortunately covered over by the nineteenth-century spa establishment. Reconstructions from drawings suggest a building with bathing wings and thermally fed *piscinae:* see M. Desnoyers, "Néris-les-bains (Allier): Ville thermale gallo-romaine," in Pelletier, *Médecine en Gaule,* 42–49; Manderscheid, 153–54, s.v. "Néris-les-Bains, Thermes Sud."

98† L. Julius Julianus, patronus municipi. Ocriculum (Regio VI). Second century (?). *CIL* 11.4090.

Iuliae Luciliae, | L. Iuli Iuliani fil., | patron[i] municipi, | cuius pater | thermas Ocricola|nis a solo extructas | sua pecunia dona|vit. | decur(iones), Aug(ustales), pleps | l(ibentes) d(ono) d(ederunt).

Trans.: "The decurions, Augustales, and plebs willingly gave (this monument) as a gift to Julia Lucilia, daughter of L. Julius Julianus, patron of the city. Her father built the baths at his own expense from the ground up and donated them to the people of Ocriculum."

NOTES: This inscription was found in the baths and is dated by letterform; see C. Pietrangeli, *Ocriculum* (Rome, 1943), 67. Nielsen (1.40 n. 25), accordingly, includes this text among her second-century material. In contrast, Gaggiotti et al. (*Umbria*, 24) prefer an Augustan date for Julianus. The remains of this bath, as described by Gaggiotti et al. (loc. cit.) and Pietrangeli (op. cit., 69–71; *Otricoli*, 64–75), are most unusual for an Augustan structure, insofar as they feature an octagonal room roofed with a dome. Unless detailed investigation of the remains suggest an Augustan construction date, the second-century attribution should stand. The wording is somewhat unclear: did Julianus build the baths, or did his father (i.e., Julia Lucilia's grandfather) do so? All in all, it seems likely that the *patronus municipi* carried out the work. Other texts from Ocriculum referring to members of this family show that it was prominent in the town for at least two generations: our benefactor (L. Julius Julianus) is reported to have had an extensive local career (*CIL* 11.4087) and is commemorated again as *patronus municipi* in *CIL* 11.4088; another relative, L. Julius Lucilianus, possibly Julianus' brother or son, is honored as *patronus municipi* in *CIL* 11.4089; and the daughter, Julia Lucilia, is honored in the present inscription, although apparently by genealogical proxy, since she is not expressly credited with any benefactions. On the local prosopography, see Pietrangeli, *Ocriculum*, 33–36. On the remains of baths at Ocriculum, see the notes to no. 124.

C. Torasius Severus, IIIIvir i(ure) d(icundo), augur. Spoletium (Regio VI). Second century (?). *CIL* 11.4815 = *ILS* 6638.   99†

C. Torasius C. f. Hor. Severus, IIIIvir i. d., | augur, suo et P. Mecloni Proculi Torasiani, pontif(icis), | fili sui, nomine, loco et pecunia sua fecit. idem | ad celebrandum natalem fili sui in publicum dedit HS *(250,000)* | ex quorum reditu III k. Sept. omnibus annis decuriones in publico | cenarent et municipes praesentes acciperent aeris octonos; item | dedit VIviris Aug(ustalibus) et Compit(alium) Larum Aug(usti) et mag(istris) vicorum HS *(120,000)* ut ex reditu | eius summae eodem die in publico vescerentur. | hunc ob merita eius | erga rem publicam ordo decurionum patronum municipi adoptavit.

Trans.: "C. Torasius Severus, son of Gaius, of the voting tribe Horatia, *quattuorvir* for administering the law, augur, in his own name and in that of his son P. Meclonius Proculus Torasianus, priest, built (the baths) at his own expense and on his own land. He also gave 250,000 sesterces into the public purse for the celebration of his son's birthday, in order that from the return on this money, on 30 August every year, the councillors might dine in public and the citizens of the town who are present might receive eight asses each. He also gave 120,000 sesterces to the priests of the Lares Compitales and Augustus and to the masters of the neighborhoods, in order that they might dine in public on the same day, funded by the return on this sum. The *ordo* of councillors, on account of his services to the city, adopted him as patron of the town."

NOTES: Nielsen (1.40 n. 25) dates this inscription to the second century. Fragmentary remains at Spoletium, tentatively dated to the second century, have been identified with these baths, but the case is more hypothetical than certain: see L. di Marco, *Spoletium: Topografia e urbanistica* (Spoleto, 1975), 62–63; Gaggiotti et al., *Umbria*, 113; C. Pietrangeli, *Spoletium* (Rome, 1939), 64–66. (Both Di Marco and Pietrangeli date this inscription by letterform.) The inscription was found among the remains of the baths, so the word *thermae* has been omitted. Cassiodorus (*Var.* 4.24) mentions the *Thermae Turasii* at Spoletium, and they are probably also the subject of the repair work carried out by Constantius and Julian that is recorded in another text; see no. 16. *Lares Augusti et Compitales* and the *magistri vicorum* were elements in local neighborhood identity in Roman towns; see Laurence, 38–42.

100   Incertus, flamen. Ager Pictonum, Aquitania. Second century (?). *CIL* 13.1169.

[—Lugu]dun[i—orna]lmenti[s] o[rnatus], | flámen [—] | balineum [cum suis orna-mentis de] | s[u]o [restituit].

NOTES: This inscription is dated by letterform. The text is fragmentary, but a *flamen,* appearing in the nominative, was clearly the benefactor. Possible mention of *[orna]menta* (it could also be *[funda]menta*) at the start of line 2 suggests at least a decoration, if not a restoration.

101†   C. Auf(idius) Vegetus, IIvir II, curat(or). Burgvillos, Baetica. Second century (?). *CIL* 2.5354 = *ILER* 2050.

in hon(orem) dom(us) divinae. | G. Auf. G. f. Gal. Vegetus | IIvir II, curat(or), bal-ineu(m) | aedifi(cavit) et G. Auf. G. f. G[al.] | Avitus f., IIvir desig(natus), | d(e) s(ua) p(ecunia) d(edit) | et editis circiens(ibus) [ded(icavit)].

Trans.: "In honor of the divine household. G. Aufidius Vegetus, son of Gaius, of the voting tribe Galeria, *duovir* twice, curator, built the bathhouse, and G. Aufidius Avitus, son of Gaius, of the voting tribe Galeria, his son, *duovir* designate, gave it at his own expense and dedicated it with the staging of circus games."

NOTES: The date is by letterform. Nielsen (1.65 n. 9) cites the date without qualification; Curchin (166 [no. 298]) assigns it to the "middle or late second century." On the stone, the last letters of line 4 are *G. f. G. M.* which is a stonecutting error, since it makes no sense. In all likelihood, the *M.* should be taken either as "AL" of "GAL." (the voting tribe of father and son) or "N." of "N[EPOS]," ("grandson of G(aius)"). There is no indication if any time elapsed between the construction and the "giving" of the baths; on the latter benefaction, see no. 212. It is therefore to be considered a single joint benefaction; compare the wording of no. 182.

102†   Senat(us) populusq(ue) Lanivinus. Lanuvium (Regio I). 198/211. *CIL* 14.2101 = *ILS* 5686.

imp. Caes. L. Septimio Severo Pio Pertinaci Aug. et imp. Caes. M. Aurelio Antonino Pio Felici Aug. | senat. populusq. Lanivinus | in locum balnearum, quae per vet-ustatem in usu esse desierant, thermas ex quantitatibus, quae | ex indulgentia dominorum | nn. principum honorariarum summarum sacerdotiorum adquisitae sunt, item ex usuris | C kalendari, ampliatis locis et cellis, a fundamentis exstruxit et dedicavit.

Trans.: "To Imperator Caesar L. Septimius Severus Pius Pertinax Augustus and Im-perator Caesar M. Aurelius Antoninus, *pius, felix,* Augustus. The senate and the people of Lanuvium, in place of the *balneae,* which through old age had ceased to be used, built from the foundations and dedicated *thermae,* with an extended area and enlarged rooms, from those sums that, by the indulgence of our masters the emperors, were acquired as *summae honorariae* for the priesthoods, and also from the interest of one-hundredth (part) per month."

NOTES: This inscription is the only one in the sample that expressly states that *summae honorariae* were used to build baths, although Pliny the Younger (*Ep.* 10.39.5) reports that the cost of the huge baths at Claudiopolis in Bithynia was to come from this very source, also granted to the city by the emperor. For the use of *summae honorariae* in local building activities, see Duncan-Jones, *Economy,* 86–87 and 147–55; id., "Who Paid?" 28–33, updated and expanded in Duncan-Jones, *Structure,* 174–84, esp. 182–83. Here the "indulgence" of the emperors consisted of allowing either the amount of existing *summae* to be raised or (as at Claudiopolis) more offices to be created, in order to cover, in part, the cost of the bath project.

M. Sattonius Ju[cun]dus, dec(urio) c(oloniae) U(lpiae) T(raianae). Coriovallum, Germania Inferior. Ca. 200 (?). *AE* 1959.9.   **103**

Fortunae [Reduci]. | M. Sattonius Iu[cun]ldus, dec(urio) c(oloniae) U(lpiae) T(raianae), bali[neo] | resstitut(o) *(sic)* v(otum) s(olvit) l(ibens) m(erito).

NOTES: The restoration is dated by Nielsen variously to ca. 200 (1.75 n. 7) or ca. 250 (2.21 [C.154]). Note that a decurion of the nearby Colonia Ulpia Trajana (Xanten) here restores the baths at Coriovallum (Heerlen), suggesting that he had property in the region of the smaller town. For the remains of these baths, originally constructed in the mid–first century, see Manderscheid, 120, s.v. "Heerlen/Coriovallum"; Nielsen, 2.21 (C.154).

L. Patric(ius) Martialis et L. Partric(ius) Marcus Ling(ones), fratr(es), omnib(us) offic(iis) civilib(us) . . . functi. Vertillium, Germania Superior. Second or third century (?). *CIL* 13.5661.   **104**

i(n) h(onorem) d(omus) d(ivinae). L. Patric(ius) Martialis et L. Patric(ius) Marcus | Ling(ones), fratr(es), omnib(us) offic(iis) civili(bus) in civiltate sua funct(i), cellam vestibulam e regiolne columnae cum suis omnib(us) commod(is) | d(e) s(ua) p(ecunia) Vikan(is) Vertillensib(us) largiti sunt.

NOTES: Ruins of baths dating to the second century are known at the site: see Manderscheid, 222, s.v. "Vertault/Vertillium"; Nielsen, 2.14 (C.96). Since they were destroyed by the end of the third century, this text (which probably refers to the building) must date to a prior period. The formula *omnibus honoribus functo* appears only after 120, at least in Spain and probably also in the western provinces in general: see Curchin, 39 (for Spain); L. Wierschowski, "AE 1980, 615 und das erste Auftreten der Formel 'omnibus honoribus in colonia sua functus' in den westlichen Provinzen," *ZPE* 64 (1986): 287–94 (for the western provinces).

Res p(ublica) muni[cipi Sigensium]. Siga, Mauretania. 211/17. *AE* 1934.80.   **105†**

pro salute d. [n. imp. Caes.] | M. Aureli Anto[nini, p(ii), f(elicis), Aug.] | thermas An[toninianas] | res p(ublica) muni[cipi Sigensium] | devot[a numini maiestatique eius—].

Trans.: "On behalf of the safety of our lord, Imperator Caesar M. Aurelius Antoninus, *pius, felix,* Augustus. The town of Siga, faithful to his spirit and majesty, [built *and/or* dedicated] the Antonine Baths."

NOTES: The date is that provided by Nielsen (1.85 n. 9). In all likelihood, this inscription records the construction of these baths and their dedication to Caracalla, although it cannot be ruled out that an existing structure was here being rededicated in honor of the ruling monarch; compare no. 90.

T. Sennius Sollemnis, IIvir, [o]mnib(us) honorib(us) [et] munerib(us) . . . [functus]. Viducasses, Gallia Lugdunensis. Ca. 220/40. *CIL* 13.3162.I = *ILTG* 341.   **106†**

This statue base is carved on three sides. The main text on the front, cited below, records the benefactions of Sollemnis; two letters of praise from imperial officals (not cited below) occupy the side panels. Unfortunately, the front face, on which the pertinent text is carved, is the most damaged. Only the opening lines and the bath-related lines, themselves fragmentary, are cited here.

T. Sennio Sollemni Sollem|nini fil., IIvir. sine sorte quater, aug(uri), | [o]mnib(us) honorib(us) [et] mun[eribusq(ue)] VII [functo] . . . *(six lines skipped)* | (10) [bal]neum quod [pop]u[lar]ibus coloniae s[uae] | pr[ofut]urum S[ollemninus—put?]ribus | funda[me]ntis inst[itutis reli]querat | consumm[av]it, [item legavit] fructum unde in perpetuum instauraretur.

Trans.: "To T. Sennius Sollemnis, son of Sollemninus, *duovir* four times without drawing lots, augur, a man who held all seven of the municipal offices . . . The bath, which was to be a benefit to the people of his colony, and which Sollemninus had abandoned since the foundations were improperly laid, Sollemnis completed; and he bequeathed in his will a trust from which the baths might be repaired in perpetuity."

NOTES: Mommsen offered the following reconstruction of the missing section following *pr[ofut]urum: S[ollemninus coeptis ope]ribus, funda[me]ntis in[stitutis inch]o[a]verat* [Sollem-ninus had begun the baths, with initial work and the laying of foundations]. However, this textual restoration is not at all sure, since the stone is heavily mutilated. At line 15 Sollemnis is said to be an *amicus* and *cliens* of Ti. Claudius Paulinus, *leg. Aug. pr. praet.* (see *PIR*[2] C 955; Thomasson, 1.41 [no. 17]); at line 20 he is identified as a *cliens probatissimus* of M. Aedinius Julianus, who was a successor of Paulinus in the provincial legateship (see *PIR*[2] A 113; Thomasson, 1.41 [no. 18]). *Exempla* of letters from both men are reproduced on the flanks of the stone. These letters date the inscription to the 220s or, possibly, the 230s.

107   Local council. Castellum Mastar, Numidia. 228. *AE* 1908.244.

genio | balineo Cast(elli) | Mas(taris) | o. m. a solo | quartum idibus Decembribus | Modesto et Probo | cos.

NOTES: This text seems to commemorate the construction of baths, especially in view of the phrase *a solo,* perhaps with *facto* understood. Where the erection of baths is recorded in the passive voice with no agent indicated, as here, a construction by the local authority ought to be assumed: compare nos. 49 and 122; Duncan-Jones, *Economy,* 91 (no. 30). The letters *o. m.* remain problematic. They can be variously restored, as *o(b) m(eritam), o(ptimi) m(aximi), o(rdine) m(aximo),* and so on. If they are restored as *o(rdine) m(aximo),* the agents of the benefaction might here be expressed. Given that the place was a *castellum,* these were probably military baths, but not necessarily so: Castellum Mattiacorum in Germania Superior boasted large city baths; see Nielsen, 2.21 (C.160).

108†   M. Tullius Venneianus, IIvir q(uin)q(uennalis), p(atronus) c(oloniae). Paestum (Regio III). Early third century. *AE* 1935.28 = *ILPaest* 100.

M. Tullius Vennelianus, IIvir q(uin)q(uennalis), p(atronus) c(oloniae), balneas | nobas a solo sua pecunia extru|xit et dedicavit. M. Tullius Cice|ro Venneianus filius balneas eas|dem, vi ignis multifaria *(sic)* corruptas, | sua pecunia restituit, curantibus | Tulliis Primigenio et Nedymo et | contutoribus eorum, et incollumes ad usum civium re-ipu|blicae tradidit.

Trans.: "M. Tullius Venneianus, *duovir* with censorial powers, patron of the colony, built from the ground up and dedicated the New Baths at his own expense. After they had been damaged in many places by the violence of a fire, his son, M. Tullius Cicero Venneianus, restored the same baths at his own expense, with Tullius Primigenius and

Tullius Nedymus and their *contutores* overseeing the work. Cicero Venneianus handed the baths over to the use of the city, safe and sound."

NOTES: Duthoy ("Profil social," 151 [nos. 366 and 367]) dates this inscription to the Severan period; Nielsen (1.40 n. 25) and Mello and Voza *(ILPaest)* posit an early third-century date. Tullius Primigenius is securely dated to 245 by the consular titles *imp. Philippo et Titiano* in another inscription *(ILPaest* 102), so the early or middle part of the third century seems an appropriate date for this benefaction. A noteworthy feature of this text is the mention of the *contutores* of the Tullii Primigenius and Nedymus. If taken literally to mean "guardians," it suggests that Primigenius and Nedymus were minors, which seems unlikely. The most plausible explanation is that the term *contutores* refers to the main benefactors, the Marci Tullii Venneiani, and thus carries the sense more of *compatroni* than of "guardians." According to this reading, the Tullii Cicerones also took a hand in overseeing the work. For a discussion of this problem, see *ILPaest,* vol. 1, p. 165. The remains of these baths, adjacent to the forum, are known but ill investigated; see Manderscheid, 166, s.v. "Paestum, Terme di M. Tullio Venneiano." They find no mention in J.G. Pedley, *Paestum: Greeks and Romans in Southern Italy* (New York, 1990).

Tib. Cl. Marcellinus, e(ques) R(omanus), dec(uriarum) III. Viminacium, Moesia Superior. 244/49. *CIL* 3.8113.   109

(the first line is missing) | [pro salute] | Marciae Otacilliae Severae, | sanctissimae Aug. | coniugis d. n. | Phillipi Aug. et | matris Philippi nobilissimi Caes. | et castrorum, | domum suam et baln(eum) | refecit et paravit | Tib. Cl. Marcellinus, eq(ues) R(omanus, dec(uriarum) III e[t ? ..6..] | *(the last three lines are very fragmentary)*.

NOTES: For Marcia Otacilia Severa, wife of Philip the Arab, see *PIR*[2] M 266. The context may imply that the baths were private, attached to a *domus;* compare *CIL* 11.1222 = *ILS* 1554 (near Placentia; Trajan/Hadrian) for a *praetorium cum balineo* built by freedpeople, where *praetorium* means "palace" or "mansion." The appearance of the word *paravit* in this instance may mean that the baths were provided for public use; alternatively, it could indicate that the facility was heated or supplied with water in readiness for use. All in all, it is unusual, but not unprecedented, for a construction of strictly private function to be commemorated in a formal inscription like this one. Despite this uncertainty as to the inscription's context, it is included here. For a comparable restoration of a *domus* and *balineum,* see no. 12, where the bath apparently did serve a public function.

L. Octavius Aur[elianus?] Didasius, c(larissimus) v(ir), pa[tr]onus. Vreu, Africa. Mid- to late third century. *AE* 1975.880.   110†

Didasi | L. Octavio Aur[eliano?] | Didasio, c. v., m[. . .]o | civi genitali, ob [sin]gu[la]|rem in protegendis [civib(us)] | fidem et paratum [er]ga [o]mn[e]s | amorem, thermas [et aquam *or* formam corrup]|tam post diluviem [..10..]|to servato recte (?) [..5..] | propria liberalitate [ex]o[r]navit] | excoluit, perfecit, dedi[c]avit. | benemerito civi et pa[tr]ono [splen]|didissimus ord[o et] populus [Mun(icipii) | V]ruensium statuam [posueru]nt d(ecreto) d(ecreto) [p(ecunia) p(ublica)].

Trans.: "(Statue) of Didasius. To Lucius Octavius Aur[elianus?] Didasius, of senatorial rank [. . .], a native citizen of this town, on account of his singular loyalty in protecting the citizens and his affection displayed toward all. The baths (and their water supply *or* appearance?), which were damaged after the flood [and were restored? . . .], since it was preserved upright (?) [. . .], because of his own generosity, he adorned, beautified, completed, and dedicated. The most eminent *ordo* and the people of the town of Vreu set up this statue to a most deserving patron, following a decree of the decurions and at public expense."

NOTES: The stone is a statue base reused in the Byzantine fort. Although the inscription is badly mutilated, it is clear that Didasius carried out extensive restoration work on the baths.

111   [Municipium S]eptimium Aurelium Severianum Antoninianum Frugiferum Concordium Liberum Thibursicensium Bure and several decurions. Thibursicum Bure, Africa. 260/68. *AE* 1913.180 = *ILAfr* 506.

(four lines have been erased) [Municipium S]eptimium Aurelium Severianum Antoninianum Frugiferum Concordium Liberum Thibursicensium Bure thermas Gal[lienianas | r]eformatas et excultas pecunia publica perfecit et dedicavit. proconsule L. Naevio Aquilino, c. v., patrono municipi, dedica[ntibus] | Naevio Balbino Aquilino, leg(ato) Karthag(inis), cc. vv., patronis pub(licis) ad cuius operis musaeum pleriq(ue) decuriones HS XLI mil. C.C. (i.e., *41,200*) conl[atis—].

NOTES: The erased opening lines contained the titles of Gallienus and of Salonina and Saloninus, his wife and son, respectively. L. Naevius Aquilinus was proconsul of Africa in 260/68, and Naevius Balbinus Aquilinus may have been his son: see *PLRE* 1.91–92, s.v. "Aquilinus 5 and 6"; Thomasson, 1.388 (no. 143). Both men were *patroni municipii*. The reference to restoration *(reformatas)* is at first glance surprising, in that it is unlikely for baths built under Gallienus to have needed restoration during his reign. Thus, these are either earlier baths that were renamed on restoration (a common practice; see Thomas and Witschel, "Constructing Reconstruction," 146) or baths that were completed on a different plan than originally conceived (i.e., *reformatas . . . perfecit* = "completed on an altered plan"). The addition of the *musaeum* is here recorded as the work of several decurions, whose names probably followed in the lost last lines of the text. Their joint contribution was probably made *ob honorem* or as a *summa honoraria;* if so, this benefaction is a single one by the local authorities, funded from different sources (compare no. 96). See also Wesch-Klein, 211–12 (no. 5).

112†   Res [p(ublica)]. Caesena (Regio VIII). Probus or Carus. *CIL* 11.556 = *ILS* 5687.

balneum Aurelianum ex liberalitate | imp. Caes. M. Aureli Pii Fel. Aug., | servata indulgentia pecuniae eius, | quam deus Aurelianus concesserat, | facta usurarum exactione | curante Statio Iuliano, v. e., curatore, | res [p(ublica)] refecit.

Trans.: "The city rebuilt the Bath of Aurelian, out of the generosity of the emperor Caesar Marcus Aurelius, *pius, felix,* Augustus. The indulgence was observed from that money that the god Aurelian had granted, after a requisition of interests was made. Statius Julianus, of equestrian rank, curator, saw to the work."

NOTES: This text is interesting for the detailed financial information it provides about how the state funded this project, even if the arrangements are more than a little unclear: Did Aurelian grant an indulgence—possibly a remission of taxes—specifically for the erection of the bath or for general public purposes? Has a figure for the amount of interest requisitioned dropped out of the text at line 5? For discussion, see G. Poma, "Osservazioni su *CIL*, XI, 556: *Liberalitates* imperiali nei confronti di *Caesena*," *AttiBol* 29–30 (1990): 29–34. A similar situation apparently pertained at Lanuvium under Caracalla. Here the town built *thermae* to replace disused *balneae,* "from those sums that, by the indulgence of our masters the emperors, were acquired as *summae honorariae* for the priesthoods" (no. 102); this latter *indulgentia* appears to have been specifically for the bath-replacement project. Statius Julianus was most likely a *curator rei publicae* (of equestrian rank), seeing to it that the imperial generosity was not abused by the local authorities: see Camodeca, "Ricerche," 518–19, s.v. "Caesena 1"; *PLRE* 1.480, s.v.

"Julianus 39." The physical remains of these baths have yet to be subjected to close study: see Mangani, Rebecchi, and Strazzulla, *Emilia,* 29–32; G.A. Mansuelli, *Caesena, Forum Popili, Forum Livi* (Rome, 1948), 59–60.

Local council. Thagora, Numidia. 290/94. *CIL* 8.4645 = *ILS* 5714 = *ILAlg* 1.1032.   113†

pro salute dd. nn. Diocletiani et Maximiani Aug. | cella unctuaria, quae per seriem annorum in usu non fuisset, saeculo | eorum restituta et dedicata est Aurel. Aristobulo procos., c. v, Macrinio Sossiano, l[eg.,] c. v.

Trans.: "For the safety of our masters Diocletian and Maximian, Augusti. The *cella unctuaria,* which for a length of years had not been in use, was restored and dedicated in their reign, when Aurelius Aristobulus, of senatorial rank, was proconsul and Macrinius Sossianus, of senatorial rank, was legate."

NOTES: For the proconsul Ti. Claudius Aurelius Aristobulus, see *PIR*[2] C 806; *PLRE* 1.106, s.v. "Aristobulus." For Sossianus, see *PLRE* 1.849, s.v. "Sossianus 2." The *cella unctuaria* seems to have been an oiling room, probably associated with the palaestra.

Q. Vetulenius Urbanus Herennianus, fl(amen) p(er)p(etuus), curator r(ei) p(ublicae),   114† cum Magnilio filio suo, florentissimo adq(ue) prudentissimo adulescenti. Turca, Africa. Late third century. *CIL* 8.828 = *ILS* 5713.

Magnílianorum. | Q. Vetulenius Urbanus Herennianus, | fl(amen) p(er)p(etuus), curator r(ei) p(ublicae), apodyterium novum | in dextera cellis exeuntibus | a solo constructum et scalas [n]ova[s], | cetera restaurata adq(ue) statuis | marmoribus, tabulis pictis, | columnis ingressu cellarum, | alisq(ue) reb(us) ornata, sumptu proprio | cum Magniliano filio suo, florentissimo adq(ue) prudentissimo | adulescenti, voto | omnium [ci]viu[m] | perfecit adq(ue) dedicavit et univer|se plevi *(sic)* epulum per tridum dedit nec | non et ludos scenicos exibuit *(sic)*.

Trans.: "(Statues) of the Magniliani. Q. Vetulenius Urbanus Herennianus, priest for life, curator of the city, constructed from the ground up the new *apodyterium*—on the right as one leaves the bathing rooms—and the new steps as well; he restored the rest of the rooms and adorned them with marble statues, paintings, columns at the entrance to the rooms, and other forms of decoration. By a vote of the entire citizen body, he completed and dedicated these works at his own expense, along with his son Magnilianus, a most distinguished and fine young man, and he gave a banquet for three days to all the commoners, and he put on theatrical games."

NOTES: The date is that ascribed by Wilmanns (*CIL* 8.828). The reading of lines 5 and 8–9 is unsure. An alternative for line 5 is *a solo constructum piscinas duas* [he constructed from the ground up the *apodyterium,* two pools], and an alternative for lines 8–9 is *columnis [al]v[ib]us cellarum,* | *cathredeb(us) ornata* [he adorned them with columns and pools for the bathing rooms and seats]. Rebuffat ("Vocabulaire thermal," 21–22) believes that the inscription is entirely concerned with the *apodyterium,* but the phrase *cetera restaurata* suggests that a more widespread renovation took place alongside the addition of the new changing room.

Resp(ublica) col(oniae) Thib(ursici) Bure. Thibursicum Bure, Africa. Late third cen-   115† tury or later. *ILS* 5712.

ex avio loco et rupe | iam minanti sta|tuas n(umero) IIII marmoreas | at cultum et splendo|rem apodyteri ther|marum resp(ublica) col(oniae) | Thib(ursici) Bure transtulit, | provisione instantia Aureli Honorat(ini) | Quietani, eq(uitis) R(omani), cur(atoris) | rei p(ublicae).

Trans.: "The authorities of the colony of Thibursicum Bure transferred four marble statues from a remote place—because the cliff was threatening to collapse—for the decoration and splendor of the changing room of the baths; (this was done) through the foresight and insistence of Aurelius Honoratinus Quietanus, Roman *eques,* curator of the city."

NOTES: The date is suggested by Quietanus' position as *curator rei publicae.* He seems to have been a local official (he finds no mention in *PIR²,* *PLRE,* or *RE*). The reading of *iam* in the second line is not secure; the word might be *ruinam.* For similar benefactions, see nos. 27 and 39. The building may be the Thermae of Gallienus mentioned in no. 111.

116　Respubl(ica). Canusium (?) (Regio II). Third century. *AE* 1987.307.

balneum publicum | a Caesidio Proculo refectum | respubl(ica) vetustate quassatum | decur(ionum) decr(eto) atplicito omni cultu | restituit.

NOTES: The date is that assigned by the editors of *AE.* The text was found in the vicinity of Canusium, so it is somewhat unsure if it originally pertained to that city. Two benefactions are recorded here: (1) the restoration by the state, which is the main benefaction being commemorated, and (2) the previous restoration by Caesidius Proculus, apparently a local benefactor (= no. 181). The term *vetustate quassatum* is an interesting variation on the standard *vetustate corruptum/conlapsum/delapsum.* Two baths are known from the center of Canusium near the forum, but the uncertainty over the inscription's provenance makes identification with either risky; see Greco, *Magna Grecia,* 260.

117†　Plautius Lupus, IIvir. Lepcis Magna, Tripolitania. Third century. *IRT* 601b.

[q]uod expostulantibus universis decurio|nibus uti Plautio Lupo, o(ptimo) o(ordinis) n(ostri) vir(o), biga de pub(lico) | collocetur q(uid) d(e) e(a) r(e) f(ieri) p(laceret), c(ensentis) L. Cassi Longini, II|vir(i) desig(nati), q(uid) p(laceret) c(irca) i(d) f(ieri) dec(uriones) i(ta) c(ensuerunt): cum Plautius Lupus, | o(ptimus) o(rdinis) n(ostri) vir, cum flamonium consensu | omnium sibi delatum libenter suscepis|set, opulentissimos ludos ediderit singu(lariter)q(ue) magnificentissima liberalitate pro|meruerit, in IIviratus quoq(ue) honore om|nia secundum splendorem natalium | [s]uorum dignitatemq(ue) col(oniae) n(ostrae) egerit et | [e]ffusissimis adfectibus iterum splen-|didissimos ludos ediderit, nec contentus | his liberalitatibus cellam thermar(um) | marmorib(us) Numidicis et opere musaeo ex|ornavit, omni deinde occasione sin-gul(ariter) | [p]romeruerit et proxime cum ad munus pub(licum) | [e]x testamento Iuni Afri, c(larissimae) m(emoriae) viri, edendum curator el|le[c]tus esset sollicitudini la-boriq(ue) suo non pe|percerit et observata amplissimi senatus voluntate splen-didissime munus edi curaveri[t] | debentque huiusmodi adfectus | remunerari ut reliqui quoque ad eamdem (*sic*) volup|[tat]em sollicitari possint placere Plautio Lupo | o(ptimo) o(rdinis) n(ostri) v(iro) [bi]gam de publ(ico) ubi volet collacari pos|[se, Plau]tius Lupus de suo collocaturum se dixit.

Trans.: "When all of the decurions were urging that a two-horsed chariot be set up at public expense in honor of Plautius Lupus, the best man of our *ordo,* and L. Cassius Longinus, *duovir* designate, moved what action should be resolved in this matter, the decurions thus decreed what action should be resolved concerning this matter: 'Since Plautius Lupus, the best man of our *ordo,* when he had willingly undertaken what was entrusted to him with the unanimous agreement of the priests, gave the most sumptuous games and was particularly deserving of merit due to his most magnificent generosity; since he carried out all his duties while in the office of *duovir* in a manner in keeping with the splendor of his family and the dignity of our colony and, with the most lavish affection, gave very splendid games on a second occasion; since, not satisfied with these bounties, he beautified the *cella thermarum* with Numidian marble and mosaics and was thereafter particularly deserving on every occasion and, recently, when he was chosen as curator to stage the public show bequeathed in the will of the late Junius Afer, of senatorial rank, he did not spare his application and effort and, having abided by the will of the most eminent senate, he saw to the staging of a very splendid show; and diligence of this sort ought to be repayed so others can be stimulated to put on the same entertainment, it was resolved that a two-horse chariot be set up at public expense in honor of Plautius Lupus, the best man of our *ordo*, wherever he wished it to be placed. Plautius Lupus said that he would put it up at his own expense.'"

NOTES: The stone, a statue base carved on three sides, was found in the west side of the Severan harbor and is dated by letterform. (Neither of the inscriptions cited under *IRT* 601 is the dedicatory inscription for the building, as cited by Fant, "*IRT* 794b," 292; for that text, see *IRT* 361.) The above text is from the left-hand face of the stone and is interesting for several reasons. The *cella thermarum* is a room of unclear function (see appendix 3). Note especially the laudatory comment that immediately follows the notice of work on the baths, which seems to imply that Lupus, despite his many honors, was especially respected for having adorned this building in particular. Finally, note the reason for honoring him: to stimulate others to act. It is not clear to which of Lepcis' baths this text refers (see the notes to no. 119). For text and discussion, see Wesch-Klein, 123–25 (no. 21).

M. Sentius Crispinus, decurialib(us) omnibus honer(ibus) functus. Interamna Lirenas   118†
(Regio I). Third century or later (?). *CIL* 10.5348 = *ILS* 5698.

M. Sentio Crispino, | decurialib(us) omnibus honer(ibus) | functo. huic ordo et u|niversus populus ob | merita et labores eius | honorem biselliatus | et ornamenta decurio|natus gratuita obtulerunt, | quod opera thermarum es|tivalium vetustate cor-rup|ta s(ua) p(ecunia) restituit exornavit|que, porticos etiam circum|cingentes col-imbum a solo | constituit, statuam ampli|ficandam memoriam eius | ponendam cen-suerunt. | l(oco) d(ato) d(ecurionum) d(ecreto).

Trans.: "To M. Sentius Crispinus, who held all the decurial offices. To this man the *ordo* and the entire people, on account of his services and efforts, offered the honor of a *bisellium* and the insignia of the decurionate free, because he restored and adorned at his own expense the structures of the summer baths, which were ruined with old age, and because he also built porticoes surrounding the *colimbum* from the ground up. They voted that a statue of him be set up to amplify his memory. Space was given by decree of the decurions."

NOTES: A *bisellium* was an honorific seat, so named because it could accommodate two people. This inscription should be read in conjunction with no. 141, which records a restoration of these baths by another member of the Sentii in 408. Nielsen (1.41 n. 26) opts for a tentative fourth-century date for the present text, and M. Cagiano de Azevedo (*Interamna Lirenas vel Sucasina* [Rome, 1947], 27) and Coarelli (*Lazio*, 215–17) consider the two inscriptions to be contem-poraneous. It is possible that the two texts commemorate different phases of the same construction project, but the present inscription, with its matter-of-fact wording and aspirated spelling of *thermae* (compare *termas* in no. 141) appears to derive from an earlier era; I date it tentatively to as early as the third century. If this earlier date is correct, the Sentii can be seen to maintain a connection with these baths over time (compare the association of the Lucilii Gamalae with the Temple of Venus at Ostia; see *CIL* 14.375 and 376). Perhaps an even earlier Sentius had built the building in the first place. *Colimbum* (from the Greek κολυμβίς) appears to be another term for *piscina,* meaning "swimming pool" (see no. 311), though the etymology might demand that the former was specifically intended for diving. Whether there was any physical difference between a *colimbum* and a *piscina* is not sure—was the former deeper? Nielsen (1.155, s.v. "kolym-betra") comments that the word is "synonymous with *natatio* and *piscina.*" For the physical remains of this building, see Cagiano de Azevedo, op. cit., 24–27; Coarelli, loc. cit.

119   P. Cornelius Attax Marcianus, L. Appius Amicus Rufinianus, cur(atores) refectionis. Lepcis Magna, Tripolitania. Third century (?). *AE* 1925.105 = *IRT* 263.

P. Cornelius Attax | Marcianus, | L. Appius Amicus | Rufinianus, | cur(atores) refectionis | thermarum ter[tium], | deo Aesculapio | v(otum) s(olverunt).

NOTES: This inscription was found in the Hadrianic Baths (for the fragmentary dedicatory inscription dated to 127, see *IRT* 361). It is dated by letterform to the third century. The restoration *ter[tium]* is more probable than *tert(iae)* and so refers to "the third set of baths," as opposed to the *curatores refectionis* or the number of restorations (however, Thomas and Witschel [162 n. 169] prefer *tert[iae]*). To my knowledge, *curator refectionis* has no parallel among local offices, although there is evidence for curators attached to specific bathhouses; see nos. 267 and 270. On curators in general, see *RE* 4.1774–1813, s.v. "curator" (Kornemann). For the remains of this facility and those of the other baths at Lepcis Magna, see R. Bartoccini, *Le terme di Lepcis* (Bergamo, 1929); Manderscheid, 136–37, s.v. "Leptis (Lepcis) Magna"; Nielsen, 2.27 (C.212–15); Yegül, 186–92 (Hadrianic Baths), 242–43 (Hunting Baths), 408 (Unfinished Baths).

120†   Vicani Petrenses. Vicus Petra, Moesia. Third or fourth century. *AE* 1935.172 = *AE* 1977.758 (see *AE* 1939.100).

q(uod) b(onum) f(austum) f(elix). | vicani Petrenses qui contul[e]runt | causa salutis corporis sui balineu(m) faciundu(m). quod opus | effectu(m) magisterio anni Nymphidi Maximi et Aeli Gemi[n]i, qu(a)estori|bus vici Ulpio Romano et Cassio Primitivo, curantibus operi N[ymp]hidio | Maximo s(upra) s(cripta) et Aelio Iulio.

Trans.: "What is good, favorable, and lucky. The villagers of Petra who contributed to the building of the bath for the sake of their bodily health. The work was carried out in the magisterial year of Nymphidius Maximus and Aelius Geminus, when Ulpius Romanus and Cassius Primitivus were quaestors of the village. Nymphidius Maximus, mentioned above, and Aelius Julius saw to the work."

NOTES: It is not clear how many villagers contributed to the erection of the baths. Had there been a limited number, we might expect a list of names, but this may have put the cost of the inscription beyond the means of such a small place as Vicus Petra. Whatever the case, it is clear from official involvement in the work that the local council was responsible for the construction.

121†   C. Sallius Pompeianus Sofronius, patronus. Amiternum (Regio IV). 325. *AE* 1937.119/20 = *SuppItal* 9 (1992): 85–90 (no. 34).

This bronze *tabula patronatus,* thirty-six lines in length, honors C. Sallius Pompeianus Sofronius. His grandfather, Sallius Proculus, is reported to have been a *patronus* of the town, as was his father, also named Sallius Proculus (lines 11–12). The text is dated to 7 December 325 (*Paulino et Iuliano coss. VII idus Dec.*, line 1). The pertinent lines (21–25) read:

. . . thermas quas *(sic)* iam olim disperier{e}ant antiquitus inpendiis et sua pecunia | cum porticis novis factis et omni ornamento at pulcridinem *(sic)* restauravit | statuisque decoravit et nomine d(omini) n(ostri) Constanti beatiss(imi) Caes(aris) natalle idibus Nob(embribus) dedicavit, quarum dedicatio{b}ne biduum teatrum et dena iuve|naliorum spectaculis exsibuit sub {v} presentia Cl(audi) Urani, v. p., corr(ectoris) n(ostri) . . .

Trans.: " . . . The baths, which had for a long time been ruined, he restored to beauty with his outlays and at his own expense, having added new porticoes and all their decoration as well; and he decorated the baths with statues and dedicated them in the name of our lord, Constantius, the most blessed Caesar, on his anniversary on 13 November. At their dedication, he gave two days of theater and ten of Juvenalia in the amphitheater, which our corrector Claudius Uranius, *vir perfectissimus*, attended . . . "

NOTES: For Claudius Uranius, see *PLRE* 1.982, s.v. "Uranius 4." For an overview of such patronal contracts, see Nicols, "*Tabulae Patronatus*." No significant remains of baths are known at Amiternum; see Coarelli and La Regina, *Abruzzo*, 17–24. The *(dies) natalis* here cannot be Constantius' birthday, since that is attested as 7 August 317; see *PLRE*, 1.226, s.v. "Constantius 8." Therefore the anniversary probably refers to his proclamation as Caesar, which is usually dated to 8 November 324: see *PLRE*, loc. cit.; T.D. Barnes, *The New Empire of Diocletian and Constantine* (Cambridge, MA, 1982), 85. If so, this inscription forces a revision of that date.

Local council. Olisipo, Lusitania. 336. *CIL* 2.191 = *ILS* 5699 = *ILER* 2049.   122†

thermae Cassiorum | renovatae a solo iuxta iussionem | Numeri Albani, v. c., p(raesidis) p(rovinciae) L(usitaniae), | curante Aur. Firmo. | Nepotiano et Facundo coss.

Trans.: "The Baths of the Cassii were renovated from the ground up, following the order of Numerius Albanus, of senatorial rank, governor of the province of Lusitania. Aurelius Firmus saw to the work, when Nepotianus and Facundus were consuls *(i.e., 336).*"

NOTES: For Albanus, see *PLRE* 1.32, s.v. "Albanus"; Firmus appears to be a local. Two benefactions are recorded here: (1) the original construction by the Cassii, of uncertain social status (= no. 147), and (2) the renovation by the local council.

C. Aurelius Stat[ianus], cur(ator) r(ei) p(ublicae), una cum omn[ibus decurionibus].   123 [?]sinsensium (modern Henchir-Haouli), northwest of Furnos Maius, Africa. 340/50. *AE* 1934.133 = *ILTun* 622.

Saeculo felic[issimo] | dd nn Fl. Constanti et Fl. Con[stantis] | administrantibus etiam | Fl. Dardanio Amp., proc., c. v., et l{a}egatis | [p]ulcerrimum factum cum porticus | [. .] turpia foedabantur ad statum I | [pisc]inalis ad restaurationem d|[..5..]s, colitumque nitent, soliar[em cellam | ..6..]oleum a fundamentis perc| [..7..]proneum aquiducti a fu[ndamentis | ..9..]ium solium vero inst[auravit?, | ..10..]t C. Aurelius Stat[ianus | ..10..] cur(ator) r(ei) p(ublicae) una cum omn[ibus decurionibus | ..11..]sinsensium perfecit et [dedicavit].

NOTES: For Flavius Dardanius, see *PLRE* 1.242, s.v. "Dardanius"; this man is attested as doing something to baths in Carthage in the fragmentary *ILTun* 1093: *[Da]rdanus thermis procon.* Although the current text is very fragmentary, enough survives to make it clear that Aurelius Statianus and the local decurions restored and extended the baths at Henchir Haouli: the portico seems to have been returned to its previous condition; some restoration was carried out in the *piscina* area; the *soliaris cella* was built from foundations (?), as was the *[—]proneum* of the aqueduct, an element that is not identifiable; and the *solium* in one of the rooms was restored. For a discussion of the meaning of *soliaris cella*, see DeLaine, "'Cella Solearis.'"

124†   Sex. Cluvius Martinus et M. Caesolius Saturninus, omnibus honoribus functi. Ocriculum (Regio VI). 341. *CIL* 11.4095 = *ILS* 5696.

provocati temporis beatitudinem dd. | impp. Constan[ti et Constantis] Augustorum[q]ue nn., | volumptatem *(sic)* thermarum hiemalium Sex. Cluvius Mar|tinus et M. Caesolius Saturninus, omnibus honori|bus functi, de sua pecunia ordini seu civibus Ocri|colanis ad meliorem pulcritudinem pro civica ad|fectione cum augmento operi novi exercientes | adsignaverunt et dedicaverunt. | (iuxta) die XVI | K[a]l. De|c[e]mbr. | Marcel|lino et | Pro|bino | con|suli|bus.

Trans.: "Sex. Cluvius Martinus and M. Caesolius Saturninus, men who held all the municipal offices, repaired the felicity of the challenged age of our lords and emperors Constantius Augustus and Constans Augustus and the pleasure of the winter baths at their own expense and, in accordance with their civic-mindedness, dedicated and handed over the baths, enlarged by new construction, to the *ordo,* or rather, to the citizens of Ocriculum for their better beauty. 16 November when Marcellinus and Probinus were consuls *(i.e., 341).*"

NOTES: This inscription stood on the building itself and was found near the baths in 1782 or early in 1783. Two other inscriptions from the town, carved on the bases of two benefactors' statues that probably stood in the forum or some other prominent place, also mention this restoration; see *CIL* 11.4096 (for Martinus) and 11.4097 = *ILS* 5697 (for Saturninus). These statue bases, also dated to 341, reveal that the two men were brothers. It seems that this work was in progress in the previous year, when Constans and Constantine II were struggling for supremacy in Italy: see Zos. 2.40–41; Eutr. 10.9. It also appears that this family had a long history of local prominence, since a Republican inscription at the site commemorates L. Caesilius and L. Clovius *(sic)* as *quattuorviri aediles;* see Pietrangeli, *Ocriculum,* 34. The two known baths at Ocriculum stood side by side, so the *thermae hiemales* were either an extension of the earlier structure (built by L. Julius Julianus [see no. 98]) or a separate construction that stood nearby: see Gaggiotti et al., *Umbria,* 24; Manderscheid, 157, s.v. "Ocriculum"; Pietrangeli, *Ocriculum,* 68–71; id., *Otricoli,* 64–75.

125†   C. Paccius Felix, omnib(us) honorib(us) et honeribus pe[r]functus, cur(ator) r(rei) p(ublicae), patron(us). Casinum (Regio I). Mid- to late fourth century. *CIL* 10.5200.

C. Pacci Felicis | C. Paccio Felici pat(ri) omnib. honor. et honeri|bus pe[r]functo, filio C. Pacci Felicis, patron(i) | coloniae Casin(atium), cuius inmensis bene|ficiis patria cognoscitur cumulata cur(atore) | r(ei) p(ublicae) nost(rae), cuius provisone semper feliciter | guvernati (sumus), cur(atori) et instauratori aedium | publicorum, cuius opera et sollicitu|dine{m} inpendiisque propriis post | seriem annorum therm⟨a⟩e Noviani | nobis in usu sunt restitutae; ob his | omnibus laboribus eius quos cir|ca patriam civesque suos exibuit | digno patrono universus | populus coloniae

Casinatilum una cum liberis nostris | statuam marmoream erigen|dam digne censuimus.

Trans.: "(Statue) of C. Paccius Felix. To C. Paccius Felix Senior, who held all of the municipal magistracies and offices, the son of C. Paccius Felix, the patron of the colony of Casinum. By his immense benefactions our city is recognized, after being enhanced by our curator; by his foresight we have always been governed successfully. To the guardian and restorer of the public temples, by whose effort and care and personal outlay the Baths of Novianus (or Novius), after a length of years, were restored to our use; on account of all these efforts of his that he has displayed toward our city and its citizens, we, the entire people of the colony of Casinum, together with our children, decreed the fitting erection of a marble statue to a worthy patron."

NOTES: This text is dated by Camodeca ("Ricerche," 494–95, s.v. "Casinum, 2") to the second half of the fourth century; Nielsen (1.41 n. 26) assigns it more broadly to the fourth century. In contrast, G. Carettoni (*Casinum* [Rome, 1940], 35) proposes a second-century date for it, on the basis of its language and terminology. However, the rhetorical effusiveness and the fact that a local man is a curator and partron of the town point to the later date.

L. Alfius Fannius Primus So[..4..], quaest(or), curator frumento, d(u)umvir, om-   126
nib(us) honerib(us) et honoribus functus, vir patronus et curator [rei publicae?].
Trebula (Regio I). Mid- to late fourth century. *CIL*10.4559.

L. Alfio Fannio Primo So[..4..] | quaest(ori), curatori frumento, | d(u)umviro om-
nib(us) honerib(us) et | honoribus functo, sacerd(oti), | viro patrono et curatori | [rei
p(ublicae)?] a Pisoni aurum atque | argentum obraetium se|rio ilustravit *(sic)*, thermas
ae|tiam Constantianas [l]on[g]a | vetustate corrupta ex virib(us) suo *(sic)* | quam etiam
e Sabinianeus ordl[..6..]rem filio Viaceni | re(stituit), statuam benemerenti patrono |
[. . .]pa [..4..]tissimo [..6..] | duoviro senatus populusque Trebu(lanorum) | me
[..8..] statuam decreverunt. | d(ecreto) d(ecurionum).

NOTES: Camodeca ("Ricerche," 500–501, s.v. "Trebula") dates this inscription to the second half of the fourth century. It is a difficult text to decipher, due to its fragmentary nature, but the main benefaction—restoration of the *Thermae Constantianae*—is clearly recorded and credited to Fannius. The mention of the *aurum atque argentum obraetium* prompts comparison with *CIL* 10.3732 = *ILS* 1216 from Grumo (between Naples and Capua), which mentions an *exactor auri et argenti provinciarum III* (i.e., Sicily, Sardinia, and Corsica) named C. Caelius Censorinus, an ex-consul of this period (see *PLRE* 1.196, s.v. "Censorinus 2"). An alternative reading of [..]a *Pisoni aurum* etc. is [. .]apis qui, where [. .]apis is the fragmentary name of a town of which Fannius was curator.

Ann[i]us Namptoius, flamen p(er)p(etuus), cur(ator) reip(ublicae), cum Thu[bur-   127†
bitan]ae urbis florentissimo sena[tu] | c[u]n[ct]aque eius p[l]e[be]. Thuburbo Maius,
Africa. 361. *AE* 1916.87/88 = *ILAfr* 273.

Presented below are two texts of the same inscription, written on two sides of the same slab.

273a: *(the first four lines are very fragmentary)* |que hu[more supe]rfluo [m]agis
f[l]eban[t qu]am prol[ue]bant vigili cura sollertique | [lab]ore inpens[o i]ntra sep-
timum mensem adiecti[s] omnibus perfectisque cunctis | quib[u]s lavacra indigebant
Ann[i]us Namptoius, fl(a)m. p. [p.,] iurisconsultus, [magister] | studi[or]um, cur. rei.

p., cum Thu[burbitan]ae urbis florentissimo sena[tu] | c[u]n[ct]aque eius p[l]e[be | per]feci[t, e]xcoluit, dedicavit.

273b: [beatissimo saeculo dd.] nn. C[onstanti Pii Fel]ici[s Maxim]i | [et invictissimi Augusti] et Iuli[ani no]bil[issimi] Cae[saris | pro]co[ns]ulatu Clo[di H]ermogenian[i, v. c., p]roc. [p. A., et le]gatione [Crepe]rei | Optatiani, v. c., leg. Karthag., [t]hermas [aes]tivales po[s]t ann[os solidos] octo | i[n]tra septimum mensem a[d]iectis omnibus perfectisq[ue] cuncti[s | qu]ibus lavacra ind[i]gebant Ann[i]us Namptoivus *(sic)* fl(a)m. [p.] p., | iurisconsultus, magister st[udiorum], cur reip., cum Thub[ur]bi[t]anae | [u]rbis ordine amplissim[o c]unct[a]que eius plebe | [per]fecit, excoluit, dedicavit.

Trans. (273b): "In the most prosperous age of our masters Constantius, *pius, felix, Maximus*, the most invincible Augustus, and Julian, the most noble Caesar, in the proconsulate of Clodius Hermogenianus, of senatorial rank, proconsul of the province of Africa, and in the legateship of Crepereus Optatianus, of senatorial rank, legate of Carthage, Annius Namptoius, perpetual priest, jurist, master of studies, curator of the city, along with the most eminent *ordo* of the city of Thuburbo and the entire plebs, after adding everything and completing everything that the *lavacra* required, completed, adorned, and dedicated the summer baths within the seventh month [of his year in office?], after eight whole years."

NOTES: For Q. Clodius Hermogenianus Olybrius, see *PLRE* 1.640–42, s.v. "Olybrius 3"; for Crepereus Optatianus, see *PLRE* 1.648–49, s.v. "Optatianus 2." This is an interesting pair of texts, of which only the more complete is translated. Both evidently refer to the same benefaction. One version (a) omits mention of the important imperial dignitaries, the provincial governor and his legate. Other than this omission, the differences in wording are minimal, save that the surviving and very fragmentary opening lines of the first version (a) appear to have contained more information on the terrible state of the baths (lines 5–6): " . . . With the liquid overflowing (the pools?) wept rather than washed; with watchful care and skillful work, and at cost, within the seventh month . . . " This version also omits mention of the "eight whole years," which might be a reference to the period when bathers used the incomplete facilities (Annius Namptoius is said to have "completed" them) unsatisfactorily. Two more points are worth making. First, the text is ambiguous as to who was reponsible for the work. It says that Annius Namptoius completed the job himself but did so in conjunction with the city's decurions and the entire plebs, which suggests that it was a joint effort on the part of Annius Namptoius and the local council. There are parallel examples of this sort of wording, where the main verbs are usually in the singular; for a discussion, see chapter 6, p. 150. In this case, note that the first version (a) mentions *inpenso*, but without an accompanying *suo* or *publico*, thus leaving the ambiguity over responsibility unresolved. Second, the meaning of *lavacra* is unclear: is it a synonym for the *thermae* mentioned earlier, or does it refer to a specific part of the baths? If the latter, what part does it refer to? Possibly, if the details in the first version (a) are taken into account, the *lavacra* were the pools (on *lavacra*, see the notes to no. 13). For the remains of these baths, originally constructed in the mid- to late second century, see L. Drappier, "Les thermes de *Thuburbo Maius*," *BAC*, 1920, 64–74; Nielsen, 2.28 (C.222); Yegül, 222–30.

128   Local council. Madaurus, Numidia. 361/63. *ILAlg* 1.2100.

Presented below are four fragments of the same text from the Large Baths at Madaurus.

Frs. a and b, as combined by Gsell *(ILAlg):* b[eatissimis temporibus florentissimoque (?) sa]eculo d. n. Iul[ian]i | per[petui Aug. thermae—in]curia paene ad in|tertitum [redactae? — ca]meris omnibus | et soliis e[t? — n]on tantum in|[f]eriorum [—]tis voragini | [— sup]e[r]io[rum] (?).

Fr. c: [—]s qui picturae grati[am | —] melioribus ornam[entis — | —] sunt proconsola[tu | —] sumtu publico [—].

Fr. d: [instantia? Ma]criani, ducen|arii, [splend]id[i] e[t] laudab[i]l[i]s v[i]ri, cur(atoris) rei p(ublicae), perfec[t]ae sun[t] et cum ordin[e] | eiusdem col[oniae no]st(rae) et populo d[e]d[ic]atae.

NOTES: The inscription comes from the ruins of the Large (or Summer) Baths at Madaurus (*ILAlg* reports it under "fouilles des grands thermes"); Nielsen, 2.30 (C.237) mistakenly assigns it to the Small (or Winter) Baths. Both buildings appear to date to the same period, since they both yielded dedications to Severus and Caracalla of the years 202–5; see *ILAlg* 1.2084–85 (Small Baths) and 1.2087–89, 2092 (Large Baths). Architecturally, they are consistent with such a date; see Yegül, 222. Despite the fragmentary condition of this inscription, enough is discernible to make out that the baths underwent restoration and adornment at public expense *(sumtu publico)*. This fact and the use of the passive forms suggest that the work was the responsibility of the local council, rather than any individual officer. Nevertheless, the precise role of the *curator rei publicae* (evidently here a local official) remains uncertain. For the remains of the Large Baths, see Manderscheid, 144, s.v. "Madaurus (Mdauorouch), Grands Thermes"; Nielsen, 2.30 (C.236). On the Small Baths, see Manderscheid, 144, s.v. "Madaurus, Petits Thermes"; Nielsen, 2.30 (C.237).

Local council. Madaurus, Numidia. 364. *ILAlg* 1.2101.   129†

pro tanta securi[tate temporum] | dd. nn. Valentiniani [et Valentis perpetuo]rum Aug[g. | therm]as aestivas, olim splen[did(issimum *or* -issimae)] coloni[ae nostrae? orn]a[mentum? | sed? tot re]tro annis ruinarum labe deformes pa[rietibusque omni?]um soli|orum ita corruptis ut gravibus damnis adficerent, [nun?]c omni idonitate con|structas et cultu splendido decoratas, sed et patinas ampliato aeris pondere | omni idonitate firmissas proconsulatu Publi Ampeli, v. c., Octavio Privatia|no, v. c., legato Numidiae, Cec. Pontilius Paulinus, ff(lamen) p(er)p(etuus), p(atronus) c(oloniae), curat[o]r rei p(ublicae), pecunia | publica perfecit porticum quo[q]ue ingredientibus ab atri[o], sed et pronaum | eidem coh(a)erentem commeantibus per viam, trabibus ti[g]nis [—] ceterisque | [—Pont]ilius Pauli[|nus—] ordine.

Trans.: "On behalf of the great security of the age of our lords Valentinian and Valens, perpetual Augusti. The summer baths, once the most splendid ornament of our colony (*or* once the ornament of our most splendid colony), but for so many years past deformed by the decay of ruins and by such destruction to the walls of all the pools that they caused serious loss, now (?) were built with all usefulness and decorated with fine ornament, but also the *patinae* were firmed up with a greater weight of bronze in all usefulness. Caecilius Pontilius Paulinus, *flamen* for life, patron of the colony, curator of the city, completed the work at public expense in the proconsulate of Publius Ampelius, of senatorial rank, when Octavius Privatianus, of senatorial rank, was legate of Numidia. Also a portico as one enters from the atrium, and likewise a porch linked to the same (portico? atrium?) as one moves down the street, with wooden beams . . . and other . . . Pontilius Paulinus . . . with the *ordo*."

NOTES: For P. Ampelius, see *PLRE* 1.56–57, s.v. "Ampelius 3"; for Privatianus, see *PLRE* 1.731, s.v. "Privatianus." This text was found in two fragments to the north of the forum and the theater and is apparently in reference to the Large (or Summer) Baths (on which, see the notes to no. 128). Although a local official is said to carry out the work, it was funded *pecunia publica* and so was the responsibility of the local council. The official is probably given prominence to highlight the last three lines of the text, which may have recorded additional work he carried out at his own expense. This is an informative inscription for naming parts of baths: the *solia, patinae* (of uncertain identification, but apparently associated with the boilers; see Pall. 1.39.3), *portico,* and *pronaum.*

130†   Q. Basilius Flaccianus, fl(amen) p(er)p(etuus), augur et cur(ator) [rei pub(licae)]. Calama, Numidia. 366/68. *CIL* 8.5335 = *ILS* 5730 = *ILAlg* 1.256.

beatissimis temporibus dd. nn. Valentiniani et Valentis perpetuorum Augg., procons[ulatu v. c. Iuli Festi Hymetii, legatio]|ne v. c. Fabii Fabiani, piscinam quae antea tenuis aquae pi[g]ra fluenta capiebat, nunc ve[ro — unda?]|rum intonantium motibus redundantem, Q. Basilius Flaccianus, fl(amen) p(er)p(etuus), augur et cur(ator) [rei pub(licae) restitut?]| et excepto[rio ..20.. exst]ructo adq(ue) perfecto cum [. . .]lio Maximo Auf[id]iano, [f(ilio) suo ded(icavit)].

Trans.: "In the most prosperous age of our lords Valentinian and Valens, perpetual Augusti, in the proconsulate of Julius Festus Hymetius, of senatorial rank, and in the legateship of Fabius Fabianus, of senatorial rank, Q. Basilius Flaccianus, priest for life, augur, and curator of the city, restored the pool, which used to be supplied with the tiny trickle of a narrow water channel but now truly overflows with the motion of thundering torrents (?); and after building and completing a cistern (?) *(and other elements?),* he dedicated the work along with his son, [?]lius Maximus Aufidianus."

NOTES: For Hymetius, see *PLRE* 1.447, s.v. "Hymetius"; for Fabianus, see *PLRE* 1.322, s.v. "Fabianus 3." Both men are attested in the province for the years 366–68. It is not made explicit that this *piscina* was part of a bathhouse, but that is its most likely context, especially given the mention of the *exceptorium,* a reservoir also associated with baths; see nos. 132 and 137. See also *CIL* 8.4291 = *ILS* 3063; *OLD,* s.v. "exceptorium"; Shaw, "Noblest Monuments," 66–67.

131†   Incertus, cur(ator) rei publicae cum ordine splendido et universo popul[o]. Madaurus, Numidia. 366/68. *ILAlg* 1.2102.

pro tanta felicitate tempo[rum invictissi]|morum principum dd. nn. per[p. Augg. Valenti]|niani et Valentis, piscinalem istam [cellam? —] | et soliarem cellam, lacuniis densis ita foed[atas ut ima pavi]|menti monstrarent, atque ita retentione[m caloris prohi]|berent, compellente religione sanctae p[— et commodo Roma?]|norum civium, exquisitis diversorum co[lorum marmoribus], | artificibus quoque peregrinis adductis et [adhibitis?, splen]dentes novoque omnino opere tes(s)ellatas, pr[oconsulatu Iuli Festi, v. c.], | Fabio Fabiano, v. c. et inlustre, legato Numidi[ae — , cur.] | rei p(ublicae), inter cetera in quibus ia(m)du[dum —], | cum ordine splendido et universo popul[o restituit et dedicavit?]. felicit[er]!

Trans.: "On behalf of the great happiness of the unconquered age of our emperors and lords, perpetual Augusti, Valentinian and Valens. [?], curator of the city, among his other benefactions by which for some time already [he has favored the city?], along with the eminent *ordo* and the entire people, restored and dedicated that pool room (?) and the *cella soliaris,* which were marred with frequent holes such that the lowest levels of the pavement were showing through and, accordingly, prevented the retention of heat; and, driven by his scrupulous regard for the sacred p[?] and by the comfort of the Roman (?) citizens, he introduced (?) choice marbles of different colors, and he also brought in foreign artisans and put them to work; and he restored the resplendent mosaics with entirely new workmanship. He did this in the proconsulate of Julius Hymetius, of senatorial rank, and when Fabius Fabianus, of senatorial rank and a distinguished gentleman, was legate of Numidia. Happily!"

NOTES: This inscription was found in the Large (or Summer) Baths at Madaurus (on the remains of which, see the notes to no. 128; see the notes to the previous entry for Hymetius and Fabianus). Responsibility for the benefaction is unclear in this case, since the *curator rei publicae* appears to be the main benefactor and the phrase *inter cetera in quibus ia(m)du[dum —]* suggests that there had been previous benefactions; compare wording of no. 35. But the *ordo* and the *populus* were somehow involved, perhaps only in the dedication; compare no. 140. On the *cella soliaris,* see the notes to no. 123. The possible mention of the Roman citizens as among the chief beneficiaries is noteworthy; compare no. 167.

[?]dius Honorati(a)nus, fl(amen) p(erpetuus), cur(ator) r(ei) p(ublicae). Thugga, Africa. Gratian. *AE* 1925.31 = *ILAfr* 573 = *ILTun* 1500.   132

atrium thermar[um Lic]inianarum ab antiquis c[oe]ptum, excep|toriis in eodem loco su[biectis], quod inperfecto opere corruptum adque | ruderibus foedatum [erat —]dius Honorati(a)nus, fl(amen) p(erpetuus), cur(ator) reip(ublicae) II, [cu]m statua | signoq(ue) felicissimi Fl. Gr[atian]i CCCRATU opere perfecit itemq[ue dedica]vit.

NOTES: This inscription was found in the Licinian Baths at Thugga, built during the reign of Gallienus (see the very fragmentary *CIL* 8.26559). The text says the atrium had been started sometime previously, "by the ancients" *(atrium . . . ab antiquis coeptum),* but had been shabbily built *(quod inperfecto opere corruptum adque ruderibus foedatum [erat]).* Merlin (*ILTun*) could not make sense of the letters *CCCRATU.* They are probably a corruption of *accurato* or some such expression aimed at contrasting the high quality of Honoratianus' work with the *inperfectum opus* of the *antiqui.* For *exceptorium,* see the notes to no. 130; see also no. 137. Nielsen (2.28–29 [C.224]) cites *ILTun* 1500 as evidence for the Gallienic construction of the baths and *ILAfr* 573 for a rebuilding under Gratian; in fact, both references are to different publications of the current text (although, to be sure, the inscription does provide evidence for both of these constructional operations). For the remains of this building, see Manderscheid, 213, s.v. "Thugga, Thermes des Licinii"; Nielsen, loc. cit.; Yegül, 206–12.

Local council and Flavianus Leontius, curator rei publicae. Abbir Maius, Africa.   133†
368/70. *AE* 1975.873.

salvis ddd. nnn. Valentiniano, Valente, Gratiano perpetuis Auggg., proconsul[a]tu Petroni Claudi, c. v,. et Mari Victoriani, l[e]gati Kartaginis, c. v., | oceanum a fundamentis coeptum et soliarem ruina conlapsum, ad perfectionem cultumque perductos ingressus novos signis adpositis decoravit | Flavianus Leontius alme *(sic)* Kart(haginis) principalis, curator rei p(ublicae), ordinis splendidissimi conlatione, cum amore populi incoav[i]t, perfecit, dedicavit.

Trans.: "When our lords Valentinian, Valens, and Gratian, perpetual Augusti, are safe and well, in the proconsulate of Petronius Claudius, of senatorial rank, and (during the tenure of office) of the legate of Carthage Marius Victorianus, of senatorial rank, Flavianus Leontius, *principalis* of nurturing Carthage, curator of the city, began, completed, and dedicated the *oceanum,* which had been started from its foundations, and the *soliaris,* which had collapsed in ruin, and he decorated the new entrances, brought to the point of perfection and beauty with statues set up alongside. He did so with contributions from the most eminent *ordo* and with the enthusiasm of the people."

NOTES: For Petronius Claudius, see *PLRE* 1.208, s.v. "Claudius 10"; Marius Victorianus is otherwise unattested. The *oceanum* is in all likelihood a pool decorated with marine scenes, as the editors of *AE* suggest, or a room named for its decoration: see HA *Alex. Sev.* 25.5; *AE* 1989.743. Leontius was from Carthage itself (rather than from Abbir Maius, which lay in its *territorium*), and he stemmed from an especially privileged class of decurions (the *principales*). The editors of *AE* propose that he may have owned land in the region of Abbir Maius, thus explaining why he was *curator* there. The funding for the operations appears to have to come from the local council; the curator is not expressly credited with contributing to the work and appears to have acted as the town's agent.

134   Incertus, cur(ator) r(ei) p(ublicae). Hr. Bu Auga (ancient name not known), Africa. 371/73. *CIL* 8.16400.

ddd. nnn.Valentiniano, Valenti, et Grat[iano —] | Sextio Rustico, v. c., proconss. p. A[fr]i[cae, et —], | v. c., legato Numidiae, balneae quae i[—] | redintegrat(a)e sunt devotione totius ordini[s —] | cur(ator) r(ei) p(ublicae) opus et sollicitudine et sumtibus adi[uvit —].

NOTES: For Rusticus (Julianus), see *PLRE* 1.479–80, s.v. "Julianus 37." The main task of restoration is expressed in the passive voice, implying that the local council was the main agent (see the notes to no. 107), although, if the last section is correctly restored, the *curator rei publicae* appears to have assisted "with his concern and at his expense."

135   Incertus, mag(ister) *or* mag(istratus). Segusio, Alpes Cottiae. 375/78. *CIL* 5.7250 = *ILS* 5701.

salvis ddd. nnn. Valente, Gratiano, et Valentiniano imp[pp. perp. Auggg.] | thermas Gratianas dudum coeptas et omissas mag. aput [—] | Alp. Cott. extruxit ornavit et usui Segusinae reddidit civit[atis, —] | formavit, fistulas dedit, aquam deduxit, ne quid vel utilitati vel us[ibus deesset].

NOTES: The benefaction appears to have been partly a construction of the baths (or at least a completion of them) and partly a decoration.

136   C. Volusius Victor, qu⟨a⟩estor r(ei) p(ublicae). Ocriculum (Regio VII). Late fourth century. *CIL* 11.4094.

C. Volusio Victor|i, qu⟨a⟩estori r(ei) p(ublicae) Oc|riculanorum; IIII|viri, aediles, IIIIviri iur|e {e}d(i)c(undo), IIII quinq., cives ei | plebei hoc emerito stat|uam huic posuerunt q|ui termas iemalis ad pristi|nam dig(nitatem) restauravit et | d(e)d(i)c(a)v(it).

On left side: p(o)s(i)t(a) | diae *(sic)* III nonas Nob.

NOTES: For a photograph of the stone, see fig. 26D. The date is that assigned by Nielsen, 1.41 n. 26; Pietrangeli (*Ocriculum,* 68; *Otricoli,* 64) dates it by letterform to the late fourth or early fifth century. The form *termas* and the designation of the building as summer baths, which only appear in the fourth century, support a late date; see above, chapter 5, n. 49. The inscription was found in the ruins of baths at the end of 1782 or early in 1783. For the physical remains, see the notes to no. 124.

137†   G. Optatianus, fl(amen) p(er)p(etuus), cur(ator) r(ei) p(ublicae). Thuburbo Maius, Africa. Late fourth century. *ILAfr* 285.

[cellam s]oliarem cum solis omni etiam refuso instrumento aeris et plumbi firma refec[it] | e⟨t⟩ solidavit, piscinam novam nomine cochleam redditis veteribus exceptoriis adiecit, | dedicavit G. Optatianus, fl(amen) p(er)p(etuus), cur(ator) r(ei) p(ublicae).

Trans.: "G. Optatianus, priest for life, curator of the city, firmly rebuilt and strengthened the *cella soliaris* along with its pools, after also recasting all the bronze and lead elements; he added a new *piscina,* called "The Cochlea," and restored the old cisterns. G. Optatianus, priest for life, curator of the city, dedicated (the work)."

NOTES: The inscription comes from the Winter Baths; the date is that proffered by Nielsen, 2.28 (C.223). In this text, the *cella soliaris* is evidently a room with *solia* (communal pools) in it; see DeLaine, "'Cella Solearis.'" On *exceptoria,* see the notes to no. 130; see also no. 132. For the remains, see Drappier, "Les thermes," 57–64; Nielsen, 2.28 (C.223); Yegül, 238. For another text recording the gift of lead to baths, see no. 251.

[Gab?]inius Salvianus Edilicius, p(atronus) a(lmae) K(arthaginis). Thuburbo Maius,   138
Africa. 395/408. *AE* 1914.57 = *ILAfr* 276.

Salviani p(atroni) a(lmae) K(arthiginis). | hortante felicitate temporum dd. Au|ggque nn. Arcadi et Honori inclytorum | principum ubique victorum proconsul[latu — | — | Gab?]inio Salviano Edilicio p(atronus) a(lmae) K(arthaginis) statuam | [vo]to [pa]triae officiorum etiam eius er|[ga e]am meritis indultam r(es) p(ublica) felix | T[h]urburbo Maius amantissimo civi | ac sui amanti quod etiam thermarum | hiemalium ex ima fundamentorum ori|gine usque [ad] fastigia culmen erexit idem | quoque[.]ioc[— te]mporis vel usus vel | [..4..]n[. propri?]o [sump?]tu omnium locorum | *(the last lines are too fragmentary to make sense of, except* [su]mptu proprio . . . inpen|sisque su[is] *in lines 16–17).*

NOTES: This is a fragmentary text found in the forum, but it expressly refers to the Winter Baths at Thuburbo Maius. The main lines are clear: "[To Salvianus] because he raised the roof of the winter baths, from the lowest levels of the foundations to the pediments." The baths, however, date to the age of M. Aurelius and so here undergo a thorough reconstruction. For the remains, see the notes to no. 137.

Maecius Paternus, curator et pa[trono] civitatis. Volsinii (Regio VII). Fourth or fifth   139†
century. *CIL* 11.7298 = *ILCV* 364 = *ICI* 1.18.

[—] | [is]tius ordinis sive c[iv]ita[ti]s et rec[t]ori omni[um] | [co]mmeantium Maecio Paterno, curatori et pa[trono | hu]uisce *(sic)* civitatis, iudicio omnium conprob[ato, | r]estauratori thermarum Tusciani, qui vix[it | a]nnis LVII, menses VIIII, d(ies) XX et fecit cum uxore su[a | Vi]rginia ann(os) XXXV Apra uxor sed et Patern[a | et M]arcellus fili patri piisimo depositio *(sic)* VI[— | Se]ptembr(es) pax tibi cum sanctis.

Trans.: "[—] of that *ordo* or the city, and to the guide of all travelers, Maecius Paternus, curator and patron of this city; he earned the respect of all, restorer of the baths of Tuscianus. He lived fifty-seven years, nine months, and twenty days and spent thirty-five years with his wife Virginia. Apra his [second?] wife, and also Paterna and Marcellus, his children, (offer?) a trust to their most holy father, on this *(date lost)* of September. Peace to you with the saints."

NOTES: Camodeca ("Ricerche," 516–17, s.v. "Volsinii 3") dates this text to the fourth or fifth century. These baths, hardly investigated, stand outside one of Volsinii's gates; see G.F. Gamurrini, "Regione V (Picenum)," *NSc,* 1896, 324.

140   Cl. S[ise]na Germanianus, curator rei p(ublicae). Madaurus, Numidia. 407/8. *ILAlg*
       1.2108.

excellens glo[ria ddd. nnn. invic]ltissimorum prin[cipum Arcadi, H]onor[i et The-
odosi] | semper Auggg., adm[inistrante [P]omp(eio) Proc[ulo], | v. c,. procons. p(ro-
vincae) A(fricae), leg[ato Num.] Q. Thersio Cr[ispino] | Meget(h)io, v. c., Cl. S[ise]na
Germanianus, | curator rei p(ublicae), ce[lla]m balnearum lon[ga] | serie temporum
ruina desolatam usi[busque] | lavacrorum den[e]gatam sumptu prop[rio et] |
camoeram cum suspensuris constructam nov[is] | ab splendido ordin[e] decretis titulis
ded[icavit].

NOTES: This inscription is from the Large (or Summer) Baths (on which, see the notes to no.
128). For Crispinus Megethius, see *PLRE* 2.752, s.v. "Megethius"; for Proculus (Porphyrius),
see *PLRE* 2.900–901, s.v. "Porphyrius 3." This benefaction is clearly the work of the curator
(*sumptu proprio* leaves little doubt). Here the *ordo* and *populus* appear to have taken part only
in the dedication.

141†   M. Sentius Redemptus, v(ir) l(audabilis), omnibus honoribus et honeribus curiae suae
       perfunctus, ex origine patronatus. Interamna Lirenas (Regio I). 408. *CIL* 10.5349.

industriae ac sapientiae. praeclaro | M. Sentio Redempto, v. l., primario civitatis |
nostrae, omnibus honoribus et honeribus culriae suae perfuncto, ex origine pa-
tronatus, | venientemque populum suum pro sua belnivolentia ab indictione auri
argentiqu(e) pop[u]llum suum liberum reddidit, termas extivas | in sordentibus ac
ruina conlabsas ex prop[rio] | ad summam{m}manum revocavit, cuius tantis |
be[ne]ficiis circa nos comulatis *(sic)* ad perpetuam falmam statuam eidem erigendam
universus | populus Interamnatium censuerunt.

On one side: d. prid. Non Iulias | Basso et Filippo, vv. cc., cons.

Trans.: "To industry and wisdom. To the outstanding M. Sentius Redemptus, *vir
laudabilis,* the principal man of our community, who held all the municipal magistracies of his *curia,* a man of patronal descent. He freed his people from the imposition of a tax on gold and silver, when his people came to him on account of his
kindness; he restored at his own expense the summer baths down to their last detail,
after they had fallen into ugliness and ruin. For such great benefactions heaped up
around us, the entire people of Interamna voted that a statue be erected to him for his
everlasting fame. *(On the side)* On 6 July when Bassus and Filippus, of senatorial
rank, were consuls *(i.e., 408)."*

NOTES: For the consuls Bassus and Filippus, see *PLRE* 2.219–20, s.v. "Bassus 7," and 2.876–
77, s.v. "Philippus 9." See also no. 118.

142   M. Aurelius Restitutus, cur(ator) r(ei) p(ublicae), cum splendido ordine suo. Mem-
       bressa, Africa. 412/14. *ILS* 5731.

salvis | dd. nn. Honorio et | Theodosio pp. Augg., | administrante Q. Senltio Fabricio
Iuliano, | v. c., iterum procos., v(ice) s(acra) i(udicans), | statuas et ornatum | piscinales
conlocavit | M. Aurelius Restiltutus ex toga., cur(ator) | r(ei) p(ublicae), cum splen-
dildo ordine suo.

NOTES: For Q. Sentius Fabricius Julianus, see *PLRE* 2.641–42, s.v. "Julianus 28." This is
another text that links the activities of the *curator rei publicae* and the *ordo* of the community;
see above, chapter 6, p. 150.

Private Benefactors

Satellia Anus. Capua (Regio I). Undated. *CIL* 10.3922f = *ILS* 5708.   143*

Satellia M. f. Anus [—] | apodyterium ad novitatem re[stituit | . .] epistylis ceterisque marmoribus o[rnavit].

NOTES: Remains of baths at Capua are known but ill investigated; see De Caro and Greco, *Campania*, 210–14.

[—] Grati pat(er) et f(ilius). San Nicola al Torone (ancient name not known; Regio   144
III). Undated. *AE* 1969/70.178.

[—] Grati pat[er] et f. | balneum sua peculnia fecerunt d(ecreto) d(ecurionum) | [p]ater epulo dato [de]dicavit.

NOTES: The remains of the baths are known "au sommet de la ville," according to the *AE* entry. Both men stemmed from the same family in the local nobility.

Tuscianus. Volsinii (Regio VII). Undated. *CIL* 11.7298 = *ILCV* 364 = *ICI* 1.18.   145

The full text is cited at no. 139. Here note the portion that reads:

. . . Maecio Paterno . . . [r]estauratori thermarum Tusciani . . .

NOTES: The restoration of these *thermae* took place in the late Empire, but the date of the initial construction of these baths is not known. Gamurrini ("Regione V," 324) posited a first-century date, but on the unconvincing basis of stucco decoration.

[Terentia Postu]mina. Novaria (Regio XI). Undated. *CIL* 5.6522.   146*

[Terentia Q. f. Postu]mina suo et | [C. Veturi L. f. Lucum]onis viri sui et | [C. Veturi C. f. Postum]ini f. sui nomine | [balineum s]olo privato et | [lavationem] gratuitam in | [perpetuum] dedit.

NOTES: If the *dedit* is taken to govern both *balineum solo privato* and *lavationem gratuitam in perpetuum,* it can be taken to mean "built" and "provided," respectively. Alternatively, *factum* could be assumed in association with *balineum,* or *dedit* could denote a transferral of ownership from Terentia to the local community. However, the construction of the bath appears the more natural interpretation.

Cassii. Olisipo, Lusitania. Undated. *CIL* 2.191 = *ILS* 5699 = *ILER* 2049.   147

The full text is cited at no. 122. Here note the portion that reads:

thermae Cassiorum | renovatae a solo . . .

NOTES: As with the baths of Tuscianus (no. 145), the original construction date of these baths, restored in the late Empire, cannot be determined. The status of the Cassii at Olisipo—whether they held local office or were private benefactors—is not known, but they are not attested among the local magistrates there; see Curchin, 174–75 (nos. 366–77). This observation is hardly conclusive, however, since the body of epigraphic data from this town is not large.

Terentius Donatus and Frumentius Longianus. Cuicul, Numidia. Undated. *AE*   148/149
1920.33.

balneum | Terenti Donati resitutu(m) | [p]er i⟨n⟩stantia(m) Frume⟨n⟩ti Longiani.

NOTES: Two benefactions are recorded here: (1) the original construction by Terentius Donatus and (2) the restoration by Frumentius Longianus. The baths are insufficiently investigated for any deductions be made about their date; see Manderscheid, 103, s.v. "Cuicul, Bains de Terentius."

150   L. Acilius Granianus. Timgad, Numidia. Undated. *CIL* 8.2340 = *ILS* 9259a and 9259b.

ILS 9259a: Aesculapiu[m] | L. Acilius | Granianus | L. Iulio Ian[u]|ario socero | suo at *(sic)* exor|natione[m] | balinei | dono dedit.

ILS 9259b: Hygiam | L. Acilius | Granianus | L. Iulio Ianua|rio socero | suo at *(sic)* exor|nationem | balinei | dono dedit.

NOTES: These inscriptions were carved onto two statue bases from Timgad, presumably set up as part of a single benefaction by the same benefactor. Since the texts were not found in situ, it is unclear if the baths were public or private.

151†*   Alfia Quart[a]. Marruvium Marsorum (Regio IV). Undated (but possibly late Republic or early Empire). *CIL* 9.3677 = *ILS* 5684.

Alfia P. f. Quart[a balneum] | muliebre a solo [fecit], | eadem lapide va[rio ex]|ornavit, labrum aen[eum cum] | foculo, sedes posu[it p(ecunia) s(ua)].

Trans.: "Alfia Quarta, daughter of Publius, built the woman's bath from the ground up; she also, at her own expense, adorned it with variously colored stone and placed in it a bronze *labrum* along with a stove and seats."

NOTES: This inscription is noteworthy for its detail about bath terminology. *Foculus* can mean "brazier," but it is expressly associated with the *labrum* here, so it probably refers to a stove for heating the *labrum*'s water supply. This text may date to the period of Marruvium's greatest growth, during the end of the Republic and the early Empire. The terse wording of the text supports this proposition. Remains of baths are known at Marruvium, but they are insufficiently investigated to allow any conclusions to be drawn about them; see Coarelli and La Regina, *Abruzzo*, 100–101.

152   Novianus or Novius. Casinum (Regio I). Undated (but possibly Hadrianic). *CIL* 10.5200.

The full text is cited at no. 125. Here note the portion that reads:

. . . therm⟨a⟩e Noviani | nobis in usu sunt restitutae . . .

NOTES: The main benefaction (a restoration) dates to the mid- to late fourth century. The builder may have been called Novius rather than Novianus, and a freedman named C. Novius Philemon is attested at the site (*CIL* 10.5269). If the Novii were indeed responsible for these baths, *Thermae Novianae* may here be corrupted to *Thermae Noviani*. Another possibility is that an adoptee out of the Novius family is denoted. The family appears to have been of decurional status. For the physical remains, apparently with a Hadrianic core, see Carettoni, *Casinum*, 99–101. Coarelli (*Lazio*, 217–25) reports no significant ruins of this building.

153   L. Cluvienus Cilo. Bergomum (Regio XI). Undated (but possibly high Imperial). *CIL* 5.5136.

L. Cluvienus L. f. Ani. | Cilo | balneum et | aquas dedit.

NOTES: The inscription is executed *litteris maximis et pulcherrimis (CIL)*, suggesting a high Imperial date. Here *dedit* most probably means "built." The identity and status of the benefactor are not known.

Montanus. Tarraco, Hispania Tarraconensis. Undated (but before the late third or   154
early fourth century). *CIL* 2.4112 = *ILER* 1306.

The full text is cited at no. 28. Here note the portion that reads:

. . . restitutori | thermarum Montanarum . . .

NOTES: These baths were probably named after their builder. One L. Numisius Montanus is
attested at Tarraco in the Hadrianic period as an *omnibus honoribus functus* (Curchin, 226 [no.
907]) but beyond the coincidence of the nomenclature, there is nothing to tie this man to the
baths. It is also conceivable that the name of the baths means "Mountain Baths," in an obscure
reference, perhaps, to some feature of the building (its size, location, decoration, or a view from
the building?).

Sabinus. Telesia (Regio II). Undated (but before 352/57). *CIL* 9.2212 = *ILS* 5690 (see   155
also *AE* 1972.150).

The full text is cited at no. 31. Here note the portion that reads:

. . . thermas | Sabinianas restituit . . .

NOTES: *Sabinus* is a very common Roman cognomen, making identification of this benefactor
all but impossible.

Frumentius. Tigava, Mauretania. Undated (but possibly late Imperial). *CIL* 8.21497   156†
= *ILS* 5705.

tu modo, Frumenti, | domito virtute | rebelli | respicis ac reparas | dumis contecta |
lavacra.

Trans.: "You, Frumentius, a rebel lately tamed by virtue, cared for and repaired the
lavacra that were covered with briars."

NOTES: This is a mosaic inscription found in the ruins of baths. If the term *lavacra* denotes the
whole complex, a late Imperial date is suggested; but the word may refer to a specific part of the
building; see notes to no. 13. The wording also suggests that Frumentius had led a dissolute life
before displaying his civic-mindedness in his bath repair.

L. Betilienus Vaarus. Aletrium (Regio I). Late second century B.C. *CIL* 1².1529 = *CIL*   157†
10.5807 = *ILS* 5348 = *ILLRP* 528.

L. Betilienus L. f. Vaarus | haec quae infera scripta | sont de senatu sententia | facienda
coiravit: semitas | in oppido omnis, porticum qua | in arcem eitur, campum ubei |
ludunt, horologium, macelum, | basilicam calecandam, seedes, | [l]acum balinearium,
lacum ad | [p]ortam, aquam in opidum adqu(e) | arduom pedes CCCXL fornicesq(ue)
| fecit, fistulas soledas fecit. | ob hasce res censorem fecere bis, | senatus filio stipendia
mereta ese iousit populusque | statuam donavit Censorino.

Trans.: "L. Betilienus Vaarus, son of Lucius, saw to the construction of the buildings
listed below, in accordance with a decree of the senate. He made all the paths in the
town, the portico that leads to the arch, the field where the people exercise, the clock,
the market, the whitewashing of the basilica, the seats, the pool of the baths, the pool
near the gate; he ran the aqueduct for 340 feet into the town and the steep, he made
the arches, and he reinforced the pipes. On account of these deeds, he was twice
censor, the senate ordered his son exempted from military service, and the people gave
a statue to Censorinus."

NOTES: This inscription is difficult but informative. It has been dated to the late second century B.C. and is certainly pre-Sullan, since Aletrium lost its senate during the Sullan campaigns of the Social War. The list of Betilienus' works is interesting in itself, but note especially the *lacus balinearius*, a feature of unclear function. It may have been some sort of *natatio*, either associated with a bathhouse (although they are more commonly found in baths of a later age) or standing independently. Alternatively, the phrase may denote a pool for supplying a bathhouse, tantamount to a well or reservoir. Since public troughs are regularly termed *lacus* in Frontinus—and one is mentioned in the present text as being near a gate of the town—perhaps the *lacus balnearius* was such a trough located in or near the bathhouse. For another Republican *lacus*, not expressly associated with a bathhouse, see *CIL* 1².2099 = *ILLRP* 615 (Interamna Naharis; post-Sullan). An undated text from Pitinum Pisaurense, documenting numerous alterations to a bathhouse or bathhouses, also mentions a *lacus* (no. 50). Another uncertainty in the present inscription is who exactly was responsible for the work. There is no formula, such as *s(ua) p(ecunia)* or *p(ecunia) p(ublica)*, to indicate who incurred the cost of the undertakings. Betilienus is said to have acted in accordance with a decree of the local authorities, which points to the agency of the local community. But for his actions, he earns great kudos: two censorships, a new name (Censorinus), exemption from military service for his son, a public statue for himself, and this commemorative inscription. Given all this, Betilienus was probably acting alone, with the decree of the local senate putting an official stamp of approval on his personal construction program. Finally, he is not credited with holding any offices before the censorships he earned for his benefactions, which suggests he was acting as a private benefactor when he undertook the various constructions listed. No remains of the baths are known, although Coarelli (*Lazio*, 196–98), who believes *lacus balnearius* means "la piscina per i bagni," speculates that the establishment may have been suburban.

158   L. Turcilius Rufus. Murcia, Hispania Tarraconensis. Augustan (?) (possibly later). *CIL* 2.3542 = *ILER* 2046.

L. Turcilius P. f. | Rufus | [ther]mas [f]ec(it).

NOTES: The inscription was found among the ruins of baths. The Augustan date, assigned on the basis of letterform by Mommsen, would make this use of the word *thermae* the earliest of which I am aware (see above, chapter 1, p. 17). Realistically, however, the inscription could date to any time in the first century.

159†*   Incertus, praefectus Aegypt[i et] Terentia A. f. mater eiu[s et] Cosconia Lentulii *(sic)* Malug[inensis f.] Gallitta uxor eius. Volsinii (Regio VII). Early to mid–first century. *CIL* 11.7285 = *ILS* 8996.

[—] | praefectus Aegypt[i, et] | Terentia A. f. mater eiu[s, et] | Cosconia Lentulii *(sic)* Malug[inensis f.] | Gallitta uxor eius, ae[dificiis] | emptis et ad solum de[iectis] | balneum cum omn[i ornatu | Volsiniens]ibus ded[erunt | ob publ]ica c[ommoda].

Trans.: "[?], prefect of Egypt, and Terentia, daughter of Aulus, his mother, and Cosconia Gallita, daughter of Lentulus Maluginensis, his wife, having purchased the buildings on the site and demolished them, gave the bathhouse with all its decoration to the Volsinians, for the sake of public convenience."

NOTES: Because the male benefactor here is reported to have been a *praefectus Aegypti*, his identity has been proposed as L. Seius Strabo, the father of L. Aelius Sejanus, the infamous native of Volsinii who was praetorian prefect under Tiberius (Tac. *Ann.* 4.1.3); see, e.g., *AE* 1983.398. G.V. Sumner ("The Family Connections of L. Aelius Seianus," *Phoenix* 19 [1965]: 134–39) makes a strong case for the identification here of C. Caecina Tuscus (praetorian prefect in 55; prefect of Egypt in 63–64). The issue remains unresolved: see M. Corbier, "La famille de

Séjan à Volsinii: la dédicace des Seii, *curatores aquae*," *MEFRA* 95 (1983): 748–53; Thomasson, 1.343 (no. 13). Whether Strabo or Caecina, the man is acting as a benefactor of his native town. The *dederunt* here clearly denotes an act of construction, as it is stated that the buildings that stood on the site were bought and demolished to make room for the baths (not an uncommon practice; see Merten, 11–15). An ill-investigated set of baths near the forum is associated with this facility: see P. Gros, *Bolsena: Guide des fouilles* (Paris, 1981), 43; Manderscheid, 82, s.v. "Bolsena/Volsinii, Thermes dits de L. Seius Strabo"; Torelli, *Etruria*, 219 (who attributes the work to Caecina Tuscus).

M. Nigidius Vaccula. Pompeii (Regio I). Mid–first century (before ca. 54). *CIL* 10.818.   160

M. Nigidius Vaccula p(ecunia) s(ua).

NOTES: This text is inscribed on braziers found in the Forum Baths and Stabian Baths in Pompeii. Vaccula appears to have died around 54, but little is known of this member of an influential local family; see Castrén, *Ordo,* 195 (no. 266.3).

T. Claudius Faustus Regi[n(us)] et Claudia Nais. Coela, Thrace. 55. *CIL* 3.7380 = *ILS* 5682.   161†*

numini domus Augustae | T. Claudius Faustus Regi[n(us)] et | Claudia Nais Fausti | balneum populo et familiai | Caesaris n(ostri) d(e) [s(ua)] p(ecunia) f(ecerunt) idemque | aquam in eius balnei usus | perduxerunt et consacrarunt | [Nerone] Caesare Aug. et Antistio Vetere | cos.

Trans.: "To the spirit of the Augustan household. T. Claudius Faustus Reginus and Claudia Nais, wife of Faustus, built the bathhouse for the people and *familia* of our Caesar at their own expense. They also supplied water for the use of this bath and consecrated it when Nero Caesar Augustus and Antistius Vetus were consuls *(i.e., 55)."*

L. Rufellius Severus, p(rimi)p(ilaris), tr(ibunus). Fanum Fortunae (Regio VI). First century or earlier (?). *CIL* 11.6225 = *ILS* 5679.   162

The full text is cited at no. 73/74. Here note the portion that reads:

. . . balineum á L. Rufellio Severo p(rimo)p(ilari), tr(ibuno), factum . . .

NOTES: The main benefaction, a restoration, is tentatively dated to the first century. Rufellius' initial construction must have taken place earlier, perhaps even in the Republic, since a total of two restorations are recorded as having been carried out on the building before the main repair.

Incertus, Pacati f(ilius). Andemantunnum, Germania Superior. First century (?). *CIL* 13.5687.   163

[—]i Pacati f. | [—]anae f. calil[darium cum s]uis ornaml[entis —] s(ua) p(ecunia) p(erfecit). l(oco) d(ato) d(ecucrionum) d(ecreto).

NOTES: Although this text is fragmentary, enough survives to make clear that a bath benefaction was involved and that the benefactor, with no identifiable offices, was probably a private citizen. Date is by letterform.

T. Flavius Mythus, Aug(usti) lib(ertus) and Flavia Diogis. Capena (Regio VII). Late first or early second century. *CIL* 11.3932 = *ILS* 5770.   164†*

T. Flavio T. f. Quir. Flaviano, | aedili, quaestori designato | municipio Capenae foederato, | T. Flavius Aug. lib. Mythus et | Flavia Diogis parentes filio piissimo |

fecerunt et sibi et suis libertis libertabusq(ue) | utriusque sexus posterisque eorum | cum balneo et aedificis quae sunt iuncta | ex utraque parte secus viam cum aquae | ductu ex fundo Cutuleniano et iugera | agri Cutuleniani p(lus) m(inus) IIII ita ut depalatum est. h(oc) m(onumentum) h(eredem) n(on) s(equitur).

Trans.: "To T. Flavius Flavianus, son of Titus, of the voting tribe Quirina, aedile, quaestor designate in the federated town of Capena. T. Flavius Mythus, freedman of the emperor, and Flavia Diogis, his parents, made (this monument) for their most dutiful son, themselves, their freedpeople of both sexes, and their descendants, along with the bath and the buildings that adjoin it on both sides fronting the street, the aqueduct that comes out of the property of Cutulenus, and the approximately four *iugera* of the farm of Cutulenus as it is staked out. This monument does not pass to the heir."

NOTES: Nielsen (1.40 n. 25) dates this inscription to the late first century; the names of the imperial freedpeople suggest a Flavian date. The wording of this inscription is odd, in that the section featuring the bathhouse is uncomfortably incorporated into what is an otherwise straightforward epitaph. The most reasonable explanation for its appearance is that Mythus and Flavia wished to remind people of their civic benefactions, namely, the bath, the buildings adjoining it, its aqueduct, and the demarcation of a certain plot of land, possibly the location of the springs that fed the aqueduct. Despite the complexity and size of some Roman funerary monuments, the baths are not likely to have been part of the tomb (see H. von Hesberg, *Römische Grabbauten* [Darmstadt, 1992], esp. 164–201); indeed, their location at Capena itself is not readily apparent, since Capena's *territorium* contained many settlements; see G. Gazzetti, *Il territorio capenate* (Rome, 1992). Furthermore, the site of Capena has not been extensively excavated and is known primarily through field surveys: see M.C. Mazzi, ed., *Capena e il suo territorio* (Bari, 1995), 23–144; Torelli, *Etruria,* 39–41. Given all this, the site of the baths referred to here remains unknown.

165†*   Voconia Avita. Tagilis, Baetica. Late first or early second century. *AE* 1979.352.

Voconia Q. f. Avita | thermas reipublicae | suae Tagilitanae s(olo) s(uo) s(ua) p(ecunia) f(ecit) | easdemque circensibus | edi(t)is e(t) epulo dato dedicavit | at quot opus tuendum usumq(ue) | perpetuum [t]hermarum praebandum | r(ei) p(ublicae) Tagilitanae d(enariorum) duo milia q(uingentos) dedi(t).

Trans.: "Voconia Avita, daughter of Quintus, built baths for her city of Tagilis on her own land and at her own expense. She dedicated the baths and gave races and a meal. Toward the maintenance of the building and the perpetual use of the baths, she gave to the city of Tagilis twenty-five hundred denarii."

NOTES: It is unclear if the "perpetual use" of the baths included a benefaction of free bathing. If so, it is unusually worded here (compare nos. 197–213).

166   Iu[rat]h⟨a⟩n [?]giaduris f[il]ius. Sabratha, Tripolitania. Late first or early second century. *AE* 1980.900.

dom(i)no Sapurno vico M[. . .]no v(oto) s(uscepto) Iu[rat]h⟨a⟩n [?]giaduris f(ilius) f(ecit).

NOTES: This inscription is found on a *labrum* discovered in 1973 and featuring two texts, one neo-Punic (on the interior) and one Latin (on the rim). The latter is cited above; for comparable *labrum* inscriptions, see nos. 68 and 75. It is clear from the nomenclature that the benefactor was of local African origin, and since no offices are listed, he seems to have been acting as a private citizen. *Sapurno* stands for *Saturno*. Iurathan's name can be postulated from the neo-Punic text, which mentions him. The *labrum* may have originated outside Sabratha proper, possibly from a sanctuary. Whatever the case, baths are the most likely context for it. For an overview of the city's development, see D.J. Mattingly, *Tripolitania* (Ann Arbor, 1994), 125–27.

Cives Romani. Sexaginta Prista, Moesia Inferior. 100. *AE* 1966.356.   167

imp. Cae[s. Nervae Traiano Aug.] | Ger., p[ont. max., tr. pot., cos., . . . p. p.] | per M.' Lab[erium Maximum Quintium?] | C[rispinu]m, [leg. Aug. pr. pr.], | cives Roman[i consistentes] Sexaginta Pri[st(is) balneum?] | cura ag[ente] | C. Anton[io . . . f(ecerunt)?].

NOTES: Laberius was *consul ordinarius* in 103 and was killed under Hadrian on suspicion of conspiracy: see *PIR*[2] L 9; Thomasson, 1.131 (no. 66). The name of this place means "Sixty Boats" and reveals the importance of the river to its economy. Here the Roman citizens of the place built a bath. The question is, was it reserved for their exclusive use (see above, chapter 8, n. 53)?

Fabius, Sergius, and Putin[ius?]. Altinum (Regio X). Post-100 (and earlier). G. Brusin,   168/169†
"Grado: Nuove epigrafi romane e cristiane," *NSc*, 1928, 283.

[—] | d(ecurionum) d(ecreto). | [h]ic rei p(ublicae) Altinatium HS *(1,600,000)* [n(ummum] ded(it) | [i]ta ut balinea Sergium et Puti[nium] | HS *(800,000)* n(ummum) refecta in usu mu[nicip(um) *or* municip(ii)] | essent et alia HS *(400,000)* n(ummum), ut ex [eorum] | reditu cale[fier]ent, et HS *(200,000)* n(ummum) [in perp(etuam)] | tutelam eo[ru]mdem *(sic)*, item HS [*(200,000)* n(ummum)] | ut ex usuris eorum VII idus [. . .] | natali ipsius et VII idus eas[dem] | natali Petroniae Magnae ma[tris] | suae, XVII kal(endas) Ian(uarias) natali L. Fabii St[ellat(ina)] | Amminiani patris sui decurio[nes | Au]g(ustales) et seviri sportulas acci[perent].

Trans.: "*(the text is missing the opening line[s])* . . . by decree of the decurions. This man gave 1,600,000 sesterces to the city of Altinum, in such a way that the Baths of Sergius and the Baths of Putinius be repaired with 800,000 sesterces and be available for the use of the town; so that from the return on another 400,000 sesterces the baths be heated and maintained in perpetuity with 200,000 sesterces. Likewise, he gave 200,000 sesterces so that from the return on this sum, the decurions, Augustales, and *seviri* receive cash handouts on the 7th (*or* 9th) of *[month missing]*, his birthday, and on the same day of that month, the birthday of Petronia Magna, his mother, and on the 16th of December, the birthday of his father, L. Fabius Amminianus, of the voting tribe Stellatina."

NOTES: For a photograph of this inscription, see fig. 26E. The date given above for this inscription follows that assigned by Duncan-Jones (*Economy*, 160 [no. 468]), on the basis of the criteria he lays out in op. cit., 362–63. Nielsen (1.122) opts for a post-160 date for the main Fabian benefactions, but she does not explain her reasoning. Two phases of benefaction are commemorated here: (1) the initial construction of the baths by Sergius and Putinius and (2) the multiple benefactions of Fabius at some later date. If Fabius' actions do indeed date to the earlier part of the second century, the original construction of the baths took place probably in the first century or possibly in the Republic. As the wording *Balinea Sergium et Puti[nium]* makes clear, two separate buildings are denoted here—i.e., a *Balineum Sergium* and a *Balineum Puti[nium]*. The identity of these men is otherwise unknown, and nothing is known of the baths themselves; see Mangani, Rebecchi, and Strazzulla, *Emilia*, 192–93.

170†   Q. Solonus Fabius Severinus, e(gregius) v(ir). Nemausus, Gallia Narbonensis. Post-100. *CIL* 12.3165b = *ILS* 5680.

honóri | Q. Solóni Fabi Severini, e. v., | ob merita eius praeterita et | praesentem liberalitatem | quo mátúrius balneum úsibus | plebis exhiberétur, fabri tign(uarii) Nem(ausenses).

Trans.: "The carpenters of Nemausus for the esteem of Q. Solonus Fabius Severinus, *egregius vir,* on account of his (giving) past services and prompt generosity, so that the bath might be opened more quickly for the use of the plebs."

NOTES: The date is suggested by the fullness of Severinus' nomenclature (see Duncan-Jones, *Economy,* 362–63). The sense of the inscription is that Solonus hastened the completion of the baths. The work may have been a restoration, but in that case we might expect a verb like *reddere* rather than *exhibere.* Given the wording, completion of a construction project already in progress is the most likely context; compare, e.g., nos. 6, 106, 111, 127, 132, 176, 184 (note also no. 133). The text can also be read as meaning that the baths were reserved for the use of plebs (see Nielsen, 1.146 n. 2). This meaning is unlikely, since mention of the plebs serves chiefly to designate the beneficiaries of Severinus' *liberalitas,* as is typical for such euergetistic commemorations, rather than to indicate the exclusive identity of the baths' clientele. Since the dedicants, the carpenters of the town, were plebs themselves, mention of the plebs in the text is hardly surprising. Moreover, there is no clear evidence for social segregation among bathing facilities; see above, chapter 8, pp. 206–12. For the epigraphic form *tignuarius,* compare *CIL* 3.611 = *ILS* 7188, 6.6365.

171†   C. Plinius Caecilius [Secundus, cos.]. Comum (Regio XI). Ca. 100/109. *CIL* 5.5262 = *ILS* 2927.

C. Plinius L. f. Ouf. Caecilius [Secundus cos.,] | augur, legat. pro pr. provinciae Pon[ti et Bithyniae] | consulari potesta[t.] in eam provinciam e[x s.c. missus ab] | imp. Caesar. Nerva Traiano Aug. German[ico Dacico p. p.,] | curator alvei Ti[b]eris et riparum e[t cloacar. urb.,] | praef. aerari Satu[r]ni, praef. aerari mil[it., pr., trib. pl.,] | quaestor imp., sevir equitum [Romanorum,] | trib. milit. leg. [III] Gallica[e, Xvir stli]ltib. iudicand., ther[mas ex HS—] adiectis in | ornatum HS *(300,000)* [— et eo ampl]lius in tutela[m] | HS *(200,000)* t(estamento) f(ieri) i(ussit), [item in alimenta] libertor(um) suorum homin(um) C. | HS *(1,866,666)* rei [p(ublicae) legavit, quorum in]crement(o) postea ad epulum | [pl]eb(is) urban(ae) voluit pertin[ere ..4.. item vivu]s dedit in aliment(a) pueror(um) | et puellar(um) pleb(is) urban(ae) HS [*(500,000),* item bybliothecam et] in tutelam bybliothecae HS *(100,000).*

Trans.: "C. Plinius Secundus, son of Lucius, of the voting tribe Oufentina, consul, augur, propraetorian legate of the province of Pontus and Bithynia who was sent to that province with consular power, following a vote of the senate, by the emperor Caesar Nerva Trajan Augustus Germanicus, conqueror of Dacia, father of his country, he was curator of the river Tiber's channel and banks and of the sewers of the city, prefect of the treasury of Saturn, prefect of the military treasury, praetor, tribune of the plebs, quaestor of the emperor, *sevir* of the Roman *equites,* military tribune of Legion III Gallica, *decemvir* for judging cases, ordered in his will that baths be constructed from *(amount lost)* sesterces and that a further 300,000 sesterces be added for their decoration and another 200,000 sesterces for their upkeep. He also bequeathed 1,866,666 sesterces to the city for the support of his one hundred freedmen, the increase of which he wished put toward a banquet for the urban plebs thereafter, *[lacuna].* While alive, he gave 500,000 sesterces for the support of boys and girls of the urban plebs, and he gave 100,000 sesterces for the library and its upkeep."

NOTES: The benefactor is Pliny the Younger. Although the inscription is fragmentary, Pliny's bath benefactions are clear. A putative bath building has been located at Comum, but it has not been adequately investigated; see Cavalieri Manasse, Massari, and Rossignani, *Piemonte,* 331.

L. Min[icius Na]talis, cos. and L. Minicius [Natalis Quadro]nius Verus, augur,   172
trib(unus) plebis desig(natus). Barcino, Hispania Tarraconensis. Ca. 120. *CIL* 2.4509
= *CIL* 2.6145 = *ILS* 1029.

L. Min[icius L. fil. Gal. Na]talis cos., procos. | provinc. [Africae, sodalis Augus]tális, lég. Aug. pr. pr. divi Traiálni Par[thici et imp. Traiani Ha]driáni Aug. provinc. Pan-|nonia[e Inf.], curator a]lvei Tiberis et ripárum et | cloacar[um urbis, leg. divi Tra]iání Parthici leg. III Aug., leg. dilvi Traia[ni Parthici leg. — doni]s donátus expeditióne Dácic[a] | prima, a[b eodem imperatore] coróná válári múráli aurea, | has[tis puris III, vexillis III, l]ég. pr. pr. provinc. Africae, pr., | trib. pl., q. p[rov. — , IIIIvi]r. viárum curandarum, et | L. Minicius L. f. [Natalis Quadro]nius Vérus f., augur, trib. plébis | desig., q. Aug. et [eodem tempore leg. p]r. pr. patris provinc. Africae, tr. | mil. leg. I Adiut. p. f., l[eg. XI Cl. p. f., leg. XIIII Ma]rt. Vic., IIIvir monetalis a(ere) a(argento) a(uro) f(lando) f(eriundo), | balineum c[um port]icibus solo suo et | du[ctus aquae] fécerunt.

NOTES: The two benefactors are father and son, who, as the inscription says, had extensive service records under Trajan and Hadrian. The father had reached the suffect consulship in 106 and the proconsulate of Africa (see *PIR*² M 619; Thomasson, 1.380 [no. 70]), while the son's highest post at the time the text was carved was *tribunus plebis designatus* (see *PIR*² M 620); the latter was later to leave one hundred thousand sesterces to Barcino in his will (*CIL* 2.4511). Clearly, both men are acting here as private benefactors, in the guise of local scions who did well in the imperial service; see the comments of H.-G. Pflaum in *REA* 76 (1974): 413 (a review of S.M. Bigorra, *Inscripciones romanas de Barcelona (lapidarias y musivas)* [Barcelona, 1973]).

[Ser. Cornelius Dolabella Metilianus Pompeius Mar]cel[l]us, IIIvir a(ere) a(rgento)   173
a(uro) f(lando) f(eriundo). Corfinium (Regio IV). Ca. 120 (?). *CIL* 9.3153.

[Ser. Cornelius Dolabella Metilianus Pompeius Mar]cel[l]us, IIIvir a(ere) a(rgento) a(uro) f(lando) f(eriundo), s[alius Palatinus, — | —] balineum solo suo s(ua) p(ec-unia) ae[dificavit — | — Ser. Co]rneli Dolabellae Metiliani in ho[norem — | —] curam agente L. Venetio L. f. [—].

NOTES: A note in *SuppItal* 3 (1987): 112 (*ad* 3153) dates this inscription to the mid–second century. Dolabella is also honored in the following entry and was suffect consul in 113 (see *PIR*² C 1350). This bathhouse may, however, have been separate from that commemorated in no. 174, since it appears to have been completed when Dolabella was still alive, and since the work was supervised by a different person (L. Venetius here, C. Alfius Maximus in no. 174). Alter-natively, the two inscriptions may commemorate different phases of the same project, as is assumed in *PIR*² (loc. cit.) and *SuppItal* (loc. cit.). If so, it is noteworthy that the baths were opened and dedicated while still some way from completion. Since the texts were not found in situ, the problem cannot be resolved with any certainty. The incompleteness of the current text leaves much of Dolabella's career missing, so it is impossible to say at what stage he undertook this particular project. However, the mention of *in honorem* in the last line may refer to Dolabella's co-option as *patronus;* if so, the project dates to after Trajan's death, perhaps around 120. Compare *CIL* 9.3154 = *ILS* 1049, which provides his full career: *IIIvir(o) a(ere) a(rgento)*

a(uro) f(lando) f(eriundo), | *salio Palat(ino), quaestori* | *divi Traiani Parthici*, | *sevir(o) equit(um)*
Rom(anorum) turm(ae) | *III, pr(aetori), co(n)s(uli), flam(eni) Quir(itum)*, | *Corfinienses publice*
patrono. If any physical remains are known, they have yet to be fully investigated; see Coarelli
and La Regina, *Abruzzo,* 118–27.

174†   Ser. Cornelius Dolabella Metilianus, cos., M. Atilius Bradua, cos., M'. Acilius Aviola,
cos. Corfinium (Regio IV). Post-122. *CIL* 9.3152 = *ILS* 5676.

Ser. Cornelius Ser. f. Dolabella Metilianus, cos., | balineum solo suo s(ua) p(ecunia)
aedificavit et contexit. | M. Atilius Bradua, cos., et M'. Acilius Aviola, cos., bonor(um)
possessor(es) | Dolabellae Metialiani, in hoc opus dederunt HS centena mil(ia) n(um-
mum) | res p(ublica) et populus Corfiniensis datis HS CLII (i.e., *152,000*) n(ummum)
consummavit, curam agente | [C. Alfio] T. f. Ser. Maximo.

Trans.: "Ser. Cornelius Dolabella Metilianus, son of Servius, consul, built and roofed
the bath on his own land at his own expense. M. Atilius Bradua, consul, and M'.'
Acilius Aviola, consul, users of the estate of Dolabella Metialianus, gave 100,000
sesterces to this work; the city and people of Corfinium spent 152,000 sesterces on it.
C. Alfius Maximus, son of Titus, of the voting tribe Sergia, supervised the work."

NOTES: This benefaction may be a continuation of the project commemorated in the previous
entry. Bradua was consul in 108 (*PIR*² A 1302), Aviola in 122 (*PIR*² A 50), so the text postdates
the latter date. C. Alfius Maximus is mentioned in another inscription (*CIL* 9.3168 = *ILS*
5417b), which records that he bequeathed money for various works. Although the local council
got involved in the completion of the baths, Dolabella is clearly credited with initiating this
project, either his second bath construction at Corfinium or a single effort that spanned many
years (see previous entry). There is a possibility that the final sum is *CIII* rather than *CLII,*
reducing the city's contribution from 152,000 sesterces to 103,000.

175†   Incertus. Tarraco, Hispania Tarraconensis. Second century (possibly Hadrianic). *CIL*
2.6102.

These fragmentary remains of a funerary eulogium of an unnamed benefactor read, in
part:

(4) [extremum hoc munus hab]ere mereris, qui per te ipse pl[enis mune]ribus cives
tuos reddid]isti, quibus tu saepe placuisti [liberalitate | balneas aedificasti, insti]tuisti
nymphas calidas, qua[drigis | forum exornasti d]uabus . . .

Trans.: "'You deserve to have this utmost tribute, you who, through your own
efforts, repaid your citizens with full services; you often pleased them with your
generosity. You built the baths, you installed the heated *nymphae,* and you adorned
the forum with two four-horsed chariots . . .'"

NOTES: Fine letter quality implies a date of high prosperity, possibly Hadrianic, but most
probably sometime in the second century. Baths can be inferred by the presence of the phrase
[insti]tuisti nymphas calidas, since *nymphae calidae* (a poetic designation for "heated water")
were most likely found in a bathhouse; nevertheless, the construction of baths is not a certainty
in this instance.

176   P. Tullius [Varro], pater, cos. and [L. Dasumius Tullius Tuscus]. Tarquinii (Regio VII).
Mid–second century (post-161?). *CIL* 11.3366.

[th]ermas municipi [—]s quas P. Tullius, | pater eius, cos., Au[g. legato, s]estertio ter.
et tr.| testamento f[ieri iussi]t adiecta pecunia | ampliatoqu[e ope]re perfecit.

NOTES: The father is the consular P. Tullius Varro. The date of his consulship is disputed: Groag (*RE* 7A.1326–29, s.v. "Tullius 57") locates it sometime in the early second century, perhaps in 108 or 109, while Degrassi (37) dates it to 127. Varro's son, probably named in the lacuna in the opening line, was adopted by a Dasumius who cannot be securely identified but who was dead by 108, since his will of that date survives in a mutilated inscription from Rome (*CIL* 6.10229 = *ILS* 8379a; see also *PIR*² D 13). The will made Varro's son Dasumius' heir in the first degree, on the condition that he adopt Dasumius' name. The problem lies in identifying the son, the main benefactor here. A body of opinion supports the identification of L. Dasumius Tullius Tuscus, consul in 152 (*PIR*² D 16); see Duncan-Jones, *Economy,* 157 (no. 445 and note). Another inscription from these baths honors this man (*CIL* 11.3365 = *ILS* 1081), making the identification seem more secure. Groag (*RE* 7A.1328), however, believes this identification to be mistaken, since, he argues, the dates do not add up: a gap of forty-four years falls between the adoption of L. Dasumius Tullius Tuscus in 108 and his consulship in 152. Instead, Groag (*PIR*² D 15) prefers an identification of the son as P. Dasumius Rusticus, consul in 119; in Groag's reconstruction, L. Dasumius Tullius Tuscus was possibly L. Dasumius Rusticus' natural son (see *PIR*² D 15). This debate bears on the date of the work, since if L. Dasumius Rusticus was indeed Varro's natural son, he would have built the bath in the early second century, while if L. Dasumius Tullius Tuscus was the son in question, a date in the middle of the century is to be preferred. The evidence, as it stands, seems to be against Groag's suggestion. The gap of forty-four years between adoption and consulship for L. Dasumius Tullius Tuscus is not insuperable: Dasumius could have adopted Varro's son while he was still a child. Furthermore, five honorary inscriptions were found together in one room of these baths. Aside from our current inscription, one honors L. Dasumius Tullius Tuscus (cited above) and dates to sometime after 161 (he is named as *sodalis Antoninianus*). The other honorands are P. Tullius Varro, the man who is reported in the current inscription as having bequeathed 330,000 sesterces for the baths in his will (*CIL* 11.3364 = *ILS* 1047); Q. Petronius Melior, who restored the baths sometime after 230 (no. 24); and Domitia Melpis, wife of Q. Petronius Melior (*CIL* 11.3368). Although an *argumentum ex silentio,* the absence of L. Dasumius Rusticus, the man Groag identifies as the main bath builder commemorated in the current inscription, is curious. I offer one final comment: as noted above, Degrassi dates Varro's consulship to 127, so his death and bequest probably date to the mid–second century and secure the identification of L. Dasumius Tullius Tuscus as Varro's natural son; if this identification is accepted, a date of the mid–second century is to be preferred for this construction work.

Arruntius Granianus (?). Tifernum Tiberinum (Regio VII). Ca. 170. *CIL* 11.5939 =   177†
ILS 5678.

[— statuas?] sibi et fil. suo Ne|[p]o[t]i ex HS *(60,000)* n(ummum) poni iussit | et ob dedicatione earum | dec(urionibus) *(denarios)* V, VIvir(is) *(denarios)* III, pleb(i) *(denarios)* II | dari iussit; item reliquit | ad balinei fabrica(m) rei p(ublicae) | Tif(er-natium) Tib(erinorum) HS *(150,000)* n(ummum), quae ex sen|tentia Aemili Front-onis, | cl. vir., postea deinde Arri | Antonini, cl. vir., rei p(ublicae) Tif(ernatium) Tib(erinorum) | ab Cipellis Profuturo et Pi|centino her(edibus) et ab Arruntia | Am-piana her(ede) Arrunti Grania|ni numerata sunt. her(edes) posuer(unt) | l(oco) d(ato) d(ecreto) d(ecurionum).

Trans.: *"(the text is missing the opening line[s])* . . . he ordered (statues?) put up to himself and his son Nepos from 60,000 sesterces, and on the occasion of their dedication, he ordered that five denarii be given to each of the councillors, three denarii to the *seviri,* and two denarii to the commoners. He also left 150,000 sesterces to the city of Tifernum Tiberinum for the building of a bath. Following the rulings of Aemilius Fronto, of senatorial rank, and afterward of Arrius Antoninus, of senatorial

rank, this sum was payed out to the city of Tifernum Tiberinum by Cipellus Pro-
futurus, Cipellus Picentinus, and Arruntia Ampiana, heirs of Arruntius Granianus.
The heirs set up this monument. Space given by decree of the councillors."

NOTES: This acephalous inscription records the provisions of the will of a benefactor whose
name is lost but who, on the basis of the closing lines, was probably named Arruntius Granianus. In his will, the benefactor bequeathed to the town 150,000 sesterces for the construction
of a bath. This provision was then contested by the heirs, and a decision on the dispute was
reached by Aemilius Fronto and Arrius Antoninus, officials under M. Aurelius (see *PIR*² A 349,
1088). Their status is unclear. Duncan-Jones (*Economy*, 157 [no. 447]), who also supplies the
date offered above, suggests that they were successive *iuridici* for this region of Italy (on *iuridici*,
see Simshäuser, "Entstehung," 426–33). Camodeca ("Ricerche," 460–61) considers them successive *curatores rei publicae* of the city, while *PIR* makes no judgment either way. In defense of
Duncan-Jones, however, it does seem odd that these men are not named here as *curatores*, a post
with special local significance as opposed to the more distant *iuridici*. Putative remains of a bath,
dated to the second century, are known at the site; see Gaggiotti et al., *Umbria*, 170.

178   Flavius Catullus. Epamanduodurum, Germania Superior. Second century (?). *CIL*
       13.5416/17.

Cited here are two fragments of the same inscription, restored as a single text (following that offered in *CIL*).

Flav[ius Ca]tullus | testam[ento ad marmora]ndum balineum legavit r(ei) p(ublicae)
(denarios) (75,000) | quod C. F[lavius Ga]llus her(es) p(erficiendum?) c(uravit) |
[vicesi]mis et tributis | legati s(upra) s(cripti) | [ad co]nsummátiónem.

NOTES: This inscription is dated by letterform. Here, seventy-five thousand denarii (three
hundred thousand sesterces) is left to the local community for decorating the baths with marble,
with the work to be overseen by Catullus' son and heir, C. F[lavius G]allus. The meaning of
tributa here is unclear, but it has some connection with the bequests, as does the *vicesima*, a five-
percent tax levied on bequests following a law of Augustus (see Dio 55.25.1–6; Pliny *Pan.* 37.1;
Simshäuser, "Entstehung," 410).

179*   Marcia Aurelia Ceionia Demetrias, stolata femina. Anagnia (Regio IV). Late second
       century. *CIL* 10.5918 = *ILS* 406.

Marciae Aurel. | Ceioniae Deme|triadi, stolatae feminae, ob dedicationem | ther-
marum, quas post mul|tum temporis ad pristinam | faciem suis sumptibus restau-
|raverunt, s(enatus) p(opulus)q(ue) Anagnin(orum) | statuam ponendam censuerunt; |
o[b] cuius dedicationim *(sic)* dedit decuri|onibus *(denarios)* V, sivir(is) *(sic) (denarios)*
II, popul(o) *(denarios)* sing(ulos), | et epulum sufficiens omnib(us).

NOTES: This inscription is on a statue base from Anagnia, commemorating the same benefaction as that recorded in no. 95. The plural *restauraverunt* makes it clear that Marcia did not act
alone in the restoration, and it probably alludes to the participation of M. Aurelius Sabinianus
Euhodus, who was probably her father (see *PIR*² M 261 for Marcia, a concubine of Commodus
later involved in his murder; see HA *Comm.* 8.6, 17.1–2). It is possible that both statues stood
side by side in their original context and so should be read together, but it is not clear why
Sabinianus' inscription makes no mention of Marcia's input, while this text implicitly links
Marcia's acts with those of her father.

180   P. Aelius Geme(l)lus, vir clarissimus. Apulum, Dacia. Late second or early third
       century. *CIL* 3.1006.

Fortunae | Aug. | sacrum. | P. Aelius Gemellus *(sic)*, vir clarissimus, | perfecto a solo balneo | consacravit.

NOTES: For Gemellus, see *PIR*[2] A 180. Apulum was the site of a legionary fortress and a civilian settlement (made a *municipium* under M. Aurelius); see no. 219. It is unclear from which of the two contexts this inscription derives. Gemellus' senatorial status tends to suggest that he was attached to the army, but such attachment would not preclude him from acting as benefactor to the civilian settlement.

Caesidius Proculus. Canusium (Regio II). Second or third century. *AE* 1987.307.   181

The full text is cited at no. 116. Here note the portion that reads:

balneum publicum | a Caesidio Proculo refectum . . .

NOTES: This restoration took place before a reconstruction by the local authorities in the third century and may date to the previous century. Caesidius Proculus' status is not clear.

Papius I[—] , Pa[pius —]anus filius eius. Mididi, Africa. Second or third century.   182
CIL 8.609 = *CIL* 8.11775.

[—]e se[m]iple[nas? —] quas Papius I[— i]n privato solo suo suis sumtibus, | [civibus? civitat]is Mididit[an(orum) a]edificavit Pa[pius —]anus, filius eius, patriae suae | [dedit et dedic(avit) lege harum?] therma[rum more urba?]n(o) lavat(ur).

NOTES: The fragmentary text presented above is a composite of three fragments of an epistyle inscription; I follow here the text and date proposed by Wesch-Klein (139–40 [no. 1]). Despite the lacuna in the text where the word *thermas* should be, it seems clear that the main benefaction was the construction of a set of baths (remains of which were visible to J. Schmidt of *CIL* in 1881); compare no. 101 for a similar "built-and-gave" benefaction by a father and son. In the present case, the wording, especially the mention of *patria sua* as the beneficiary, suggests that the son gave the baths over to public ownership rather than offered free bathing in them. The last line of the inscription, a restoration suggested by Mommsen and adopted by Wesch-Klein, would translate: " . . . gave (the bath) to his homeland and dedicated it; by a regulation of these baths, people bathed in the urban manner." The phrase is odd, to say the least.

[—] Stulinus, generosa familia progenitus. Villa Magna, Africa. Second or third   183
century. *CIL* 8.897.

[tempore (*or* iussu) fortissim|orum] piisimor[u]mq(ue) princip(um) | s[ub ad]minis-tratione procons(ulis) p(rovinciae) A(fricae), | [perfecto dedicatoque | baln(eo)?,] institutis nunc solio uno i⟨n⟩fimo | [—] congestioni et [. . .] parieti in | [—] Stulinus generosa familia progenitus perfecit, excoluit, ludos dedit dedicavit.

NOTES: This mutilated text was in service as a threshhold stone when discovered. As a result, the precise nature and extent of all of Stulinus' work is not recoverable. It is clear enough, however, that he was responsible at least for the completion of one of the *solia* (the communal bathing pools) and perhaps for the completion and decoration of some other part—or possibly the whole—of a bath building. *Dedit* here probably means that the baths were handed over to public ownership at their dedication.

M. Valerius Bradua Mauricus, c(larissimae) m(emoriae) v(ir), cos., and Q. Vi[r]ius   184†
Egnatius Sulpicius Priscus, consularis. Albingaunum (Regio IX). Post-211. *CIL* 5.7783 = *ILS* 1128.

M. Valerius Bradua Mauricus, c. m. v., | cos., pont., sodalis Hadrianalis, | curator operum publicorum, | curator aquarum sacrae urbis et Miniciae, | censitor provinciae

Aquetanicae, | procos. provinciae Africae, | balneum quod vivos inchoaverat, | Q. Vi[r]ius Egnatius Sulpicius Priscus, | consularis, pontifex et flamen divi Severi, | curator aquarum sacrae urbis et Miniciae | eodemque tempore praefectus alimentorum, | perfectum Albi[n]ga[u]nensibus a[t]signavit.

Trans.: "The late M. Valerius Bradua Mauricus, of senatorial rank, consul, pontifex, priest of Hadrian, curator of public works, curator of the waters of the sacred city and of the Minicia, *censitor* of the province of Aquitania, proconsul of the province of Africa—the bath that he started while still alive, Q. Virius Egnatius Sulpicius Priscus, of consular rank, pontifex and priest of the divine Severus, curator of the waters of the sacred city and of the Minicia, and at the same time prefect of the *alimenta,* completed and handed over to the people of Albingaunum."

NOTES: Valerius was consul in 191: see *RE* 7A.2347, s.v. "Valerius 113" (Hanslik); Degrassi, 53. Virius, or Vibius, was consul at some indeterminate time: see *RE* 9A.235–36, s.v. "Virius 4" (Hanslik); Degrassi, 138. Thomasson (1.386 [no. 121]) dates Valerius' African proconsulship to between 198 and 208. Why Virius finished the work begun by Valerius is not sure, but they may have been friends, since Valerius Bradua and Q. Virius Larcius Sulpicius Pr(iscus?) (the present Virius' father?) had cooperated on the erection of an arch at Rome (*CIL* 6.1541). Alternatively, both may have owned property in the region of Albingaunum (Bradua, for one, is honored in another text found here in the 1960s; see *SupplItal* 4 [1988]: 257–58 [no. 6]). The remains of these baths are very fragmentary; see Cavalieri Manasse, Massari, and Rossignani., *Piemonte,* 203.

185   M. Tullius Cicero Venneianus, filius. Paestum (Regio III). Early third century. *AE* 1935.28 = *ILPaest* 100.

The full text is cited at no. 108. Here note the portion that reads:

. . . M. Tullius Cice|ro Venneianus filius balneas eas|dem, vi ignis multifaria *(sic)* corruptas, | sua pecunia restituit . . .

NOTES: This passage mentions the son of the man who built the baths; see no. 108. Although his father had been a *duovir quinquennalis* and *patronus coloniae,* there is no indication that his son held any posts or titles.

186   C. Arrius Pacatus. Cirta, Numidia. Early third century. *CIL* 8.7031.

C. Arrius Paca|tus balineum | Pacatianum | sibi mensib(us) XIV.

NOTES: For Pacatus, see *PIR*² A 1102 and the stemma ibid., p. 214, where he appears as a grandson of C. Arrius Antoninus, consul in 170. Note the short time in which the baths were built. Wilmanns *(CIL)* reports that the remains of the baths are known; Manderscheid (101, s.v. "Constantine/Cirta") lists them as unpublished.

187†*   [Jul]iae Me[m]mia [Pris?]ca Ruf[a] Aemil[iana] Fidia[na], claris[sima et nobilissima f]emina. Bulla Regia, Africa. 220–40. *AE* 1921.45 = *ILAfr* 454a.

[Iul]iae Me[m]mia[e] | [Pris?]cae Ruf[ae] Aemill[iana]e Fidia[nae], claris|[simae et nobilis]s[imae f]eminae, | [C. Memmi I]ul. Albi consularis | [viri patr]oni et alumni fil(iae), ob | [praecipu]am operis sui thermarum | [magnifi]centiam qua et patriam | [suam e]xornavit et saluti civium | [..10..]ico consulere | [dignata] est | [—] bene et eius | [— pa]tronae et *(the text continues on another side of the stone, but in a very fragmentary form).*

Trans.: "To Julia Memmia Prisca Rufa Aemiliana Fidiana, a woman of most noble senatorial family, daughter of C. Memmius [Fidus] Julius Albius, a man of consular rank and patron and native of the city, on account of the outstanding magnificence of her work, the baths, by which she both beautified her hometown and looked after the health of the citizens [?]ico, she was worthy [—] well and her [—] to the patroness and . . . "

NOTES: The inscription was found in the ruins of these baths. Julia Memmia was the daughter of C. Memmius Fidus Julius Albius, consul in 191 or 192 (see *PIR*² M 462; see M 487 for Julia Memmia). An inscription honoring Albius was also found in these baths; see *ILAfr* 453. The complex has been excavated and is a large and impressive establishment, as is only to be expected of a consular benefaction. A recent and systematic analysis of the ruins suggests a date of 220–40 for their initial construction: see Broise and Thébert, *Les thermes memmiens,* esp. 107 and 271 on the date, 347–51 on this inscription; see also Wesch-Klein, 73–74 (no. 5). For some useful items absent from Broise and Thébert's bibliography, see Manderscheid, 86, s.v. "Thermes des Iulia Memmia"; Nielsen, 2.26–27 (C.207); Yegül, 217–19.

Vibia Galla. Alba Fucens (Regio IV). Mid–third century. *AE* 1962.30 (see *AE* 1952.19).

Vibia C. f. Galla baln[ea] | de sua pecunia ref(iciunda) cur[avit].

NOTES: This is a mosaic inscription from one entrance to the baths; an almost identical text from another entrance calls the building a *balne[u]m* (*AE* 1952.19). Vibia Galla is possibly the daughter of the emperor Trebonian (251–53); see *RE* 8A.1999, s.v. "Vibia 71" (Hanslik). An inscription honoring Trebonian (*CIL* 9.3916) was found at Alba Fucens, strengthening the identification with Vibia here. Compare the bath benefaction at Miletus that may have been the work of the empress Faustina; see no. 315. For the remains, see Coarelli and La Regina, *Abruzzo,* 83–84 (they suggest, on the basis of the style of the inscription, that this Vibia Gallia may be a female ancestor of Trebonian, possibly of the first or second century); Manderscheid, 50, s.v. "Alba Fucens"; J. Mertens, *Alba Fucens* (Brussels, 1969), 1.69–72.

M. Aur(elius) Valerius, v. p., ducen[ari]us, ex protectorrib(us) lateri[s] divini. Narona,   189
Dalmatia. 280. *CIL* 3.1805 = *ILS* 5695.

thermas rei p(ublicae) h[i]ema[les rog]a[nte] | populo in ruinam [de]lap[sas] | M. Aur. Valerius, v. p., ducen[ari]us, ex protectorib(us) lateri[s] | divini, de frugalitate sua CTE|[—]orum sa[..8.. | ..11.. aedifi]cavit et lava|ntes rei p(ublicae) tradidit, epulu|m quoque c[i]vibus suis ea | die praebu[i]t Messala et | Grato cos., dedicante M. Aur. | Tiberiano, v. p., praes(ide) prov(inciae) Del(matiae).

NOTES: Valerius was a native of this town in Dalmatia and thus is acting here as a local benefactor: see *PIR*² A 1625; *PLRE* 1.941, s.v "Valerius 8." For M. Aurelius Tiberianus, see *PIR*² A 1620; Thomasson, 1.95 (no. 55). The unintelligible letters *CTE* may also read *OTE.*

Q. Aemilius Victo[r] Saxonianus. Grumentum (Regio III). Late third century. *CIL*   190
10.222 = *ILS* 586.

balnea | ex disciplin[a d. n.] | L. Domiti Aur[eliani in]|victi Aug. po[st longam] | seriem ann[orum resti]|tuit | Q. Aemilius Victo[r] | Saxonianus.

NOTES: What precisely is meant by *balnea ex disciplina d(omini) n(ostri) L. Domiti Aureliani* is not clear. Mommsen *(CIL),* on the basis of HA *Aurel.* 45.2, suggested that it referred to a more severe mode of bathing preferred by the emperor. It seems unlikely, however, that an emperor would be so concerned with regulating methods of bathing. Also, because the meaning of *thermae hiemales* is not clear (what does the term actually denote?), Mommsen's proposition is doubly difficult. Poma ("Osservazioni," 30, 32–33) more plausibly suggests that the phrase in question refers to closer imperial regulation of how the construction was financed and administered (see no. 112). On *thermae hiemales/aestivales*, see above, chapter 5, n. 49.

191   L. Julius Pompilius Betulenus Apronianus, c(larissimus) i(uvenis). Amiternum (Regio IV). Third century. *CIL* 9.4196.

L. Iulius Pompilius | Betulenus Apronianus, c. i., | balneas Amiterninis | patriae sue *(sic)* dedit.

NOTES: The date is provided by *SupplItal* 9 (1992): 33 (*ad* 4196). In all likelihood, the text records the construction of a bathhouse—it is so understood by, e.g., Coarelli and La Regina (*Abruzzo*, 20)—but this reading is not completely secure. No significant remains of baths are known at the site; see the notes to no. 121.

192   Nonius Marcell[us] Herculius. Thubursicum Numidarum, Numidia. 324. *CIL* 8.4878 = *ILS* 2943.

beatissimo sa[eculo d. n. | C]onstantini ma[ximi] | semper Aug. et [Crispi] | et Constantin[i nobb. Caess.], | plateam v[e]terem [omni] | lapid[e] spoliatam | Nonius Marcell[us] | Herculius so[lide?] | construavit [et ther]|mas et ce[tera rui]na dilap[sa aedificia] . . . *(the text breaks off)*

NOTES: The man mentioned in this inscription is the same Nonius Marcellus who wrote the ancient dictionary and who stemmed from a noted Thubursican family: see *RE* 17.882–97, s.v. "Nonius 38" (Strzelecki); *PLRE* 1.552, s.v. "Marcellus 11." Although the word *restituit* or its synonym is missing, the surviving text makes it clear that a restoration was being commemorated. Remains of two public baths are known at Thubursicum, but it is unclear which facility is referred to here: see Manderscheid, 212, s.v. "Thubursicum Numidarum"; Nielsen, 2.31–32 (C.251); Yegül, 247–49.

193   Valentius B[ae]bianus Junior. Asola (Regio X). 336. *AE* 1972.202.

Valentius B[ae]lbianus Iunior | balneum a sollo fecit Nepotilano et Faculndo cons.

NOTES: No significant remains of baths are known at the site; see Cavalieri Manasse, Massari, and Rossignani, *Piemonte*, 266–67.

194† Incertus. Satafis, Mauretania. 359/88. *CIL* 8.20267 = *CLE* 1802 = *CLE* 1911 = *ILCV* 229 = *ML* 41.

[post fla]mmas cinere[sque] suos nova surgere foenix | [scit; nu]nc ut pulcra r[e]novetur fabrica mole | [—]ne, facis, cui la[u]dem nobile corpus, | [nomen, op?]es peperere suae quibus omnia polles, | [—] Romuleo genitum quem stem[m]ate p[atru]m | [—]m Mauris claro [p]ermisit honore. | [surrec?]turis thermis [h]onos iste resurget | [— per te? que]m gaudet sibimet [n]utrisse Satafis. | [a(nno)] pr(ovinciae) CCCXX[—]II.

Trans. (adapted from *ML*): "The phoenix knows how to rise anew following the flames and its own ashes; now you, *[name lost]*, see to it that the construction is renewed in a handsome heap, you for whom your fine body and the appropriate [fame and resources?], with which you can achieve anything, have evoked praise. You were born of a family tree of Roman fathers, and [the emperor] placed you over the Moors in a position of high honor. That honor will rise again from the baths, which themselves will rise again through your agency; Satafis rejoices that it nurtured you for itself. In the *[figure fragmentary]* year of the province."

NOTES: This text was found among the ruins of baths at Satafis. The date is that adopted in *CIL, ILCV,* and *ML.* I have adopted the supplements suggested by Courtney (*ML,* p. 265), which differ somewhat from those proposed by Bücheler *(CLE)* and Diehl *(ILCV).* It is clear that the text commemorates the reconstruction of baths by a local man who had served in the imperial administration, apparently without distinction, since there is much talk here of restoring pride and honor. Unfortunately, the benefactor cannot be identified securely. For another verse commemoration of a constructional bath benefaction, this time of an unclear nature and uncertain benefactor, see *CIL* 3.6306 = *CIL* 3.8153 = *CLE* 273 = *ML* 39 (Singidinum, Moesia).

Incertus. Beneventum (Regio II). Late Imperial. *CIL* 9.1596 = *ILS* 5511.   195

[—] spect⎟ [—⎟ —] ⎟ iustitia [admir]abili, castita⎟te conspic[uo, repar]atori fori pro ⎟ magna [parte co]nlapsi in ruín(a) ⎟ cotidie [auctas], restitutori ba⎟silicae [. . . cu]m porticibus sagit⎟ta[riorum et] regionis viae novae, ⎟ repar[atori] thermarum Commo-diana⎟rum, re[para]tori collegiorum, repa⎟ratori [porti]cus Dianae, reparatori ⎟ basil-icae [L]ongini ac totius prope civitatis [post h]ostile incendium, conditori, [ob] insignia eius in omnem pro⎟[v]in[ciam] praecipuaque in se et patriam ⎟ [urbem m]erita populus Beneven⎟[tanu]s ad aeternam memoriam ⎟ [..4..] statuam conlocavit.

NOTES: This inscription is dated by Nielsen (1.41 n. 26) to the fourth or fifth century; on these baths, see the notes to nos. 10 and 27. The present text is a long acephalous commemoration of the deeds of a benefactor who is listed as *restitutor* or *reparator* of a host of buildings, including the forum, a basilica, porticoes, roads, collegia, a portico of Diana, a basilica of Longinus—indeed, *totius prope civi⎟tatis [post h]ostile incendium,* "of nearly the entire city after the enemy burned it." This statement might be hoped to place a firmer date on the text, but there is little solid information on burnings of Beneventum in the fourth and fifth centuries: see *PECS,* 149, s.v. "Beneventum" (Salmon); *RE* 3.273–75, s.v. "Beneventum 2" (Hülsen) and Suppl. 1.248 (id.); Zazo, "Benevento." The city certainly suffered devastation in the Gothic wars of Justinian, between 536 and 547 (Procop. *Goth.* 7.15.11), which renders the notice of enemy action here curious, since it is unlikely (although not impossible) that a sixth-century benefactor would be restoring so many public buildings.

Maria Anthusa. Cures Sabini (Regio IV). Late Imperial (?). *CIL* 9.4974 = *ILS* 5709.   196*

Maria Anthúsa et P. M[—] ⎟ baptistérium et cella[m—] ⎟ de sua pecunia ma[rmoribus ornavit?].

NOTES: Both Maria and Anthusa are late Imperial Roman names, though they are known in earlier Greek sources. The *cella* mentioned here is possibly the *cella frigida,* where *baptisteria* (pools) were to be found (see Pliny *Ep.* 2.17.11, 5.6.25; Nielsen, 1.155, s.v. "baptisterium"). The restoration of the last line is my own and seems plausible given what survives of the rest of the text. Mention of decoration "with marble" *(marmoribus)* is quite common in bath-related inscriptions; compare esp. no. 143, but see also nos. 51, 58, 79, 114, 117, 131. It is unclear if this building is the one referred to in no. 96.

Part B

Nonconstructional Benefactions

Free Bathing

197† L. Urvineius Philomusus, l(ibertus), mag(ister) conl(egii) libert(orum). Praeneste (Regio I). Undated. *CIL* 14.3015 = *ILS* 6256.

L. Urvineio L. l. Philomuso, | mag(istro) conl(egii) libert(orum), | publice sepulturae et statuae in foro locus | datus est, quod is testamento suo lavationem populo gratis | per triennium gladiatorumque paria X et Fortunae Primig(eniae) | coronam auream p(ondo) I dari, idemque ludos ex HS *(200,000)* per dies V fieri iussit. | Philippus l(ibertus) monumentum de suo fecit.

Trans.: "Space was given for a public tomb and a statue in the forum to L. Urvineius Philomusus, freedman of Lucius, *magister* of the collegium of freedmen, because he ordered in his will that free bathing be given to the people for three years and that ten pairs of gladiators be given and a gold crown weighing one pound be given to Fortuna Primigenia, and he also ordered that games be held over five days from two hundred thousand sesterces. Philippus, his freedman, made this monument at his own expense."

NOTES: A collegium of freedmen is an unusual institution. Another may have existed at Pompeii (*CIL* 4.117 = *ILS* 6419g), and at Ephesos *collegia libertorum et servorum domini n. Augusti* find mention (*CIL* 3.6077 = *ILS* 1505), but they are something of a rarity; see M.S. Ginsburg, "*Princeps Libertinorum*," *TAPA* 65 (1934): 198–206. Evidently, heads of such collegia could be affluent people, as Urvineius' generous benefactions indicate.

198 Incertus. Ocriculum (Regio VII). Undated. *CIL* 11.4100.

[—] dedit [— lavationem ? i]ncolis, hospitib[us, fa]milleisque *(sic)* eorum.

NOTES: Despite its fragmentary nature, this text probably commemorates an offer of free bathing; compare the wording of nos. 199, 201, 204–6, 208. That the inscription was found in the ruins of the baths at Ocriculum only supports this interpretation: see Pietrangeli, *Ocriculum,* 68; id., *Otricoli,* 64.

199† Decuriones. Buie, near Histria (ancient name not known; Regio X). Undated. *CIL* 5.376 = *InscrIt* 10.3.71.

colonis, incolis, | peregrinis, | lavandis gratis d(ecreto) d(ecurionum) p(ecunia) p(ublica) p(ositum).

Trans.: "It was ordained by decree of the decurions that colonists, inhabitants, and foreigners bathe for free at public expense."

[Terentia Postu]mina. Novaria (Regio XI) . Undated. *CIL* 5.6522.   200*

The full text is cited at no. 146. Here note the portion that reads:

. . . [lavationem] gratuitam in | [perpetuum] dedit.

Incertus. Vercellae (Regio XI). Undated. *CIL* 5.6668.   201

[lavationem gratuitam | in perpetuu]m munic[ipibus, incolis, | hospitibus, a]dven-torib[us dedit].

NOTES: Despite the fragmentary nature of this text, that it records a free bath benefaction seems plausible, given the list of the different classes of beneficiaries; see notes to no. 198.

T. Aviasius Servandus. Bononia (Regio VIII). Undated (but probably first or second   202
century). *CIL* 11.720 = *ILS* 5674.

The full text is cited at no. 1/2. Here note the portion that reads:

in huius balinei lavation(em) HS *(400,000)* . . . Servandus | pater testament(o) legavit, ut ex reditu eius summ(ae) | in perpetuum viri et impuberes utriusq(ue) sexsus | gratis laventur.

NOTES: This inscription was carved in different lettering below the main commemoration of the constructional efforts of Augustus and Gaius, and it cut into the ornamental border of the original text. The fine quality of the letters suggests a date in the first or second century. Here a fund of four hundred thousand sesterces is set up, the interest from which is to pay for the free entry of men and *impuberes* of both sexes into the bathhouse. Duncan-Jones (*Economy,* 173 [no. 647], 215 [no. 1308]) calculates the interest at twenty thousand sesterces per annum at a rate of 5 percent; see ibid., 116–17 n. 258 and 132–38 on Roman interest rates, which alternate between 5 and 6 percent.

M. Helvius Anthus, IIIIIvir Aug(ustalis). Lucurgentum, Baetica. Undated (but some-   203†
time in the Principate). *AE* 1953.21 = *ILER* 1732.

M. Helvius Anthus Lucurg(entinus), | IIIIIvir Aug., edito spec|taculo per quad-ridulum ludorum scaeni|corum et dato gym|nasio per eosdem | dies, item mulie|ribus balineum gra|tis (dedit). huic ordo splen|didissimus Lucurgentin|orum petente populo orna|menta decurionatus decrevit. Helvius Anthus ob honorem | statuam tan(t)i pa-tris cum basi s(ua) p(ecunia) d(ono) d(edit). | p(opulos)q(ue) f(ecit).

Trans.: "M. Helvius Anthus, of Lucurgentum, *sevir Augustalis,* staged a spectacle of theatrical games that lasted four days and gave a *gymnasium* throughout those same days; he also gave free baths to the women. To this man, the most eminent *ordo* of Lucurgentum decreed the insignia of the decurionate, since the people demanded it. Helvius Anthus, on account of this honor, gave as a gift at his own expense a statue of his great father, along with its base. The people made (this monument)."

C. Aurunceiu[s] Cotta. Praeneste (Regio I). First century B.C. or later (?). *CIL*   204
14.2979 = *ILS* 5672.

C. Aurunceiu[s C. f.] | Cotta | colonis, incolis, hospit[ibus], | adventoribus servisqu[e] | eorum | lavationem ex sua pecunia | gratuitam in perpetuom dedit.

NOTES: Nielsen (1.132–33) dates this inscription to the early Imperial period, as does Cenerini ("Evergetismo," 210–12; she does not provide an exact date but includes it among the early

Imperial material). It may be of late Republican date, however: note the spelling of *perpetuom* (compare nos. 205 and 206); A.R. Hands (*Charities and Social Aid*, 207 [D.75]) dates it to the "late first century B.C."

205   Q. and C. Poppaeei, patron(i) municipi et coloniai. Interamnia Praetuttiorum (Regio V). First century B.C. or Augustan (?). *CIL* 1².1903a = *CIL* 9.5074 = *ILS* 5671 = *ILLRP* 617.

Q., C. Poppaeei Q. f., patron(i) | municipi et coloniai, | municipibus, coloneis, in-coleis, | hospitibus, adventoribus, | lavationem in perpetuom de | sua pecunia dant.

NOTES: For a photograph of the stone, see fig. 26F. If the two Poppaei are identified with the brothers C. Poppaeus Sabinus and Q. Poppaeus Secundus who were consuls in A.D. 9, an Augustan date for the benefaction is to be preferred: see T.P. Wiseman, *New Men in the Roman Senate, 139 B.C.–A.D. 14* [Oxford, 1971], 254 (nos. 340 and 341); Cenerini, "Evergetismo," 206. The absence of any mention of their consulships here indicates a date before 9, but it is not clear how much earlier. If, however, the identification is inaccurate, the text may date to the late Republic (note the archaic spellings of *perpetuom* and *coloniai;* Degrassi includes the text in his *ILLRP,* while Nielsen [1.132] muses that it belongs "presumably in the Late Republican period").

206† L. Octavius Rufus, trib(unus) mil(itum), duomvir quinq(uennalis), publ(icus) pa-tronus. Suasa (Regio VI). Augustan (?). *CIL* 11.6167 = *ILS* 5673.

L. Octavio L. f. Cam. | Rufo, trib. mil. leg. IIII | Scythicae, praef(ecto) fabr(um) | bis, duomviro quinq(uennali) ex | s(enatus) c(onsulto) et d(ecreto) d(ecurionum), auguri ex d(ecreto) d(ecurionum) | creato, | qui lavationem gratuitam | municipib(us), in-coleis, | hospitib(us) et adventorib(us), | uxsorib(us), serveis ancilleis|que eor(um) in perpetuom | dedit, d(ecreto) d(ecurionum) publ(ice) patrono.

Trans.: "To L. Octavius Rufus, son of Lucius, of the voting tribe Camilia, military tribune of Legion IIII Scythica, *praefectus fabrum* twice, *duovir* with censorial powers by senatorial decree and by decree of the decurions, appointed augur by decree of the decurions, who gave in perpetuity free bathing to the citizens of the town, the inhabi-tants, guests and visitors, their wives, their slaves, and their maids. (This monument was built) in honor of our patron by decree of the decurions from public funds."

NOTES: The Augustan date is suggested by a combination of several features of the text. That Rufus served as a tribune in Legion IIII Scythica is a useful indicator, since the legion was raised under Augustus; a *terminus post quem* for the inscription is thus set. However, the legion continued to exist into the third and fourth centuries, and no precise date can be put on Rufus' service in it; see *RE* 12.1556–64, s.v. "Legio IIII Scythica" (Ritterling), esp. 1563 on the undatable Rufus. As to Rufus' *prefectura fabrum*, it is not clear which of the two forms of the office he held—the Republican military post or the post-Augustan municipal one; see the notes to no. 82. The location of the office in his *cursus*, sandwiched between his military tribuneship and his quinquennalate, is not helpful, since it can be read either as the culmination of his military service or as the start of his municipal career. The archaic orthography of the words *perpetuom, incoleis, serveis,* and *ancilleis* (compare nos. 204 and 205) points to an early date. The appearance of all of these features is consistent with an Augustan context for the inscrip-tion, with the orthography indicating the earlier part of that period (see Mouritsen, *Elections,* 91). The physical remains at Suasa are extremely sparse; see Gaggiotti et al., *Umbria,* 216–17.

Decuriones. Nemausus, Gallia Narbonensis. Ca. 14. *CIL* 12.3179 = *ILS* 2267.   207†

Ti. Caesaris | díví Aug. f. Augusti | miles missicius, T. Iulius | Féstus, militávit annos XXV | in legióne XVI, decreto decurion(um) | accepit frumenti m(odios) L., balneum et | sui *(sic)* gratuitum in perp(etuum) et aream in|ter duós *(sic)* turrés per P. Pusonium Pere|grinum IIIIvir. et XIvir. adsignátam.

Trans.: "T. Julius Festus, a veteran discharged by Ti. Caesar Augustus, son of the deified Augustus, who served twenty-five years in Legion XVI, received by decree of the decurions fifty *modii* of wheat, free use of the baths for life, and the vacant lot between the two towers, which was assigned to him by P. Pusonius Peregrinus, *quattuorvir* and *undecimvir.*

NOTES: Dessau reports that he cannot make sense of the phrase *balneum et sui;* it may be a miscarving of *et balnei usum* (as suggested by Dessau). The beneficiary, Festus, may well have been a soldier discharged without dishonor after the mutinies on the Rhine in 14, in which Legion XVI Gallica participated—it was stationed at Moguntiacum in Germania Superior when disorder erupted (see Tac. *Ann.* 1.37.4; *RE* 12.1761–65, s.v. "Legio XVI" [Ritterling]). *Un-decemviri* are only attested at Nemausus in this inscription, which prompted Hirschfeld (*CIL,* vol. 12, p. 382) to suggest that they were abolished in the early Empire.

M. Helvius Rufus Civica, prim(i)pil(aris). Vallis Digentiae (near Tibur; Regio I). After   208
20. *CIL* 14.3472 = *ILS* 2637.

M. Helvius M. f. Cam. Rufus | Civica, prim(i)pil(aris), | balneum | municipibus et incolis | dedit.

NOTES: This appears to be the Helvius Rufus who won the *corona civica* in North Africa against Tacfarinas in 20 (see Tac. *Ann.* 3.21.3–4). If so, he adopted the title *civica* as his *signum;* see *PIR*[2] H 75. This text, from the mention of the beneficiaries, appears to denote an offer of free bathing, rather than the construction of the baths; see the notes to no. 198.

Incertus. Urbs Salvia (Regio V). Second half of first or early second century. *AE*   209
1979.202.

(the first line is fragmentary) [. . . balneum muli]ebre [— | — ite]mque lava[tionem . . . | . . . gratuitam in per]petuum [de sua pecunia ? dedit].

NOTES: Although the text is very fragmentary, enough survives to suggest that the unnamed benefactor did something for the women's baths (built, restored, adorned, dedicated them?) and then provided free baths *in perpetuum.* See also nos. 203 and 213, where free baths are provided for women only (though not specifically in a *balneum muliebre*). No substantial remains of baths are known at the site; see Gaggiotti et al., *Umbria,* 260–64.

M. Valerius Proculinus, IIvir. Singilia Barba, Baetica. 109. *AE* 1989.420.   210†

M. Valerio M. f., | M. n., G. pron., Quir. | Proculino, IIvir(o) m(unicipum) m(unicipii) | Liberi Singiliensis | cives et incolae ex aere conlato | hic in IIviratu publicos ludos et | totidem dierum privatos dedit, | item | populum universum in municipio | habitantem et incolas oleo et balineo | gratuito dato pervocavit, | item quo die ludos iu(v)enum in theatro | dedit gymnasium et balinea viris et | mulieribus gratuita praestitit. | huic cives et incolae pr(idie) k(alendas) Ianuarias | abeunti e IIviratu ob rem publicam | bene atministratam consensu omnium | in foro publice gratias egerunt et | hostias quas inmolaret, item | statuam ex aere conlato dederunt. | ordo decreto locum eligere | permisit | IIvir(atu) A(ulo) Cornelio Palma Frontiano II | P(ublio) Calvisio Tullo cos.

Trans.: "To M. Valerius Proculinus, son of Marcus, grandson of Marcus, great-grandson of Gaius, of the voting tribe Quirina, *duovir* of the citizens of the town of Liberum Singiliense, the citizens and inhabitants (dedicated this monument) from the money collected. This man, during his duovirate, gave public games and, on just as many days, private games. In addition, he gave oil and free bathing and invited all the people living in the town and the inhabitants; likewise, on the day he gave games for the young men in the theater, he presented a *gymnasium* and free baths to the adult men and women. To this man, when he was laying down the duovirate on 31 December, on account of his having administered the city well, the citizens and inhabitants in unanimous agreement gave thanks publicly in the forum, and from the money collected, they gave him victims for his sacrifices and a statue. The *ordo*, by decree, allowed him to choose the location for the statue. His duovirate was when Aulus Cornelius Palma Frontianus was consul for the second time, with Publius Calvisius Tullus *(i.e., 109)*."

NOTES: Valerius Proculinus can now be added to the local magistrates of this town; see Curchin, 162 (nos. 249–51). The text is closely analyzed by Le Roux in "Cité et culture municipale." Le Roux (271) translates *pervocavit* as "il a . . . addressé une convocation générale," which squeezes a lot of meaning out of a single word, especially one that is otherwise unattested in classical Latin. In fact, the prefix *per-* probably acts here as an intensifier and should not be translated at all. If so, the meaning is more mundane: Valerius Proculinus made a benefaction and then invited the urban *populus* and *incolae* to enjoy it, perhaps by means of cryers, as Le Roux (275–76) suggests elsewhere.

211† Not specified. Pagus Lucretius in the Ager Arelatensis, Gallia Narbonensis. Antoninus Pius. *CIL* 12.594 = *ILS* 6988.

[p]agáni pági Lucreti, quí sunt fini|bus Arelátensium locó Gargario, Q. Cor. | Marcellí lib. Zosimo, IIIIIIvir(o) Aug. Col. Iul. | Paterná Areláte, ob honorem eius, qui nótum *(sic)* fecit | iniuriam nostram omnium sáec[ulor]um sacrá|tissimó principi T. Áelio Antónino [Pio], [patiente]r Rómae | m[an]sit (?), per multós annós ad práesides pr[ovinci]áe perse|cútús est iniúriam nostram suis in[pendiis e]t ob hoc | dónavit nóbis inpendia quaé fecit, ut omnium sáecul|lórum sacrátissimí principis imp. Caes. Antónini Aug. Pii | beneficia dúrárent permanérentqué quibus fruerémur, | [oleo?] et balineo gratúitó quod ablatúm erat paganís | [Pagi Lucreti], quód usi fuerant amplius annis XXXX.

Trans.: "The villagers of Pagus Lucretius, who are within the territory of Arelate in the Gargarian quarter, to Q. Cornelius Zosimus, freedman of Marcellus, *sevir Augustalis* at Colonia Julia Paterna Arelate, on account of his office. He made known our grievance to the most revered *princeps* of all ages T. Aelius Antoninus [Pius] and patiently waited (?) at Rome; for many years he sought requital of our grievance with the governors of the province at his own expense and, on account of this, presented to us the expenses he incurred, in order that the benefits of the most revered *princeps* of all ages Imperator Caesar Antoninus Augustus Pius might endure and remain for us to enjoy, [namely, oil?] and free bathing, which was withdrawn from the villagers of Pagus Lucretius, and of which they had made use for more than forty years."

NOTES: This inscription is most interesting. The phrase *patienter Romae mansit* in lines 6–7 is an emendation suggested by Hirschfeld in *CIL; oleo* in line 12 is my own suggestion. The situation behind the inscription appears to have been as follows. Pagus Lucretius had enjoyed a benefaction of free bathing (and oil?) for forty years, and the benefit had been cut off for some unstated reason. This appears to have been the *iniuria* that so occupied Zosimus. Zosimus, an official at the colony of Arelate, in the *territorium* of which Pagus Lucretius stood, then petitioned the emperor in Rome and pestered the governors of the province, all at his own expense, to restore these lost *beneficia*. It is noteworthy that the inscription does not state that Zosimus was successful in his petitions. Several questions remain. Who had bestowed the benefaction in the first place? The petitioning of the emperor and imperial officials and the wording of the closing lines of the inscription may point to a member of the central administration as the agent, but this identification is far from certain. The emperor's subjects were not averse to bringing local grievances to his attention or to that of his provincial agents; and mention of the *beneficia* of Pius that are to endure probably refers to the hoped-for restoration of the original benefaction, not its inception. Further, the last sentence suggests that the original *beneficia* had been of limited duration (as is the case in many examples of free-bathing inscriptions, see above) but that the villagers had come to expect their free bath as a right. Yet another question is, where was the pertinent bathhouse located, in Pagus Lucretius or at Arelate? The actions of Zosimus appear to foreshadow those of the late Imperial *defensor civitatis,* officially established by Valentinian, whose main duty was to protect the lower classes from oppression and maltreatment by the rich; see Jones, *Later Roman Empire,* 144–45, 279–80, 726–27.

C. Auf(idius) Avitus, IIvir desig(natus). Burgvillos, Baetica. Second century (?). *CIL*   212
2.5354 = *ILER* 2050.

The full text is cited at no. 101. Here note the portion that reads:

. . . balineu(m) . . . d(e) s(ua) p(ecunia) dedit | et editis circiens(ibus) [ded(icavit)].

NOTES: Since the inscription also records that Avitus' father built the baths for the town, *dedit* cannot here mean "built." It may denote the transferral of the building to public ownership (compare no. 182), but if so, it is difficult to see the relevance of the formula *de sua pecunia* in this act. As a result, an offer of free bathing upon the opening of the baths seems the most likely benefaction here.

Caesia Sabina. Veii (Regio VII). Third century (?). *CIL* 11.3811 = *ILS* 6583.   213†*

Caesiae Sabinae | Cn. Caesi Athicti. | haec sola omnium | feminarum | matribus c(larissimorum) vir(orum) et | sororib(us) et filiab(us) | et omnis ordinis | mulieribus municipib(us) | epulum dedit, diebusq(ue) | ludorum et epuli | viri sui balneum | cum oleo gratuito | dedit. | sorores piissimae.

Trans.: "To Caesia Sabina, wife of Cn. Caesus Athictus. This woman, alone of all women, gave a banquet to the mothers of men of senatorial rank, to their sisters and daughters, and to female citizens of the town of all ranks, and on the days of the games and the banquet given by her husband, she offered bathing and free oil. The most loyal sisters (made this monument to her)."

NOTES: The date is that assigned by Nielsen (1.133). It is not perfectly clear whether Caesia restricted the free baths and oil to the same groups as had enjoyed the meal (i.e., the women of the town), but the sense would seem to suggest that this was the case, especially since the dedication was made by Caesia's *sorores piissimae,* which presumably denotes the beneficiaries.

Oil Distributions[1]

214 M. Annius, sacerdos, eq(ues) R(omanus), p(atronus) m(unicipii). Satafis, Mauretania. Undated. *CIL* 8.8396 = *ILS* 5728.

M. Annius, | sacerdos, | eq(ues) R(omanus), p(atronus) m(unicipii), cur|ator et dis-|punctor, | conchas de suo posuit.

NOTES: *Conchae* were vessels for holding or measuring out oil (see *OLD*, s.v.).

215† L. Caecilius Cilo, IIIIvir a(edilicia) p(otestate). Comum (Regio XI). Pre-100. *CIL* 5.5279 = *ILS* 6728.

L. Caecilius L. f. Cilo, | IIIIvir a(edilicia) p(otestate), | qui testamento suo HS n(um-mum) *(40,000)* municipibus Comensibus | legavit, ex quorum reditu quot annis per Neptunalia oleum | in campo et in thermis et balineis omnibus quae sunt | Comi populo praeberetur, t(estamento) f(ieri) i(iussit) et L. Caecilio L. f. Valenti et P. Caecilio L. f. Secundo et Lutullae Picti f. contubernali. | aetas properavit, faciundum fuit, noli plangere, mater, mater | rogat quam primum ducatis se ad vos.

Trans.: "L. Caecilius Cilo, son of Lucius, *quattuorvir* with the power of aedile, who bequeathed in his will forty thousand sesterces to the citizens of Comum, in order that, from the return on this sum, every year, throughout the Neptunalia, oil might be provided to the people in the Campus and in all the *thermae* and *balineae* that are in Comum; he ordered in his will that (this monument) be built also for L. Caecilius Valens and P. Caecilius Secundus, the sons of Lucius, and Lutulla, daughter of Pictus, the *contubernalis*. Time hastened by; it had to happen. Do not mourn, mother. Mother asks that you bring her to yourselves as quickly as possible."

NOTES: Duncan-Jones (*Economy,* 202 [no. 1088]) reckons a return of twenty-four hundred sesterces per annum if the interest rate were 6 percent. It is possible, as suggested in *PIR*[2] C 30, that this man was an ancestor of Pliny the Younger. If so, the first-century date is confirmed, and the inscription probably dates to the first half of that century. The precise status of Lutulla is somewhat mysterious. When applied to females, *contubernalis* usually means a "companion" for a male slave (compare no. 261), but here she is apparently attached to the benefactor. If so, she may have been a slave concubine: see J.F. Gardner, *Women in Roman Law and Society* (London, 1986), 56–60; S.M. Treggiari, "*Contubernales* in CIL 6," *Phoenix* 35 (1981): 42–69; id., *Roman Marriage:* Iusti Coniuges *from the Time of Cicero to the Time of Ulpian* (Oxford, 1991), 52–54.

216† Quinquennalis of the Collegium Dianae et Antinoi. Lanuvium (Regio I). 136. *CIL* 14.2112 = *ILS* 7212.II.29–31.

Item placuit: ut quinquennalis sui cuiusque temporis diebus sollemn[ibus ture] | et vino supplicet et ceterís officiís albatus fungatur, et die[bus natalibus] | Dianae et Antinoí oleum collegio in balinio *(sic)* publico po[nat antequam] epulentur.

---

1. I do not include here a series of inscriptions from Africa, Spain, and Germany that record the exhibition of *gymnasia* to the people, sometimes specified as taking place in the baths. Such texts may denote distributions of oil, but the *gymnasia* may also be gymnastic displays of some sort (see, e.g., nos. 203 and 210); the meaning may even have varied by context. See my paper, "Gifts of *Gymnasia*: A Test Case for Reading Quasi-Technical Jargon in Latin Inscriptions," *ZPE* 124 (1999): 263–75.

Trans.: "It was likewise resolved that on the festival days during his term of office, the *quinquennalis* should worship with incense and wine and carry out his other duties in white, and that on the birthdays of Diana and Antinoos, he place oil for the society in the public baths before they stage their banquet."

C. Aufidius Verus, pont(ifex), q(uaestor), IIvir q(uin)q(uennalis). Pisaurum (Regio VI). Early to mid–second century. *CIL* 11.6360.   217†

C. Aufidio C. f. Cam. | Véro, pont(ifici), q(uaestori), IIvir(o) q(uin)q(uennali), | plebs urbana ob merit(a) eius | ex aére conlato cuius dicatione | dedit decurionibus singul(is) HS n(ummos) XL, | Augustal(ibus) HS n(ummos) XX, plebei HS n(ummos) XII, adiecto | pane et vino et oleum in balineis. l(oco) d(ato) d(ecreto) d(ecurionum).

Trans.: "The city's plebs (dedicated this monument) from money collected to C. Aufidius Verus, son of Gaius, of the voting tribe Camilia, priest, quaestor, *duovir* with censorial powers, on account of his services. At his declaration of citizenship, he gave forty sesterces to each of the decurions, twenty to the Augustales, and twelve to the plebs, and he added bread and wine and oil in the baths. Space given by decree of the decurions."

NOTES: This inscription is carved onto a statue base. Nielsen (1.40 n. 25) dates it to the Julio-Claudian period. However, the stemma attached to *CIL* 11.6335 includes this Aufidius as the father of C. Aufidius Victorinus, consul II in 183 (see also *PIR*[2] A 1393), in which case the benefactor of this text would date to the early or mid–second century. He seems to have declared himself a citizen of Pisaurum, and the ceremony accompanying this act was the occasion for the benefactions.

L. Caecilius Optatus, c(enturio) missus honesta missione, atlectus inter immunes, IIvir III. Barcino, Hispania Tarraconensis. 161/69. *CIL* 2.4514 = *ILS* 6957 = *ILER* 5838.   218†

L. Caecilius L. f. | Páp. Optatus, | *(centurio)* leg. VII G. Fel., | et *(centurio)* leg. XV Apollin., | missus honestá | missione ab imp. M. | Aur. Antonino et Aur. | Vero Aug., atlectus a Bar[c(inonensibus)] | inter immunes, consecut(us) | in honores aedilicios, | IIvir III, flam. Romae | divorum et Augustorum, | qui r(ei) p(ublicae) Barc(inonensium) ita leg(avit): do, lego, | darique volo *(denarios) (7,500),* ex | quorum usuris semissibus | edi volo quodannis spectac(ula) | pugilum die IIII iduum Iuni | usque at *(denarios) (250)* et eadem die ex *(denariis) (200)* oleum in thermas publi[c(as)] | populo praeberi et [l]ecta praes|tari ea condicione volo, ut | liberti mei, item libertorum meorum | libertarumque liberti, quos honor(em) *(on the side)* seviratus contiger|it, ab omnibus mulneribus seviratus ex|cusati sint. Quot si quis | eorum at munera | vocitus fuerit, | tum ea *(denarios) (7,500)* at | rem pub(licam) Tarrac(onensium) | transferri iubeo, | sub eadem forma | spectaculorum, quot | s(upra) s(criptum) est, edendorum | Tarracone. l(oco) d(ato) d(ecreto) (decurionum).

Trans.: "L. Caecilius Optatus, son of Lucius, of the voting tribe Papiria, centurion of Legion VII Gemina Felix and centurion of Legion XV Apollinaris, honorably discharged by the emperors M. Aurelius Antoninus Augustus and Aurelius Verus Augustus. He was granted tax-exempt status by the people of Barcino, and he won the offices of aedile, *duovir* three times, and the priesthood of Rome and the deified Augusti; he bequeathed to the city of Barcino as follows: 'I give, bequeath, and want given 7,500 denarii; from the 6 percent interest on this sum, I want boxing matches staged on 10 June every year up to a cost of 250 denarii. Also, on the same day, I want 200 denarii spent on supplying oil to the public baths for the people. I want the bequests provided on the condition that my freedmen and the freedmen of my freedmen and freedwomen who have attained the office of the sevirate be excused from all the duties of the sevirate. But if any of them should be called to the duties of office, then I order that the 7,500 denarii be transferred to Tarraco, subject to the staging of games at Tarraco of the same type as described above.' Space given by decree of the decurions."

NOTES: The mathematics add up: 6 percent of 7,500 is 450, the amount Optatus wanted spent every year. This man is a fine example of a soldier who did well in the local magistracies following his retirement; see Curchin, 45–47 and 185 (no. 445). Note the threat to transfer the benecation to Tarraco, Barcino's neighboring and rival community, if the prescriptions of Optatus are not adhered to. See also S. Dardaine, "L'évergétisme *ob honorem* en Bétique," *Ktema* 16 (1991): 281–91.

219   Incertus. Apulum, Dacia. M. Aurelius. *CIL* 3.7805 = *ILS* 7145.

Two fragmentary lines, in which three letters can be read, are followed by

| (3) [—i]n balne|[o] populo pu|blice oleum | posuit. | l(oco) d(ato) d(ecreto) d(ecurionum).

On the side: [—]rarissim[o]. | Sex. Sentinas Maxi|mus anno primo | [f]acti municipi | posuit.

NOTES: Apulum was a double settlement, a fortress and a civilian village that was granted municipal status under M. Aurelius (see *PECS*, 74–75, s.v. "Apulum" [Marinescu]). This text is expressly from the latter. The benefactor who distributed the oil is not named, but Sextus Sentinas Maximus is a good candidate, if we assume a connection between the two inscriptions.

220   [P. Alfius Max]imus Numerius Av[itus], sevi]r eq(uitum) R(omanorum), allectus in[ter tribunicios praetori]. Rome. Severan. *CIL* 6.1474.

[P. Alfio Max]imo Numerio Av[ito, | sevi]r(o), eq(uiti) R(omanorum), allecto in[ter tribunicios, | praetori] cand(idato), leg(ato) prov(inciae) Ba[eticae, | praef(ecto) frum(enti) d]andi, sacerd(oti) Iun[onis? — | lu]perco, cur(atori) civitate [— quod balneo vetustate | collapso] in eor. min. usui id [reddiderit et non | m]odo calchidicum [— | c]ollapsam renova[rit sed etiam | cell]am hypocaustam n[— | i]nstante extrui c[uraverit | — vetustate conla[psam | re]fomari et excoli [praeceperit | et divisionem] oleariam pecun[ia sua —] | instituere enisus s(it) . . . *(the rest is irrelevant)*.

NOTES: This inscription is from a Christian cemetery on the Esquiline Hill. Despite the very fragmentary condition of the text, its main thrust is clear enough. This Numerius lived in the Severan period, serving under Severus Alexander; see *PIR*² N 202. Since Numerius carried out extensive work on the baths, the formulation *oleariam divisionem* is undoubtedly a reference to an oil distribution in baths.

221*   Caesia Sabina. Veii (Regio VII). Third century (?). *CIL* 11.3811 = *ILS* 6583.

The full text is cited at no. 213. Here note the portion that reads:

. . . balneum | cum oleo gratuito | dedit.

Water Supply

[—] Chrysanthus [VIvir Aug.] et Clodia Agatha uxor. Narbo, Gallia Narbonensis.   222
Undated (but sometime in the Principate). *CIL* 12.4388.

The full text is cited at no. 58. Here note the portion that reads:

. . . [balineum —] et marmoribus exstructum et ductu(m) | [aquae? — feceru?]nt . . .

L. Cluvienus Cilo. Bergomum (Regio XI). Undated (but possibly high Imperial). *CIL*   223
5.5136.

The full text is cited at no. 153. Here note the portion that reads:

. . . balneum et | aquas dedit.

Local council. Praeneste (Regio I). Ca. 80 B.C. *CIL* 1².1473 = *CIL* 14.3013 = *ILS*   224
5667 = *ILLRP* 659.

The full is text cited at no. 63. Here note the portion that reads:

. . . aquam per publicum | ducendum d(e) d(ecurionum) s(ententia) | coeravere.

Ti. Claudius Faustus Regi[n(us)] and Claudia Nais. Coela, Thrace. 55. *CIL* 3.7380 =   225*
ILS 5682.

The full text is cited at no. 161. Here note the portion that reads:

. . . idemque | aquam in eius balnei usus | perduxerunt et consacrarunt . . .

P. Faianius P[le]beius, IIvir. Forum Novum (Regio IV). First century. *CIL* 9.4786 =   226†
ILS 5767 (see also *SuppItal* 5 [1989]: 181–82 [no. 14]).

P. Faianius P[le]beius, IIvir. iter., | aquam ex ag[ro] suo in municipium | Forum Novom
[pe]cunia sua adduxit, | et lacus om[ne]s [f]ecit, et in piscinam | quae in Campo est
saliendam | curavit idemque probavit; | et cum venditor soli in quo balneum est |
parum cavisset emptori de aqua, | ut posset in balneo fluere, | aquam suam in id
balneum ne carerent | commodo municipes | P. Faianius Plebeius dedit.

Trans.: "P. Faianius Plebeius, *duovir* for the second time, brought water from his own
land into the town of Forum Novum at his own expense, built all the troughs, and
oversaw the discharge of the water into the *piscina* that is in the Campus; he also
approved the work. Also, since the seller of the lot on which the bath stands offered
the buyer no guarantee concerning the water supply, P. Faianius Plebeius, in order
that water would flow in the bathhouse, gave his own water to that bathhouse, so that
the citizens of the town might not be deprived of its convenience."

NOTES: The date is provided by *SuppItal,* which also presents a newly discovered copy of the
text, albeit more fragmentary in form. The inscription offers an interesting insight into the sharp
practices surrounding bath transactions. It seems that the person who sold the ground for the
town's baths had made no provision for their water supply and that the buyer had failed to
demand sufficient sureties in this regard. Thus, Faianius gave water to the baths, as well as to the
troughs and the *piscina.* It is not clear who the buyer was in this case; the tone of the inscription
suggests that it may have been the town and that this bathhouse was Forum Novum's main
bathing facility.

227* C. Sempronius Sempronianus, IIvir, pontufex *(sic)* perpet(uus) and Sempronia Fusca Fibia Anicilla, filia. Aurgi, Hispania Tarraconensis. Trajan (?). *CIL* 2.3361 = *ILS* 5688 = *ILER* 2040.

The full text is cited at no. 78. Here note the portion that reads:

. . . thermas aqua perducta . . . | . . . pecunia impensaque sua omni d(ederunt) d(edicaverunt).

228* T. Flavius Mythus, Aug(usti) lib(ertus) and Flavia Diogis. Capena (Regio VII). Late first or early second century. *CIL* 11.3932 = *ILS* 5770.

The full text is cited at no. 164. Here note the portion that reads:

. . . cum balneo . . . cum aquae | ductu ex fundo Cuteleniano et iugera | agri Cuteleniani p(lus) m(inus) IIII ita ut depalatum est . . .

229 L. Min[icius Na]talis, cos. and L. Minicius [Natalis Quadro]nius Verus, augur, trib(unus) plebis desig(natus). Barcino, Hispania Tarraconensis. Ca. 120. *CIL* 2.4509 = *CIL* 2,6145 = *ILS* 1029.

The full text is cited at no. 172. Here note the portion that reads:

. . . balineum c[um port]icibus solo suo et | du[ctus aquae] fécerunt.

230 C. Sennius Sabinus, praef(ectus) fabr(um). Vicus Albinnensis, Gallia Narbonensis. Hadrian/Antoninus Pius. *CIL* 12.2494 = *ILS* 5768.

The full text is cited at no. 82. Here note the portion that reads:

. . . aquás iúsque | eárum aquarum tubo ducendarum, ita ut récte | perfluere possint, vicanis Albinnensibus d(e) s(uo) d(edit).

231 Incertus. Carthage, Africa. 148/61. *CIL* 8.12513 = *ILS* 345.

[e]x permissu [—] optimi maximique principis imp. Caes. | T. Aelii Hadria[ni Antonini A]ug. Pii [Britt.?] [Ge]rmanici, Dacici, [po]nt. | maximi, cos. IIII, t[ribunicia]e potesta[t ..4.. I]I, p. p., pro[cos.], | et M. Aelii [Aurelii Veri Cae]s. ceterorum[q]ue liberorum [eius — | — aquam magno u]sui futuram thermis [— | — [cir]cuitum marm[oribus] *(the remaining six lines are very fragmentary).*

NOTES: This inscription probably recorded the construction of an aqueduct for the Antonine Baths at Carthage, but the agent of the work cannot be determined from the text. If the aqueduct was erected in the same operation as the baths, the agent was probably the local authorities (compare no. 86). But the last two lines (not cited above) strongly suggest that an individual benefactor is at work here, since they mention *beneficiis eius au[cta]* and the possible name of the benefactor, *[—]us Val[—].* His identity will remain a mystery unless another inscription with his complete name is found.

232 L. Octavius Aur[elianus?] Didasius, c(larissimus) v(ir), pa[tr]onus. Vreu, Africa. Mid-to late third century. *AE* 1975.880.

The full text is cited at no. 110. Here note the portion that reads:

. . . thermas [et aquam *or* formam corrup]|tam post diluviem [..10..]|to servato recte (?) [..5..] | propria liberalitate [ex]o[rnavit] | excoluit, perfecit, dedi[c]avit.

NOTES: Uncertainty over the restoration of the text makes it possible that it may not refer to a water-supply restoration.

Incertus. Municipium Tubernuc, Africa. 364/75. *CIL* 8.948.   233

[— dd nn. Valente et Valen]tiniano Augg. solium estibalium therm[arum — | —]is ut puro fonte pulcrior redderetur aspe[—].

NOTES: Here the water supply to the *solium* of the summer baths was improved by tapping a better source.

Q. Basilius Flaccianus, fl(amen) p(er)p(etuus), augur et cur(ator) [rei pub(licae)].   234
Calama, Numidia. 366/68. *CIL* 8.5335 = *ILS* 5730 = *ILAlg* 1.256.

The full text is cited at no. 130. Here note the portion that reads:

. . . piscinam quae antea tenuis aquae pi[g]ra fluenta capiebat, nunc ve[ro — unda?]|rum intonantium motibus redundantem, Q. Basilius Flaccianus, fl(amen) p(er)p(etuus), augur et cur(ator) [rei pub(licae) restituit?]| et excepto[rio ..20.. exst]ructo adq(ue) perfecto . . .

Incertus, mag(ister) *or* mag(istratus). Segusio, Alpes Cottiae. 375/78. *CIL* 5.7250 =   235
ILS 5701.

The full text is cited at no. 135. Here note the portion that reads:

. . . fistulas dedit, aquam deduxit, ne quid vel utilitati vel us[ibus deesset].

NOTES: The local magistrate who completed and adorned the *Thermae Gratianae* also improved its water supply. *Fistulae* were pipes that, as a fragmentary inscription from Lucus Feroniae (Regio VII) specifies, were fed by a water *castellum* (*AE* 1978.296): *fistula . . . in balneo ad castellum quod est . . . pedes CCXXIIII . . .*

[F]l(avius) Felix Gentilis, v. p., pr(a)es[es prov(inciae), patr]onus. Satafis, Mauretania.   236
379/83. *CIL* 8.8393 = *CIL* 8.20266.

The full text is cited at no. 38. Here note the portion that reads:

. . . [aquae?]ductum therma[rum | nup]er lignis putrib(us) constitutum at [nunc] mirabili opere agpera[— | constr]uctum ins[ti]tuit, perfecit, dedicavitq(ue) . . .

NOTES: Here the governor restores the aqueduct, previously made out of wood that was now rotting, with "marvellous work." *Agpera[—]* appears to be *ac pera[—]*, perhaps to be restored to *ac pera[cute]*.

Local authorities (and Geminus?). Thignica, Africa. 393. *CIL* 8.1412 = *CIL* 8.15204.   237

[aquae]ductos taetra ac deformi caligine mersos et nullo felici aspect[u gaudentes | — proconsulatu Ae]mili Flori Paterni, v. c. et inlustris, et Eri Fani Geminiani, v. c., leg. c. vib[—] | [—] valet in sple[ndidissimo municipio? [—]m et Fl. P (?) Gemino provisionis [—] beneficio quae usui [privato ero]gabatur lavacris praestitit quae hac viduata on[eribus illis? iussit f]ieri civibus | / / / / / / n [— k]andido f.f. l.l. p.p.p. d.d. [—] sumtu public[o restituit] / / / / / et dedicavit.

NOTES: For Aemilius Florus Paternus, see *PLRE* 1.671–72, s.v. "Paternus 6"; for Geminianus, see *PLRE* 1.389, s.v. "Geminianus." The text is fragmentary, and determining the agent is difficult. The phrase *sumtu publico* at the end clearly indicates that the main work (restoration of an aqueduct) was the responsibility of the local authorities. The word *gemino* is more problematic. If the preceding letters are correctly restored (which is far from certain), it may be part of a man's name, but his role in the benefaction remains unclear. Alternatively, *gemino* may modify *beneficio,* in reference to the double nature of the benefaction, since not only were the aqueducts repaired, but also (line 3) "[the water?] that used to be put to private use, he gave over to the baths as a matching benefaction of his foresight" *(gemino provisonis [aquam?] beneficio quae usui [privato ero]gabatur lavacris praestit).* The reading in either case is difficult, which is hardly surprising, since the text was found in fifteen fragments.

238†   Furius C. l(ibertus) Togius Quintil[l]us. Tarentum (Regio II). Second half of the fourth century. *ILS* 5700.

Pentascinensibus thermis, quae longo temporis | trac[tu] intercepto aquae meatu lavacris fre|[que]ntari desierant, undis largioribus afluen|[tem ny]mphalem aquam in meliores usus sua [impensa —] Furius C. l(ibertus) Togius Quintil[l]us | induxit, | [curante Aure?]lio Petrio, v. p.

Trans.: "Furius Togius Quintillus, freedman of Gaius, brought flowing nymphal water in more copious surges to the *Thermae Pentascinenses* at his own expense and for their better use. For a long time the baths had ceased to be visited in their *lavacra,* owing to the interruption of the water supply by an earthquake. [Aure?]lius Petrius, *vir perfectissimus,* saw to the work."

NOTES: The date is that assigned by Lippolis ("Thermae Pentascinenses," 140–41); Nielsen (1.41 n. 26) assigns it more broadly to the fourth century. Furius Togius Quintillus appears to have been a freedman; the proposed identification of the benefactor with Furius Cl. Togius Quintillus (as in *PLRE* 1.760, s.v. "Quintillus 2"), a corrector of Apulia and Calabria (see *CIL* 9.1127), is less likely, given the state of the stone (see Lippolis, loc. cit.). *Lavacra* here evidently denotes some part of the *thermae* (see below, appendix 3, s.v. "lavacrum") that had fallen into disuse. The baths have been excavated and are poorly preserved; they may date originally to the Augustan period. For a full discussion of the remains and the associated inscriptions, see Lippolis, op. cit. See also, Manderscheid, 201, s.v. "Taranto/Tarentum"; Nielsen, 1.45 n. 64 (see also 1.49 n. 91).

Baths Heated

239†   T. Fl(avius?) Avitus Forensis, IIvir iter., q(uin)q(ennalis), omnib(us) munerib(us) functus. Misenum (Regio I). Late second/early third century (?). *CIL* 10.3678 = *ILS* 5689.

T. Fl. Avito | Forensi, IIIvir. iter., qq., omnib. | munerib. functo. hic | idem ad lavacrum bal|near(um) publicar(um) ligni | duri vehes n(umero) *(400)* en|thecae nomine in per|petuum obtulit, ita | tamen ut magistratuus | quodannis successorib(us) | suis tradant; filio | T. Fl. Aviti, v. e., patron(i) col(oniae), | ordo et popul(us) Misenat(ium).

Trans.: "To T. Flavius Avitus Forensis, *duovir* for the second time, censor, having completed all the duties of office. This same man supplied four hundred cartloads of hardwood to the *lavacrum* of the public baths in perpetuity as an appurtenance of his estate, in such a way that the magistrates pass them on each year to their successors. The *ordo* and people of Misenum (dedicated this monument) to the son of T. Flavius Avitus, *vir egregius,* patron of the colony."

NOTES: This interesting benefaction is dated by the form of the nomenclature. The ex-magistrate set up a foundation of four hundred wagonloads of hardwood as fuel for the *lavacrum* of the baths and passed the administration of the benefaction on to his successors in office.

Fabius. Altinum (Regio X). Post-100. Brusin, "Grado," 283.   240

The full text is cited at no. 168/69. Here note the portion that reads:

. . . et alia HS *(400,000)* n(ummum), ut ex [eorum] | reditu cale[fier]ent . . .

NOTES: This figure would yield twenty thousand sesterces per annum if the rate was 5 percent; see Duncan-Jones, *Economy*, 215 (no. 1307). At 6 percent the yield would be twenty-four thousand sesterces per annum. This inscription makes explicit the difference between the benefaction of providing for the upkeep *(tutela)* of baths and that of heating them *(calefactio)*; compare nos. 242–47.

C. Sempronius Sempronianus, IIvir, pontufex *(sic)* perpet(uus) and Sempronia Fusca   241*
Fibia Anicilla, filia. Aurgi, Hispania Tarraconensis. Trajan (?). *CIL* 2.3361 = *ILS* 5688 = *ILER* 2040.

The full text is cited at no. 78. Here note the portion that reads:

. . . thermas aqua perducta cum silvis agnuar(um) | trecentarum pecunia impensaque sua omni d(ederunt) d(edicaverunt).

NOTES: Here an area of three hundred *agnuae* of woodland is given to the baths. The woodland was to provide fuel for the baths, a practice known from other sources; see R. Meiggs, *Trees and Timber in the Ancient Mediterranean World* (Oxford, 1982), 257–38 and 329. An *agnua* was about 120 meters[2]: see Varro *Rust.* 1.10.2; Columella *Rust.* 5.1.5.

Funds for the Maintenance of Baths

L. Aemilius Daphnus, sevir. Murgi, Baetica. Flavian (?). *CIL* 2.5489 = *ILER* 2045.   242

The full text is cited at no. 72. Here note the portion that reads:

. . . in | [tutc]lam earundem thermarum quam|diu ipse vixisset annuos *(denarios) (150)* | pollicitus est.

NOTES: Daphnus had built these baths for the town and here provides 150 denarii (= 600 sesterces) for their upkeep. This sum is consistent with another benefaction of this type (see no. 243) but is small in comparison to others known (see nos. 244–46). The divergences in the amounts probably reflect the relative size and luxury of the buildings in question. *Tutela* means "upkeep" in the sense of cleaning and so forth.

Voconia Avita. Tagilis, Baetica. Late first or early second century. *AE* 1979.352   243*

The full text is cited at no. 165. Here note the portion that reads:

. . . at quot opus tuendum usumq(ue) | perpetuum [t]hermarum praebandum | r(ei) p(ublicae) Tagilitanae d(enariorum) duo milia q(uingentos) ded(it).

NOTES: This woman had built the *thermae* for the town. Here 2,500 denarii (= 10,000 sesterces) is donated to the town as a foundation for the perpetual maintenance of the structure. This amount would yield 500 sesterces per annum if the rate was 5 percent, 600 if it was 6 percent (these are the two most common rates proposed by Duncan-Jones; see notes to no. 202). Presumably, the *usus* of the baths would flow from their being properly maintained, although the phrase conceivably denotes a benefaction of free bathing.

Fabius. Altinum (Regio X). Post-100. Brusin, "Grado," 283.   244

The full text is cited at no. 168/69. Here note the portion that reads:

. . . et HS *(200,000)* n(ummum) [in perp(etuam)] | tutelam eo[ru]mdem *(sic)* . . .

245   C. Plinius Caecilius [Secundus, cos.]. Comum (Regio XI). Ca. 100/109. *CIL* 5.5262 = *ILS* 2927.

The full text is cited at no. 171. Here note the portion that reads:

. . . [— et eo amp]lius in tutela[m] | HS *(200,000)* t(estamento) f(ieri) i(ussit) . . .

246   Q. Avelius Priscus Severius Severus Annavus Rufus, flamen divi Aug(usti), patronus municipi, IIIIvir quinq(uennalis). Corfinium (Regio IV). 180 or later. *AE* 1961.109 = *SupplItal* 3 (1987): 144–45 (no. 8).

The full text is cited at no. 88. Here note the portion that reads:

. . . et balineum Avelianum | muliebre cum HS XXX m(ilia) n(ummum) donavit . . .

NOTES: The 30,000 sesterces was probably for the upkeep of the establishment, which had been either built by Avelius or donated as an existing structure to the local community. Duncan-Jones (*Economy,* 215 [no. 1308a]) calculates the yield of the foundation at 1,800 sesterces per annum if the interest rate was 6 percent, at 5 percent the yield would be 1,500 sesterces per annum.

247   T. Sennius Sollemnis, IIvir, [o]mnib(us) honorib(us) [et] munerib(us) . . . [functus]. Viducasses, Gallia Lugdunensis. Ca. 220/40. *CIL* 13.3162.I = *ILTG* 341.

The full text is cited at no. 106. Here note the portion that reads:

. . . [item legavit] fructum unde in perpetuum instauraretur.

NOTES: The amount of the *fructus* is not specified, but it is tantamount to funds assigned *in tutelam.*

Miscellaneous

Ground Given for Baths

248*   Junia Rustica, sacerdos perpetua, et prima in municipio Cartimitan[o]. Cartima Baetica. Flavian (?). *CIL* 2.1956 = *ILS* 5512 = *ILER* 2054.

The full text is cited at no. 71. Here note the portion that reads:

. . . solum | balinei dedit . . .

NOTES: Here ground is given for the bath, but the text does not say Junia built the actual facility on her ground, as do, for instance, nos. 99, 146, 159, 172–74, and 182.

249†   Q. Torius Culleo, proc(urator) Aug(usti) provinc(iae) Baet(icae). Castulo, Hispania Tarraconensis. First to third centuries. *CIL* 2.3270 = *ILS* 5513 = *ILER* 1417.

Q. Torio Q. f. Culleoni, | proc. Aug. provinc. Baet., | quod muros vetustate | collapsos d(e) s(ua) p(ecunia) refecit, solum | ad balineum aedificandum | dedit, viam quae per Castul. | saltum Sisaponem ducit | adsiduis imbribus corrup|tam munivit, signa Ve|ne|ris Gen[e]tricis et Cupidi|nis ad theatrum posuit, | HS centies, quae illi summa | publice debebatur, addito | etiam epulo populo remisit: | municipes Castulonenses | editis per biduum circens(ibus) d(ederunt) d(edicaverunt).

Trans.: "After two days of circus games, the citizens of Castulo gave and dedicated (this monument) to Q. Torius Culleo, son of Quintus, imperial procurator of the province of Baetica, because he rebuilt at his own expense the walls that had fallen down with old age, gave ground for the construction of baths, strengthened the road that runs through Castulo to the Saltus Sisaponis after it had been undermined by heavy rains, set up statues of Venus Genetrix and Cupid at the theater, and, after staging a public banquet, remitted a debt of ten million sesterces that was owed to him by the city."

NOTES: The massive benefactions of Culleo to Castulo were, in all likelihood, to his home-town; for a full discussion, see Duncan-Jones, "Procurator as Civic Benefactor." The date is uncertain but reckoned by Duncan-Jones (op. cit., 84) to lie within the broad limits of 20–160; J.H. Humphrey (*Roman Circuses: Arenas for Chariot Racing* [London, 1986], 668 n. 27) prefers a date of the third century. Thomas and Witschel ("Constructing Reconstruction," 144) suggest that the damage to the walls might have been caused by the Frankish invasion in ca. 260. If so, Culleo's date is firmly fixed in the third century.

Private Baths Bought and Made Public Property

Local council. Teanum Sidicinum (Regio I). First century (?). *CIL* 10.4792 = *ILS*   250
5677.

s. c. Balneum Clodianum | emptum cum suis aedificis | ex pecunia Augustal. HS *(60,000)* *(six names follow)*.

NOTES: Nielsen (1.40 n. 25) includes this inscription among her first-century material. It seems that a private bath was bought by the town to be made a public facility. Duncan-Jones (*Economy*, 157 [nos. 450–51]) considers the amount mentioned in the inscription a construction cost, but there is no mention of building activity in the text. It is likely that the sixty thousand sesterces was the cost of the *balneum* divided equally among the six Augustales named, probably as *summae honorariae* of ten thousand sesterces each. Compare *AE* 1979.156 (dated to 29 March 151) for a fragmentary inscription from this town that mentions *thermae*, but there is no reason to suspect a connection with the present text.

Lead to Baths

Incertus. Nemus Dianae (Regio I). Undated. *CIL* 14.4190 = *ILS* 5727.   251

[—] | ad horrea Sempron. | ad balneum vetus | in quattuor, | plumb(i) pondo 8,662 | et labella IV, idem | donus pro se et suis.

NOTES: Here an anonymous benefactor gives a remarkable 8,662 pounds of lead to the baths. The lead would be used perhaps for the four *labella* (bowls or basins of uncertain function) mentioned at the end of the citation (the lead is given *in quattuor*) or possibly for pipes and/or pool lining (the King's Bath at Bath was lined with lead). Lead was evidently a much needed commodity for the baths (see no. 137). Other inscriptions report the presence of pipes in baths: see, e.g., nos. 50, 82, 135; no. 46 contains the words *fistulas reposuit*, though the pipes in question may not have been part of the baths. Note also the inscription found on the pipe from the Baths of Agrippina at Rome (*CIL* 15.7247): *in lavacro Agrippinae* | *Imp. Caes. Traj. Hadriani Aug. sub cur(a) Tre\belli Marini Martialis serv. fecit.* Here a slave on the staff of a *procurator aquarum* makes the pipe that goes into the bath (see *RE* 6A.2265, s.v. "Trebellius 12" [Stein]). It can be surmised that the laying of pipes was a major benefaction in itself.

Sportulae Distributed at the Baths (?)

Incertus. Bisica, Africa. Date uncertain (possibly late Imperial). *CIL* 8.23880.   252†

This list of benefactions of an unknown benefactor (the inscription is acephalous and in two fragments) ends (lines 3–4):

. . . thermas quoque | [d]ecuriones sportulis muneravit, civesque et populos universos non solum propriae urbis verum etiam vicinarum epulis quam largissime ministravit.

Trans.: " . . . He presented the baths and also the decurions with *sportulae* and served the citizens and the whole people not only of his own city but of the neighboring towns with the most lavish banquets possible."

NOTES: The wording is unusual, but it is clear from other sources that *sportulae* could be distributed at the baths (see above, chapter 8, p. 217). The wording could also mean that the benefactor presented the baths (i.e., built them) and then gave *sportulae* to the decurions, but this reading would require an unusual use of *quoque* to mean *et* (the inscription is not included in Wesch-Klein's list of African liberalities). Compare no. 58, where baths are dedicated with a distribution of *sportulae*, which may have taken place in the building. It should be noted that there may be a lacuna before "[d]ecuriones," in which case the bath benefaction and the gifts of *sportulae* may not be directly unrelated.

Nonbenefactory Texts

Omitted here for reasons of space is a large body of mosaic texts—usually in Greek verse, of late Imperial date—that praise various facets of the bathing experience. The collection and analysis of such texts has already been partially carried out by Robert ("Épigrammes, 76–84) and Dunbabin ("*Baiarum Grata Voluptas*").

Advertisements

A bath. Suessa (Regio I). Undated. *CIL* 10.4754.   253†

L. Maeci Polli Iunoris | [—]? balneum.

Trans.: "The bath of L. Maecius Pollius Junior."

NOTES: It is possible that there is no lacuna between the lines, making this text a straightforward advertisement.

Bath *in praedis*. Bononia (Regio VIII). Undated. *CIL* 11.721 = *ILS* 5721.   254†

in praedis | C. Legianni Veri | [b]alineum, more urbico lavat(ur) | [et] omnia commoda praestantur.

Trans.: "In the premises of C. Legiannus Verus is the bath, where you can bathe in the manner of the city and where every convenience is available."

NOTES: *Urbicus* probably denotes here *the* city, meaning Rome. For a variation, see the fragmentary *CIL* 8.20579 (Thamalla, Mauretania; undated): *in his praed[iis]* | *fl. Auggg p. p.* | *balneum cy[—]* | *more prep[—]*. The text cannot be adequately reconstructed, but it can be postulated that *cy[—]* was possibly the name of the bath and *prep[—]* may have been some adjective (*praeparatus? praepollens?*) that advertised the baths' pleasures.

Bath *in praedis*. Lugdunum, Gallia Lugdunensis. Undated. *CIL* 13.1926 = *ILS* 5722.   255†

in his prae[dis] | C. Auli Apri sa[cerdotalis] | thermulae s[alutares] | aqua font[is] . . .

Trans.: "In these premises of C. Aulus Aper, priest, are the healthy little baths with springwater . . . "

Bath *in praedis*. Lecourbe, Numidia (ancient name not known). Undated. *AE*   256†
1933.49.

in his praediis Cominiorum | Montani et Feliciani Iun(ioris) | et Feliciani patris eorum, | balneu[m et] omnis humani|tas urbico more praebetur.

Trans.: "In these premises of Cominius Montanus and Cominius Felicianus Junior and Cominius Felicianus, their father, is the bath, and every refinement in the manner of the city is on offer."

257†   *Thermae* of Crassus Frugi. Pompeii (Regio I). First century. *CIL* 10.1063 = *ILS* 5742.

thermae | M. Crassi Frúgi | aqua marina et baln(eae?) | aqua dulci. Ianuarius l(ibertus).

Trans.: "The Thermae of M. Crassus Frugi with seawater and the Baln(eae) with freshwater (*or* with bathing in freshwater). Januarius the freedman."

NOTES: This text is carved on a marble slab found outside the walls of Pompeii. The freedman Januarius was presumably the *conductor* or *balneator* of the establishment and may also have set up the inscription. For discussion, see above, chapter 2, pp. 62–63.

258†   Bath *in praedis*. Pompeii (Regio I). First century. *CIL* 4.1136 = *ILS* 5723.

in praedis Iuliae Sp. f. Felicis | locantur | balneum Venerium et nongentum, tabernae, pergulae, | cenácula ex idibus Aug. primis in idus Aug. sextás annós continuos quinque. | S(i) q(uinquennium) d(ecurrerit) l(ocatio) e(rit) n(udo) c(onsensu).

Trans.: "In the premises of Julia Felix, daughter of Spurius, are leased the *Balneum Venerium et Nongentum,* taverns, *pergulae,* and upper-story apartments, available from the first 13 August to the sixth 13 August on a five-year continual lease. If the five years pass, the lease will be by agreement alone."

NOTES: The meaning of the epithets *Venerium* and *nongentum* are disputed. R. Étienne (*La vie quotidienne à Pompéi*[2] [Paris, 1977], 366) believes that *Venerium* was the name of a group of youths who used the baths, while *nongentum* means "gentlemanly." As a result, he sees the facility as a club for well-to-do young men. This position has recently been supported by P. Ginestet (*Organisations de la jeunesse,* 99, 225 [no. 42]) who argues for a *collegium iuvenum Veneriorum* at Pompeii; but for him *nongentus* (meaning "nine hundred") is the number of members of the Pompeian *iuventus*. Richardson (*Pompeii,* 292–93) concedes that *Venerium* may denote the people who frequented the baths, but he does not think they comprised a club, since there is no mention of a collegium in the text. Dunbabin (*"Baiarum Grata Voluptas,"* 16) includes the *Balneum Venerium et Nongentum* among baths named after deities and suggests that statues of the pertinent divinities (in this case Venus) probably stood in prominent positions in such establishments. More recently, A. Varone ("Voices of the Ancients: A Stroll through Public and Private Pompeii," in *Rediscovering Pompeii* [Rome, 1990], 31) translates the term as "the baths of the Venerii and the judges" but offers no explanation as to what this reading may signify. Koloski-Ostrow (58 nn. 92, 93) believes that the name indicates the exclusiveness of the establishment and its clientele, with *Venerium* meaning "elegant" and *nongentum* meaning "the best people"; a recent translation of the inscription follows Koloski-Ostrow's lead and renders the phrase "an elegant bath suitable for the best people" (E. Fantham et al., *Women in the Classical World* [Oxford, 1994], 334). Surprisingly, Parslow (*"Praedia Iuliae Felicis"*) does not address the problem of the bath's name directly. It is perhaps worth noting that Venus was the patron goddess of Pompeii but, that said, a *Balneum Veneris* is attested at Liternum (no. 43) and a *cistern(am) Veneri(s)* at Lepcis Magna (*IRT* 314; see also ibid., 315a). Venus bore associations with luxury and comfort, so the reference may be to the elegance of the establishment, while simultaneously evoking the patronage of the city's chief goddess. *Nongentum* is more difficult. Pliny (*HN* 33.31) reports that *nongenti* were equestrians who supervised ballot boxes at elections. Since there were elections in progress in Pompeii when the inscription was painted, *nongentum* may well have had some connection with that event, possibly as a topical reference (it is worth remembering that this text was a temporary advertisement, not a permanent commemoration). There may have been a collegium of *nongenti* who frequented these baths, though there is no corroborative evidence for the existence of such a collegium at Pompeii. Alternatively, the term may mean something like "a bath fit for the use of *nongenti*," i.e., important and high-ranking officials at election time. Whatever the case, both epithets appear ultimately to have emphasized the pleasantness of the baths. Other texts advertising baths in *praediae* (for which, see nos. 254–56 and 259) all make a point of highlighting the comfort of their amenities.

Bath *in praedis*. Ficulea (Regio I). Second century (?). *CIL* 14.4015 = *ILS* 5720.   259†

in [h]is praedis Aurelliae Faustinianae | balineus, lavat(ur) mo|re urbico, et omnis | humanitas praesta|tur.

Trans.: "In these premises of Aurelia Faustiniana is the bath, where you can bathe in the manner of the city and where every refinement is available."

NOTES: The date is suggested by the form of Aurelia's name. Note the unusual form *balineus* for *balineum*.

Epitaphs

A drowned child. Rome. Undated. *CIL* 6.16740 = *ILS* 8518.   260†

Daphnus et | Chryseis, | Laconis liberti, | Fortunato suo. v(ixit) a(nnis) VIII, | balneo Martis piscina | perit.

Trans.: "Daphnus and Chryseis, freedpeople of Laco, to their Fortunatus. He lived eight years. He died in a pool in the Baths of Mars."

NOTES: The *Balneum Martis* is otherwise unknown. See also chapter 8, no. 20.

The corrupting effect of baths. Rome. Julio-Claudian *CIL* 6.15258 = *CLE* 1499 =   261† *ILS* 8157 = *ML* 170a.

v(ixit) a(nnis) LII. | D(is) M(anibus) | Ti. Claudi Secundi. | hic secum habet omnia. | balnea, vina, Venus | corrumpunt corpora | nostra, | set vitam faciunt | b(alnea), v(ina), V(enus). | Karo contubernal(i) | fec(it) Merope Caes(aris liberta) | et sibi et suis p(osteris) e(ius).

Trans. (adapted from *ML*): "He lived fifty-two years. To the spirit of the departed Ti. Claudius Secundus. Here he has everything with him. Baths, wine, and sex ruin our bodies, but they are the essence of life—baths, wine, and sex. Merope, freedwoman of Caesar, made (this tomb), for her dear companion, herself, and their family and descendants."

NOTES: Since Merope is an imperial freedwoman and the *contubernalis* of Secundus, he was undoubtedly himself an imperial freedman; his name therefore dates him to the Julio-Claudian period (probably under Claudius or Nero). Similar sentiments are expressed on an inscribed spoon found near Gallipoli (*CIL* 3.12274c = *CLE* 1923 = *ML* 170b), which states that *balnea, vina, Venus faciunt pro|perantia fata* [Baths, wine, and sex make the Fates hasten], and in a Greek epigram (*Anth. Pal.* 10.112) that reads: οἶνος καὶ τὰ λοετρὰ καὶ ἡ περὶ Κύπριν ἐρωὴ / 'ὀξυτέρην πέμπει τὴν ὁδὸν εἰς Ἀίδην [Wine, baths, and the impulse for Cypris [i.e., Aphrodite] send you on a shortcut to Hades!]. See also the parallels cited in *ML*, pp. 369–70.

The dead miss the baths. Ostia (Regio I). Second century (?). *CIL* 14.914 = *ML* 171.   262†

D(is) M(anibus) | C. Domiti Primi. | hoc ego su(m) in tumulo Primus notissi|mus ille. vixi Lucrinis; potabi saepe Fa|lernum; balnia, vina, Venus mecum | senuere per annos.

hec *(sic)* ego si potui, | sit mihi terra lebis. set tamen ad Ma|nes foenix me serbat in ara, qui me|cum properat se reparare sibi. | L(ocus) d(atus) fun[e]ri C. Domiti Primi a tribus Messis, Hermerote, Pia et Pio.

Trans. (adapted from *ML*): "To the spirit of the departed C. Domitius Primus. I, the well-known and famous Primus, am in this tomb. I lived on Lucrine oysters; I often drank Falernian wine. Baths, wine, and sex aged with me through the years. If I managed this, may the earth be light on me. Yet among the spirits, the phoenix, which rushes to renew itself along with me, saves me on the altar. Space given for the burial of C. Domitius Primus by the three Messii—Hermeros, Pia, and Pius."

NOTES: Courtney (*ML*, p. 370) suggests that Primus was a freedman, although on what basis he does so is not made clear. Falernian was a high-grade wine, as attested by its being the most expensive wine available in a price list from a tavern on the Via degli Augusali at Pompeii (*CIL* 4.1679). The phoenix was quite possibly represented on the man's tomb, which would explain the reference to it here. Comparable sentiments are found in a text cited by L. Robert ("Aphrodisias," *Hellenica* 13 [1965]: 189): Ἄνθος τοῖς παροδείταις χαίριν· λοῦσαι, πίε, φάγε, βείνησον· τούτων γὰρ ὧδα κάτω [οὐ]δε[ν] ἔχις [The flower is dear to travelers. bathe, drink, eat, fuck, for you bring none of these below [to Hades]].

263† A dear wife. Ostia (Regio I). Second or third century. *AE* 1987.179.

[D(is) M(anibus) | . . .]nia P. f(ilia) Sebotis, | Q. Minucius Q. f. Pal. Marcellus | coniugi carissimae, pientissim(ae), castissim(ae), | coniugali, quae numquam sine me in publlicum aut in balineum aut ubicumq(ue) ire volet, | quem virgine(m) duxi ann(orum) XIIII, ex qua filia(m) habeo, | cum qua tempus dulce{m} luminis vidi quae me | felicem fecit, set ego mallebam viveres; illa erat | mea felicitas si te superstite(m) reliquisse(m); v(ixit) ann(is) XXI, m(ensibus) II, d(iebus) XXI.

Trans.: "To the spirits of the departed. [?]nia Sebotis, daughter of Publius. Q. Minucius Marcellus, son of Quintus, of the voting tribe Palatina, to his most beloved wife, loyal, chaste, a good wife, who never wanted to go out in public without me, either to the baths or anywhere else. I married her a virgin at fourteen; I had a daughter by her; I saw with her a sweet time of light; she made me happy. Yet I would prefer that you were alive—it would have been my good fortune, if you had survived me. She lived twenty-one years, two months, and twenty-one days."

264† A dear wife. Lugdunum, Gallia Lugdunensis. Second or third century. *CIL* 13.1983 = *ILS* 8158.

D(is) et M(anibus)| memoriae aetern(ae) | Blandiniae Martiolae puellae | innocentissimae, quae vixit | ann(os) XVIII, m(enses) VIIII, d(ies) V. Pompeius | Catussa cives Sequanus tec|tor coniugi incomparabili | et sibi benignissime, quae me|cum vixit an(nis) V, m(ensibus) VI, d(iebus) XVIII | sine ula *(sic)* criminis sorde; vi⟨v⟩us | sibi et coniugi ponendum cu|ravit et sub ascia dedicavit. tu qui legis, vade in Apolinis *(sic)* lavari, quod ego cum coniu|ge feci; vellem si aduc *(sic)* possem.

Trans.: "To the spirits of the departed. To the eternal memory of Blandinia Martiola, a most blameless girl who lived eighteen years, nine months, and five days. Pompeius Catussa, a Sequanian citizen, a plasterer, to his incomparable wife, who was very good to him. She lived with me for five years, six months, and eighteen days without a hint of a nasty reproach. While alive, Catussa saw to the setting up (of this monument) for himself and his wife, and he dedicated it while it was still under construction. You who reads this, go to be washed in the baths of Apollo, which I did with my wife; I would wish to, if I still could."

Bath Officials

Balneator. Rome. Undated. *CIL* 6.9395/96 = *ILS* 7718a.   265

Two related epitaphs.

CIL 6.9395: Asiniae C(ai) l(ibertae) Ammiae, | matri Felicis Fabri | balneatoris.

CIL 6.9396: C. Asinio Fe[lici] | Fabro balnea|tori. vixit | annos XXXIV.

NOTES: These epitaphs offer an interesting and rare look at the social status of an occupant of the elusive and versatile post of *balneator* (see Nielsen, 1.127–28). His mother was a freedwoman, so he was freeborn. Many other epitaphs from Rome commemorate *balneatores,* usually in an unremarkable manner—e.g., as *Felix balneator* (*CIL* 6.9216). See also *CIL* 6.6243 = *ILS* 7412, chapter 2, n. 77.

Arcarius thermarum. Brundisium (Regio II). Undated. *AE* 1978.217.   266

Qeranus *(sic),* publ(icus) | arcarius ther|marum, v(ixit) a(nnos) [—].

NOTES: A *publicus arcarius* was a slave in charge of a municipal treasury (see *AE* 1978.194), but this individual is expressly stated to have been attached to the baths. The best explanation for his duties is that they focused on the income from the publicly owned *thermae* of the city. No substantial remains of baths are known at the site; see Greco, *Magna Grecia,* 206–8.

Curator balinei. Baetulo, Hispania Tarraconensis. Undated. *CIL* 2.4610.   267†

M. Fabio Gal. Nepot[i]| Iessonensi, aed(ili), IIvir II, | fl(ameni) Romae et Augustor(um), | curatori balinei novi ob | curam et innocentiam | ex d(ecreto) d(ecurionum).

Trans.: "To M. Fabius Nepos, of the voting tribe Galeria, from the town of Iesso, aedile, *duovir* twice, priest of Rome and the Augusti, curator of the *Balneum Novum,* on account of his diligence and blamelessness. By decree of the decurions."

NOTES: Iesso was a town about ninety kilometers inland from Baetulo. Apparently Nepos had moved to Baetulo and became a leading citizen there. Precisely what his duties were as "curator of the Balneum Novum" is not clear, but, following a recent suggestion (Poma, "Osservazioni," 31–32), they possibly involved monitoring the financial aspects of the construction—and perhaps also of the operation—of these baths.

Vilicus thermarum. Rome. Post-Neronian (?). *CIL* 6.8679.   268†

D(is) M(anibus). | Onesimus Cae[s. n.], | vilic(us) therma[r(um), et a?] | bibliothec(a) gra[ec(a)], | Crescenti alu|mno suo. vix(it) | ann(is) VIIII, me(n)s(ibus) I. | b(onae) m(emoriae) fecit.

Trans.: "To the spirits of the departed. Onesimus, slave of our Caesar, *vilicus* of the baths, secretary of the Greek library, made this for Crescens, his charge, for his good remembrance. He lived nine years, one month."

NOTES: A *vilicus* was any steward or manager, and the term was often applied to an overseer on a country estate or to a supervisor in the imperial service; see *OLD,* s.v. We can only speculate what the duties of a *vilicus* at the baths were; see Nielsen, 1.126. This text has been cited as proof of the existence of libraries at baths (see, e.g., Nielsen, 1.165–66; Yegül, 179, 448 n. 132), but caution is required. It is quite possible that Onesimus was *vilicus* of the baths and secretary of an unrelated Greek library (i.e., one not located at the baths). Other inscriptions from Rome record officials termed *a bibliotheca* (e.g., *CIL* 6.4431 = *ILS* 1971, *CIL* 6.5188 = *ILS* 1589, *CIL* 6.5189 = *ILS* 1588, *CIL* 6.5884), and there is room for *et a* in the lacuna after *therma[r.—]*: see T.K. Dix and G.W. Houston, "Libraries in Roman Baths?" *Balnearia* 4, no. 1 (1996): 2–4; G.W. Houston, "Onesimus the Librarian," *ZPE* 114 (1996): 205–8. The deceased, Crescens, was a slave apprentice under Onesimus.

269†   *Vilicus thermarum.* Rome. Flavian (?). *CIL* 6.8676.

Petronia Secund[a—] | sibi et Flavio Aug[(usti) lib.?], | vilico thermar(um) N[eron-ianarum?] | num coniugi pientis[simo cum] | quo vixit annis XL sine qu[erella] | et Flavio filio Quir. Valeri[ano et libertis] | libertabus posterisquae *(sic)* eor[um]. | in fronte pedes XI, in agro ped[—].

Trans.: "Petronia Secunda, (built this tomb) for herself and Flavius, freedman of the emperor (?), *vilicus* of the Thermae Neronianae (?), surely the most loyal husband, with whom she lived for forty years without a quarrel, and for her son Flavius Valerianus, of the voting tribe Quirina, and for their freedmen and freedwomen and their descendants. Its front is eleven feet high, its area [?] feet . . .

NOTES: This inscription mentions yet another *vilicus thermarum;* see also the previous entry. The names of these freedpeople (if line 2 is correctly restored) suggest a Flavian date for the text. Flavius' status as an imperial freedman confirms that the imperial *thermae* were the emperor's concern, not public property.

270†   *Curator operis thermarum.* Aequum Tuticum (Regio II). Hadrian. *CIL* 9.1419 = *ILS* 6489.

I(ovi) o(ptimo) m(aximo). | C. Ennius C. f. Firmus, | permissu decurion(um) c(oloniae) B(eneventanae), | Benevento aedilis, | IIvir i. d., quaestor, | curator operis thermarum | datus ab | imp. Caesare Hadriano Aug.

Trans.: "To Jupiter, best and greatest. C. Ennius Firmus, son of Gaius, by permission of the decurions of the colony of Beneventum, who was aedile at Beneventum, *duovir* for administering the law, quaestor, curator of the building of the baths, appointed by the emperor Caesar Hadrian Augustus."

NOTES: This text is interesting because it throws light on the relationship between Aequum Tuticum and Beneventum, which lay some thirty kilometers apart on the Via Traiana. Ennius had been sent from Beneventum, probably upon a request from the authorities at Aequum Tuticum, to carry out some task at the latter. Unfortunately, the wording is vague. Did Ennius hold the listed offices at Beneventum or at Aequum Tuticum? If at the latter, since his appointment as curator of the baths is attributed to Hadrian, what was the role of the decurions at Beneventum in granting permission, and to what end did they do so? Zazo ("Benevento," 102) links Ennius with the attested *Thermae Commodianae* at Beneventum, which are thereby lent an earlier construction date; this proposition is most tentative, however.

271   *Exactor thermarum.* Rome. After early second century. *CIL* 6.8677 = *ILS* 1628.

D. Philetus Aug. | libertus, exactor the|rmarum Traianarum. | P. Pompeius fecit sibi et | suis libertis libertabusove *(sic)* | posterisove *(sic)* eorum | et Balera Tertylai *(sic)* co⟨n⟩iugi | optimai.

NOTES: As with the *vilici,* the duties of an *exactor thermarum* are unknown.

Adiutor thermarum. Rome. M. Aurelius or slightly later. *CIL* 6.8678.   272

M. Aurelius Aug. lib. | Ireneus, adiutor | termarum Traia(narum).

NOTES: This inscription is from a tomb that depicts a togate figure. The duties of this official are unknown.

Capsararius. Rome. After early third century. *CIL* 6.9232 = *ILS* 7621.   273†

Cucumio et Victoria | se vivos fecerunt | capsararius *(sic)* de Antonianas *(sic).*

Trans.: "Cucumio and Victoria, a *capsarius* from the Antonine Baths, made this for themselves while they were alive."

NOTES: This inscription is from a tomb. A *capsarius* was an official in charge of guarding clothes and/or collecting entrance fees: see *Dig.* 1.15.3.5; Nielsen, 1.129–30.

Miscellaneous

Avoidance of (mixed?) baths. Thuburbo Maius, Africa. Undated. *AE* 1916.112.   274†

iussu domini | Aesculapi | L. Numisius L. f. | Vitalis | podium de | suo fecit. | quis intra | podium ad|scendere vollet a mulilere, a suilla, | a faba, a ton|sore, a bali|neo commu|ne custodi|at triduo; | cancellos | calciatus | intrare nollito.

Trans.: "By order of our lord Aesculapius, L. Numisius Vitalis, son of Lucius, built the podium with his own money. Anyone wishing to enter the podium area is to abstain from women, pork, beans, the barber, and communal baths for three days; do not enter the confines with shoes on."

NOTES: The podium had a fence or wall around it (the *cancelli*), forming a sort of *temenos* sacred to Asclepius. The restriction on attending "communal" baths may refer to mixed, rather than merely "public," establishments (compare Mart. 3.51.3), which would accord with the injunction to avoid women.

Gaming board, carved onto the pavement at the forum at Timgad, Numidia. Un-   275†
dated. *CIL* 8.17938 = *ILS* 8626f.

venari, lavari, | ludere, ridere: | occ (= hoc) est vivere.

Trans.: "Hunting, bathing, gambling, laughing—that's living!"

NOTES: On such gaming boards, see Balsdon, *Life and Lesiure,* 157–58; Toner, 90–91.

Graffito: advertisement for eggs. Herculaneum (Regio I). First century. *CIL* 4.10603.   276†

Nicanor ovas.

Trans.: "Nicanor, eggs."

NOTES: This graffito is from a small podium in *opus signinum* outside an entrance to the Forum Baths. Apparently, it marked the stand of Nicanor, an egg seller.

Graffito: price list or tally. Herculaneum (Regio I). First century. *CIL* 4.10674.   277†

nuc(es) biber(ia) XIIII; | singa II; | panem III; | offellas III XII; | thymatla IIII VIII; | LI.

Trans.: "Nuts, drinks—14; | hog's fat—2; | bread—3; | cutlets, for 3—12; | sausage, for 4—8; | 51."

NOTES: This graffito and the following four entries were found in a small room off the vestibule and flanking the main entrance to the Suburban Baths; see A. Maiuri, *Ercolano: I nuovi scavi (1927–1958)* (Rome, 1959), 1.153–54. The list is either a price list for a seller of food in this room or a tally of food and drink enjoyed by literate customers (as suggested, e.g., by J.J. Deiss in *Herculaneum: Italy's Buried Treasure²* [New York, 1985], 147). In view of the provision of two numbers for some items, the price list seems the more plausible explanation. The prices are in *asses*. The last figure (LI) probably represents a price for a combination of all the items listed and some unspecified service(s) (all the items listed carry a combined price of thirty-nine *asses*).

278†   Graffito: lunch and sex. Herculaneum (Regio I). First century. *CIL* 4.10677.

Apelles cubicularius | Caesar(is) | cum Dextro | pranderunt hic iucundissime et | futuere simul.

Trans.: "Apelles, chamberlain of the emperor, and Dexter had lunch here most pleasantly and fucked at the same time."

NOTES: This graffito is from the same room in the Suburban Baths as no. 277. Given the details provided by this entry and the following two entries, it is possible that this room served as a brothel attached to the baths.

279†   Graffito: sex. Herculaneum (Regio I). First century. *CIL* 4.10678.

Apelles Mus cum fratre Dextro | amabiliter futuimus bis bina(s).

Trans.: "We, Apelles the Mouse and his brother Dexter, lovingly fucked two women twice."

NOTES: This graffito is from the same room in the Suburban Baths as no. 277. Deiss (*Herculaneum,* 147) erroneously omits mention of the women and takes the passage to mean that the two men engaged in homosexual sex.

280†   Graffito: message to a lover. Herculaneum (Regio I). First century. *CIL* 4.10676.

Hermeros Primigeniae dominae: | veni Puteolos in vico Tim(i)niano et quaere | a Messio num(m)ulario Hermerotem Phoebi.

Trans.: "Hermeros to his mistress Primigenia: come to Puteoli and in the Timinian district ask the banker Messius for Hermeros, son (*or* slave) of Phoebus."

NOTES: This graffito is from the same room in the Suburban Baths as no. 277.

281†   Graffito: service and sex. Herculaneum (Regio I). First century. *CIL* 4.10675.

duo sodales hic fuerunt et, cum diu malum | ministrum in omnia haberent | nomine Epaphroditum, vix tarde | eum foras exigerunt. | consumpserunt persuavissime cum futuere HS CVS.

Trans.: "Two companions were here and, since they had a thoroughly terrible attendant called Epaphroditus, threw him out onto the street not a moment too soon. They then spent 105½ sesterces most agreeably while they fucked."

NOTES: This graffito is from the same room in the Suburban Baths as no. 277.

282†   Regulations for operating a bathhouse. Metallum Vipascense, Lusitania. Hadrian. *CIL* 2.5181 = *ILS* 6891.

Only the pertinent lines (19–31) of this lengthy charter of an imperial mining facility are cited below.

(19) balinei fruendi. conductor balinei sociusve eius omnia sua inpensa balineum [quod ita conductum habe]bit in | pr. k. Iul. primas omnibus diebus calfacere et praestare debeto a prima luce in horam septim[am diei mulieribus] et ab hora octava | in horam secundum noctis viris arbitratu proc(uratoris) qui metallis praeerit. aquam in [balineum usque ad] summam ranam hypo|caustis et labrum tam mulieribus quam viris profluentem recte praestare debeto. conductor a viris sing(ulis) | aeris semisses et a mulieribus singulis aeris asses exigito. excipiuntur liberti et servi [Caes(aris) qui proc(uratoris)] in offi[c]is erunt vel | commoda percipient, item inpuberes et milites. conductor socius actorve eius [instrumentum balinei et e]a omnia quae | (25) ei adsignata erunt integra conductione peracta reddere debeto nisi siqua vestutate c[orrupta erunt]. aena quibus | utetur lavare tergere unguereque adipe e recenti tricensima quaque die recte debeto. [si vis maior damnumque fatale inpedi]lerit, quo minus lavare recte possit, eius temporis pro rata pensionem conductor reputare debe[to. praeter] haec et siquid | aliut eiusdem balinei exercendi causa fecerit reputare nihil debebit. conductori ve[ndere ligna] nisi ex recisamini|bus ramorum quae ostili idonea non erunt ne liceto. si adversus hoc quid fecerit in singul[as vehes HS] centenos n(ummos) fisco d(are) d(ebeto). | si id balineum recte praebitum non erit, tum proc(urator) metallorum multam conductori quotiens recte praebitum non erit | usque ad HS CC dicere liceto. lignum conductor repositum omni tempori habeto, quod diebus . . . *(the text breaks off)*.

Trans.: "(Regulations) for operating the baths. The *conductor* of the bath or his partner is to heat the bath every day and keep it open for use, entirely at his own expense, as stipulated in the lease for the bath that runs until 30 June next, for women from first light to the seventh hour of day, and for men from the eighth hour to the second hour of night, in accordance with the decision of the procurator who runs the mines. He is to provide a properly flowing water supply for the bath up to the highest water-level marker in the boilers (?) and for the *labrum,* for both men and women. The *conductor* is to charge one half *as* for men and one full *as* for women. Exempt from charge are those imperial slaves and freedmen who work for the procurator or who enjoy privileges, likewise minors and soldiers. When the lease has expired, the *conductor,* his partner, or his agent is to return in good order all the instruments of the bath entrusted to him, unless some have dilapidated through old age. Once a month he should properly wash, scrub, and polish with fresh fat the bronzes that he uses. If some greater power or serious loss impedes the proper running of the bath, the *conductor* is to reckon compensation, prorated for the number of days the bath is closed. Besides this, if he does anything else to keep the bath running, he ought to reckon no compensation. The *conductor* is not allowed to sell wood, except such pruned branches as are unsuitable for burning. If he disobeys this, he is to pay one hundred sesterces for every wagonload of wood into the *fiscus.* If the bath is not run properly, let the procurator of the mines fine the *conductor* for every day the bath is not properly running, up to a maximum of two hundred sesterces. The *conductor* is to keep at all times a supply of wood, which on days . . . *(the rest of the section is missing)."*

NOTES: This fascinating, behind-the-scenes look at the baths contains much useful information. As a whole, the law deals with the activities of various *conductores,* i.e., people who obtain government contracts to perform certain tasks. This inscription has often been used to generalize about such matters as bath economics, entrance fees, opening hours, and mixed bathing (see, e.g., Heinz, 146, 150; Nielsen, 1.126–27, 132, 137; Yegül, 45, 46–47). But caution is required. In the first place, its context is something of a special case: an imperially owned and run mining facility. The very long opening hours of these baths, for instance, might therefore be peculiar, since mining, then as now, was especially dirty work. Similarly, depending on the shifts of the workers, the reservation of the baths for women early in the day could be a dictate of necessity rather than of morality. Noteworthy is the prohibition on selling combustible wood—to earn special mention, this must have been a sharp practice on the part of some bathmen, who probably sold wood provided to them by the authorities.

283†   The glass ball game. Rome. Second century (?). *CIL* 6.9797 = *ILS* 5173 = *ML* 124.

Ursus, togátus vitreá quí prímus pila | lúsi decenter cum meís lúsóribus, | laudante populó maximís clámóribus, | thermis Traiiáni *(sic)*, thermís Agrippae et Titi, | multum et Nerónis, si tamen mihi créditis, | ego sum. ovantés veníte, pilicrepí, | statuamque amíci, floribus, violís, rosís, | folióque multó adque unguentó marcidó | oneráte amantés, et merum prófundite | nigrum Falernum aut Sétínum aut Caecubum, | vivó ac volentí dé apothécá dominicá, | Ursumque canite vóce concórdi senem hilarem, | iocósum, pilicrepum, scholasticum, | qui vicit omnes antecessorís suós | sénsú decóre adque arte suptílissimá. | nunc véra versu verba dícamus senés: | sum victus ipse, fateor, á ter cónsule | Véró patrónó, nec semel sed saepius, | cuius libenter dicor exodiarius.

Trans.: "Ursus am I, who was the first citizen to play gracefully the glass ball game with my fellow players, while the people approved with clamorous applause in the Thermae of Trajan, in the Thermae of Agrippa and of Titus, and frequently in Nero's (if only you believe me). Come together rejoicing, ballplayers, and lovingly cover the statue of your friend with blossoms, roses, and violets and many a leaf, and with languid perfume; pour forth the dark Falernian wine, or Setian, or Caecuban, from the master's cellar to one who is alive and willing; and sing with harmonious voice of the old man Ursus, a merry fellow, full of jest, a ballplayer, a scholar, who surpassed all of his predecessors in tact, dignity, and subtle skill. Now let us old men speak the truth in verse: I have been defeated, I confess it, by the patron Verus, thrice consul—not once but many times; I am gladly called his clown."

NOTES: For discussion of this text, see above, chapter 8, p. 195–96.

284†   A *familia thermensis*. Patavium (Regio X). Late second century or later. *CIL* 5.2886.

[pro salute et per|p]etuitate dominorum | familiae thermensi | Thermarum Urban{i}a[r(um)].

Trans.: "For the health and perpetuity of our lords (*or* masters), to the *familia thermensis* of the Urbane Baths."

NOTES: Mommsen suggests that these baths may be the famed hot springs in the Field of Apon: see Suet. *Tib.* 14.3 and Mart. 6.42.4; compare Pliny *HN* 2.227, 31.61. These sources, however, call those springs *fons Aponi,* not *thermae urbanae*; the connection seems tenuous. The name Urbane Baths probably refers to a particular kind of bath, in the *more urbico* mold (see nos. 254, 256, 259). Mention of the *familia*—i.e., the slave attendants—of the Urbane Baths is of particular interest (such use of the word *familia* was common: see Frontin. *Aq.* 116–19; *CIL* 5.2541, *CIL* 6.33469 = *ILS* 9028). Who set up the text is not clear.

Baths and health. Bu-Ngem (ancient name not known), Tripolitania. Before 238. *AE*   285†
1929.7b = *IRT* 918 = *ML* 40.

Quaesii multum quot | memoriae tradere(m), | **A**gens prae cunctos in | hac castra
milites, | **V**otum communem, pro|que reditu exercitus | **I**nter priores et futuros red-
dere(m). | **D**um quaero mecum dig|na divom nomina, | **I**nveni tandem nomen | et
numen deae | **V**otis perennem quem | dicare(m) in hoc loco. | **S**alutis igitur quan|dium
cultores sient, | **Q**ua potui sanxi nomen, | et cunctis dedi | **V**eras salutis lymphas, |
tantis ignibus | **I**n istis semper ha|renacis collibus | **N**utantis Austri solis | flammas
fervidas | **T**ranquille ut nando | delenirent corpora. | **I**ta tu qui sentis mag|nam facti
gratiam | **A**estuantis animae | fucilari spiritum, | **N**oli pigere laudem | voce reddere |
Veram, qui voluit | esse te sanum tib[i], | **S**et prostare vel | salutis gratia.

Trans. (adapted from *ML*): "I, in charge of all the soldiers in this camp, pondered at
length what vow for the common interest, for the return of the army, I should
discharge and put on record, among previous and future vows. While I was pondering
names of worthy gods, I at last found the name and spirit of a goddess to consecrate
with my vows forever in this place. Therefore, to the best of my ability, I have
consecrated the name of Health for as long as there be worshipers, and I have given to
everyone the waters that truly belong to Health, so that in this great heat, in these
ever-sandy dunes of the shifting south, their bodies, swimming at leisure, may soothe
the burning flames of the sun. So you who feel great gratitude for the fact that the
breath of your panting respiration is refreshed, do not feel shy about offering vocal
and accurate praise to the man who desired you to be healthy; on the contrary, at least
bear witness because of Health."

NOTES: This text was found in the baths in the fortress at Bu-Ngem, on the Tripolitanian
frontier. Reynolds and Ward-Perkins *(IRT)* associate it with *IRT* 919, which is a stele recording,
simply, *centurio* | *[Leg. III Aug.]* | *faciendum* | *curavit*, with the name of the legion erased
following its *damnatio* in 238 (see *RE* 12.1493–1505, s.v. "Legio III Augusta"] [Ritterling]).
Thus a date of the early third century is provided for both texts (they are both executed in third-
century rustic lettering, and the baths were completed in 203; see the comments of Courtney in
ML, pp. 263–65). Every two lines of the above inscription constitute one line of verse, the
beginning of which forms an acrostic (indicated above in bold capital letters) that spells out Q.
Avidius Quintianus, thereby giving a name to the dedicator. Although this inscription is from a
military bathhouse, it provides interesting testimony of the association of baths and health and
of the soothing qualities of the baths in the extreme climate of the North African desert.

Price for services. Diocletian's price edict. 301. *CIL,* vol. 3, p. 1936; 7.75–66.   286†

capsario in signulis labantibus: *(denarios)* duos; | balneatori privatario in singulis
lavantibus: *(denarios)* duos.

Trans.: "To the *capsarius* 2 denarii per bather; to the private bathman, two denarii per
bather."

NOTES: For *capsarius,* see the notes to no. 273. The *balneator* here is specifically designated
privatarius and so was apparently in charge of a privately leased public bathhouse. On the price
edict in general, see S. Lauffer, *Diokletians Preisedikt* (Berlin, 1971).

Baths as proof of city status. Orcistus, Phrygia. 325–31. *CIL* 3.352 = *CIL* 3.7000 =   287†
ILS 6091 = *AE* 1981.779.

This lengthy text contains several elements (a petition to Constantine and two imperial rescripts concerning the status of Orcistus). Cited below are lines 16–31 of panel I, from the first imperial rescript.

(16) adseruerunt enim vicum suum | spatiis prioris aetatis oppidi splendore florulisse ut et annuis magistratu⟨u⟩m fascibus orn[a]|retur essetque curialibus celebre et popul[o] | civium plenum. ita enim ei situ ad[q]ue ingenio | locus opportunus esse perhib[e]tur ut ex qu|attuor partibu[s e]o totidem in sese confluan[t] | viae, quibus omnibus publicis mansio tamen [u]|tilis adque accomo[da] esse dicatur, aquaru[m] | ibi abundantem aflu[en]tiam, labacra quoqu[e] | publica priva[taqu]e, forum {i}statuis veterum | principum ornatum, populum comm[a]nentium | adeo celebrem [ut se]dilia [qu]ae ibidem sunt [fa]|cile conpleantur, pr[aeter]ea ex decursibus | praeterfluentium [a]quarum aquimolin[a]|rum numerum copiosum.

Trans.: "They [the Orcistans] affirmed that their *vicus* had flourished with the luster of an *oppidum* for the duration of a previous era, so that it was dignified with the annual fasces of magistrates, abounded in *curiales*, and had a full population of citizens. It is endowed with a location so opportune, both in its situation and natural quality, that four roads converge on it from as many regions, for which there is a *mansio* for all public needs that is said to be functional as well as comfortable. There is an abundance of water that flows there, public and private baths, a forum adorned with the statues of emperors of old, a sedentary population so numerous that all the seats as are there are easily filled up, and, in addition, a great quantity of water mills, by virtue of the water that flows by from the hills."

NOTES: It is noteworthy that baths, both public and private (the latter meaning, presumably, privately owned but publicly accessible), are cited among the claims the Orcistans made to justify their city status. For a full discussion of this text, see A. Chastagnol, "L'inscription constantinienne d'Orcistus," *MEFRA* 93 (1981): 381–416.

Part D

Greek Texts

Constructional Benefactions

Emperors

Vespasian. Cadyanda, Lycia. Precise date uncertain. *IGRR* 3.507 = *TAM* 2.651.   288†

αὐτοκράτωρ Καῖσαρ Φλάουιος Οὐασπασιανὸς (*sic*) Σεβαστὸς | κατεσκεύασεν τὸ βαλανεῖον ἐκ τῶν ἀνασοθέντων χρημάτων ὑπ' αὐτοῦ | τῇ πόλει.

Trans.: "The emperor Caesar Flavius Vespasianus Augustus built the bath from the money saved by him for the city."

NOTES: The last phrase of the inscription reports that Vespasian used funds that were under imperial control to erect these baths. Cagnat *(IGRR)* comments on ἀνασοθέντων: "Ita lapis." The form, however, derives from ἀνασῴζω, which raises interesting questions as to how exactly Vespasian "saved" money for Cadyanda (see next entry). The baths have been partially excavated: see Farrington, *Roman Baths of Lycia,* 151–52 (no. 14); E. Frézouls, M.-J. Morans, and D. Longpierre, "Urbanisme et principaux monuments de Kadyanda," *Ktema* 11 (1986): 236; Yegül, 299–300.

Vespasian. Patara, Lycia. 68/69. *IGRR* 3.659 = *TAM* 2.396.   289†

αὐτοκράτωρ Καῖσαρ Φλάο[υι]ος Οὐεσπασιανὸς | Σεβαστὸς τὸ βαλανεῖον κατεσκεύασεν | [ἐκ] θεμελίων σὺν τοῖς ἐν αὐτῷ προσκοσμήμασιν καὶ ταῖς κολυμβήθραις διὰ Σέξτου Μαρκίου Πρείσκου πρεσβευτοῦ | [τ]οῦ ἀντιστρατήγου, [ἐ]κ [τ]ῶν συν[τ]η[ρ]ηθέντων χρημάτων κ[οι]νῶν τ]οῦ ἔθνους δηναρίων [—] καὶ τῶν ἀπὸ τῆς Παταρέων πόλεως | συντελειώσαντος καὶ ἀφιερώσαντος τὰ ἔργα.

Trans.: "The emperor Caesar Flavius Vespasianus Augustus built the bath from its foundations, along with the adornments in it and the diving pools, from the preserved communal funds of the province, denarii *(amount missing),* and the money of the city of Patara. Sex. Marcius Priscus, the propraetorian legate, completed and dedicated the work."

NOTES: For Sextus Marcius, see *PIR*[2] M 242; Thomasson, 1.276 (no. 5). Vespasian's name has been inserted over an erasure, probably the name of Nero. The text credits the emperor with the work, yet it reports that the funding came from provincial and local sources. The best explanation is that the provincial money was considerd the emperor's property or, at least, that it was not released without his permission. Vespasian's "saving" of money for Cadyanda in the previous entry is probably also to be read in this sense. For the remains, see Farrington, *Roman Baths of Lycia,* 72–73, 156–57 (no. 38); Yegül, 299.

Trajan (?). Arykanda, Lycia. 98/99 (?). *IK* 48 (Arykanda) 24.   290†

[αὐτοκράτωρ Καῖσαρ Νέρ|ουας Τραιανὸς Σεβαστὸς | Γερμανικὸς κατεσκεύ|ασε]ν τὸ
βαλ[ανεῖον ἐκ θεμε|λίων|] διὰ πρ[εσβ]ε[υτοῦ | αὐτο]ῦ καὶ ἀντιστρ[ατήγου | Λουκίου]
Ἰουλίου [Μαρεί|νου Καικιλ]ίου Σ[ίνπλικος].

Trans.: "The emperor Caesar Nerva Trajan Augustus Germanicus built the bath from
its foundations, through his propraetorian legate Lucius Marinus Caecilius Simplex."

NOTES: For L. Julius Marinus Caecilius Simplex, see *PIR*² I 408; Thomasson, 1.278 (no. 15).
Although heavily restored, a good case can be made for restoring Trajan's name and his agency
in the work; see *IK* 48 (Arykanda), pp. 25–29. The remains of these modest baths have been
excavated: see Farrington, *Roman Baths of Lycia,* 150–51 (no. 10); Yegül, 258, 299.

Imperial Officials

291   Flavius Octavius Victor (?), praefectus annonae. Ostia (Regio I). 328 or later. *AE*
1984.150 (see *SEG* 33 [1983] 773) = Cicerchia and Marinucci, *Scavi di Ostia*
11.219–22 (no. C 107).

λουτρον αλεξιπον|ον ~~~~~~~~~|ιξεν [—] Βίκτωρ ἀρχὸς ἐών κύδιμος Αὐσονίης.

NOTES: This Greek verse inscription in three fragments was found in the Forum Baths; it
survives only in transcript. It records that a certain Victor—probably the *praefectus annonae* ca.
328 or later, as suggested in the article in *AE*—carried out some work on the baths. Unfortunately the verb is missing, so the nature of that work (restoration, extension, or adornment) is
not recoverable. *RE* (Suppl. 15.293–94, s.v. "Octavius 90a" [Eck]) prefers a date in the second
half of the fourth century for the text, while Nielsen (2.6 [C.27]) omits mention of the
benefaction.

Local Authorities

292†   Λ. Οὐάκκιος Λαβέων, γυμνασίαρχος. Kyme, Asia. 2 B.C.–A.D. 14. *IGRR* 4.1302 = *IK*
5 (Kyme) 19.

In this lengthy honorary inscription, Labeo is praised by the people for a range of
benefactions presented while he held various posts. The lines cited below represent
part of an inscription cited within this text as having accompanied statues of Labeo
set up in the gymnasium.

|(37) . . . ὁ δᾶμος ἐτείμασεν Λεύκιον Οὐάκκιον Λευκίω | υἱὸν Αἰμιλία Λαβέωνα,
φιλοκύμαιον εὐεργέταν, γυμνασι|αρχήσαντα καλῶς καὶ μεγαλοδόξως, ὀνθέντα δὲ | καὶ
τὸ βαλανῆον τοῖς νεοῖσι καὶ πρὸς τὰν εἰς αὐτὸ χοραγί|αν ταῖς ὑπαρχοίσαις αὐτῶ κτή-
σαις ἐν Ζμαραγήῳ . . .

Trans.: " . . . The people honored Lucius Vaccius Labeo, son of Lucius, of the voting
tribe Aemilia, friend of Kyme and benefactor, who was a good and well-respected
gymnasiarch, who set up the bath for the young and his properties in Zmarageos for
its upkeep . . . "

NOTES: Engelmann (the editor of *IK* 5) states that these are the baths near the Gymnasium of
the Neoi at Kyme. The text implies that they were reserved for the use of the Neoi only. For the
work of gymnasiarchs in giving money for baths, see Delorme, *Gymnasion;* L. Robert, "Inscriptions d'Aiolide," *BCH,* 1933, 502–4 (= id., *Opera Minora Selecta* 1.446–48); id., *Études
Anatoliennes* (Amsterdam, 1970), 315–18; A.H.M. Jones, *The Greek City from Alexander to
Justinian* (Oxford, 1940), 221–22.

Ἀπερλειτῶν καὶ τῶν συνπολιτυομένων ἡ βουλὴ καὶ ὁ δῆμος. Aperlae, Lycia. 80/81.   293†
IGRR 3.690 = *ILS* 8796.

αὐτοκράτορι Τίτῳ Θεοῦ Οὐεσπασιανοῦ υἱῷ Καίσαρι | [Οὐεσ]πασιανῷ Σεβαστῷ
ἀρχιερεῖ μεγίστῳ, δημαρχικῆς | [ἐξου]σίας τὸ ι', αὐτοκράτορι τὸ [ι]ε', ὑπάτῳ τὸ η',
πατρὶ πατρίδος, | τειμητῇ / / / / / / / / / / / | ἐπὶ Τίτου Αὐρηλίου Κυήτου πρεσβευτοῦ καὶ
ἀντιστρα[τή]γο]υ τοῦ Σεβαστοῦ καὶ Γαίου Βιήνου Λόγγου ἐπιτρόπου [τοῦ] | Σεβαστοῦ,
Ἀπερλειτῶν καὶ τῶν συνπολιτευομένων | ἡ βουλὴ καὶ ὁ δῆμος τὸ βαλανεῖον καὶ τὸ
πρόστοον κατε|σκεύασεν ἐκ θεμελίων.

Trans.: "To the emperor Titus Caesar Vespasianus Augustus, son of the god Vespasian, chief priest, holder of the tribunician power for the tenth year, imperator for the
fifteenth time, consul for the sixth time, father of his country, to the censor *(Domitian's name erased)*. When T. Aurelius Quietus was propraetorian legate and
C. Bienus Longus was procurator, the council and people of Aperlae and the con-
federacy built the bath and its *prostoon* from the foundations."

NOTES: For T. Aurelius Quietus, see *PIR²* A 1592; Thomasson, 1.277 (no. 10). For C. Bienus
Longus, see *PIR²* B 127.

[—] Νίγερ. Birbeth, Egypt. Flavian (?). *IGRR* 1.1162.   294

ἔτους γ' αὐτοκράτορος [Οὐεσπασιανοῦ *or* Τίτου Καίσαρος] | μηνὸς Ἐπεὶφ κε' [—] |
Νίγερ Γλυβερίνου [—] | ἀνέθηκεν βωμό[ν τοῖς ἐν ὀνείροις ἐπιφανέσι θε[οῖς
ἐπιστᾶσι] | ὑπὲρ τῶν εὐεργῶς κ[ατεσκευασμένων?] | ἐν μησὶ β' λουτήρων [—λιθίνων?] |
καὶ τοῦ περιλειπομέ[νου χρόνου] | τοῦ αὐτοῦ ἔτους ὧν ἄλλων [δεήσει] | στύλ(ων) β' ἀνὰ
πόδες λ' καὶ [—] | καὶ δ' πόδ(ες) κδ' καὶ ζ' πό[δ(ες).] | καὶ ληνῶν β' καὶ μακρ[—] | καὶ
τριστίκων πᾶσι στ[ύλοις] | καὶ πλακῶν κατεργασθ[εισῶν | —] καθιδροῖ βωμ(ὸν) τῷ
ἀνδ[— | —].

NOTES: The fragmentary nature of the text makes even the reconstruction of Vespasian's or
Titus' name in the opening line uncertain. It is clear, however, that although Niger's offices are
missing from the text, he was a local magistrate: there is mention of work completed within a
certain number of months "of the same year" (τοῦ αὐτοῦ ἔτους), i.e., the year he held office
(compare no. 296). Despite the difficulty of reading, Niger's benefactions can be discerned in
outline, and they included setting up stone (?) bathtubs, erecting two pillars fifty feet in height,
and possibly also erecting four pillars twenty-four feet high, and seven others at a height now
lost. He also provided varioius fixtures associated with the pillars.

Κένδεος, στρατηγός. Iotapa, Cilicia. 176 or later. *IGRR* 3.833.   295

This lengthy inscription honors Kendeos and members of his family, in particular
Mas, his wife. Only the opening and the pertinent lines are provided here.

[ἡ βουλὴ καὶ ὁ δῆμος ἐτ]εί[μ]ησαν Κένδ[εο]ιν Ἀ[π]α[τ]ουρ[ί]ου, ἄνδρα εὐσχη]μ[ονέ-
στατον, τάγματ]ος [βουλευτικοῦ, πατέρα] | Κενδέου φ[ιλοπάτριδος], ἀν[δρὸς πολλὰ
πε]|φιλοτειμ[ημένου περὶ τὴν πατρίδα . . . *(eight lines skipped)* | (13) . . . ἐ[πι]δοὺς καὶ
εἰς [τὸ κοι]νὸν βαλανεῖον κατασκευα[ζ]όμενο[ν οἴκ]οθεν δηνάρια ‚ακε' (i.e., *1025)*
. . . *(five lines skipped)* | (20) . . . καὶ [α]ὐτὴ δὲ ἡ Μᾶς ἀ[ρχ]ιερασαμένη θεᾶς
[Σ]ε[β]αστῆς Φ[αυ]στείνης . . .

NOTES: Faustina, whose cult is mentioned in this text, died suddenly in the East in 176; see
PIR² A 716. Two small baths are known at Iotapa, but one cannot be securely dated (see

Farrington, *Roman Baths of Lycia,* 168 [no. 93]), and the other appears to date to the third century: see ibid., 168, (no. 94); Nielsen, 2.39 (C.321); Yegül, 301.

296 T. Φλ(άουιος) Δαμιανός, γραμματεύς. Ephesos, Asia. Mid- to late second century. *IK* 13 (Ephesos 3) 672 (see 17.1 [Ephesos 7.1] 3080).

This lengthy text honors T. Flavius Damianus. The pertinent lines read:

T. Φλάουιον Δαμιανόν, | γραμματεύσαντα ἐ[πι]|φανῶς καὶ μετρήσαν[τα], . . . *(eight lines skipped)* | (12) . . . ἔργον ὑπο|σχόμενον ἐν τῷ αὐτῷ ἐνιαυτῷ οἶ|κον ἐν τῷ Οὐαρίῳ βαλανείῳ μ[ε]|τὰ οἰκοδομῆς καὶ παντὸς κόσ|μου . . .

NOTES: This text is on a statue base. For Damianus, a native of Ephesos and a recognized sophist, see *PIR*² F 253. *IK* 17.1 (Ephesos 7.1) 3080 is also a statue base that contains precisely the same wording concerning the baths, at lines 13–17. For the remains of these baths, see Manderscheid, 109, s.v. "Ephesos, Thermen der Scholastikia"; Nielsen, 2.36–37 (C. 296); Yegül, 288–91. For the inscription recording their construction, see no. 308.

297† [Γ. Λικίννιος Φλα(ουιανὸς) Ἰάσων], γυμνασίαρχος. Xanthos, Lycia. Second century. *ΑΕ* 1981.834.

[—]π[. . .]ων Τραιναίων, πατρὸ[ς ἀρχιερέ]ος τῶν Σεβα]στῶν καὶ γραμματέος Λυκίω[ν | — Μ]ενεδήμου, ἐξάδελφον Φλαυίου [—|—]υ ἀρχιερέων τῶν Σεβαστῶν καὶ γραμμα]τέ|ων] Λυκίων, ἀπόγονον στρατηγῶν ναυάρχων, γυ|μνασιαρχήσαντα τῶν νέων ἐν ἐθνίκῃ πανηγύ|ρει ἐν ᾧ ἔτει ἠρχιέρατο ὁ πατὴρ αὐτοῦ, γυμνασιαρχή|σαντα τῶν γ[ε]ραίων καὶ ἐν πάσαις ἀρχαῖς φιλοδο|ξ|ήσαντα δεδωκότα δὲ καὶ ἰς τὴν καθ'ἔτος πα|νήγυριν μετὰ πατρὸς (δραχμὰς) μυρίας καὶ ἰς βαλανείου κατα[σ]κευ[ὴν] (δραχμὰς) πεντακισχειλίας, τετειμημένον πεντάκις ὑπὸ Λυκίων τοῦ κοινοῦ καὶ ὑ|πὸ τῆς πατρί|δος ταῖς καθ'ἔτος τειμαῖς, | Ξανθίων τῆς τοῦ Λυκίων ἔθνους μητρο|πόλεος ἡ βουλὴ καὶ ὁ δῆμος | τὸν ἴδιον πολείτην.

Trans.: "([Statues] of Jason and Cratippos), the (priests?) of Trajan, of his father, chief priest of the Augusti and secretary of the Lycians. (Jason, father?) of Menedemos and cousin of Flavius *[section missing],* who were chief priests of the Augusti and secretaries of Lycia, descendant of generals and admirals. He was gymnasiarch of the young at the provincial festival in the year in which his father was chief priest; he was gymnasiarch of the elderly and mindful of his reputation in all his offices, and along with his father he has given ten thousand drachmas toward the annual festival and five thousand drachmas toward the construction of the bathhouse. He has been honored five times by the commonwealth of Lycia and by his home city in the annual honors. The council and the people of Xanthos, the metropolis of the province of Lycia (honored) their own citizen."

NOTES: This inscription is on the base of a double statue, almost certainly of C. Licinnius Flavius Jason and his father, Licinnius Cratippos. Jason's name is missing here but can be reconstructed from comparison with other texts found in the city (see *AE* 1981.835; *TAM* 2.381). The editors of *AE* suggest that the figures may be *summae honorarie* (five thousand drachmas per person per office); whatever the case, the amount of money would not be enough to build an entire bathhouse.

298† ἡ Ὀλβιοπολειτῶν πόλις. Olbia, Sarmatia. 198/211. *IGRR* 1.854.

ἀγαθῇ [τ]ύ[χῃ]. | Θεοῖς πατρῴοις καὶ ὑπὲρ τῆς τοῦ [αὐτοκράτο|ρ]ος Λουκίου Σεπτιμίου Σεουήρου Πε[ρτίνακος] | καὶ Μάρκου Αὐρηλίου Ἀντωνείνου Κα[ίσαρος Σεβ]αστοῦ καὶ τοῦ σύμπαντος αὐτῶν οἴκ[ου αἰωνίου δι|α]μονῆς, ἡ Ὀλβιοπολειτῶν πόλις τὸ βα[λανεῖον? ἀνέσ|τη]σεν σὺν καὶ τῇ σκουτλώσει ἐκ τῶν δημο[σίων καὶ | κα]θιέ-ρωσ[ε]ν, διέποντος τὴν ἐπάρχειον Κο[—|—]ου, πατρὸς δὲ πόλεως Καλλισθένου Κα[λλισθένου? ἐπὶ | ἀρ]χόντων τῶν περὶ Καλλισθένην Δάδου *(a fragmentary list of names follows)*.

Trans.: "With good fortune. To the ancestral gods and for the everlasting permanence of the emperor Lucius Septimius Severus Pertinax and Marcus Aurelius Antoninus Caesar Augustus and their entire house. The city of the Olbians built from public funds the bath, along with its checkered decoration, and dedicated it. This was done when *[name lost]* was governing the province, and Kallisthenes, son of Kallisthenes (?), was father of his city, and the friends of Kallisthenes, son of Dado, were archons . . . "

NOTES: Although the word βαλανεῖον is mostly restored, mention of the checkered decoration, σκούτλωσις, makes its presence likely (see nos. 313 and 319); the phrase is reminiscent of σὺν παντὶ τῷ κόσμῳ or the like found in other bath-construction texts; see, e.g., nos. 302, 324; see also, chapter 7, n. 6. The missing governor is perhaps Cosconius Gentianus, who was in charge of Moesia Inferior in 193–97 or, possibly, in 197–98; see *PIR²* C 1526; Thomasson, 1.138–39 (no. 106).

М. Ἰούλιος Γαουείνιος, ἄρχων, ἀγοράνομος. Prusias-ad-Hypium, Bithynia et Pontus.   299†
202/211. *IGRR* 3.66 = *IK* 27 (Prusias-ad-Hypium) 20.

This lengthy text honors M. Julius Gavinius, a local magnate who presented numerous benefactions to Prusias-ad-Hypium in the Severan period. The pertinent lines read:

τὸν ἱερέα τῶν Σεβαστῶν καὶ φιλό|πατριν καὶ φιλότ[ι]μον, δὶς ἄρξαντα | καὶ πρῶτον ἄρχοντα καὶ ἱερέα | καὶ ἀγωνοθέτιν Διὸς Ὀλυμπίου | καὶ πατέρα δὶς χειλιάρχου | καὶ τιμητήν, ἀγορανομήσαντα ὑπὲρ τοῦ υἱοῦ μῆνας τρεῖς | ἐπιφανῶς, δόντα καὶ ὑπὲρ ἰδίας | ἀγορανομίας ἀργύριον εἰς ἀνάληψιν τοῦ Δομιτείου βαλανείου . . . *(twelve lines skipped)* | (24) Μᾶρκον Ἰούλιον Γαουείνιον, | σακέρδωτα . . .

Trans.: "The priest of the Augusti and a munificent man who loves his native city; he was twice archon, and the first archon, priest, and president of the games of Zeus Olympios, twice father of a military tribune, and censor. He was an exemplary aedile for three months on behalf of his son, and on behalf of his own aedileship he gave money for the restoration of the Baths of Domitius . . . Marcus Julius Gavinius, priest . . . "

NOTES: Two benefactions are commemorated here: (1) the original construction by a man called Domitius and (2) the restoration by the local official Julius Gavinius. The original construction cannot be dated securely but was probably the work of one of the local Domitii: see *IK* 27 (Prusias-ad-Hypium) 19 for a Domitius Julianos; ibid., p. 85, for discussion of the identity of the Domitius of the current inscription. It is most unlikely that the emperor Domitian was the benefactor (as suggested by Delorme, *Gymnasion*, 244–45 n. 4). Three sons of Julius Gavinius are attested in this text: two who reached equestrian status as *tribuni militum* and a third who was perhaps a minor and on whose behalf Gavinius assumed the aedileship. His payment of money for his own aedileship was undoubtedly a *summa honoraria*.

Γλύκων [καὶ —]κος, οἱ Παμφί[λου? λ]ογιστεύσαντες. Ἀπατειρηνῶν κατοικία, near   300
Ephesos, Asia. 211/12. *IK* 17.1 (Ephesos 7.1) 3249.

αὐτοκράτορσι Και|[σ]άρσι Μ. Αὐρ. Ἀντω|[ν]εί[νῳ [καὶ Λ. Σεπτ. Γέτᾳ] | ἔτους σνθ' *(i.e.,*
259), Γλύκων | [καὶ . . .]κος, οἱ Παμφί|[λου? —| . . . λ]ογιστεύσαντες | [τῆς]
Ἀπατειρηνῶν κα|[τοικ]ίας ἐν τῷ σνδ' *(i.e., 254).* | [ἔτει] ἐπὶ μιᾷ φιλοτειμί|ᾳ [καὶ] δό-
ντες τὸν λόγ[ον, κ]ατὰ τὴν προτροπὴν | το[ῦ] ἀξιολογωτάτου Τ. | Φλ. Λευκίου Ἱέρακος |
ἔδωκαν παρ' ἑαυτῶν | ἔξωθεν εἰς τὴν ἐπισ|κευὴν τοῦ μεγάλου βα|λανίου ἀργυρίου
(δηνάρια) σν' *(i.e., 250).*

NOTES: This village, in the hinterland of Ephesos, cannot be securely located. These men are
clearly of local origin and hold local magistracies; λογιστής was the Greek equivalent of *curator*
(see Mason, *Greek Terms for Roman Institutions,* 66, s.v.). For T. Flavius Leucius Hierax, see
*PIR*² F 308. The money for the baths was an additional benefaction, performed after the men
had carried out an accounting at the village.

301   Local authorities. Mitylene, Asia. 413. *AE* 1971.454.

ἐκτίσθη | τὸ βαλανῖον |ἐπὶ ὑπατίας | Φλ(αβίου) Λουκίου, | δεσποτεύοντος | Εὐλωγίου
τοῦ Λα|λαγριωνίο[υ], ἐ|πιτροπεύοντος | [Ἀ]υξεντίου.

NOTES: For Flavius Lucius, see *PLRE* 2.692, s.v. "Lucius 3"; Eulogius and Auxentius are not in
PLRE.

Private Benefactors

302†   [Πρ]όκλ[ος Βί]των. Smyrna Asia. Undated. *IGRR* 4.1440.

Ἀπόλλων[ος] | καὶ Σε[ράπιδος] | Σεβαστῶν εἰ[ργ]ά[σατο] | τὸ [βα]λανεῖον [σὺν] | παντὶ
[τῷ κ]όσμ[ῳ Πρ]ό|κλο[ς Βί]των, ψηφ[ί]|σαντος Τίτου Κα|τίου τοῦ [εὐεργέτου καὶ |
π]άτρωνος [αὐ]τοῦ, λ(υκάβαντος) γ '.

Trans.: "Proklos Bito, in three years, built the Bath of Imperial Apollo and Serapis,
along with all its decoration, after Titus Catius, the benefactor and patron, proposed
it."

NOTES: This inscription is strange; much of the reading remains uncertain. Especially noteworthy here is the coupling of Apollo and Serapis, gods who evoked both healthful and imperial
associations. For baths named after gods, see above, chapter 6, p. 172; see also Nielsen, 1.146–
47 n. 9. Titus Catius appears to have proposed the construction of the baths in a council
meeting, hence the legal verb ψηφίζω, "to propose a vote," occurs here. The appearance of this
verb may indicate that the local authorities were responsible for the bath, but if so, the text does
not make this responsibility clear.

303   [Ἄππι?]ος Κλαύδιος Μ]ενέλαος. Labraunda, Asia. Undated. *Bull. ép.* 1965.368, no.
9 (see also loc. cit., no. 4).

ὁ δῆμος [Ἄππι?]ον Κλαύδιον Χρυσά[ορος υ]ἰὸν Κυρείνα Μενέ[λαον, πολλ]ὰ μὲν καὶ
ἄλ[λα παρεσ]χημένον ἀνα[τεθη]κότα δὲ Θεοῖς Σε[βαστ]οῖς καὶ Διὶ Λαβραι[ύνδ]ωι καὶ
τῷ Δήμωι [ἐκ τ]ῶν ἰδίων καὶ τὸ βαλανεῖον.

NOTES: *Bull. ép.,* loc. cit., no. 4 is a more fragmentary record of this man's activities and also
mentions the bath.

304†*   Πώλλα Λαμπία. Isthmos, Cos. Undated. *Bull. ép.* 1967.439.

Πώλλα Λαμπία, Κῷα, Σεβαστῷ βαλανείῳ καὶ τῷ δήμῳ τῷ Ἰσθμιωτῶν τὴν Ἀφροδείτην
ἐκ τῶν ἰδίων ἀνέθηκεν.

Trans.: "Polla Lampia, of Cos, set up the statue of Aphrodite for the Augustan Bath and for the people of Isthmos at her own expense."

NOTES: This inscription is on the base of a statue of Aphrodite. The text assumes that the "people of Isthmos" would be using the baths, so they could see the statue.

Διόδοτος κτλ. Meiros, Phrygia. Undated. *Bull. ép.* 1972.461.   305

ὅσοι ἐπανγε[ιλάμενοι ἐπέ]δωκαν ἰς τ[ὸ ἐν τῷ βα]λανείωι ἀπροδ[υτήριον] Διόδοτος *(a list of names follows).*

NOTES: This nondescript text from this small place lists the contributors to the construction of a changing room in a bathhouse.

Τι. Κλαύδιος Ἅλυς, Σεβαστοῦ ἀπελεύθερος κ[αὶ ἡ γυνὴ αὐτοῦ]. Beujuk Tepekeui   306*
(ancient name not known), Asia. Julio-Claudian. *IGRR* 4.228.

ὑπὲρ τῆς τῶν Σεβαστῶν σωτηρίας κα[ὶ αἰωνίου διανομῆς] | Τι. Κλαύδιος Σεβαστοῦ ἀπελεύθερος Ἅλυς κ[αὶ ἡ γυνὴ αὐτοῦ—] | καὶ τὰ τέκνα αὐτῶν [Τι. Κ]λαύδιος Κυρίνα Ἰοῦσ[τ(ος?)—καὶ—] | Ἀρτεμίδι Σεβαστῇ Βαιιανῇ τὸν ναὸν καὶ τὰ [βαλανεῖα—] | ἐκ θεμελίων κατασκευάσαντες ἐ[κ τῶν ἰδίων], | ἐπιμελείᾳ Τίτου Φλαουίου Σεβαστοῦ ἀπελ[ευθέρου—].

NOTES: The benefactors are an imperial freedman and his wife. Although the word βαλανεῖα is missing, its presence seems likely not only due to τὰ immediately preceding the lacuna but also since the dedication is Ἀρτεμίδι Σεβαστῇ Βαιιανῇ, a goddess with healing powers associated with baths (compare the *mater dea Baiana, CIL* 10.3698 = *ILS* 4175). As there is mention of a temple built along with the baths, this establishment may possibly have had strong religious associations.

Λεπούσκλα. Asopos, Laconia. First or second century. *SEG* 39 (1989) 372 = *AE*   307†*
1991.1443.

θεοῖς Σεβαστοῖ[ς καὶ τᾷ] | Ἀσωπειτῶν πόλ[ει—] | Λεπούσκλα τὸ βαλανεῖ[ον] | ἐκ θεμελίων κατα|σκευάσασα [ταῖς ἰδίαις] | δαπάναι[ς].

Trans.: "To the divine Augusti and the city of Asopos. Lepouskla built the bath from its foundations at her own expense."

NOTES: This text was found in the ruins of baths. The date may be second century (the multiple Augusti possibly indicate this date), unless the dedication is to dead Augusti.

Πόπλιος Κυιντίλιος Οὐάλης Οὐάριος. Ephesos, Asia. Hadrian. *SEG* 28 (1978) 862 =   308
IK 12 (Ephesos 2) 500.

[—Σεβαστ]ῷ Πόπλιος Κυιντίλιο[ς (Ποπλίου υἱὸς) Οὐάλης Οὐάριος —|—]ρυ [. .]αδ[.]τα[.] ὑπὸ τὸ βαλαν[εῖον].

NOTES: This inscription is very fragmentary, but it clearly commemorates Quintilius Varius' construction of the Varius or Scholastikia Baths, among the ruins of which it was found. That Varius built the baths is confirmed not only by the findspot but also by the testimony of other inscriptions found at Ephesos: one, also found in the baths, honors his daughter Quintilla Varia and describes her as θυγατέρα Πο. Κυιντιλίου Ο[ὐ]ἰάλεντο[ς] Οὐαρίου τοῦ [τὰ] | ἔργα [τ]αῦ[τ]α κα[τ]ασκευα|σαμ[ένου ἐκ τῶ]ν ἰ[δ]ίων | τῇ ἑαυ[τοῦ πα]τ[ρί]δ[ι] (*IK* 13 [Ephesos 3] 986); see also the next entry and *IK* 13 (Ephesos 3) 962.

[Πόπλιος Κυιντίλιος Οὐάλης Οὐάριος (?) σὺν γυναικὶ καὶ Οὐαρίλληι, θυγ]ατρί.   309*
Ephesos, Asia. Hadrian. *SEG* 16 (1959) 719 = *IK* 12 (Ephesos 2) 455.

['Αρτέμιδι Έφεσίαι καὶ αὐτοκράτορι Τραιανῶι Ἀδριανῶι Καίσ]αρι Σ[εβαστῶι καὶ τῶι
νεωκόρωι Ἐφεσίων δήμωι Πόπλιος Κυιντίλιος Ποπλίου υἱὸς Γαλερία Οὐάλης Οὐάριος
σὺν — γυναικὶ καὶ Οὐαρίλληι θυγ]ατρὶ φιλοσέ[βαστος ἀποκαταστήσας ἐκ θε]μελίων
τὸν θᾶκον σὺ[ν τοῖς κα]τ' αὐτοῦ ἐπικειμένοις παιδισκήοις καὶ κοσμήσας πα[ντὶ κό-
σμωι — ἐκ τῶν ἰδίων ἀνέθηκεν].

NOTES: This very fragmentary inscription is from the architrave of the latrine in the Varius
Baths and is reconstructed by comparison with *IK* 12 (Ephesos 2) 429. The line breaks, however,
cannot be securely established. A θᾶκος was a latrine, and a παιδισκεῖον was a brothel. The *IK*
commentary denies the possibility of a brothel here but offers no alternative explanation for the
appearance of the word παιδισκήοις. In light of the sexual functions of baths, I see no real reason
to doubt the existence of a brothel here, especially given that the definition of a brothel keeper in
the *Digest* (3.2.4.2) includes any *balneator* who hires slaves to guard clothing and also to
practice prostitution; see above, chapter 1, pp. 34–36 on sex at the baths. For the remains, see
the notes to no. 296.

310†* Ἰάσων, ἀνὴρ ἀξιόλογος, μετὰ καὶ τῆς θ[υ]γατρὸς αὐτοῦ Λυ[κί]ας. Cyaneae, Lycia.
143/46. *IGRR* 3.704.

This lengthy inscription, running to 125 lines in several columns, honors Jason, son of
Nikostratos, and includes the following decree from the town of Myra, dated 13
October 146. The pertinent text, IIa.1–13, reads:

[ψήφ]ισμα [Μυρέ]ων· | ἔδοξε Μυρέων τῆς μητροπόλεος | τοῦ Λυκίων ἔθνους τῇ βουλῇ
καὶ τῷ δ[ήμ]ῳ· | ἐπ(ε)ὶ Ἰάσων Νεικοστράτου, πολείτης ἡμῶ[ν], | ἀνὴρ ἀξιόλογος,
πρ[ω]τεύων ἔν τε τῷ ἔθνει | καὶ τῆς πόλε[ω]ς ἡμῶν, γεγον[ὼ]ς ἀρχιερεὺς [τῶν] |
Σ[εβ]αστῶν καὶ γραμματεὺς Λυκίων, ἐ[ξ] αρχῆς ἀγαθὴν | δ[ιάθ]ε[σ]ι[ν] ἔχει πρὸς [τὴ]ν
πόλιν ἡμῶν [καὶ] ἠγ[ω]νοθέτησεν | τῆς πανηγύρεος τῆς ἀρχηγέτιδος [θ]εᾶς Ἐλευθέρας
φιλο|τείμως κ[α]ὶ με[γα]λο{συ}ψύχως, δωρεάς τε μεγαλοπρεπεῖς | πεποίηται εἴς τε
κατασκευὴ[ν] στοᾶς πρὸ τοῦ κατα[σκευασμένου βαλανείου [πρ]ὸς τῇ [π]λ[α]τείᾳ
δηνάρια μύρια | μετὰ καὶ τῆς θ[υ]γατρὸς αὐτοῦ Λυ[κί]ας . . .

Trans.: "Decree of Myra. It was decreed by the council and people of Myra, metropolis of the province of Lycia: since Jason, son of Nikostratos, our citizen, a worthy
man, a leading man both in the province and of our city, having become the chief
priest of the Augusti and secretary of the Lycians, has been from the start well-
disposed toward our city and gave generous and liberal games at the festival of our
founding goddess Eleutheria, and made magnificent gifts for the construction of a
portico in front of the bath already built by the piazza, ten thousand denarii along
with his daughter Lycia . . . *(the text goes on to thank Jason, who is named as
Lyciarch).*"

NOTES: Jason was *Lyciarch* in 143–44. It is clear enough that the portico, or stoa, in question
was part of the baths, like the προστῷον of the baths at Aperlae; see no. 293. The text reports
that the baths had already been constructed (κατασκευασμένου) but does not indicate who was
responsible for that operation.

311 Ὀπραμόας. Rhodiapolis, Lycia et Pamphylia. Before 149. *IGRR* 3.739 = *TAM* 2.905,
XIX B–D.

This huge inscription running to several hundred lines is carved on the walls of
Opromoas' mausoleum at Rhodiapolis. Included in the inscription are the texts of
letters and rescripts from emperors, imperial officials, and others honoring the great

benefactor. Here listed are his benefactions to three communities commemorated as part of document 63, a decree of the Lycian council sent to Antoninus Pius and dated to 149.

Telmessos (XIX B.7–10): . . . τῇ δὲ Τελμησ|σέων πόλει εἰς κατασκευὴν βαλανείου καὶ ἐ|ξέδρας *(denarii)* τρισμύρια καὶ δηναρία πεντάκις | χείλια *(35,000)* . . .

Oenoanda (XIX B.13–14): . . . τῇ Οἰνοαν[δέ]ων εἰς κατασκευ|[ὴν] βαλανείου *(denarii)* μύρια *(10,000)* . . .

Gagae (XIX D.2–5): . . . [καὶ τῇ Γαγ]ατῶν εἰς κατασκευὴν βαλανείου | κα[ὶ τοῦ κολύ]νβου καὶ τῶν λοιπῶν χρηστηρίων | ἤ[δη *(denarii)* μύρια] ὠκτάκις χείλια *(8,000)* ὑποσχόμενος | π[ληρώσειν] . . .

NOTES: In all, thirty-two cities are listed (some as multiple beneficiaries), with a total outlay of some eight hundred thousand denarii, i.e., 3.2 million sesterces. For a translation and discussion of this text, see F.W. Danker, *Benefactor: Epigraphic Study of a Greco-Roman and New Testament Semantic Field* (St. Louis, 1982), 104–51 (no. 19). For Opromoas, a citizen of Rhodiapolis who died ca. 152, see R. Heberdey, *Opromoas: Inschriften vom Heroon zu Rhodiapolis* (Vienna, 1897); *RE* 18.748–49, s.v. "Opramoas" (Miller). The baths at both Telmessos and Gagae are unknown; those at Oenoanda may be Baths MK 1 at the site. See Farrington, *Roman Baths of Lycia,* 78 (Telmessos and Gagae), 156 (no. 35 [Oenoanda]).

Τι. Φλαούιος Κλειτοσθένης Κλαυδιανός. Thera. Before 149/50. *IG* 12.3.326 (see *SIG*³ 852).   312†

This lengthy decree honors Ti. Flavius Kleitosthenes Claudianus. Only the pertinent lines are cited.

| (6) ἐπειδὴ Τ. Φλάουιος Κλειτοσθένης Κλαυδιανός, | ἀνὴρ γένους τε ἐπιφανείᾳ διάσημος, κἀπὶ ταῖς εἰς | τὴν πατρίδα λιτουργίαις διαβόητος, ἃ μὲν βαλαν|είων κατασκευαῖς τὰ ἐπίνεια τῆς πόλεως κοσμήσ|ας, ἃ δὲ καὶ τὸ τῆς Εἰλειθυίης ἱερὸν ἀλέκτῳ πολυ|τελείᾳ κατειργασμένον ἔργον πατρῷον ἀπαράφ[θ]ο|ρον πρὸς [ἀπ]όλαυσιν πο[λ]ι[τ]ῶν τε καὶ τῶν ἐπιδημούν|των [ξ]έν[ω]ν διαφυλάσσων.

Trans.: "Since T. Flavius Kleitosthenes Claudianus, a man noteworthy for the prominence of his family, famous on account of his liturgies toward the city, embellished the city's harbors with the construction of baths and, for the enjoyment of the citizens and the resident foreigners, carefully maintained undamaged the Temple of Eileithuia, a building erected by his father in indescribable extravagance."

NOTES: In a decree dated to 149/50 and made in honor of Claudianus (*SIG*³ 852), his previous benefactions are mentioned, probably those listed in the earlier (undated) text cited in this entry. The location of these baths has not been identified.

Incertus. Xanthos, Lycia. 140s. *SEG* 30 (1980) 1535.   313†

The relevant lines of this lengthy inscription are

| (1) δωρεὰς ἔδωκεν . . . | (6) Ξανθίοις . . . | (7) . . . εἰς γυναικεῖον βαλανεῖον *(10,000) (denarii)*, εἰς τὰ ἐν τῶι | ἱερῶι ἔργα *(125,000) (denarii)*, εἰς τὸ γυμνάσιον | καὶ τὸ ἐν αὐτῶι βαλανεῖον *(40,500) (denarii)*; . . . | (16) Μυρεῦσιν εἰς τὴν περίστυλον τοῦ | γυμνασίου καὶ τὴν σκούτλωσιν | αὐτοῦ καὶ τοὺς κείονας *(50,000) (denarii)*; | Τλωεῦσιν εἰς μὲν βαλανεῖον *(30,000) (denarii)* | εἰς δὲ τὴν ἀγορὰν *(50,000) (denarii)* . . .

Trans.: "He has given gifts: . . . To Xanthos, 10,000 denarii for the women's bath, 125,000 denarii for the projects in the temple, and 45,000 denarii for the gymnasium and the bath in it . . . To Myra, 50,000 denarii for the peristyle of the gymnasium and its checkered decoration and columns. To Tlos, 30,000 denarii for the bath and 50,000 denarii for the agora . . . "

NOTES: The editors of *SEG* comment, "Though Opramoas is not mentioned, it is virtually certain that he is the benefactor." This view follows that of the inscription's original publisher (see A. Balland, *Fouilles de Xanthos,* vol. 7, *Inscriptions d'époque impériale du Létoon* [Paris, 1981], 185–214), but it has recently been decisively challenged, so an otherwise unattested benefactor is to be considered the subject; see J.J. Coulton, "Opromoas and the Anonymous Benefactor," *JHS* 107 (1987): 171–78. Coulton (174–75) argues that many of these benefactions took place in the 140s, following the earthquake of 140/41, and so are contemporaneous with Opromoas' actions, against which they can be compared. The text offers interesting evidence for bath terminology in Asia, since it distinguishes gymnasia from βαλανεῖα, in one instance specifying a βαλανεῖον in a gymnasium, for which, see Delorme, *Gymnasion,* 246–47. None of the bath buildings mentioned here can be identified with any degree of certainty; see Farrington, *Roman Baths of Lycia,* 163 (nos. 63–67 [Xanthos]), 154 (nos. 27–30 [Myra]), and 161–62 (nos. 58–62 [Tlos]). Note, however, ibid., 74, where the East Baths at Xanthos are tentatively identified as the γυμνάσιον καὶ τὸ ἐν αὐτῶι βαλανεῖον.

314   Ὀπραμόας. Tlos, Lycia. Ca. 152 or before. *IGRR* 3.679 = *TAM* 2.578.

Of this lengthy inscription, only the opening is pertinent.

Τλωέων τῆς μητροπόλ[εως] | τοῦ Λυκίων ἔθνους ἡ βουλὴ | καὶ] ὁ δῆμος καὶ ἡ γερουσ[ία] (ἐτίμησαν) | Ὀπραμόαν Ἀπολλωνίο[υ] | δὶς τοῦ Καλλιάδου Τλ[ωέα] | καὶ Ῥοδιαπολεί-την, πο[λει]|τευόμενον δὲ καὶ ἐν τ[αῖς] | κατὰ Λυκίων πόλεσι [πά]|σαις, τὸν ἀρχιερέα τ[ῶν] | Σεβαστῶν καὶ γραμμα[τέα] | Λυκίων τοῦ κοινοῦ, [δι' ἃ πα]|ρέσχεν καὶ τῇ ἡμετέ[ρᾳ πό]|λει, χαρισάμενον καὶ [ἀργυ]|ρίου δηναρίου μυριάδα[ς ἓξ] | εἰς τὴν τοῦ θεάτρου κα[τα]|σκευὴν καὶ ἐξέδρας [τῆς] ἐν τῷ βαλανείῳ . . .

NOTES: This benefaction took place at Tlos, as the text makes clear, so the attribution in *IGRR* to Patara is erroneous. The text appears to be posthumous and so dates to after ca. 152; however, Opromoas' actions at Tlos must predate his death, since they are not a bequest (see Coulton, "Opromoas," 174). There are no signs of such an exedra in the surviving baths at the site; see Farrington, *Roman Baths of Lycia,* 68–69.

315/316†*   Incertus, Μακάριος, and Εὐχαρία. Miletus, Asia. Incertus, before 176; Makarios and Eucharia, third century (?). *AE* 1906.177/78 = A. von Gerkan and F. Krischen, *Thermen und Palaestren* (Berlin, 1928), 164–66 (no. 339).

[εὐτυχῶς | —] | Μακάριος [δ]ηίων δ[ῆριν ἀλεξάμενος] | ἀνδροφόνων· τὸ δὲ κῦδο[ς ἐ]ν ἀ[στοῖσιν μέγ' ἀέξων] | ἀντ' ἀσιαρχίης λουτρὸν ἔτευ[ξε νέον] |
εὐτυχῶς | οὗτος ὁ Μακαρίοιο πελώριος ἐνθάδε κόσμο[ς,] | ὃν κάμεν ἧ πάτρη θρέπτρα χαριζόμενος, | ἀντ' ἀσιαρχίης ὕπατον κλέος ἄστει τεύξας | Εὐχαρίης ἀλόχου ταῖς ἀγανοφροσύναις |
εὐτυχῶς | Μακάριος τὸ λοετρὸν ἐς ἀρχαῖον θέτο κάλλος | Φαυστείνης καμάτων δεύτερος ἀθλοθέτης. | Τατιανὸς δὲ πόνοιο δικασπόλος εὕρατο τέρμα | τὰς νύμφας καλέων τὰς πυρὶ μισγομένας. | ἄστει δ' ὤπασε κόσμον· [ἐλ]αφρίζουσι δὲ μόχθων | πάντες λυσιπόνοις χεύ[μασι] τερπομένοι{ς} | Φαυστίνης τὸ παλαιὸν ἐπ[ώνυμον] ἦσθα, λοετρόν, | ἀλλά σε Μακαρίου νῦν κα[λέσει πατρ]ιά, | οὕνεκ' ἀφειδήσας κτεάν[ων] μεγαλαύχ[έϊ θ]υμῷ | γῆρας ἀποξύσας αὖθί [σ' ἔ]θηκε νέον.

Trans.: "In good fortune; *[text missing]* Makarios, ravaging, warded off battle with killers and, as he increased his renown greatly in the cities, he built a new bath in return for his Asiarchy.

"In good fortune; this is the mighty ornament of Makarios in this place, which he built for his native city in willing gratitude for its nurture; in return for his Asiarchy, he furnished an esteemed reputation for the city with the generosities of his wife, Eucharia.

"In good fortune; Makarios, the second steward of labors, restored the Bath of Faustina to its ancient beauty. Tatianos, the judge, found an end of the work when he summoned the fire-wedded nymphs. He gave an ornament to the city: all are relieved from their toils as they take their delights in the labor-lightening streams. Bath, in the distant past, you were Faustina's by name but now our city will call you Makarios', because he was unstinting with his property and, with a proud spirit, he scraped off old age and made you new again."

NOTES: This verse inscription is from the Baths of Faustina at Miletus. From the opening lines, Makarios appears to have taken part in some imperial campaigns, but it is not clear when and where. The description of his role as defensive may indicate that the context is to be found in the troubles of Asia Minor in the mid–third century, but since the inscription is not securely dated, this reading is largely conjectural. The building was dedicated to and named after Faustina, undoubtedly the wife of M. Aurelius (see *PIR*² A 716), who visited Asia in 164 and died while in Asia in 176 (the other Faustina was the wife of Antoninus Pius; see *PIR*² A 715). The wording of the inscription—with its designation of Makarios as "the second steward of labors"—suggests that an individual was responsible for the original construction. Faustina is as good a candidate for initial constructor as any, but her actions would represent a break with the immediate past, when imperial women made no known financial outlays for public purposes; see M.T. Boatwright, "The Imperial Women of the Early Second Century A.C.," *AJP* 112 (1991): 518–25. In any case, the name of a bath alone is insufficient grounds for deducing imperial agency in its construction; chapter 6, p. 171. Note how the building is renamed following Makarios and Eucharia's actions. Tatianos appears to have been a local official who approved the restored bath and made it operational, which would explain the references to the "fire-wedded [water] nymphs." For the remains of these baths, see Manderscheid, 149–50, s.v. "Miletos, Thermen der Faustina"; Nielsen, 2.38 (C.306); Yegül, 291.

Θομαλλαχίς. Palmyra, Syria. 182. H. Ingholt, "Inscriptions and Sculptures from Palmyra," *Berytus* 3 (1936): 109–12 (no. 11).   317†*

Θομαλλαχὶς Ἀδδουδάνου τοῦ Ἰαριβωλέου[ς] | τοῦ Ἀδδουδάνου τοῦ Φιρμωνὸς οἱ | ἀπὸ φυλῆς Χωνειτῶν τειμῆς ἕνε|κεν φειλοτειμησαμένην | δηνάρια δισχείλια πεντακό|σια εἰς οἰκοδομὴν βα|λανείου Ἀγιλβώλου καὶ | Μαλαχιβήλου θεῶν | ἔτους γθυ Λώου.

Trans. (Ingholt): "Thomallakhis, daughter of Haddûdan, son of Yarhibôlê, son of Haddûdan, son of Firmôn, those of the tribe Khônites in her honor, she having presented 2,500 denarii towards the building of the bath of the gods Agilbol and Malakbel. Year 493, August (= A.D. 182)."

NOTES: This inscription documents an interesting example of bathing culture operating on the very edge of the empire. The remains of baths at Palmyra have yet to be closely studied (an establishment of Diocletianic date is known from the city: see Manderscheid, 166–67, s.v. "Palmyra, Baths of Diocletian"; Nielsen, 2.46 [C.382]). The bath may have stood in the "Sacred Garden" of these deities, mentioned in inscriptions but yet to be located on the ground; see J. Teixidor, "Religion und Kult in Palmyra," in *Palmyra: Geschichte, Kunst und Kultur der syrischen Oasenstadt* (Linz, 1987), 37–38. This woman was evidently a member of an important local family and can trace her genealogy back some four generations. Here she contributes 2,500 denarii (= 10,000 sesterces) toward the erection of the baths, but this amount is not enough to cover the entire cost of the construction. Ingholt (op. cit., 111–12) maintains that the baths were public but belonged to the temple of the two gods mentioned (the tribe Khonites may be sacerdotal), as is the case with other public buildings at Palmyra. See above, chapter 6, p. 172, for baths named after gods.

318   ? Δομίτιος. Prusias-ad-Hypium, Bithynia et Pontus. Before late second century. *IGRR* 3.66 = *IK* 27 (Prusias-ad-Hypium) 20.

The full text is cited at no. 299. Here note the portion that reads:

. . . δόντα καὶ ὑπὲρ ἰδίας | ἀγορανομίας ἀργύριον εἰς ἀνάληψιν τοῦ Δομιτείου βαλανείου . . .

319   Incertus. Comama, Pisidia. Not before second century. *SEG* 19 (1963) 830.

— | . . . ἄρξαντα τήν τε πρώτην δυανδρ[ί]|αν, ἀλλὰ καὶ τὴν ἐπώνυμον πενταετηρι|[κ]ὴν δυανδρίαν, ἀρχιερασά[μ]ενον τῶν Σεβα[σ]|τῶν εὐθύζως καὶ φιλοτίμως, εἰρηναρχή|σαν|τα, καὶ πάσας τὰς πρεπούσας τῷ ἀξιώματι αὐτο[ῦ] | ἀρχὰς καὶ λειτουργίας ἐκτελέσαντα μεγαλοπρε|πῶς, ἔτι καὶ ἐπιδόντα καὶ εἰς αἰωνίαν νέμησ[ιν] | τῇ πατρίδι αὐτοῦ ἀργυρίου κεφαλαίου δηναρίω[ν] | μυριάδας τρεῖς, ἔτι τε εἰς ἐπισκευὴν καὶ σκού|τλωσιν τοῦ ἐν Κρητωπόλει βαλανείου δηνάρια τετρα|κισχείλια, ἀλλὰ μὴν καὶ εἰς νέμησιν τῇ ἑτέρᾳ αὐτοῦ π[α]|τρίδι —].

NOTES: The date is supplied by *SEG*. Note again the appearance of checkered decoration (σκούτλωσις) in the baths. What exactly the "first duumvirate" was is unclear. These baths are reported as being in Cretopolis, a city of unsure location near Comama, which seems to have been the second "fatherland" of the benefactor, if the last lines are restored correctly; see the comments of G.E. Bean in "Notes and Inscriptions from Pisidia," part 2, *AnatSt* 10 (1960): 50–53.

320*   Τρύφων μετὰ τῆς γυναικός, Ἄμμας. Tacina, Asia. 202/3. *IGRR* 4.881.

ἀγαθῇ τύχῃ· [ὑπὲρ σωτηρ]ίας καὶ [νείκης κ]αὶ [αἰων]ίου διανομῆς τῶν μεγίστων καὶ α[νεικήτ]ων αὐτοκρατόρων | [Λ. Σεπτιμίου] Σεουήρο[υ καὶ] Μ. Αὐρ. Ἀντωνείνου [καὶ] | Νέας Ἥρας Ἰουλίας [καὶ Π. Σεπτιμίου Γέτα—] καὶ τοῦ | σύνπαντος οἴκου τῶν Σεβαστῶν καὶ ἱερᾶς συνκλήτου καὶ δήμου τοῦ Ῥωμαίων, ἐπὶ ἀνθυπάτου τοῦ λαμπροτάτου | Ταρίου Τιτιάνου, τῇ γλυκυτάτῃ πατρίδι, τῷ Τακινέων δήμῳ μετὰ πάσας ἀρχάς τε καὶ λειτουργίας καὶ διαποντίου[ς] | πρεσβείας, ἅς ἤνυσεν ἐπὶ θεοῦ Κομμόδου, Τρύφων Ἀπολλωνίδου ὑποσχόμενος ἀπὸ προικὸς Ἰάδος θυγα|τρὸς ἰδίας ἡρω[ίδ]ος, καὶ προσφιλοτειμησάμενος μετὰ τῆς γυναικὸς Ἄμμας Δάου καὶ εἰς τὸν Βασιλῶ τῆς | [θυγατρὸς αὐτ]ῶν λό(γ)ον, ἐπὶ τῷ καὶ αὐτὰς διὰ βίου μετέχειν, ἐκτελέσ(ας) τὸ βαλανεῖον παρέδωκεν.

NOTES: Tarius Titianus was prococonsul of Asia and served there in 202/3; see *RE* 2.2323, s.v. "Tarius 4" (Fluss); Thomasson, 1.233 (no. 168).

321†*   [Κουρ]τία Ἰουλία [Οὐαλ]έντιλλα, ὑπα[τικ]ή. Tabila, Asia. Septimius Severus or later. *IGRR* 4.1378.

[Κουρ]τίαν Ἰουλίαν | [Οὐαλ]έντιλλαν, ὑπα|[τικὴ]ν, τὴν κυρίαν, | [ἐ]νχειρίσασαν | [τ]ὴν ἐπιμέλειαν | [τῆς] κατασκευῆς | [τοῦ] βαλανείου καὶ | [τῶν] περὶ τὸν τόπο[ν | οἰκο]δομημάτων [—].

Trans.: "Curtia Julia Valentilla, of consular family, the mistress, saw to the construction of the baths and of the buildings around the site *(the text breaks off)*."

NOTES: This woman was of a consular family, daughter of the consular Julius Curtius Crispus; see *PIR*² C 1596 (father) and 1622 (daughter). The appearance of the word ἐπιμέλειαν may suggest that Valentilla, as a prominent and affluent person, was asked to carry out the work. The *lacuna* at the end of the text makes unclear her treatment of the buildings around the site: she may have demolished them to make room for the baths (compare no. 159) or built them along with the baths (compare no. 164).

Τι. Ἰούλιος Ἰοῦστος Ἰουνιανός. Ancyra, Galatia. Caracalla. *SEG* 27 (1977) 842 = *AE* 1981.782.

322†

Τι(βέριον) Ἰούλιον Ἰοῦστον Ἰουνια|νόν, γ' ἀρχιερέα, κτιστὴν | τῆς μητροπόλεως, πορφύραι | κὲ στεφάνωι διὰ βίου τετιμημένον, φιλόπατριν, πάσαις | διενεγκόντα φιλοτιμί|αις κὲ ἔν τε διανομαῖς πλου|τίσαντα τὴν πατρίδα, ἔργοις | τε περικαλλεστά-τοις κο|σμήσαντα, κὲ μόνον τῶν | πρὸ αὐτοῦ δι' ὅλης ἐλαιοθε|τήσαντα τῆς ἡμέρας, ἐπι|μεληθέντα δὲ κὲ τῆς κατα|σκευῆς τοῦ βαλανείου, | φυλὴ Διὸς Τραπεζῶν ἐτίμη|σεν

Trans.: "The tribe of Zeus Trapezon honored Tiberius Julius Justus Junianus, three times chief priest and founder of the metropolis, honored with the purple and crown for life, friend of his native city, who excelled in all his munificences and distributions, who enriched his native city and beautified it with absolutely splendid works, who, alone of those who came before, provided oil throughout the whole day, and who took charge of the construction of the baths."

NOTES: Justus most likely constructed the baths at personal expense, as part of his "absolutely splendid works." *AE* (1981.782) reports that the baths have been located and are dated by coin finds to the reign of Caracalla: see also Manderscheid, 55–56, s.v. "Ankara/Ancyra"; Nielsen, 2.41 (C.336); Yegül, 279.

[οἱ ἀπὸ μητρο]κωμίας Ζοραουηνῶν. Zorava, Syria. Severus Alexander. *IGRR* 3.1155.

323†

ἀγαθῇ τύχῃ. | ὑπὲρ σωτηρίας καὶ νείκης τοῦ κυρίου ἡμῶν αὐτοκ[ράτορος Καίσαρος Μάρκου] | Αὐρηλίου Σεουήρου [Ἀλ[εξάνδρο]υ] Εὐσεβοῦς Εὐτυχ[οῦς Σεβαστοῦ, οἱ ἀπὸ μητρο]|κωμίας Ζοραουηνῶν ἔκτισαν τὸ βαλανεῖον ἰ[δίαις δαπάναις].

Trans.: "With good fortune. For the safety and victory of our lord, the emperor Caesar Marcus Aurelius Severus Alexander, *pius, felix,* Augustus, the people of the chief village of Zorava built the bath with their own money."

NOTES: If the restoration of οἱ ἀπὸ μητροκωμίας is correct, the wording might imply that the bath was the work of the local authority, except that the closing phrase, again if correctly restored, says that the money came from private pockets, which would mean that a group of unnamed private benefactors who came from the μητροκωμία carried out the work.

Αὐρ(ηλία) Αἰλ(ία) Φοίβη. Julia Gordos, Asia. 230/31. *AE* 1974.618 (see also *Bull. ép.* 1971.601) = *TAM* 5.758.

324†*

Ἀγαθῇ τύχῃ. | θεοῖς πατρίοις καὶ αὐτοκράτορι Καίσαρι Μ. Αυρ. Σεουή|ρῳ [Ἀλεξά-νδρῳ] Εὐσεβεῖ Εὐτυχεῖ Σεβ(αστῷ) καὶ τῷ σύμπαντι | οἴκῳ αὐτοῦ καὶ τῇ γλυκυτάτῃ Ὑσσηνῶν κατοικίᾳ Αὐρ(ηλία) Αἰλ(ία) | Φοίβη, θυγάτηρ Αὐρ(ηλίου) Ἰόλλα Εφε-σιανοῦ ἑκατοντάρχου, |ἐγγόνη δὲ Αἰλ(ίας) Φοίβης ματρώνης στολάτης, κατεσκεύα|σεν ἐκ ⟨β⟩άθ(ρ)ων τὸ | περίστῳον τοῦ βαλανείου σὺν παντὶ τῷ | κόσμῳ αὐτοῦ ἐκ τῶν ἰδίων σὺν καὶ τοῖς τροφεῖσιν αὐτῆς | Τ. Αἰλ. Ἐπαφροδείτῳ καὶ Αἰλ. Καλλιτύχῃ, προνοησαμέ-νων τῆς | τοῦ ἔργου κατασκευῆς Τ. Αἰλ(ίου) Ἀλεξάνδρου, τοῦ συντρόφου | αὐτῆς, καὶ Αὐρηλίων Διοδώρου Τυράννου καὶ Μητροφάνους | Λύδου καὶ Διονυσίου β', συντελεσθέντος τοῦ ἔργου ἐπὶ ἀνθυ|πάτου Ἀμείκου, ἔτους τιε', μη(νὸς) Ὑπερβερταίου β'. τῆς ἐπιγραφῆς ταύτης ἀντίγραφον ἀπε[τέθη] εἰς τὸ ἐν Ἰουλίᾳ Γόρδῳ | ἀρχεῖον, ἧς καὶ ἀντίγρ[αφον ἀπόκειτα]ι παρ' αὐτῇ.

Trans.: "With good fortune. For the ancestral gods and the emperor M. Aurelius Severus *[Alexander], pius, felix,* Augustus, and to his entire house and to the very pleasant village of the Hussenans. Aurelia Aelia Phoebe, daughter of Aurelius Iolla Ephesianus, centurion, and granddaughter of Aelia Phoebe, noble matron, built from the foundations the colonnade of the baths with all its decoration, at her own ex-pense, along with her foster parents, T. Aelius Epaphroditus and Aelia Kallituche. Her foster brother T. Aelius Alexander superintended the work along with Aurelius Diodorus and Aurelius Tyrannus and Aurelius Metrophanes Ludos and Aurelius Dionysius II. The work was completed when Amicus was proconsul, in the 315th year (of the province), on the twelfth day of the month of Hyperberetaios. A copy of this inscription was sent for storage to the archive at Julia Gordos, a copy of which was kept in reserve beside it."

NOTES: This text comes from a small town called Ὑσσηνῶν κατοικία (line 3) about twenty kilometers northwest of Julia Gordos. The village lay in the *territorium* of the city, as the deposition of a copy in the archives at Julia Gordos makes clear (compare the inscription from a village near Ephesos; see no. 300). For village baths in Asia Minor, see L. Robert, "Inscriptions de Lydie," *Hellenica* 9 (1950): 30–31 n. 5. In this case, the woman benefactor was of a high-ranking local family: her father was a centurion (ἐκατόνταρχος) and her mother a μάτρωνα στολάτη. Descendants of the family went on to become knights and senators under Valerian and Gallienus; see the commentary to the *AE* entry. Aelia's position is interesting. She was appar-ently raised by the Aelii, despite being born of the Aurelii. Both families took part in the benefaction: Aelia's foster parents appear to have contributed money to the project; her foster brother and some members of her birth family (her brothers [?]) oversaw the work—assuming that all the Aurelii mentioned as overseeing the work were relatives of Aelia's father, Aurelius Iolla Ephesianus. For Amicus, who is otherwise unattested, see *RE* Suppl. 14.44, s.v. "Amicus 1a" (Eck); Thomasson, 1.235 (no. 185).

325†*   Σχολαστικία. Ephesos, Asia. Fourth century. *AE* 1957.13 = *SEG* 16 (1959) 718 = *IK* 12 (Ephesos 2) 453.

τύπον γυναικὸς εὐσεβοῦς λίαν | σοφῆς Σχολαστικίας μοι τοῦτο(ν) | ὦ ξένε βλέπεις ἣ καὶ κλιθέν|τος ἐνθαδί τινος μέρους χρυ|σοῦ παρέσχε πλῆθος ἐς καινουργίαν.

Trans.: "Stranger, you are looking at a statue here of a faithful, exceedingly wise wife, my Scholastikia. When a part leaned within, she gave most of the money for renovation."

NOTES: This inscription was carved on a statue base found in an apsed room of the Varius Baths, also called the Scholastikia Baths due to this text. The text is rather vague as to what was wrong with the building, but the remains show evidence of extensive renovation in the fourth century: see Nielsen, 2.36–37 (C.296); Yegül, 288–91.

326†   Εὐστόλιος. Kourion, Cyprus. Late fourth century. *SEG* 26 (1976/77) 1474.

[Κουριέας] τὸ πάροιθε ἐν [ὄλβ]ῳ παντὶ πέλοντας | [νῦν ἐν δίῃ ἰδ]ὼν ἐκ ποδὸς Εὐστόλιος | [οὐ πατρίης χώ]ρης ἐπελήσατο, ἀλλ᾽ ἄρα καὶ τῆς | [ἐμνήσθη φιλί]ως, λουτρὰ χαρισσά-μενος· | [ἦ ῥ᾽ αὐτὸς δὴ] δίζετο Κούριον, ὥς ποτε Φοῖβος, | [γαίην δὲ β]ρυχίην θῆκεν ὑπηνεμίην.

Trans.: "Seeing the people of Kourion, who in the past existed in complete happiness, now existing in a divine state, Eustolios did not immediately neglect his home country but rather remembered it and freely gave the baths. Surely, he sought out Kourion, as Phoebus once did, and made the sea-covered earth (to be) blown by the winds."

NOTES: This mosaic verse inscription from the fourth-century baths at Kourion makes it clear that Eustolios was responsible for the building. The exact reading of the inscription, however, is extremely difficult, due to its mutilated condition. The original text and comments of T.B. Mitford (*The Inscriptions of Kourion* [Philadelphia, 1971], no. 204) have been severely crit-icized and cannot be taken as reliable: see R.S. Bagnall and Th. Drew-Bear, "Documents from Kourion: A Review Article," part 2, "Individual Inscriptions," *Phoenix* 27 (1973): 239–41; W. Peek, "Metrische Mosaik-Inschrift aus Kourion," *ZPE* 23 (1976): 97–98. Peek's text is that reproduced above, but even it must be considered largely speculative. Peek (loc. cit.) suggests that the last lines lyrically commemorate the work of Eustolios in restoring the lower city at Kourion after it had been covered by the sea in an earthquake. (The mythological reference appears to be to Apollo fixing Delos in the sea.)

Ἰουλιανὸς Δόμνῃ σὺν ἀλόχωι. Serdjilla, Syria. 473. *IGLS* 4.1490.   327†*

Ἰουλιανὸς | μὲν ἔτευξεν, | χάριν δ᾽ ἔχι ἄπασα | κώμη, Δόμνῃ σὺν ἀλόχωι, κ|αὶ ἀσπέτον ὤπασεν ὄλβον, | πάτρην κυδαίνων· ἀλλὰ | φθόνον ἐκτὸς ἐλαύνοι δόξα | καὶ κῦδος ὔμμιν ἐπὶ πλίον | αἰὲν ἀΐροι. ἐτελιώθη τὸ λου|τρὸν μηνὶ Πανέμου τοῦ δπψ᾽ | ἔτους ἰνδικτιόνος ια᾽. | Θαλλασίου ἐσθλὸς παῖς Ἰουλιανὸς τόδ᾽ ἔτευξ[εν | βου]λῇ κ(αὶ) πραπίδεσσ[ιν δό-]ξαν ἔχων συνέ[ρι]|θον.

Trans.: "Julianus built (these baths)—and the whole town enjoys their charm—with his wife Domna. He gave immense joy, glorifying his hometown. But let glory drive envy away, and let the praise increase for you more and more forever. The bath was finished in the month of Panemos in the 784th year in the eleventh indiction *(i.e., 470; the month is unclear)*. Julianus, the noble son of Thalassios, built this bath with glory as his helper, by virtue of his counsel and intellect."

NOTES: This mosaic inscription found in the baths at this site is typical of late Imperial bath texts from the Greek East that praise the pleasantness of the baths and the greatness of the benefactor: compare Robert, "Epigrammes," 76–87, and, above, nos. 315/16 and 326. There are certainly difficulties of interpretation with this text. For example, does χάριν δ᾽ ἔχι ἄπασα κώμη mean that the village was grateful to Julianus (which is the natural reading of χάριν ἔχειν; it is thus translated in *IGLS*), or does it mean that the villagers had access to the grace of the baths, as suggested by Robert (loc. cit.) and Russell (*Mosaic Inscriptions of Anemurium*, 41–43)? What was the role of Domna? Did she help build the baths, or is she reported only to have felt gratitude along with the rest of the village? The wording of the inscription appears ambig-uous on these points, perhaps deliberately so. For the remains, see Nielsen, 2.46–47 (C.385); Yegül, 329–33.

Διογένης κόμης. Megara, Achaea. Late fifth century. *SIG*³ 909 = *CIG* 8622 = *SEG* 14   328†
(1957) 379.

ἔργον καὶ τοῦτο τοῦ μεγαλοπρεπεστάτου κόμητος Διογένους τοῦ παιδὸς | Ἀρχελάου, ὃς τῶν Ἑλληνίδων πόλεων ὡς τῆς ἰδίας οἰκίας κηδόμενος | παρέσχεν καὶ τῇ Μεγαρ(έ)ων εἰς μὲν πύργων κατασκευὴν ἑκατὸν χρυσίνους, | πεντήκοντα δὲ καὶ ἑκατὸν ἑτέρους δισχιλίους τε καὶ διακοσίους | πόδας μαρμάρου εἰς τὴν ἀνανέωσιν τοῦ λουτροῦ, τιμιώτερον | οὐδὲν ἡγούμενος τοῦ τοὺς Ἕλληνας εὐεργετεῖν | ἀνανεοῦν τε τὰς πόλεις.

Trans.: "This too is the work of the most magnificent Diogenes, *comes,* son of Archelaos, who, caring for the cities of the Greeks as he would his own house, gave one hundred gold pieces to the city of Megara toward the construction of ramparts, also 2,200 feet of marble for the renovation of the bathhouse, believing nothing more valuable than the benefaction of the Greeks and the renovation of their cities."

NOTES: Diogenes, although named a *comes,* did not hold office in Achaea, and so he seems to be acting here as a private benefactor; *PLRE* (2.360–61, s.v. "Diogenes 5") suggests he may have been a native of the area. If he is the same Diogenes as that, also a *comes,* named in another text (*CIG* 8621), he can be dated to the late fifth century; see *PLRE* 2.361, s.v. "Diogenes 7."

Nonconstructional Benefactions

Free Bathing

329† [Με]νέλα[ος], στεφανηφό[ρ]ος, γραμματεύς, γυμνασίαρχος. Ancyra, Galatia. Augustan (?). *IGRR* 4.555.

Of this lengthy honorary inscription, only the pertinent lines (1–6) are cited.

[ἡ βουλὴ καὶ ὁ δῆμος ὁ Ἀ]ν[κυρα]νῶν ἐτίμησ[εν | Με]νέλα[ον Μητρ]οτίμου τὸν στεφανηφόl[ρ]ον καὶ γραμματέα, γυμνασιαρχήσαντα | καὶ ἀλίψαντα τὸν δῆμον ἐκ λουτήρω[ν] | καὶ λούσαντα ἐκ τῶν ἰδίων . . .

Trans.: "The council and people of Ankyra honored Menelaos, son of Metrotimos, a crowned magistrate and secretary, who was gymnasiarch and gave oil to the people from large vessels and offered baths at his own expense . . . "

NOTES: Possible mention of νέ[οι ὁμοβωμίοι?] in the last line of the inscription is perhaps in references to Augustus and Livia, as Lafaye (*IGRR*) suggests. Menelaos, a local magistrate, provided bathing out of his own pocket. He also gave oil to the people (see no. 332).

330 (οἱ ἐπιμεληταὶ τῶν συστημάτων τῶν ἐριοπ[ώλ]ων τε καὶ λινύφων). Hypaipa, Lydia. 301. *SEG* 30 (1980) 1382.

This lengthy inscription is mostly unrelated to baths. Note, however, the portion that reads:

| (14) . . . τὸ βαλανεῖον λούειν μελέτω τοῖς ἐπιμελη[ταῖς ..7..] | τοὺς κατοίκους

NOTES: This text is part of a long inscription outlining the rules for an association of wool sellers and linen weavers as laid down by an unnamed founder; see Th. Drew-Bear, "An Act of Foundation at Hypaipa," *Chiron* 10 (1980): 509–36. The lines preceding those cited here deal with the management of property given for the association's use. The editors of *SEG* translate the phrase cited above as follows: "Provide for the functioning without charge of the public baths for the inhabitants." This translation, however, omits mention of the men charged with seeing to the baths, the managers (ἐπιμεληταί). The expression λούειν τὸ βαλανεῖον means "to provide free baths"; see Drew-Bear," op. cit., 523 (esp. n. 70). Presumably the baths were located either in Hypaipa or on the association's property.

Oil Distributions

Κοῖντος Πομπώνιος [Φλάκκος], στράτηγος, ἀγορανόμος. Laodicea, Asia. Undated.   331†
IGRR 4.860.

Of this lengthy honorary inscription, only the pertinent lines are cited.

οἱ ἐπὶ τῆς Ἀσίας Ῥωμαῖοι καὶ Ἕλληνες καὶ ὁ δῆμος ὁ Λαοδικέων ἐτείμησαν Κοῖντον
Πομπώ|νιον Κοίντου υἱὸν, Γαλερίᾳ Φλάκκον ἥρωα, στρατηγήσαντα τῆς πόλεως
δημοφελῶς (sic) καὶ γενόμενον ἐπὶ τῶν δημοσίίων προσόδων, ἀγορανομήσαντά τε
πολυτε|λῶς καὶ ἑκατέρους τοὺς θερμοὺς περιπάτους καύσαντ[α] | πρῶτον καὶ μόνον,
ἀλείψαντά τε ἐν ταῖς ἐπισήμοις ἡμέ|ραις παρ' ἑαυτοῦ κατὰ μῆνα . . . *(three lines
skipped)* | *(12)* στρώσαντά τε παρ' ἑαυτοῦ ἔνπροσθεν τοῦ Διὸς [ἀ]|κολ[ού]θω[ς] καὶ
ἀλείψαντα τὴν πόλιν πάλιν παρ' ἑαυτο[ῦ] | τοῖς κατ' ἄνδρα δρακτοῖς ἐγ λουτήρων . . .

Trans.: "The Romans and Greeks of Asia and the people of Laodicea honored
Quintus Pomponius Flaccus, son of Quintus, of the voting tribe Galeria, the hero. He
was a people-loving general of the city and was supervisor of public revenues; he was
a lavish aedile and was the first and only man to heat each of the hot ambulatories; he
also provided oil (for the people) on appointed days every month at his own expense
. . . *(line 12)* He also evenly paved the area in front of the statue (*or* Temple) of Zeus at
his own expense and provided oil for the city, again at his own expense, from large
vessels, in individual vials for each man . . . "

NOTES: Two separate oil provisions are recorded here: (1) as aedile Flaccus supplied oil on set
days every month, and (2) he marked his paving of the area in front of the statue, or Temple, of
Zeus with a second oil distribution. The term λουτῆρες refers to large containers of oil from
which disbursements took place; the smaller vessels (δράκτα) could be used to hand out the oil to
each individual from the larger λουτῆρες.

[Με]νέλα[ος], στεφανηφό[ρ]ος, γραμματεύς, γυμνασίαρχος. Ancyra, Galatia. Au-   332
gustan (?). *IGRR* 4.555.

A fuller citation of the text is provided at no. 329. Here note the portion that reads:

. . . καὶ ἀλίψαντα τὸν δῆμον ἐκ λουτήρω[ν] . . .

Γάϊος Ἰούλιος Σακέρδως, ἱερεύς Τιβερίου Κλαυδίου Νέρωνος, γυμνασίαρχος. Per-   333†
gamum, Asia. 16 or post-26. *IGRR* 4.454.

οἱ νέοι ἐτίμησαν | Γάϊον Ἰούλιον Σακέρδωτα, τὸν | νεωκόρον θεᾶς Ῥώμης καὶ θεοῦ |
Σεβαστοῦ Καίσαρος καὶ ἱερέα | Τιβερίου Κλαυδίου Νέρωνος καὶ | γυμνασίαρχον τῶν
δωδεκάτων | Σεβαστῶν Ῥωμαίων τῶν πέντε | γυμνασίων, ἀλείφοντα ἐγ λουτήρων | δι'
ὅλης ἡμέρας ἐκ τῶν ἰδίων, | προνοήσαντα τῆς τε αὐτῶν καὶ τῶν | [ἐφ]ήβων ἀγωγῆς, νό-
μους τε πατρίους | [καὶ ἤ]θη κατὰ τὸ κάλλιστον | [ἀν]εωσάμενον.

Trans.: "The young men honored Gaius Julius Sacerdos, the warden of the temple of
the goddess Rome and the god Augustus Caesar, and priest of Tiberius Claudius
Nero, and gymnasiarch of the five gymnasia for the twelfth games of Rome and
Augustus. He provided oil from large vessels throughout the whole day at his own
expense; he provided for the education of his own sons and the ephebes; and he
renewed our ancestral laws and customs in accordance with what was best."

NOTES: This text is dated by Sacerdos' holding the priesthood of Tiberius, which was not
instituted at Pergamum until 26 (see Tac. *Ann.* 4.55–56), even though the twelfth games for

Rome and Augustus, instituted in 29 B.C., were celebrated in A.D. 16. As a result, there is some uncertainty as to exactly when the provision of oil was presented, whether when Sacerdos was gymnasiarch (in 16) or when he was priest of Tiberius (in 26 or later).

334†   Σέξτος Ἰούλιος Φίλων, γυμνασίαρχος. Ilium, Asia. After 69. *IGRR* 4.216 = *IK* 3 (Ilion) 121 (see also 122–24, esp. 123).

ἡ Ἀτταλὶς φυλὴ | Σέξτον Ἰούλιον Φί[λων]α, τὸν κόσμον τῆς π[ό|λ]εως, ἔπαρχον σπεί-ρης | Φλαβιανῆς, γυμνασιαρ|χήσαντα λαμπρῶς καὶ φιλοτείμως, καὶ πρῶτον | τῶν ἀπ᾽ αἰῶνος καὶ | μέχρι νῦν μόνον ἐλαι|ομετρήσαντα τούς | τε βουλευτὰς καὶ πολείτας πά-ντας καὶ ἀλ[εί]ψαντα ἐκ λουτήρων [παν]|δημεί.

Trans.: "The tribe Attalis (honored) Sextus Julius Philo, the ornament of the city, prefect of the Flavian cohort, who was a prominent and munificent gymnasiarch and was the first ever and, to date, the only man to measure out oil for the councillors and all the citizens and bestow oil on the whole people from large vessels."

NOTES: This inscription is on a statue base. It is often not clear from such inscriptions whether the context of the benefaction was gymnasial baths or strictly Roman-style facilities, which, in this part of the empire, may have served identical purposes anyway. Some texts (e.g., no. 336) specify the placing of the oil in the baths (βαλανεῖα), but most, like this one, do not. For the term ἐκ λουτήρων, see the notes to no. 331.

335   Ἀσκληπιάδης, ἐπιστάτης, γυμνασίαρχος. Dorylaeum, Asia. Hadrian (?). *IGRR* 4.522.

Of this lengthy, acephalous text with fragmentary opening lines, only the pertinent lines are cited.

[—]βου υἱῶι Διὶ Πατρώ[ιωι —] . . . | (5) . . . Ἀσκληπιάδης Στρατονί|[κου ..5..]ένης σεβαστοφάντης δία βίου καὶ ἱερεὺς . . . | (8) γυμνα|σίαρχος ἐκ τῶν ἰδίων ἐλευθέρων καὶ δούλων ἀπὸ | ἀρχομένης ἡμέρας ἕως νυκτὸς δρακτοῖς ἐκ λου[τήρ]ων.

NOTES: The word ἀλείψας is understood here, apparently subsumed into the title "gym-nasiarch." Notice how Asklepiades provides slaves and freedmen for the distribution of the oil, again in little oil flasks drawn from the larger λουτῆρες. The fragmentary imperial titles in the opening line may be those of Hadrian.

336†   Διονύσιος, γραμματεύς. Ephesos, Asia. Ca. 140/50. *IK* 13 (Ephesos 3) 661.

Of this lengthy honorary inscription, only the pertinent lines are cited.

. . . | (4) Ἐφεσίων | πόλεως ἡ βουλὴ καὶ ὁ δῆμος | ἐτείμησεν | Διονύσιον Νεικηφόρου . . . *(ten lines skipped)* | (14) ἐλαιοθετήσαντα διὰ τοῦ υἱοῦ Διονυσίου μῆνας τέσσαρες ἐκ τῶν | ἰδίων ἄνευ τάγματος ἐν τῷ ἄνω | γυμνασίῳ, καὶ ἐν τῷ τῆς πρυτανείας ἐνι[αυ]τῷ ἐν ταῖς ἐθίμοις ἡμέραις | θέντα ἔλαιον ἐν πᾶσι τοῖς γυμνα|σίοις, καὶ τῇ τῶν Καταγωγίων | ἡμέρᾳ ἀγοραίας ἀγομένης ἔλαιον θέντα δρακτῷ ἔν τε τοῖς γυμνασί|οις καὶ ἐν τοῖς βαλανείοις τοῖς οὖ|σιν ἐν Ἐφέσῳ πᾶσιν . . .

Trans.: " . . . The council and people of Ephesos honored Dionysius, son of Nikephoros . . . *(line 14)* He [Dionysius] voluntarily provided oil at his own expense through his son Dionysius for four months in the upper gymnasium; and during the year of his *prytany,* he provided oil on the usual days in all the gymnasia; and on the day of the Katagogia, when a market was being held, he provided oil in vials in the gymnasia and all the baths in Ephesos . . . "

NOTES: This inscription is from a statue base in the agora. What is most interesting about this text is the manner in which the locations of the various oil provisions are listed, in ascending order of generosity. Ephesos had many baths and bath-gymnasia, but it seems that the building now called the "East Bath-Gymnasium" should be identified as the "upper" gymnasium: see *IK* 13 (Ephesos 3) 839; Nielsen, 2.37 (C.298); Yegül, 279–82. Dionysius also provided oil in all the gymnasia, of which at least four can be identified at Ephesos: see Manderscheid 108–10, s.vv. "Ephesos," "Hafengymnasium," "Ostgymnasium," "Theatergymnasium," and "Vediusgymnasium"; Nielsen, 2.36–37 (C.295, 297, 298, 300); Yegül, 272 (fig. 335). He also provided oil in all the other baths in the city, which cannot now be numbered. The wording seems to imply that the baths (βαλανεῖα) were more numerous than the gymnasia in the city, which would make sense. These details reveal the variety of possible contexts for those briefer and more vague commemorations of "oiling" the people.

Water Supply

Incertus Argos, Achaea. Third century (?). *SEG* 28 (1978) 396.   337

. . . [ἀγ]ορὰν καὶ τοὺς ἐν αὐτ[ῆ | σε]βαστοὺς καὶ ἥρωας | [καὶ ?] βαλανεῖα τρία μετὰ |
[τῶν τ]έκνων Τιβ. Κλαυδί[ου] Μενεκλέους καὶ Τι[β. | Κλ]αυδίου Ἀντιγόνου, τὸ |
[ἄνωθ?]ε ὕδωρ καταγαγόντα.

NOTES: This text was found in the remains of a palaestra. The editors of *SEG* suggest a third-century date for it, since it appears associated with another third-century dedication, *SEG* 28 (1978) 397. It is not exactly clear if the water was for the baths, but that is the implication. The inscription is acephalous, so the identity of the benefactor is not known.

Baths Heated

Κοῖντος Πομπώνιος [Φλάκκος], στρατηγός, ἀγορανόμος. Laodicea, Asia. Undated.   338
IGRR 4.860.

A fuller version of the text is cited at no. 331. Here note the portion that reads:

. . . ἀγορανομήσαντά τε πολυτελ[ῶς καὶ ἑκατέρους τοὺς θερμοὺς περιπάτους καύσαν[τα] . . .

NOTES: Here Flaccus heats two ambulatories, the most likely location for which is as part of a bath building, although this location is not explicitly stated.

Trusts for the Maintenance of Baths

Λ. Οὐάκκιος Λαβέων, γυμνασίαρχος. Kyme, Asia. 2 B.C.–A.D. 14. *IGRR* 4.1302 = *IK*   339
5 (Kyme) 19.

A fuller citation of the text is provided at no. 292. Here note the portion that reads:

. . . πρὸς τὰν εἰς αὐτὸ χοραγίαν ταῖς ὑπαρχοίσαις αὐτῶ κτήσαις ἐν Ζμαραγήῳ . . .

NOTES: The assignation of plots of land to support baths is attested in other sources: see nos. 228 and 241; HA *Alex. Sev.* 24.5. In most of these cases, the land is woodland, supposedly assigned to provide the baths with fuel. At least one other attested instance, however, the land was to generate income for their operation; see Dio 54.29.4.

Appendixes

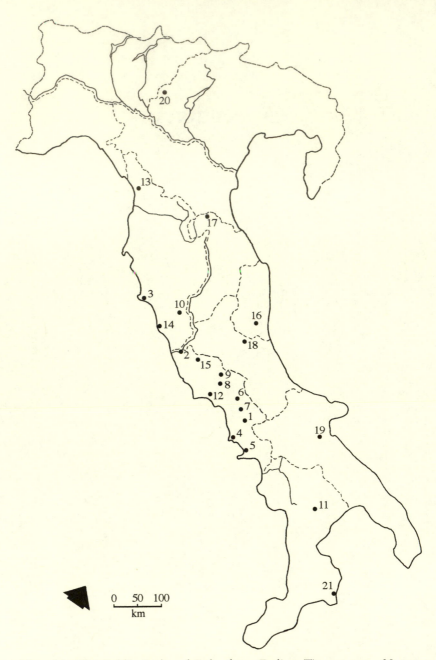

Map A1. The Public Baths of Italy, from Earliest Times to ca. 30 B.C.
(G. Fagan after Jouffroy, *Construction publique;* with permission.)

Appendix 1

The Spread of Public Bathing in the Italian Peninsula to ca. A.D. 100

Only "Roman-style" baths are indicated.

The sites on the maps are numbered according to the entries in the lists attached to each map.

Specific information about each site is to be found in the appropriate list entry.

Naturally, the baths listed here are only those for which a definite geographical location can be provided.

Numbered entries reflect the first appearance of baths at each site, that is, their construction dates (when physical remains are available for inspection) or their earliest mention in an author or inscription (which, of course, does not necessarily correspond to the date[s] of construction).

In map A2, the squares represent those sites listed in map A1 that are not attested as having had new baths in the period covered by map A2. In many cases, the Republican baths at these places continued in use throughout the period covered by map A2.

Sites are listed chronologically.

Multiple entries for single sites are indicated by bullets (•).

Map A1. The Public Baths of the Italian Peninsula, from Earliest Times to ca. 30 B.C.

Site no.	Place	Comments and references
1	Capua	216 B.C. One bath mentioned by Livy (23.7.3).
2	Rome	• Late third/early second century B.C. Baths referred to by Plautus (see above, chapter 2, pp. 45–46, for discussion); early baths mentioned in Varro *Ling.* 9.68. • Second century B.C. Caecilius Statius mentions baths, see frag. 98R (cited in Non. 194M [285L], s.v. "balneae").

		• First century B.C. Baths mentioned in several late Republican authors; see above, chapter 2, pp. 48–51, for discussion. Note specifically those named in Cic. *Rosc. Am.* 18 *(Balneae Pallicinae)* and *Cael.* 61–67 *(Balneae Seniae).*
3	Cosa	Second century B.C. (?). See *PECS,* 245–46, s.v. "Cosa" (Brown).
4	Cumae	ca. 180 B.C. Central Baths built; see Nielsen, 1.29 n. 24.
5	Pompeii	• ca. 140–120 B.C. Stabian Baths built; see above, chapter 2, pp. 57–58. • ca. 100–90 B.C. Republican Baths built; see above, chapter 2, pp. 59–60. • ca. 80 B.C. Forum Baths built; see above, chapter 2, pp. 58–59.
6	Teanum Sidicinum	ca. 130–21 B.C. One bath, probably a double building, mentioned by Aulus Gellius (*NA* 10.3.3).
7	Cales	• ca. 130–21 B.C. Indeterminate number; see Gell. *NA* 10.3.3. • ca. 90–70 B.C. Central Baths built; see Nielsen, 2.7 (C.35).
8	Ferentinum	ca. 130–21 B.C. Indeterminate number; see Gell. *NA* 10.3.3.
9	Aletrium	Late second century. *Lacus balnearius;* see no. 157.
10	Musarna	Late second/early first century B.C. Baths built; see Broise and Jolivet, "Le bain en Étrurie," 89–92; Nielsen, 2.10 (C.62).
11	Grumentum	Sullan? *Balneum* built; see no. 64.
12	Fondi	First century B.C. Baths built; see Jouffroy, *Construction publique,* 52.
13	Massarosa	First century B.C. Baths built; see ibid., 53.
14	Centumcellae	First century B.C. Baths built; see ibid., 53.
15	Praeneste	• First century B.C. Baths near entrance to Sanctuary of Fortuna Primigenia; see Coarelli, *Lazio,* 155 • First century B.C. or later (?). Offer of free bathing, see no. 204.
16	Interamnia Praetuttiorum	First century B.C. or Augustan (?). Offer of free bathing; see no. 205.
17	Mevaniola	ca. 50 B.C. Baths built; see Jouffroy, *Construction publique,* 53.

18	Alba Fucens	Mid–first century B.C. Baths built; see Nielsen, 1.35.
19	Herdonia	Caesarian. Baths built; see no. 65.
20	Brixia	49–ca. 27 B.C. Baths built or extended; see no. 66.
21	Croton	Late Republic. *Balneum* built; see no. 67.

Map A2: The Public Baths of the Italian Peninsula, ca. 30 B.C. to ca. A.D. 100

Site no.	Place	Comments and references
1	Rome	• 33 B.C. 170 *gratuita balinea* offered in city; see Pliny *HN* 36.121. • 25–19 B.C. Thermae of Agrippa built; see above, chapter 5, pp. 107–10, for discussion. • ca. 20 B.C. Horace (*Epist.* 1.1.91–93) mentions baths in Rome. • ca. 2–1 B.C. "Many baths" mentioned by Ovid (*Ars Am.* 3.638–40). • Mid–first century A.D. Baths feature in the writings of Celsus, the Elder and Younger Seneca, the Elder and Younger Pliny, and Petronius; see above, chapter 2, pp. 51–53, for discussion. • A.D. 60–66. Thermae of Nero built; see above, chapter 5, pp. 110–12, for discussion. • A.D. 79–80. Thermae of Titus built; see above, chapter 5, pp. 112–13, for discussion. • Late first century A.D. Baths feature heavily in writings of Martial and other authors; see above, chapter 1, passim; chapter 2, pp. 51–53.
2	Velia	Late first century B.C. Vignale Baths built; see Nielsen, 2.9 (C.52).
3	Pisa	A.D. 4. An indeterminate number of baths closed in Pisa to mark the death of C. Caesar; see *CIL* 11.1421 = *ILS* 140, lines 20–24.
4	Aeclanum	Augustan? Remains of baths; see *PECS*, 11, s.v. "Aeclanum" (Ward-Perkins).
5	Aquinum	Augustan. Remains of apsidal structure, perhaps baths; see Jouffroy, *Construction publique*, 95.
6	Arretium	Augustan? Remains near the theater, see ibid., 95.
7	Bononia	Augustan. Bath built by Augustus, restored by Gaius; see no. 1/2.
8	Faesulae	Augustan? Baths built; see Nielsen, 2.9–10 (C.58).
9	Herculaneum	• Augustan. Forum Baths built; see ibid. 2.7 (C.38).

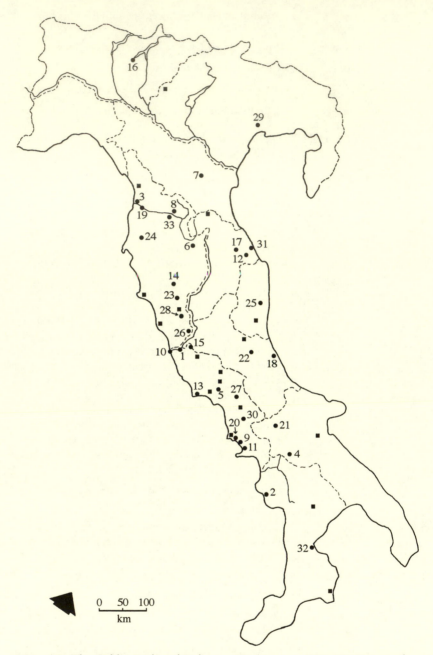

Map A2. The Public Baths of Italy, ca. 30 B.C.–A.D. 100. (G. Fagan after Jouffroy, *Construction publique*; with permission.)

		• Julio-Claudian. Suburban Baths built; see ibid., 2.7 (C.39).
10	Ostia	• Augustan. *Balneum* mentioned; see *CIL* 14.4711. • Mid–first century A.D. Baths of Invidiosus built; see Nielsen, 2.6 (C.28). • A.D. 80–90. Baths of the Swimmer built; see ibid., 2.4 (C.15).
11	Pompeii	• Augustan? *Balneus Agrippae* mentioned (may not be a bathhouse); see *CIL* 4.3878. • Tiberian? Suburban Baths built; see above, chapter 2, p. 61, for discussion. • Tiberian? *Thermae et Baln(eae?) Crassi Frugi*; see no. 257. • A.D. 62–79. Central Baths built; see above, chapter 2, p. 65, for discussion. • A.D. 62–79. *Balneum Venerium et Nongentum*; see no. 258. • A.D. 62–79. Sarno/Palaestra Baths; see above, chapter 2, pp. 61–62, 67, for discussion.
12	Suasa	Augustan (?). Offer of free bathing; see no. 206.
13	Terracina	• Augustan. Baths of Neptune built; see Jouffroy, *Construction publique*, 95. • Flavian. Baths of the Arenas; see ibid., 95.
14	Volsinii	Post–A.D. 17/18 or later. *Balneum* built; see no. 159.
15	Vallis Digentiae (near Tibur)	Tiberian (post–A.D. 20). Free baths given; see no. 208.
16	Comum	First half of the first century A.D. Multiple *balneae* and *thermae* in the town; see no. 215.
17	Forum Sempronii	First half of first century A.D. Double baths built; see Nielsen, 2.9 (C.57).
18	Teate Marrucinorum	Mid–first century A.D. Baths built; see ibid., 2.9 (C.53).
19	Massaciuccoli	Mid–first century A.D. "Baths of Nero" built; see ibid., 2.10 (C.61).
20	Naples	Nero and/or earlier. Baths near the theater; see Suet. *Ner.* 20.2.
21	Ligures Baebiani	Post–A.D. 62 (?). *Balneum* restored after earthquake; see no. 69.
22	Furfo	Julio-Claudian. Bath built; see no. 70.
23	Ferentum	Flavian? Double baths built; see Nielsen, 2.10 (C.59).

24	San Gaetano di Vada	Second half of first century A.D. Baths built; see ibid., 2.10 (C.63).
25	Urbs Salvia	Second half of first century/early second century A.D. *Balneum muliebre* (?) mentioned; see no. 209.
26	Capena	Late first century/early second century A.D. *Balneum* built; see no. 164.
27	Teanum Sidicinum	First century A.D. *Balneum Clodianum* bought by local council (presumably to be made public); see no. 250.
28	Ager Viterbiensis	First century A.D. (?) *Balneum* attested; see *CIL* 11.3010.
29	Altinum	First century A.D. (?). Two baths built; see no. 168/69.
30	Capua	First century A.D. Northeast baths, see Jouffroy, *Construction publique*, 95.
31	Fanum Fortunae	First century A.D. *Balneum* restored; see no. 73/74.
32	Copia Thurii	First century A.D. Edge of *labrum* inscribed by *duoviri*; see no. 75.
33	Florentia	First century A.D. Capitol Baths built; see Nielsen, 2.10 (C.60).

Appendix 2

The Distribution of Nonimperial Baths in Rome (and Some Possible Builders or Owners)

Introduction

The figures given below for the baths of Rome and the data plotted on the attached map are drawn from the information supplied by the Regionaries (the *Curiosum* and *Notitia*), supplemented by literary and epigraphic evidence where applicable. Grave uncertainty surrounds these numbers. Even a superficial glance at the totals of *balnea* in each region reveals that certain figures (e.g., eighty-six, seventy-five, and sixty-three) recur with suspicious regularity, suggesting that a complex reality has been simplified and systematized in the Regionaries. Further, the occurrence of the total of seventy-five (LXXV) *balnea*, which comes together in groups of regions in both lists—in Regiones IV–VII in the *Notitia* and Regiones V–VII in the *Curiosum*—further suggests systematization; a figure of sixty-five (LXV) is given for Regio IV in the *Curiosum*, one "X" short of agreement with the *Notitia*, quite possibly the result of a corruption in the manuscript tradition. Also, it is noticeable that even within the individual Regionaries the totals for *balnea* in the city do not agree: the overall total for the city is given as 856 in both lists, but the addition of the region-by-region figures leads to a total of 967 in the *Notitia* and a total of 942 in the *Curiosum*. All of this disagreement must lead to the conclusion that the numbers should not be read as wholly reliable.

Region-by-Region Listing (see map A3)[1]

Regio I (Porta Capena)

Curiosum	*Notitia*
Balnea LXXXVI	Balinea LXXXVI

---

1. It must be stressed that most of the specific identifications of builders or owners offered in this section are tentative. Very few names are known from the ancient world, especially from among the lower social orders. Because building a bath required substantial financial resources, however, it can be assumed that bath benefactors would not normally hail from among the penurious and anonymous. Figures for the baths as listed per region in the *Curiosum* and *Notitia* are those cited in H. Jordan, *Topographie der Stadt Rom im Alterthum,* vol. 2 (Berlin, 1871; reprint, Rome, 1970), 541–74.

357

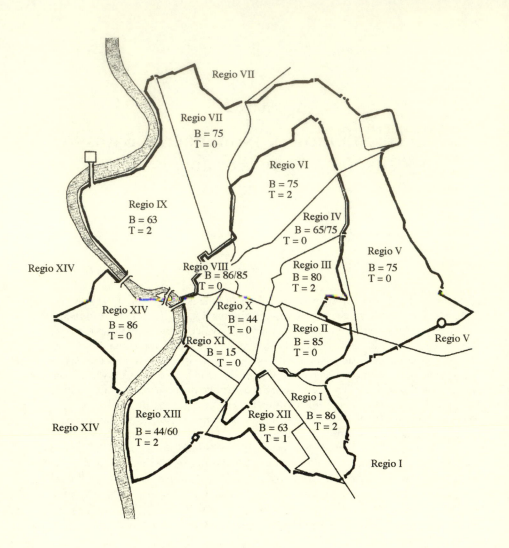

Regio VII

Regio VII
B = 75
T = 0

Regio VI
B = 75
T = 2

Regio IX
B = 63
T = 2

Regio IV
B = 65/75
T = 0

Regio V
B = 75
T = 0

Regio XIV

Regio VIII
B = 86/85
T = 0

Regio III
B = 80
T = 2

Regio XIV
B = 86
T = 0

Regio X
B = 44
T = 0

Regio II
B = 85
T = 0

Regio V

Regio XI
B = 15
T = 0

Regio I

Regio XIV

Regio XIII
B = 44/60
T = 2

Regio XII
B = 63
T = 1

Regio II B = 86
T = 2

Regio I

0 ———— 1
km

B = *Balnea* (two numbers denote conflicting totals in the *Curiosum/Notitia*
T = *Thermae*

Map A3. The Regiones of the City of Rome with the Number of *Thermae* and
Balnea per Regio Indicated. (G. Fagan after F. Coarelli, *Guida archeologia di
Roma* [Verona, 1974], 14; with permission.)

Named baths:
The Thermae of Severus and of Commodus stood in this Regio and are named in both the *Curiosum* and the *Notitia*. The following *balnea* are also named.

Balneum Abascantis et Mamertini (as named in the *Curiosum*), **Balneum Abascanti et Antiochiani** (as named in the *Notitia*), **Balneum Bolani et Mamertini** (as named in the *Notitia*).

> The confusion among these names suggests that something has gone amiss in the transmission, so it is impossible to determine with certainty in each case whether the name denotes a single building with multiple owners or separate establishments; see above, chapter 5, p. 124. As to the individuals named, various possibilities can be entertained. A freedman of Domitian was named Abascantus (see *PIR*² F 194), but the name could equally apply to any freedman of the Claudii or Flavii, see *LTUR* 1.155, s.v. "Balneum Abascanti" (D. Palombi). The praetorian prefect of 139–43 was Petronius Mamertinus; see *RE* 19.1217–19, s.v. "Petronius 44" (Hoffman). An Antiochianus was praetorian prefect in 221 (see *PIR*² A 738), and Flavius Antiochianus was consul II in 270 and urban prefect in 269–70 and 272 (see *PIR*² F 203; *PLRE* 1.70, s.v. "Flavius Antiochianus"); see *LTUR* 1.156, s.v. "Balneum Antiochiani" (D. Palombi). Finally, two consuls bore the name Vettius Bolanus, in 66 (see *RE* 8A.1857–58, s.v. "Vettius 25" [Stattmann]) and 111 (ibid., s.v. "Vettius 26" [Stattmann]); see *LTUR* 1.156–57, s.v. "Balneum Bolani" (C. Lega). All of these identifications, however, are tenuous in the extreme. The evidence is just too scrappy, so the appearance of Mamertinus, for instance, could denote an otherwise unknown person attached to the Aelii or Claudii; see *LTUR* 1.161, s.v. "Balneum Mamertini" (D. Palombi).

Balneum Torquati (as named in the *Curiosum*), **Balneum Torquati et Vespasiani** (as named in the *Notitia*).

> Again, whether these names denote a single building or two separate structures is not clear from the Regionaries; see above, chapter 5, p. 125. The appearance of Vespasian's name seems significant, assuming it bears on the original builder or owner of the building. D. Junius Silanus Torquatus was consul in 53 (see *PIR*² I 837), and L. Junius Silanus Torquatus was a senator under the Julio-Claudians (see *PIR*² I 838), but, realistically, the name could apply to anyone attached to the Silanii or Calpurnii; see *LTUR* 1.166, s.v. "Balneum Torquati" (D. Palombi). Note that Martial (10.79.2–3) reports that a Torquatus built *thermae* at Rome.

Regio II (Caelemontum)

Curiosum	*Notitia*
Balnea LXXXV	Balinea LXXXV

Named baths:
No named baths are known in this Regio.

Regio III (Isis et Serapis)

Curiosum	*Notitia*
Balnea LXXX	Balinea LXXX

Named baths:
The Thermae of Titus and of Trajan stood in this Regio and are named in both the
Curiosum and the *Notitia*. No named *balnea* are known in this Regio.

Regio IV (Templum Pacis)

Curiosum	*Notitia*
Balnea LXV	Balinea LXXV

Named baths:

Balneum Dafnidis (named in the *Curiosum* and the *Notitia*).
  This bath is otherwise unattested. The name may derive from an artistic represen-
  tation of Daphne. See above, chapter 6, p. 172, on baths named after gods; see also
  LTUR 1.159, s.v. (E. Rodríguez Almeida).
Balneum Phoebi (Juv. 7.233).
  This bath is named by Juvenal as located in the Subura, where the poet lived. It is
  probably named after a statue of Apollo that stood inside. E. Rodríguez Almeida
  (*LTUR* 1.162, s.v.), following a scholiast on the line, suggests that perhaps this
  bath is identical to the *Balneum Dafnidis,* with the whole named after representa-
  tions of Apollo and Daphne in its decorative scheme.

Regio V (Esquiliae)

Curiosum	*Notitia*
Balnea LXXV	Balinea LXXV

Named baths:

Thermae Helenianae (*CIL* 6.1136 = *CIL* 6.31244).
  These baths were probably private; see above, chapter 5, p. 117.

Bal(neum) Verul(ani or **-ianum)** (*CIL* 6.182 = *CIL* 6.30708 = *ILS* 3720).
  The inscription was found in Regio V; see *LTUR* 1.166, s.v. "Balneum Verul(ani,
  -anianum)" (L. Chioffi). Possible builders/owners include L. Verulanus Severus,
  suffect consul between 63 and 68 (see *RE* Suppl. 14.840, s.v. "Verulanus 1" [Eck])
  or Verulana Gratilla (see Tac. *Hist.* 3.69; *RE* Suppl. 14.840, s.v. "Verulanus 2"
  [Eck]).

Regio VI (Alta Semita)

Curiosum	*Notitia*
Balnea LXXV	Balinea LXXV

Named baths:
The Thermae of Constantine and of Diocletian stood in this Regio and are named in
both the *Curiosum* and the *Notitia*. The following *balnea* are also named.

Balineum Claudianum (*CIL* 6.29767).

This bath may have been privately owned by the Claudii, for whose presence in this Regio there is ample evidence: see *LTUR* 1.157–58, s.v. (E. Rodríguez Almeida); Richardson, *Dictionary*, 48, s.v.

?Balneum/Thermulae Claudi Etrusci (Mart. 6.42; Stat. *Silv.* 1.5).

E. Rodríguez Almeida (*LTUR* 1.158, s.v.) argues for the location of this facility in this Regio and even suggests that it may be identical with the preceding entry, but see the challenge of W.V. Harris ("The Heir to 'Platner-Ashby,'" *JRA* 8 [1995]: 373), who prefers a location in the Campus Martius (and so somewhere in Regiones VII or IX). The leading candidate for builder/owner is Claudius Etruscus, a Vespasianic *eques* (see *PIR*² C 860).

Thermae Olympiadis (*FTUR* 4.13.430–38).

There is no clear candidate for this Olympias. The most prominent person in Roman history with this name was a wet-nurse of Severus Alexander (see *PIR*² O 98), but she is an unlikely bath builder. Further, the name appears eighty-seven times at Rome, and in the majority of those appearances, it denotes someone of uncertain status; most occurrences date from the third century and later (see Solin, 1.219–20, s.v.). These and some other named baths in this Regio—*Thermae Sallustianae, Thermae Tiberianae*—may have been private facilities.

Balneum Stephani (Mart. 11.52.4, 14.60).

This bath was located near Martial's townhouse and so probably in Regio VI (see Sullivan, 26–30). A possible builder/owner is the imperially connected procurator who served Flavia Domitilla, niece of Domitian (see Suet. *Dom.* 17.2; *LTUR* 1.164, s.v. [E. Rodríguez Almeida]). However, with 236 attested occurrences (see Solin, 3.1182–86, s.v.), the name *Stephanus* was very common in Rome, rendering this suggestion little more than putative.

Balneum Timothinum, Thermae Novati (named in late sources listed in *FTUR* 4.13.421–29 and *LTUR* 1.165–66, s.v. "Balneum Timothinum" [G. De Spirito]).

The location of this bath is hard to pin down from the written sources. However, excavations at the site of the Church of Santa Pudenziana (into which the baths, or part thereof, were converted) revealed a simple bath of the Antonine period; see Richardson, *Dictionary*, 395, s.v. "Thermae Novati." They may also have been termed *Balneum in Subura* (for which, see *LTUR* 1.164–65, s.v. [G. De Spirito]). The owner/builder cannot be identified.

?Lavacrum Agrippinae (*CIL* 6.29765 = *CIL* 15.7247).

This bath is attested on stamped lead pipes found on the Viminal Hill. Assuming the name is not a confusion with the Thermae of Agrippa—which seems unlikely, given the distance between the findspot and Agrippa's baths—the facility can be identified as a possibly private bath associated with one of the Agrippinas; see Richardson, *Dictionary*, 234, s.v.

Regio VII (Via Lata)

Curiosum	*Notitia*
Balnea LXXV	Balinea LXXV

Named baths:
No named baths are known in this Regio.

Regio VIII (Forum Romanum Magnum)

Curiosum   *Notitia*
Balnea LXXXVI   Balinea LXXXV

Named baths:
No named baths are known in this Regio.

Regio IX (Circus Flaminius)

Curiosum   *Notitia*
Balnea LXIII   Balinea LXIII

Named baths:
The Thermae of Nero and of Agrippa stood in this Regio and are named in both the *Curiosum* and the *Notitia*, the Thermae of Nero by its later name of *Thermae Alexandrinae*. The following *balnea* are also named.

Balneae Pallacinae (Cic. *Rosc. Am.* 18).
These baths were named after the district in which they stood; see *RE* 18.156–57, s.v. "Pallacinae vicus" (Welin). Whether these baths were operating in the imperial period is not known.
Balneum Tigillini (Mart. 3.20.16; *CGL* 3.657.14).
The location is that suggested by E. Rodríguez Almeida (see *LTUR* 1.165, s.v.). The strongest possibility for builder/owner is the dissolute praetorian prefect under Nero (see *PIR*² O 91).

Regio X (Palatium)

Curiosum   *Notitia*
Balnea XLIIII   Balinea XLIIII

Named baths:

[Ba]lneum [Ca]esaris (*FUR* fr. 43).
E. Rodríguez Almeida (*LTUR* 1.157, s.v.) plausibly suggests that this bath may have been part of the imperial palace complex on the Palatine.
Lavacrum Plauti⟨a⟩ni (HA *Heliogab.* 8.6).
The name may be a corruption of *Thermae Palatini* and so may denote baths in the palace; see Richardson, *Dictionary,* 234, s.v. If the name of the baths was *Balneum Plautini,* the owner is not otherwise unattested. If the name was *Balneum Plautiani,* a possible candidate is the Severan praetorian prefect C. Fulvius Plautianus (see *PIR*² F 554); see the Teubner edition of *vita Elagabali* (ed. E. Hohl, 1971).
[Ther]mae Falerianae (*CIL* 6.29806).
An inscription, found on the Palatine, reads in part *[ex the]rmis Falerianis.* Even assuming that the restoration of the text is correct and that the findspot reflects the location of the building, neither the bath nor its builder/owner can be identified.

Regio XI (Circus Maximus)

Curiosum	Notitia
Balnea XV	Balinea XV

Named baths:
No named baths are known in this Regio.

Regio XII (Piscina Publica)

Curiosum	Notitia
Balnea LXIII	Balinea LXIII

Named baths:
The Thermae of Caracalla stood in this Regio and are named (as *Thermae Antinoni-nianae*) in both the *Curiosum* and the *Notitia*. The following *balnea* are also named.

Balineum Gratiarum (*IG* 14.1034 = *IGUR* 203).
The inscription was found in Regio XII, but it is not clear that this was its original context. The bath was named after the Graces; see *LTUR* 1.160–61, s.v. "Balneum Gratiarum" (L. Chioffi).

Balin(eum) Scriboniolum (*CIL* 15.7188 = *ILCV* 786).
This facility is attested on a fourth-century slave collar found in Regio XII. The collar reads: *Hilarionis | so* (sic). *tene me et revolca me quia fugi de r(egione) | XII a(d) balin(eum) Scrib|oniolum Rom(a)e* [I belong to Hilario. Grab me and hale me back to the *Balneum Scriboniolum* at Rome, since I have run away from Regio XII]. The slave who wore it may have been attached to the baths, but other collars mention public buildings as landmarks to locate the owner; see, e.g., *CIL* 15.7189 *(Basilica Paulli)* or *CIL* 15.7191 = *ILS* 8729 *(Forum Traiani)*. L. Chioffi (*LTUR* 1.163, s.v.) suggests that the baths may have stood in neighboring Regio I, where several privately owned establishments are attested (see above, s.v. "Regio I"). Any member of the Scribonii clan or their dependents could have built this bath. It is worth noting that (L. Scribonius?) Libo Frugi, suffect consul in 96/98 (see *RE* 2A.887–88, s.v. "Scribonius (Libo) 24" [Groag]), received an imperial water concession; see *AE* 1940.39.

Regio XIII (Aventinus)

Curiosum	Notitia
Balnea XLIIII	Balinea LX

Named baths:
The Thermae of Sura and of Decius stood in this Regio and are named in both the *Curiosum* and the *Notitia*. The following *balnea* are also named.

Balenum Mercuri (mentioned in the ninth-century Einsiedeln Itinerary; see *LTUR* 1.161–62, s.v. [D. Palombi]).
The itinerary locates these baths as lying to the southwest of the Aventine Hill. Richardson (*Dictionary*, 49, s.v.) suggests that the structure, no longer visible, may have been a fountain.

Regio XIV (Transtiberim)

Curiosum   *Notitia*
Balnea LXXXVI   Balinea LXXXVI

Named baths:

[B]alineum Ampeli[dis] (*FUR* fr. 47), **Balineum Ampelidis et Dianes** (as named in the
Curiosum), **Balineum Ampelidis, Prisci et Dianae** (as named in the *Notitia*).
  As with the named baths of Regio I, it is difficult to know whether the confusing
entries of the *Curiosum* and *Notitia* denote multiple, separate establishments or a
single structure known by different names. That a fragment of the Marble Map
refers to the *Balineum Ampelidis* alone suggests each may have been an indepen-
dent entity. Another possibility is that *Prisci* is part of the name *Ampelidis;* see
LTUR 1.156, s.v. "Balneum Ampelidis (Prisci) et Dianae" (E. Rodríguez Almeida).
There are only twenty occurrences of the name "Ampelis" known from Rome (see
Solin, 2.1074, s.v.).
?Balne(um) Cotini (*FUR* fr. 48).
  E. Rodríguez Almeida (*LTUR* 1.158–59, s.v.) places this fragment and the *Balneum Ampelidis* fragment in the same part of the Marble Map. If so, both estab-
lishments stood in the Transtiberina. Richardson (*Dictionary*, 48) offers no
location.

Named Baths of Uncertain Location

(Balneum) A. C[—] C[—] (*Syll.* 902; *LTUR* 1.157, s.v. [E.M. Steinby]).
Balneu(m) Augustae (*CIL* 6.33765 = *ILCV* 347).
  This bath is otherwise unattested.
Balin(eum) Caenidianum (inscription cited in Houston, "Onesimus the Librarian,"
and in Weaver and Wilkins, "A Lost Alumna.")
  A funerary inscription, found in Regio VI, mentions this bath, but it is not clear,
first, where the bath stood and, second, whether the bath was public or private. It
was possibly attached to the house of Caenis, Vespasian's concubine, since the
inscription is dedicated by Onesimus, a slave in the imperial household; see
R. Friggeri, "La Domus di Antonia Caenis e il *Balineum Caenidianum*," *Rend
PontAcc* 50 (1977–78): 145–54; Richardson, *Dictionary*, 48, s.v. Neither the bath
nor the house is included in *LTUR*.
Balneum Charini (Mart. 7.34; *LTUR* 1.157, s.v. [D. Palombi])
  Stein notes that *Charinus* is a common name used by Martial for perverts, so it
may be a joke—"The Pervert's Bath"; see *RE* 3.2143–44, s.v. "Charinos 7"
(Stein). That the name is attested only three times in Rome would tend to support
this suggestion; see Solin, 3.1298, s.v.
Balneum Cl(audii) T[—] (*Syll.* 903; *LTUR* 1.158, s.v. [E.M. Steinby]).
Balneum Crispini (Persius 5.126).
  R.A. Harvey (*A Commentary on Persius* [Leiden, 1981], 161) suggests that this
verse is a derivative of Hor. *Sat.* 1.3.137–39. If so, the bath may not have existed at
all. Assuming it was a real facility, the owner may have been a person attached to
the Quincti or the Caepiones; see *LTUR* 1.159, s.v. (D. Palombi).

(Balneum) L. Domiti Primig(eni) (*Syll.* 895; *LTUR* 1.159, s.v. [E.M. Steinby]).

Balneum Fausti (Mart. 2.14.11).

This bath was located somewhere in the Campus Martius and hence in Regiones VII or IX. Several identifications are possible, but all are tentative; see *RE* 6.2091–92, s.v. "Faustus 1–16" (Seeck).

?Bal(neae) Faustines (*CIL* 6.29830).

This inscription serves to label one of several edifices depicted apparently standing on an island in a copy of an ancient picture, now lost; the picture was published by Giovanni Pietro Bellori in his *Iconographia Veteris Romae* (Rome, 1764). Assuming that Bellori's picture was indeed ancient, there is still some uncertainty as to whether the buildings stood on the banks of the Tiber or on the Latian or Campanian coasts; see G. Lugli and G. Filibeck, *Il porto di Roma imperiale e l'Argo Portuense* (Rome, 1935), 40–41 (fig. 24). As a result, the *Balneae Faustines* may not have been in Rome at all.

Bal(neum) Fel(icis) (*Syll.* 890; *LTUR* 1.160, s.v. [E.M. Steinby]).

The *cognomen* Felix was associated with several noble families, but was also a popular slave name, so this may just as easily refer to a freedman as to a senator, see the entries between *PIR*[2] F 143 and 144; *RE* 6.2166–71, s.v "Felix."

Balneum Fortunati (Mart. 2.14.11).

This bath was located somewhere in the Campus Martius, and hence in Regiones VII or IX. Several Fortunati are known at Rome, but none are securely identifiable with this establishment: (1) Fortunatus, freedman of L. Antistius Vetus, consul A.D. 55 (*PIR*[2] F 480); (2) Fortunatus, freedman of Vespasian (*PIR*[2] F 481); (3) an otherwise unattested Fortunatus (*PIR*[2] F 482).

Balneum Germani (*Syll.* 886; *LTUR* 1.160, s.v. [W. Eck]).

This bath is otherwise unattested. Several late Imperial Germani are known, see *RE* 7.1258–61, s.v. "Germanus."

Balneum Grylli (Mart. 2.14.12).

This bath was located somewhere in the Campus Martius, and hence in Regiones VII or IX. The name is otherwise unattested.

Bal(neum) Imo[.]ranes (*Syll.* 889; *LTUR* 1.166, s.v. [E.M. Steinby]).

Bal(neum) Iu[—] (*Syll.* 891; *LTUR* 1.161, s.v. [E.M. Steinby]).

Bal(neum) Iul[—] (*Syll.* 892; *LTUR* 1.161, s.v. [E.M. Steinby]).

Possibly identical to previous entry.

Balneum Iuliorum Akariorum (*CIL* 6.29764; *LTUR* 1.161, s.v. [L. Chioffi]).

If the name is emended to Akakiorum, it may refer to the prominent fourth-century family of the Acacii (*PLRE* 1.6–8, s.v. "Acacius"). The letterform of the inscription also supports a late Imperial date.

Bal(neum) Lorus (*LTUR* 1.161, s.v. [E.M. Steinby]).

Balneum Lupi (Mart. 2.14.12).

This bath was located somewhere in the Campus Martius and hence in Regiones VII or IX. Several Lupi are attested at Rome, but none can be securely identified with this building. Those attested are (1) an Augustan poet (see *PIR*[2] L 419), (2) a friend of Martial (see *PIR*[2] L 421), and (3) a man who had a place reserved for him at the Colosseum (see *RE* 13.1852, s.v. "Lupus 9" [Seeck]).

Balneum Martis (no. 260).

(Balneum) M. O[—] F [—] (*Syll.* 897; *LTUR* 1.162, s.v. [E.M. Steinby]).

Bal(neum) No(v)um (*Syll.* 887; *LTUR* 1.162, s.v. [E.M. Steinby]).

Balneum Polycleti (Schol. *ad* Hor. *Sat.* 5.32).

According to the scholiast Porphyrion, this bath had originally been the *ludus Aemilii*. On the basis of this identification, Richardson (*Dictionary,* 236, s.v. "Ludus Aemilius") suggests that it may have stood in the Campus Martius, and hence it was in Regiones VII or IX. The name *Polyclitus* occurs only ten times in Rome; see Solin, 1.138, s.v.

Balneum P. V[—] R[—] (*Syll.* 898; *LTUR* 1.166, s.v. [E.M. Steinby]).

Balnea Quattuor (Mart. 5.70.4).

Martial names these baths and suggests that they were somewhere in the Campus Martius and hence in Regiones VII or IX. E. Rodríguez Almeida (*LTUR* 1.162–63, s.v.) suggests that they may be identical to the *Balnea Fausti, Fortunati, Lupi,* and *Grylli* also mentioned in Martial (q.v., above, p. 365). See also Rodríguez Almeida, "Due note marziliane: I 'balnea quattuor in Campo' e le 'sellae Paterclianae' subcapitoline," *MEFRA* 101 (1989): 243–49.

(Balneum) R[—] F[—] (*Syll.* 894; *LTUR* 1.163, s.v. [E.M. Steinby]).

(Balneum) S[—] (*Syll.* 899; *LTUR* 1.163, s.v. [E.M. Steinby]).

Balneae Seniae. (Cic. *Cael.* 61–67; *LTUR* 1.163–64, s.v. [D. Palombi]).

The builder/owner was possibly associated with the Saenii, a senatorial family attested for the mid–first century B.C. but otherwise unknown: see Sall. *Cat.* 30.1; *MRR* 2.496, s.v. "L. Saenius." For a full discussion, see A. Vassileiou, "Note sur un établissement de bains romain," *MEFRA* 97 (1985): 325–28.

Bal(neum) Sub[—] (*Syll.* 893; *LTUR* 1.164, s.v. [E.M. Steinby]).

Balneum et Thermae Tuccae (Mart. 9.75).

This might have been a suburban bathhouse. The rival epigrammist of Martial is a possible builder/owner, but this identification is most unsure; see *RE* 7A.765, s.v. "Tucca 4" (Frank).

Unnamed Baths

Unnamed bath (*CIL* 6.354 = *ILS* 2218).

An inscription on a statue base, of Severan date, was found near the Church of Santa Maria in Navicella on the Caelian Hill, and so in Regio II. The text reads, in part: *L. Ceius L. fil. Privatus | quod, cum exampliaretur | balneum subprinceps | voverat princeps castr(orum) | perigrinorum v(otum) s(olvit) l(ibens) m(erito).* Whether the baths stood in this region is not immediately apparent. Privatus is otherwise unattested.

Unnamed bath (no. 220).

Bath restored by P. Alfius Maximus Numerius Avitus, *sevir.* The inscription was found on the Esquiline Hill and so in either Regio III, IV, or V.

Unnamed bath (*CIL* 6.1744, 1744a = *CIL* 6.31916 = *ILS* 5718).

The fourth-century Naeratius Cerealis (see *PLRE* 1.197–99, s.v. "Cerealis 2") is described on a statue base as the "founder of the baths": *Naeratius Cerealis v. c., | cons. ord., | conditor | balnearum | censuit.* The inscription was found near the Basilica of Maria Maggiore and so in Regio IV. Hasty excavations in 1873 revealed parts of the foundations and some statuary; see Richardson, *Dictionary,* 49, s.v. "Balneum Nereatii Cerealis." F. Guidobaldi (*LTUR* 2.79, s.v. "Domus: Naeratius Cerealis") considers the baths public in nature. See also above, chapter 2, n. 4.

Unnamed bath (*CIL* 6.1179 = *ILS* 5732).

The fourth-century Fl. Antigonus (see *PLRE* 1.70, s.v. "Antigonus") is named as the restorer and adorner of part of this unnamed bath: *Fl. Antigonus, v. p., p(rae)p(ositus)* | *colymbum, nemus vetustate lap|sum testacio picturis ac statuis* | *cum omni cultu ador[navit]*. For a *colymbum* in a bathhouse, see no. 118.

Unnamed bath (*FUR* fr. 25)

This small corner bath is depicted on the Marble Map near the Horrea Lolliana and so in Regio XIII.

Appendix 3

Parts of Baths Mentioned in the Epigraphic Sample

Part of bath	Reference to Sample
aena (bronze fittings/instruments)	no. 282 (mentioned)
apodyterium (changing room)	nos. 114 (built); 305 (built or restored); 90 (restored?); 115 (adorned); 59, 143 (both restored and adorned)
aquaeductum (?) thermarum (aqueduct for baths)	nos. 38 (built), 58 (built?)
assa (heating device)	no. 21 (built)
atrium thermarum (entrance hall)	nos. 29 (built and adorned), 132 (completed)
baptisterium (cold pool or cold room)	no. 196 (adorned?)
basilica (hall)	nos. 8 (restored), 18 (restored and adorned)
cal(i)darium (hot room)	nos. 83, 163 (both built and adorned)
cam(o)erae (unidentifiable rooms)	nos. 140 (built and adorned); 128 (restored? and adorned)
cella balnearum (unidentifiable room)	no. 140 (restored)
cella frigidarii (cold room)	no. 90 (built and adorned)

cella natatoria
(room with a cold plunge
pool)

no. 60 (built)

(cella?) piscinalis
(room with a cold pool)

nos. 123 (restored), 142 (adorned), 131
(restored and adorned)

cella soliaris
(room with heated pools)

nos. 123 (?), 133, 137 (all restored); 131
(restored and adorned)

cella thermarum
(unidentifiable room)

no. 117 (adorned)

cella unctuaria
(anointing room)

no. 113 (restored)

cella vestibula
(entrance room)

no. 104 (built and adorned)

cohors
(exercise yard?)

no. 83 (built and adorned)

colimbum/colymbum
(plunge pool)

nos. 311 (built), 118 (extended by addition of porticus)

crypta (?)
(recesses?)

no. 90 (built and adorned)

destrictarium
(scraping-off room)

nos. 21, 61 (both built)

exceptorium
(cisterns)

nos. 130, 137 (both built); 132
(demolished)

ἐξέδραί
(recesses for relaxation)

nos. 311, 314 (built)

foculus
(stove, brazier?)

nos. 151, 160 (?) (both built)

hypocausta
(boilers)

no. 282 (mentioned)

labrum
(basin in caldarium)

nos. 59, 68, 75, 151, 166 (all built); 282
(mentioned)

laconicum
(sweat room)

no. 61 (built)

lacus
(cistern? pool?)

no. 50 (?), 157 (both built)

lavacrum (thermarum or
balnearum)
(heated section?)

nos. 127 (built); 13, 140 (restored); 237,
238 (restored water supply); 239 (heated)

musaeum
(art gallery)

no. 111 (built); see also no. 117 for *opus
musaeum,* denoting mosaic decoration

nymphae calidae
(heated pools?)

no. 175 (built)

oceanum
(pool room)

no. 133 (built)

paganicum
(ball court?)

no. 83 (built and adorned)

παιδισκεῖον
(bordello)

no. 309 (built and adorned)

palaestra
(exercise yard)

no. 61 (restored)

patinae
(parts of boilers?)

no. 129 (restored)

περίστῳον
(colonnade)

no. 324 (built and adorned)

piscina
(cold pool)

nos. 50, 59, 71, 114 (?), 137 (all built);
130 (improved water supply); 260 (mentioned)

porticus
(portico)

nos. 18, 71, 82, 118, 121, 129, 172
(built); 5, 8, 61, 87, 123 (restored); 79
(adorned); 83, 97 (built and adorned)

proneum
(porch, entrance room?)

nos. 129 (built), 123 (of an aqueduct; restored)

προστῷον
(porch)

no. 293 (built)

scalae
(stairs)

no. 114 (built)

sedes
(benches)

no. 151 (built); see also no. 114 for possible mention of *cathedrae*

solarium (sundial or terrace)	no. 21 (built)
solia (heated pools)	nos. 123, 183 (built); 128, 129, 137 (repaired); 233 (improved)
sphaeristerium	nos. 54, 55 (built); 5 (restored)
στόα (portico)	no. 310 (built)
suspensurae (hypocaust)	no. 140 (built); possibly the word here denotes tubulation in vaults
tepidarium (medium-hot room)	no. 50 (restored)
θᾶκον (latrine)	no. 309 (built and adorned)
unspecified rooms, denoted by such words as *cellae, opera,* etc.	nos. 73/74, 84, 102, 124 (built); 19, 90 (restored); 114, 196 (adorned); 296 (built and adorned)

Bibliography

Here listed are the modern works referred to in the notes. Where a collection of essays is cited more than once, I have provided an abbreviated form for that collection, which is then given its own entry. For frequently cited items, see the list of abbreviations at the beginning of the book.

Abbot, F.F., and A.C. Johnson. *Municipal Administration in the Roman Empire.* Princeton, 1926.

Adam, J.-P. *Roman Building: Materials and Techniques.* Bloomington, IN, 1994.

Aicher, P.J. *Guide to the Aqueducts of Ancient Rome.* Wauconda, 1995.

Adkins, L., and R.A. Adkins. *Handbook to Life in Ancient Rome.* New York, 1994.

Alföldy, G. *The Social History of Rome*[3]. Baltimore, 1988.

Amulree, Lord. "Hygienic Conditions in Ancient Rome and Modern London." *Medical History* 17 (1975): 244–55.

Anderson, J.C., Jr. *The Historical Topography of the Imperial Fora.* Brussels, 1984.

———. "The Date of the *Thermae Traiani* and the Topography of the *Oppius Mons.*" *AJA* 89 (1985): 499–509.

———. *Roman Architecture and Society.* Baltimore, 1997.

Anderson, W.S. *Barbarian Play: Plautus' Roman Comedy.* Toronto, 1993.

Andreau, J. "Histoire des séismes et histoire économique: Le tremblement de terre de Pompéi (62 ap. J.-C.)." *AnnEconSocCiv* 28 (1973): 369–95.

Ashby, T. *The Aqueducts of Ancient Rome.* Oxford, 1935.

Aubert, J.-J. *Business Managers in Ancient Rome: A Social and Economic Study of Institores 200 B.C.–A.D. 250.* Leiden, 1994.

Avi-Yonah, M. "The Bath of the Lepers at Scythopolis." *IEJ* 13 (1963): 325–26.

Badian, E. *Roman Imperialism in the Late Republic*[2]. Ithaca, 1968.

Bagnall R.S., and Th. Drew-Bear. "Documents from Kourion: A Review Article." Part 2, "Individual Inscriptions." *Phoenix* 27 (1973): 213–44.

Baldwin, B. "The Date, Identity, and Career of Vitruvius." *Latomus* 49 (1990): 425–34.

———. "The Career and Work of Scribonius Largus." *RhM* 135 (1992): 74–82.

Balland, A. *Fouilles de Xanthos.* Vol. 7, *Inscriptions d'époque impériale du Létôon.* Paris, 1981.

Balsdon, J.P.V.D. *Life and Leisure in Ancient Rome.* London, 1969.

———. *Romans and Aliens.* London, 1979.

Bargellini, P. "Le Terme centrali di Pompei." In *Thermes,* 115–28.

Barnes, T.D. *The New Empire of Diocletian and Constantine.* Cambridge, MA, 1982.

Barrett, A.A. *Caligula: The Corruption of Power.* New Haven, 1989.

————. *Agrippina: Sex, Power, and Politics in the Early Empire.* New Haven, 1996.

Bartoccini, R. *Le terme di Lepcis.* Bergamo, 1929.

Barton, I.M., ed. *Roman Public Buildings*². Exeter, 1995.

————. "Palaces." In *Roman Domestic Buildings,* edited by I.M. Barton, 91–120. Exeter, 1996.

Beacham, R.C. *The Roman Theatre and Its Audience.* Cambridge, MA, 1992.

Bean, G.E. "Notes and Inscriptions from Pisidia." Part 2. *AnatSt* 10 (1960): 43–82.

Beard, M., and M.H. Crawford. *Rome in the Late Republic.* London, 1985.

Benedum, J. "Die *Balnea Pensilia* des Asklepiades von Prusa." *Gesnerus* 24 (1967): 93–107.

————. "Der Badearzt Asklepiades und seine bithynische Heimat." *Gesnerus* 35 (1978): 20–43.

Bérard, F., D. Feissel, P. Petitmengin, and M. Sève. *Guide de l'épigraphiste: Bibliographie choisie des épigraphies antiques et médiévales.*² Paris, 1989.

Berry, J. "Household Artefacts: Towards a Re-interpretation of Roman Domestic Space." In Laurence and Wallace-Hadrill, *Domestic Space in the Roman World,* 183–95.

Bickerman, E.J. *Chronology of the Ancient World*². London, 1980.

Black, E.W. *The Roman Villas of South-East England.* Oxford, 1987.

Blagg, T.F.C. "Architectural Munificence in Britain: The Evidence of Inscriptions." *Britannia* 21 (1990): 13–31.

Blake, M.E. *Ancient Roman Construction in Italy from the Prehistoric Period to Augustus.* Washington, DC, 1947.

Blümner, H. *Die römischen Privataltertümer.* Munich, 1911.

Boatwright, M.T. *Hadrian and the City of Rome.* Princeton, 1987.

————. "The Imperial Women of the Early Second Century A.C." *AJP* 112 (1991): 513–40.

Boersma, J. Amoenissima Civitas: *Block V.ii at Ostia—Description and Analysis of Its Visible Remains.* Assen, 1985.

————. "Le terme tardoromane di Valesio (Salento)." In *Thermes,* 161–73.

————. Mutatio Valentia: *The Late Roman Baths at Valesio, Salento.* Amsterdam, 1995.

Boethius, A. *Etruscan and Early Roman Architecture*². London, 1978.

Bonfante, L. "Nudity as a Costume in Classical Art." *AJA* 93 (1989): 543–70.

Boulvert, G. *Esclaves et affranchis impériaux sous le Haut-Empire romain: Rôle politique et administratif.* Naples, 1970.

Bourgeois, C., and E. Sikora. "Médecine des yeux dans la sanctuaire de l'eau de Pouillé (Loir-et-Cher)." In Pelletier, *Médecine en Gaule,* 103–10.

Bourne, F.C. *The Public Works of the Julio-Claudians and Flavians.* Princeton, 1946.

Bowen Ward, R. "Women in Roman Baths." *HThR* 85 (1992): 125–47.

Bowersock, G.W. *Greek Sophists in the Roman Empire.* Oxford, 1969.

Bowman, A.K. "Public Buildings in Roman Egypt." *JRA* 5 (1992): 495–503.

Bradley, K.R. *Slavery and Rebellion in the Roman World, 140 B.C.–70 B.C.* Bloomington, 1989.

————. *Slavery and Society at Rome.* Cambridge, 1994.

Bremer, C., and A. Raevuori. *The World of the Sauna.* Helsinki, 1986.

Broise, H., and V. Jolivet. "Le bain en Étrurie à l'époque Hellénistique." In *Thermes,* 79–95.

Broise, H., and J. Scheid. *Recherches archéologiques à la Magliana: Le balneum des frères Arvales.* Rome, 1987.

Broise, H., and Y. Thébert. *Recherches archéologiques franco-tunisiennes à Bulla Regia.* Vol. 2, *Les architectures,* pt. 1, *Les thermes memmiens: Étude architecturale et histoire urbaine.* Rome, 1993.

Brundrett, N.G.R., and C.J. Simpson. "Innovation and the Baths of Agrippa." *Athenaeum* 85 (1997): 220–27.

Brunt, P.A. *Italian Manpower.* Oxford, 1971.

———. "The Roman Mob." In *Studies in Ancient Society,* edited by M.I. Finley, 74–102. London, 1974.

———. *The Fall of the Roman Republic and Related Essays.* Oxford, 1988.

Brusin, G. "Grado: Nuove epigrafi romane e cristiane." *NSc,* 1928, 282–86.

Bruun, Ch. *The Water Supply of Ancient Rome: A Study of Roman Imperial Administration.* Helsinki, 1991.

———. "Lotores: Roman Bath-Attendants." *ZPE* 98 (1993): 222–28.

———. "Private Munificence in Italy and the Evidence of Lead Pipe Stamps." In *Acta Colloquii Epigraphici Latini Helsingiae 1991 Habiti,* edited by H. Solin, O. Salomies, and U.-M. Liertz, 41–58. Helsinki, 1995.

———. "Ownership of Baths in Rome: The Evidence from Lead Pipe Installations." In Johnston and DeLaine, *Roman Baths and Bathing,* forthcoming.

Burnham, B.C., and J. Wacher. *The "Small Towns" of Roman Britain.* Berkeley, 1990.

Burton, G.P. "The Curator Rei Publicae: Towards a Reappraisal." *Chiron* 9 (1979): 465–87.

Butler, A.J. *The Arab Conquest of Egypt².* Oxford, 1978.

Cagiano de Azevedo, M. *Interamna Lirenas vel Sucasina.* Rome, 1947.

Calderini, A. *Aquileia romana: Ricerche di storia e di epigrafia.* Milan, 1930. Reprint, Rome, 1973.

Calza, G. "Die Taverne der Sieben Weisen in Ostia." *Die Antike* 15 (1939): 99–115.

Camodeca, G. "Ricerche sui *curatores rei publicae.*" ANRW 2.13 (1980): 453–534.

Carcopino, J. *Daily Life in Ancient Rome.* London, 1956.

Carducci, C. *Tibur.* Rome, 1940.

Carettoni, G. *Casinum.* Rome, 1940.

———. "Terme di Settimio Severo e Terme di Massenzio in Palatio." *ArchCl* 24 (1972): 96–104.

Carter, J. "Civic and Other Buildings." In Barton, *Roman Public Buildings,* 31–65.

Caruso, G., A. Ceccherelli, P. Giusberti, L. Maestri, and C. Vannicola. "Scavi alle Terme di Tito." *ArchLaz* 10 (1990): 58–67.

Cassatella, A., and I. Iacopi. "Il balneum presso le Scalae Caci sul Palatino." In *Thermes,* 129–38.

Castagnoli, F., C. Ceccheli, G. Giovannoni, and M. Zocca. *Topografia e urbanistica di Roma antica.* Bologna, 1958.

Castrén, P. Ordo Populusque Pompeianus: *Polity and Society in Roman Pompeii.* Rome, 1975.

Cavalieri Manasse, G., G. Massari, and M. P. Rossignani. *Piemonte, Valle d'Aosta, Liguria, Lombardia*. Guide archeologiche Laterza. Bari, 1982.

Cenerini, F. "Evergetismo ed epigrafia: *Lavationem in perpetuom*." *RivStorAnt* 17–18 (1987–88): 199–220.

Champlin, E. "The Glass Ball Game." *ZPE* 60 (1985): 159–63.

Charlesworth, M.P. "The Virtues of a Roman Emperor: The Creation of Belief." *PBA* 23 (1937): 105–33.

Chastagnol, A. "L'inscription constantinienne d'Orcistus." *MEFRA* 93 (1981): 381–416.

Cherry, D. "Re-Figuring the Roman Epigraphic Habit." *AHB* 9 (1995): 143–56.

Cicerchia, P., and A. Marinucci. *Scavi di Ostia*. Vol. 11, *Le Terme del Foro o di Gavio Massimo*. Rome, 1992.

Claridge, A. "Il vicus di epoca imperiale nella tenuta presidenziale di Castelporziano: Indagini archeologiche 1984." In *Castelporziano*. Vol. 1, *Campagna di scavo e restauro 1985*, 71–78. Rome, 1985.

———. "Il Vicus di epoca imperiale: Indagini archeologiche nel 1985 e 1986." In *Castelporziano*. Vol. 2, *Campagna di scavo e restauro 1985–1986*, 61–73. Rome, 1988.

———. *Rome*. Oxford Archaeological Guides. Oxford, 1998.

Coarelli, F. "Public Building in Rome between the Second Punic War and Sulla." *BSR* 45 (1977): 1–23.

———. *Dintorni di Roma*. Guide archeologiche Laterza. Bari, 1981.

———. *Lazio*. Guide archeologiche Laterza. Bari, 1982.

———. *Roma*⁷. Guide archeologiche Laterza. Bari, 1995.

Coarelli, F., and A. La Regina. *Abruzzo, Molise*. Guide archeologiche Laterza. Bari, 1984.

Coleman, K.M. "Fatal Charades: Roman Executions Staged as Mythological Enactments." *JRS* 80 (1990): 44–73.

———. "Launching into History: Aquatic Displays in the Early Empire." *JRS* 83 (1993): 48–74.

Colini, A.M., G.P. Sartorio, C. Buzzetti, M.N. Santi, and P. Virgili. "Notiziario di scavi e scoperte in Roma e Suburbio, 1946–60." Part 2. *BullCom* 90 (1985): 307–440.

Conte, G.B. *Latin Literature: A History*. Baltimore, 1994.

Corbier, M. "La familie de Séjan à Volsinii: La dédicace des Seii, *curatores aquae*." *MEFRA* 95 (1983): 719–56.

Corell, J. "Drei *defixionum tabellae* aus Sagunt (Valencia)." *ZPE* 101 (1994): 280–86.

Cornell, T.J., and K. Lomas, eds. *Urban Society in Roman Italy*. New York, 1995.

Coulton, J.J. "Opromoas and the Anonymous Benefactor." *JHS* 107 (1987): 171–78.

Cunliffe, B. *Roman Bath Discovered*². London, 1984.

Daly, L.W. *Aesop without Morals*. New York, 1961.

Danker, F.W. *Benefactor: Epigraphic Study of a Greco-Roman and New Testament Semantic Field*. St. Louis, 1982.

Dardaine, S. "L'évergétisme *ob honorem* en Bétique." *Ktema* 16 (1991): 281–91.

D'Arms, J.H. *Romans on the Bay of Naples: A Social and Cultural Study of the Villas and Their Owners from 150 B.C. to A.D. 400*. Cambridge, MA, 1970.

———. "Control, Companionship, and *Clientela*: Some Social Functions of the Roman Communal Meal." *EchCl* 28 (1984): 327–48.

———. "The Roman *Convivium* and the Idea of Equality." In *Sympotica: A Symposium on the* Symposion, edited by O. Murray, 308–20. Oxford, 1990.

Dauphin, C. "Brothels, Baths, and Babes: Prostitution in the Byzantine Holy Land." *Classics Ireland* 3 (1996): 47–72.

De Caro, S., and A. Greco. *Campania*². Guide archeologiche Laterza. Bari, 1981.

De Fine Licht, K. *Untersuchungen an den Trajansthermen zu Rom.* Vol. 1. Copenhagen, 1974.

———. *Untersuchungen an den Trajansthermen zu Rom.* Vol. 2, *Sette Sale.* Rome, 1990.

De Haan, N. "Privatbäder in Pompeji und Herkulaneum und die städtische Wasserleitung." *Mitteilungen des Leichtweiss-instituts für Wasserbau der Technischen Universität Braunschweig* 117 (1992): 423–45.

———. "Dekoration und Funktion in den Privatbädern von Pompeji und Herculaneum." In *Functional and Spatial Analysis of Wall Painting,* edited by E.M. Moormann, 34–37. Leiden, 1993.

———. "Roman Private Baths." *Balnearia* 2, no. 2 (1994): 8–9.

De Haan, N., and G.C.M. Jansen, eds. *Cura Aquarum in Campania.* Leiden, 1996.

Deiss, J.J. *Herculaneum: Italy's Buried Treasure*². New York, 1985.

DeLaine, J. "The 'Cella Solearis' of the Baths of Caracalla: A Reappraisal." *BSR* 55 (1987): 147–56.

———. "Recent Research on Roman Baths." *JRA* 1 (1988): 11–31.

———. "Some Observations on the Transition from Greek to Roman Baths in Hellenistic Italy." *MeditArch* 2 (1989): 111–25.

———. "The *Balneum* of the Arval Brethren." *JRA* 3 (1990): 321–24.

———. "New Models, Old Modes: Continuity and Change in the Design of Public Baths." In *Die römische Stadt im 2. Jahrhundert n. Chr.: Der Funktionswandel des öffentlichen Raumes,* edited by H.-J. Schalles, H. von Hesberg, and P. Zanker, 257–75. Bonn, 1992.

———. "Roman Baths and Bathing." *JRA* 6 (1993): 348–58.

———. "The Insula of the Paintings at Ostia I.4.2–4: Paradigm for a City in Flux." In Cornell and Lomas, *Urban Society,* 79–106.

———. *The Baths of Caracalla: A Study in the Design, Construction, and Economics of Large-Scale Building Projects in Imperial Rome.* Portsmouth, RI, 1997.

De Ligt, L., and P.W. de Neeve. "Ancient Periodic Markets: Festivals and Fairs." *Athenaeum* 66 (1988): 391–416.

Delorme, J. *Gymnasion: Étude sur les monuments consacrés à l'éducation en Grèce.* Paris, 1960.

De Ruggiero, E. *Dizionario epigrafico di antichità romane.* Rome, 1895. Reprint 1961–62. 5 vols. to date.

Desnoyers, M. "Néris-les-Bains (Allier): Ville thermale gallo-romaine." In Pelletier, *Médecine en Gaule,* 39–62.

De Ste. Croix, G.E.M. *The Class Struggle in the Ancient Greek World.* London, 1981.

Di Marco, L. *Spoletium: Topografia e urbanistica.* Spoleto, 1975.

Dionisotti, A.C. "From Ausonius's Schooldays? A Schoolbook and Its Relatives." *JRS* 72 (1982): 83–125.

Di Vita-Évrard, G. "Lepcis Magna: Contribution à la terminologie des thermes." In *Thermes,* 35–42.

Dix, T.K., and G.W. Houston. "Libraries in Roman Baths?" *Balnearia* 4, no. 1 (1996): 2–4.

Donahue, J.F. *"Epula Publica:* The Roman Community at Table during the Principate." Ph.D. dissertation, University of North Carolina at Chapel Hill, 1996.

Dosi, A., and F. Schnell. *A tavola con i Romani antichi.* Rome, 1984.

Drappier, L. "Les thermes de *Thuburbo Maius." BAC,* 1920, 55–75.

Drerup, H. "Bildraum und Realraum in der römischen Architektur." *RM* 66 (1959): 147–74.

Drew-Bear, Th. "An Act of Foundation at Hypaipa." *Chiron* 10 (1980): 509–36.

Duckworth, G.E. *The Nature of Roman Comedy: A Study in Popular Entertainment.* Princeton, 1952.

Dunbabin, K.M.D. *"Baiarum Grata Voluptas:* Pleasures and Dangers of the Baths." *BSR* 57 (1989): 6–46.

———. "Wine and Water at the Roman *Convivium." JRA* 6 (1993): 116–41.

Duncan-Jones, R. "Wealth and Munificence in Roman Africa." *BSR* 31 (1963): 159–77.

———. "The Procurator as Civic Benefactor." *JRS* 64 (1974): 79–85.

———. "Who Paid for Public Buildings in Roman Cities?" In *Roman Urban Topography in Britain and the Western Empire,* edited by F. Grew and B. Hobley, 28–33. London, 1985.

Dupont, F. *Daily Life in Ancient Rome.* Oxford, 1992.

Duthoy, R. "Les Augustales." *ANRW* 2.16.2 (1978): 1254–1309.

———. "Curatores rei publicae en Occident durant le Principat." *AncSoc* 10 (1979): 171–238.

———. "Le profil social des patrons municipaux en Italie sous le Haut-Empire." *AncSoc* 15–17 (1984–86): 121–54.

Dyson, S.L. *Community and Society in Roman Italy.* Baltimore, 1992.

Eck, W. *Die staatliche Organisation Italiens in der hohen Kaiserzeit.* Munich, 1979.

Ecochard M., and C. Le Coeur. *Les bains de Damas: Monographies architecturales.* 2 vols. Beirut, 1942–43.

Edelstein, E.J., and L. Edelstein. *Asclepius: A Collection and Interpretation of the Testimonies.* 2 vols. Baltimore, 1945.

Edelstein, L. "The Dietetics of Antiquity." In *Ancient Medicine: Selected Papers of Ludwig Edelstein,* edited by O. Temkin and C.L. Temkin, 303–16. Baltimore, 1967.

Eschebach, H. " . . . *Laconicum et destrictarium faciund.* . . . *locarunt* . . . : Untersuchungen in den Stabianer Thermen zu Pompeji." *RM* 80 (1973): 235–42.

———. *Die Stabianer Thermen in Pompeji.* Berlin, 1979.

———. "Die innerstädtische Gebrauchswasserversorgung dargestellt am Beispiel Pompejis." In *Journées d'études sur les aqueducs romains,* edited by J.-P. Boucher, 81–132. Paris, 1983.

———. *Die Arzthäuser in Pompeji. AntW* Special Issue 15, 1984.

Eschebach, L. "Die Forumsthermen in Pompeji, Regio VII, Insula 5." *AntW* 22 (1991): 257–87.

Eschebach, L., and J. Müller-Trollius, eds. *Gebäudeverzeichnis und Stadtplan der antiken Stadt Pompeji.* Cologne, 1993.

Étienne, R. "La naissance de l'amphithéâtre: Le mot et la chose." *REL* 43 (1966): 213–20.

———. *La vie quotidienne à Pompei².* Paris, 1977.

Evans, H.B. "Water Distribution: *Quorsum et cui bono?*" In Hodge, *Future Currents,* 21–27.

———. *Water Distribution in Ancient Rome: The Evidence of Frontinus.* Ann Arbor, 1994.

Evans, J.K. "*Plebs Rustica:* The Peasantry of Classical Italy." Part 2. "The Peasant Economy." *AJAH* 5 (1980): 134–73.

Fagan, G.G. Review of Nielsen, *Hermathena* 152 (1992): 100–105 .

———. "Pliny *Naturalis Historia* 36.121 and the Number of *Balnea* in Early Augustan Rome." *CP* 88 (1993): 333–35.

———. "The Reliability of Roman Rebuilding Inscriptions." *BSR* 64 (1996): 81–93.

———. "Sergius Orata: Inventor of the Hypocaust?" *Phoenix* 50 (1996): 56–66.

———. "Bathing in the Backwaters." *JRA* 10 (1997): 520–23.

———. "Gifts of *Gymnasia:* A Test Case for Reading Quasi-Technical Jargon in Latin Inscriptions." *ZPE* 124 (1999): 263–75.

———. "Interpreting the Evidence." In Johnston and DeLaine, *Roman Baths and Bathing,* forthcoming.

Fant, J.C. "*IRT* 794b and the Building History of the Hadrianic Baths at Lepcis Magna." *ZPE* 75 (1988): 291–94.

Fantham, E., H.P. Foley, N.B. Kampen, S.B. Pomeroy, and H.A. Shapiro. *Women in the Classical World.* Oxford, 1994.

Farrington, A. "Imperial Bath Buildings in South-West Asia Minor." In *Roman Architecture in the Greek World,* edited by S. Macready and F.H. Thompson, 50–59. London, 1987.

———. *The Roman Baths of Lycia: An Architectural Study.* Ankara, 1995.

Feissel, D., and J. Gascou. "Documents d'archives romains inédits au Moyen Euphrate (IIIe siècle après J.-C.)." *CRAI,* 1989, 535–61.

Ferrary, J.-L. *Philhellénisme et impérialisme: Aspects idéologiques de la conquête romaine du monde hellénistique.* Rome, 1988.

Fontanille, M.-T. "Les bains dans la médecine gréco-romaine." In Pelletier, *Médecine en Gaule,* 15–24.

Forbes, R.J. *Studies in Ancient Technology².* 9 vols. Leiden, 1964–72.

Foss, P.W. "Watchful *Lares:* Roman Household Organization and the Rituals of Cooking and Eating." In Laurence and Wallace-Hadrill, *Domestic Space in the Roman World,* 196–218.

Franklin, J.L., Jr. *Pompeii: The Electoral Programmata: Campaigns and Politics,* A.D. 71–79. Rome, 1980.

Frayn, J.M. *Markets and Fairs in Roman Italy.* Oxford, 1993.

Frederiksen, M. *Campania.* Edited by N. Purcell. Rome, 1984.

Frere, S. *Britannia: A History of Roman Britain³.* London, 1987.

Frézouls, E., M.-J. Morant, and D. Longpierre. "Urbanisme et principaux monuments de Kadyanda." *Ktema* 11 (1986): 225–38.

Friedländer, L. *Darstellungen aus der Sittengeschichte Roms*[10]. 4 vols. Leipzig, 1922. Reprint, Aalen, 1964.

Friggeri, R. "La Domus di Antonia Caenis e il *Balineum Caenidianum.*" *Rend PontAcc* 50 (1977–78): 145–54.

Gagé, J. *Les classes sociales dans l'empire romaine.* Paris, 1964.

Gager, J.G. *Curse Tablets and Binding Spells from the Ancient World.* Oxford, 1992.

Gaggiotti, M. "Frammenti epigrafici inediti da Saepinum pertinenti alla gens Neratia." *AnnPerugia* 25 (1987/88): 129–40.

Gaggiotti, M., D. Manconi, L. Mercando, and M. Verzar. *Umbria, Marche.* Guide archeologiche Laterza. Bari, 1980.

Gaiser, K. "Zur Eigenart der römischen Komödie: Plautus und Terenz gegenüber ihren griechischen Vorbildern." *ANRW* 1.2 (1972): 1027–113.

Gamurrini, G.F. "Regione V (Picenum)." *NSc,* 1896, 322–25.

Gardner, J.F. *Women in Roman Law and Society.* London, 1986.

Gargola, D.J. *Lands, Laws, and Gods: Magistrates and Ceremony in the Regulation of Public Lands in Republican Rome.* Chapel Hill, 1995.

Garnsey, P. *Social Status and Legal Privilege in the Roman Empire.* Oxford, 1970.

Garnsey, P., and R. Saller. *The Roman Empire: Economy, Society, and Culture.* Berkeley, 1987.

Gazzetti, G. *Il territorio capenate.* Rome, 1992.

Geagan, D.J. "Imperial Visits to Athens: The Epigraphic Evidence." In Πρακτικα του Η Διεθνους Συνεδριου Ελλενικης και Λατινικης Επιγραφικης, Αθηνα, 3–9 Οκτωβριου 1982, 69–78. Athens, 1984.

Gentili, G.V. *La villa erculia di Piazza Armerina: I mosaici figurati.* Milan, 1959.

Gerkan, A. von, and F. Krischen. *Thermen und Palaestren.* Berlin, 1928.

Ghini, G. "Le Terme Alessandrine nel Campo Marzio." *MonAnt,* Occasional Papers, 3, no. 4 (1988): 121–77.

Gibbs, J.P. *Control: Sociology's Central Notion.* Urbana, 1989.

Ginestet, P. *Les organisations de la jeunesse dans l'Occident romain.* Brussels, 1991.

Ginouvès, R. *Balaneutikè: Recherches sur le bain dans l'antiquité grecque.* Paris, 1962.

Ginsburg, M.S. "*Princeps Libertinorum.*" *TAPA* 65 (1934): 198–206.

Golden, M. "The Uses of Cross-Cultural Comparison in Ancient Social History." *EchCl* 11 (1992): 309–31.

Gonzalez, J. "The *Lex Irnitana:* A New Copy of the Flavian Municipal Law." *JRS* 76 (1986): 147–243.

Goodman, M. *State and Society in Roman Galilee,* A.D. 132–212. Totowa, 1983.

Gorrie, C.L. "The Building Programme of Septimius Severus in the City of Rome." Ph.D. dissertation, University of British Columbia, 1997.

Gourevitch, D. "Asclépiade de Bithynie dans Pline: Problèmes de chronologie." In *Pline l'ancien: Témoin de son temps,* edited by J. Pigeaud and J. Oroz-Reta, 67–81. Salamanca-Nantes, 1987.

Gowers, E. "The Anatomy of Rome from Capitol to Cloaca." *JRS* 85 (1995): 23–32.

Gratwick, A.S. "Drama." In *The Cambridge History of Classical Literature,* vol. 2, *Latin Literature,* edited by E.J. Kenney, 77–137. Cambridge, 1982.

Gray, E.V. "The *Imperium* of M. Agrippa." *ZPE* 6 (1970): 227–38.

Greco, E. *Magna Grecia*[2]. Guide archeologiche Laterza. Bari, 1981.

Green, R.M. *A Translation of Galen's Hygiene* (De Sanitate Tuenda). Springfield, 1951.

———. *Asclepiades: His Life and Writings.* New Haven, 1955.

Greenhalgh, P. *Pompey: The Republican Prince.* London, 1981.

Griffin, J. *Latin Poets and Roman Life.* London, 1985.

Griffin, M.T. *Seneca: A Philosopher in Politics.* Oxford, 1976.

———. *Nero: The End of a Dynasty.* New Haven, 1984.

Grilli, P., and D. Levy. *Furo: The Japanese Bath.* Tokyo, 1985.

Gros, P. *Bolsena: Guide des fouilles.* Paris, 1981.

Gros, R. "Les thermes dans la Rome antique." *HSMed* 21 (1987): 45–50.

Grotzfeld, H. *Das Bad im arabischen-islamischen Mittelalter: Eine kulturgeschichtliche Studie.* Wiesbaden, 1970.

Gruen, E.S. *The Last Generation of the Roman Republic.* Berkeley, 1974.

———. *The Hellenistic World and the Coming of Rome.* Berkeley, 1984.

Hallett, C.H. "The Roman Heroic Portrait." Ph.D. dissertation, University of California at Berkeley, 1993.

Hands, A.R. *Charities and Social Aid in Greece and Rome.* Ithaca, 1968.

Hannestad, N. *Roman Art and Imperial Policy.* Århus, 1988.

Harig, G. "Die philosophischen Grundlagen des medizinischen Systems des Asklepiades von Bithynien." *Philologus* 127 (1983): 43–60.

Harig, R. "Zum Problem 'Krankenhaus' in der Antike." *Klio* 53 (1971): 179–195.

Harris, W.V. "The Heir to 'Platner-Ashby.'" *JRA* 8 (1995): 365–75.

Harvey, R.A. *A Commentary on Persius.* Leiden, 1981.

Heberdey, R. *Opromoas: Inschriften vom Heroon zu Rhodiapolis.* Vienna, 1897.

Heinz, W. "Antike Balneologie in späthellisticher und römischer Zeit: Zur medizinischen Wirkung römischer Bäder." *ANRW* 2.37.3 (1996): 2411–32.

Henig, M. "The Gemstones from the Main Drain." In *Roman Bath,* edited by B. Cunliffe, 71–88. Oxford, 1969.

Henzen, G. *Acta Fratrum Arvalium Quae Supersunt.* Berlin, 1874.

Hermann, J.J., Jr. "Observations on the Baths of Maxentius in the Palace." *RM* 83 (1976): 403–24.

Hermansen, G. "The Population of Imperial Rome: The Regionaries." *Historia* 27 (1978): 129–68.

———. *Ostia: Aspects of Roman City Life.* Edmonton, 1981.

Hesberg, H. von. *Römische Grabbauten.* Darmstadt, 1992.

Hill, P.V. *The Monuments of Ancient Rome as Coin Types.* London, 1989.

Hirschfeld, Y. *The Roman Baths of Hammat Gader.* Jerusalem, 1997.

Hodge, A.T., ed. *Future Currents in Aqueduct Studies.* Leeds, 1991.

———. *Roman Aqueducts and Water Supply.* London, 1992.

———. "Aqueducts." In Barton, *Roman Public Buildings,* 127–49.

Homo, L. *Vespasien: L'empereur du bon sens.* Paris, 1949.

Hopkins, K. *Conquerors and Slaves.* Cambridge, 1978.

———. *Death and Renewal.* Cambridge, 1983.

Houston, G.W. "Onesimus the Librarian." *ZPE* 114 (1996): 205–8.

Howell, P. *A Commentary on Book One of the* Epigrams *of Martial.* London, 1980.

Hülsen, Ch. *Die Thermen des Agrippa in Rom: Ein Beitrag zur Topographie des Marsfeldes in Rom.* Rome, 1910.

Humphrey, J.H. *Roman Circuses: Arenas for Chariot Racing.* London, 1986.

Hunink, V. "Lucan's Last Words." In *Studies in Latin Literature and Roman History,* vol. 6, edited by C. Deroux, 390–407. Brussels, 1992.

Ingholt, H. "Inscriptions and Sculptures from Palmyra." *Berytus* 3 (1936): 83–125.

Ioppolo, G. *Le Terme del Sarno a Pompei.* Rome, 1992.

Jackson, R. "Roman Doctors and Their Instruments: Recent Research into Ancient Practice." *JRA* 3 (1990): 5–27.

———. "Waters and Spas in the Classical World." In *The Medical History of Waters and Spas,* edited by R. Porter, 1–13. London, 1990.

———. "Roman Medicine: The Practitioners and Their Practices." *ANRW* 2.37.1 (1993): 79–101.

Jacobelli, L. "Lo scavo delle Terme Suburbane: Notizie preliminari." *RStPomp* 1 (1987): 151–54.

———. "Terme Suburbane: Stato attuale delle conoscenze." *RStPomp* 2 (1988): 202–8.

———. "Die Suburbanen Thermen in Pompei: Architektur, Raumfunktion und Ausstattung." *ArchKorrBl* 23 (1993): 327–35.

———. *Le pitture erotiche delle Terme Suburbane di Pompei.* Rome, 1995.

Jacques, F. *Les curateurs des cités dans l'Occident romain de Trajan à Gallien: Études prosopographiques.* Paris, 1983.

———. *Le privilège de liberté: Politique impériale et autonomie municipale dans les cités de l'Occident romain (161–244).* Rome, 1984.

Jaczynowska, M. "Le culte de l'Hercule romain au temps du Haut-Empire." *ANRW* 2.17.2 (1981): 631–61.

Jansen, G.C.M. "Private Toilets at Pompeii: Appearance and Operation." In *Sequence and Space in Pompeii,* edited by S.E. Bon and R. Jones, 121–34. Oxford, 1997.

Johannowsky, W. "Relazione preliminare sugli scavi di Cales." *BdA* 46 (1961): 258–68.

Johnston, D.E., and J. DeLaine, eds. *Roman Baths and Bathing.* Portsmouth, RI, forthcoming.

Jones, A.H.M. *The Greek City from Alexander to Justinian.* Oxford, 1940.

———. *The Later Roman Empire, 284–602: A Social, Economic, and Administrative Survey.* Oxford, 1964. Reprint, Baltimore, 1986.

Jordan, D.R. "Curses from the Waters of Sulis." *JRA* 3 (1990): 437–41.

Jordan, H. *Topographie der Stadt Rom im Alterthum.* 2 vols. Berlin, 1871–1907. Reprint, Rome, 1970.

Jouffroy, H. "Le financement des constructions publiques en Italie: Initiative municipale, initiative impériale, évergétisme privé." *Ktema* 2 (1977): 329–37.

———. *La construction publique en Italie et dans l'Afrique romaine.* Strasbourg, 1986.

Kajanto, I. *A Study of the Greek Epitaphs of Rome.* Helsinki, 1963.

Karmi, G. "The Colonisation of Traditional Arabic Medicine." In Porter, *Patients and Practitioners,* 315–39.

Keppie, L. *Colonisation and Veteran Settlement in Italy, 47–14 B.C.* London, 1983.

Kleberg, T. *Hôtels, restaurants et cabarets dans l'antiquité romaine.* Uppsala, 1957.

Kleiner, D.E.E. *Roman Sculpture.* New Haven, 1992.

Knapp, R.C. *Latin Inscriptions from Central Spain.* Berkeley, 1992.

Kneissl, P. "Entstehung und Bedeutung der Augustalität: Zur Inschrift der ara Narbonensis (*CIL* XII 4333)." *Chiron* 10 (1980): 291–326.

Koebling, H.M. *Arzt und Patient in der Antiken Welt.* Zurich, 1977.

———. "Le médecin dans la cité grecque." *Gesnerus* 46 (1989): 29–43.

Kolb, F. "Zur Statussymbolik im antiken Rom." *Chiron* 7 (1977): 239–59.

Kolendo, J. "La répartition des places aux spectacles et la stratification sociale dans l'empire romaine." *Ktema* 6 (1981): 305–14.

Kollesch, J. "Ärztliche Ausbildung in der Antike." *Klio* 61 (1979): 507–13.

Kollesch, J., and D. Nickel. "Bibliographia Galeniana, 1900–1993." *ANRW* 2.37.2 (1994): 1351–1420.

Koloski-Ostrow, A.O. "Finding Social Meaning in the Public Latrines of Pompeii." In De Haan and Jansen, *Cura Aquarum,* 79–86.

Koloski-Ostrow, A.O., N. de Haan, G. de Klaijn, and S. Piras. "Water in the Roman Town: New Research from *Cura Aquarum* and the *Frontinus Society.*" *JRA* 10 (1997): 181–91.

Kroeber, F.V. *Public Swimming Pools: A Manual of Operation.* New York, 1976.

Kudlien, F. "Schaustellerei und Heilmittelvertrieb in der Antike." *Gesnerus* 40 (1983): 91–98.

Kühnert, B. *Die Plebs Urbana der späten römischen Republik: Ihre ökonomische Situation und soziale Struktur.* Berlin, 1991.

Kunze, E., and H. Schleif. *IV. Bericht über die Ausgrabungen in Olympia.* Berlin, 1944.

Künzl, E. "Operationsräume in römischen Thermen." *BJb* 186 (1986): 491–509.

———. "Forschungsbericht zu den antiken medizinischen Instrumenten." *ANRW* 2.37.3 (1996): 2433–639.

Kyle, D.G. *Athletics in Ancient Athens.* Leiden, 1987.

La Follete, L.A. "The Baths of Trajan Decius on the Aventine." In *Rome Papers,* edited by J.H. Humphrey, 9–88. Ann Arbor, 1994.

Lamprecht, H.-O. Opus Caementitium: *Bautechnik der Römer*[4]. Dusseldorf, 1993.

Lauffer, S. *Diokletians Preisedikt.* Berlin, 1971.

Laurence, R. "The Organization of Space in Pompeii." In Cornell and Lomas, *Urban Society,* 63–78.

Laurence, R., and A. Wallace-Hadrill, eds. *Domestic Space in the Roman World: Pompeii and Beyond.* Portsmouth, RI, 1997.

Lendon, J.E. "Social Control at Rome." *CJ* 93 (1997): 83–92.

Leon, H.J. *The Jews of Ancient Rome.* Philadephia, 1960.

Le Roux, P. "Cité et culture municipale en Bétique sous Trajan." *Ktema* 12 (1987): 271–84.

Levick, B. *Tiberius the Politician.* London, 1976.

———. *Claudius.* New Haven, 1990.

Lewis, D. *The Drawings of Andrea Palladio.* Washington, DC, 1981.

Lézine, A. *Architecture romaine d'Afrique.* Tunis, 1961.

———. *Les thermes d'Antonin à Carthage.* Tunis, 1969.

Lintott, A. Imperium Romanum: *Politics and Administration.* London, 1993.

Lippolis, E. "Le Thermae Pentascinenses di Taranto." *Taras* 4 (1984): 119–53.

Lombardi, L., and A. Corazza. *Le Terme di Caracalla.* Rome, 1995.

Lugli, G. *I monumenti antichi di Roma e Surburbio.* 3 vols. Rome, 1930–38. Supplement, 1940.

Lugli, G., and G. Filibeck. *Il porto di Roma imperiale e l'Argo Portuense.* Rome, 1935.

MacDonald, W.L. *The Architecture of the Roman Empire.* 2 vols. New Haven, 1982, 1986.

MacDonald, W.L., and J.A. Pinto. *Hadrian's Villa and Its Legacy.* New Haven, 1995.

MacMullen, R. "Market-Days in the Roman Empire." *Phoenix* 24 (1970): 333–41.

———. *Roman Social Relations, 50 B.C. to A.D. 284.* New Haven, 1974.

———. "Woman in Public in the Roman Empire." *Historia* 29 (1980): 208–18 (= id., *Changes in the Roman Empire,* 162–68).

———. "The Epigraphic Habit in the Roman Empire." *AJP* 103 (1982): 233–46.

———. "Personal Power in the Roman Empire." *AJP* 107 (1986): 512–24 (= id., *Changes in the Roman Empire,* 190–97).

———. *Corruption and the Decline of Rome.* New Haven, 1988.

———. *Changes in the Roman Empire: Essays in the Ordinary.* Princeton, 1990.

Magoulias, H.J. "Bathhouse, Inn, Tavern, Prostitution, and the Stage as Seen in the Lives of the Saints of the Sixth and Seventh Centuries." *EpetByz* 38 (1971): 233–52.

Maiuri, A. *L'ultima fase edilizia di Pompei.* Rome, 1942.

———. "Scoperta di un edificio termale nella Regio VIII, Insula 5, Nr. 36." *NSc,* 1950, 116–36.

———. "Significato e natura del *solium* nelle terme romane." *PP* 5 (1950): 223–27.

———. *Ercolano: I nuovi scavi (1927–1958).* 2 vols. Rome, 1959.

———. "Note di topografia pompeiana." *RendNap* 34 (1959): 73–88.

Manderscheid, H. "Römische Thermen: Aspekte von Architektur, Technik und Ausstattung." In *Geschichte der Wasserversorgung,* vol. 3, *Die Wasserversorgung antiker Städte,* 99–125. Mainz, 1988.

Mangani, E., F. Rebecchi, and M.J. Strazzulla. *Emilia, Venezie.* Guide archeologiche Laterza. Bari, 1981.

Manni, E. *Per la storia dei municipii fino alla guerra sociale.* Rome, 1947.

Mansuelli, G.A. *Caesena, Forum Popili, Forum Livi.* Rome, 1948.

Mar, R. "Santuarios e inversion inmobiliaria en la urbanística ostiense del siglo II." In *"Roman Ostia" Revisited: Archaeological and Historical Papers in Memory of Russell Meiggs,* edited by A.G. Zevi and A. Claridge, 115–64. London, 1996.

Mari, Z. *Tibur.* Vol. 4. Florence, 1991.

Marvin, M. "Freestanding Sculptures from the Baths of Caracalla." *AJA* 87 (1983): 347–84.

Mason, H.J. *Greek Terms for Roman Institutions: A Lexicon and Analysis.* Toronto, 1974.

Mattingly, D.J. *Tripolitania.* Ann Arbor, 1994.

Mazzi, M.C., ed. *Capena e il suo territorio.* Bari, 1995.

McGing, B.C. *The Foreign Policy of Mithridates VI Eupator, King of Pontus.* Leiden, 1986.

Mead, W.R. *An Experience of Finland.* London, 1993.

Meiggs, R. *Trees and Timber in the Ancient Mediterranean World.* Oxford, 1982.

Mertens, J. *Alba Fucens.* 3 vols. Brussels, 1969–82.

——, ed. *Herdonia: Scoperta di una città*. Brussels, 1995.

Meusel, H. *Die Verwaltung und Finanzierung der öffentlichen Bäder zur römischen Kaiserzeit*. Cologne, 1960.

Meyer, E.A. "Explaining the Epigraphic Habit in the Roman Empire: The Evidence of Epitaphs." *JRS* 80 (1990): 74–96.

Michler, M. "*Principis Medicus*: Antonius Musa." *ANRW* 2.37.1 (1993): 757–85.

Millar, F. *The Emperor in the Roman World*. London, 1977.

——. *The Roman Empire and Its Neighbours*[2]. London, 1981.

——. "The World of the *Golden Ass*." *JRS* 71 (1981): 63–75.

——. "The Last Century of the Republic: Whose History?" *JRS* 85 (1995): 236–43.

——. "Popular Politics at Rome in the Late Republic." In *Leaders and Masses in the Roman World: Studies in Honor of Zvi Yavetz*, edited by I. Malkin and Z.W. Rubinsohn, 91–113. Leiden, 1995.

Mioni, E. "Il Pratum Spirituale di Giovanni Mosco: Gli episodi inediti del Cod. Marciano greco II, 21." *OCP* 17 (1951): 61–94.

Mitford, T.B. *The Inscriptions of Kourion*. Philadelphia, 1971.

Morris, I. *Death-Ritual and Social Structure in Classical Antiquity*. Cambridge, 1992.

Mouritsen, H. *Elections, Magistrates, and Municipal Elite: Studies in Pompeian Epigraphy*. Rome, 1988.

Mrozek, S. "Á propos de la répartition chronologique des inscriptions latines dans le Haut-Empire." *Epigraphica* 35 (1973): 113–18.

——. *Les distributions d'argent et de nourriture dans les villes italiennes du Haut-Empire romain*. Brussels, 1987.

——. "Á propos de la répartition chronologique des inscriptions latines dans le Haut-Empire." *Epigraphica* 50 (1988): 61–64.

Musurillo, H. *The Acts of the Christian Martyrs*. Oxford, 1972.

Nash, E. *Pictorial Dictionary of Ancient Rome*[2]. 2 vols. London, 1968.

Neudecker, R. *Die Pracht der Latrine: Zum Wandel öffentlicher Bedürfnisanstalten in der kaiserzeitlichen Stadt*. Munich, 1994.

Nicolet, C. *Rome et la conquête du monde méditerranéen*. Paris, 1977.

——. *The World of the Citizen in Republican Rome*. Berkeley, 1980.

Nicols, J. *Vespasian and the* Partes Flavianae. Wiesbaden, 1978.

——. "*Tabulae Patronatus*: A Study of the Agreement between Patron and Client-Community." *ANRW* 2.13 (1980): 535–61.

——. "*Patrona Civitatis*: Gender and Civic Patronage." In *Studies in Latin Literature and Roman History*, vol. 5, edited by C. Deroux, 117–42. Brussels, 1989.

Nutton, V. "Murders and Miracles: Lay Attitudes towards Medicine in Classical Antiquity." In Porter, *Patients and Practitioners*, 23–53.

——. "The Perils of Patriotism: Pliny and Roman Medicine." In *Science in the Early Roman Empire: Pliny the Elder, His Sources and Influence*, edited by R. French and F. Greenaway, 30–58. London, 1986.

Oleson, J.P. *Greek and Roman Mechanical Water-Lifting Devices: The History of a Technology*. Toronto, 1984.

——. "Water-Lifting Devices at Herculaneum and Pompeii in the Context of Roman Technology." In De Haan and Jansen, *Cura Aquarum*, 67–77.

Onorato, G.O. "La data del terremoto di Pompei, 5 Febbraio 62 d. Cr." *RendLinc*, 1949, 644–61.

Orsi, P. "Prima campagna di scavi al santuario di Hera Lacinia." *NSc* Suppl., 1911, 77–124.

Ostrow, S.E. "The Augustales in the Augustan System." In *Between Republic and Empire: Interpretations of Augustus and His Principate,* edited by K. Raaflaub and M. Toher, 364–79. Berkeley, 1990.

Paasilinna, A., and T. Ovaska. *A Businessman's Guide to the Finnish Sauna.* Helsinki, 1984.

Packer, J.E. *The Insulae of Imperial Ostia.* Rome, 1971.

———. "Middle and Lower Class Housing in Pompeii and Herculaneum: A Preliminary Survey." In *Neue Forschungen in Pompeji,* edited by B. Andreae and H. Kyrielis, 133–46. Recklinghausen, 1975.

Parslow, C.C. "The *Praedia Iuliae Felicis* in Pompeii." Ph.D. dissertation, Duke University, 1989.

Paul, G.M. "Symposia and Deipna in Plutarch's Lives and in Other Historical Writings." In *Dining in a Classical Context,* edited by W.J. Slater, 157–69. Ann Arbor, 1991.

Pavolini, C. *Ostia.* Guide archeologiche Laterza. Bari, 1983.

Pedley, J.G. *Paestum: Greeks and Romans in Southern Italy.* New York, 1990.

Peek, W. "Metrische Mosaik-Inschrift aus Kourion." *ZPE* 23 (1976): 97–98.

Pelletier, A., ed. *La Médecine en Gaule: Villes d'eaux, sanctuaires des eaux.* Paris, 1985.

Perry, B.E. *Aesopica.* Urbana, 1952.

Pflaum, H.-G. "Titulature et rang social sous le Haut-Empire." In *Recherches sur les structures sociales dans l'antiquité classique,* edited by C. Nicolet, 159–85. Paris, 1970.

Phillips, E.D. *Aspects of Greek Medicine.* New York, 1973.

Phillips, J.H. "The Emergence of the Greek Medical Profession in the Roman Republic." *Transactions and Studies of the College of Physicians of Philadelphia,* n.s., 3 (1980): 267–75.

Pietrangeli, C. *Spoletium.* Rome, 1939.

———. *Ocriculum.* Rome, 1943.

———. *Otricoli: Un lembo dell'Umbria alle porte di Roma.* Rome, 1978.

Pigeaud, J. "L'introduction du Méthodisme à Rome." *ANRW* 2.37.1 (1993): 565–99.

Pirson, F. "Rented Accommodation at Pompeii: The Evidence of the *Insula Arriana Polliana* VI.6." In Laurence and Wallace-Hadrill, *Domestic Space in the Roman World,* 165–81.

Poma, G. "Osservazioni su *CIL,* XI, 556: *Liberalitates* imperiali nei confronti di *Caesena.*" *AttiBol* 29–30 (1990): 29–34.

Porter, R., ed. *Patients and Practitioners: Lay Perceptions of Medicine in Pre-Industrial Society.* Cambridge, 1985.

Potter, T.W. *Roman Italy.* Berkeley, 1987.

Price, M.J., and B.L. Trell. *Coins and Their Cities.* Detroit, 1977.

Price, S.R.F. *Rituals and Power: The Roman Imperial Cult in Asia Minor.* Cambridge, 1984.

Purcell, N. "The *Apparitores:* A Study in Social Mobility." *BSR* 51 (1983): 125–73.

———. "Wine and Wealth in Ancient Italy." *JRS* 75 (1985): 1–19.

Ramage, E.S. *The Nature and Purpose of Augustus's* Res Gestae. Stuttgart, 1987.

Rawson, E. "The Life and Death of Asclepiades of Bithynia." *CQ* 32 (1982): 358–70.

———. *Intellectual Life in the Late Roman Republic.* London, 1985.

———. "*Discrimina Ordinum:* The *Lex Julia Theatralis.*" *BSR* 55 (1987): 83–114.

Rebuffat, R. "Vocabulaire thermal: Documents sur le bain romain." In *Thermes,* 1–34.

Reinhold, M. "Usurpation of Status and Status Symbols in the Roman Empire." *Historia* 20 (1971): 275–302.

Reynolds, J. "Four Inscriptions from Roman Cyrene." *JRS* 49 (1959): 95–101.

Riddle, J.M. "High Medicine and Low Medicine in the Roman Empire." *ANRW* 2.37.1 (1993): 102–20.

Riggsby, A.M. "'Public' and 'Private' in Roman Culture: The Case of the *Cubiculum.*" *JRA* 10 (1997): 36–56.

Robert, L. "Inscriptions d'Aiolide." *BCH,* 1933, 492–504 (= id., *Opera Minora Selecta* 1.436–48).

———. *Études Anatoliennes.* Amsterdam, 1939. Reprint, 1970.

———. "Adeimantos et la ligue de Corinthe: Sur une inscription de Delphes." *Hellenica* 2 (1946): 15–33.

———. "Épigrammes relatives à des gouverneurs." *Hellenica* 4 (1948): 35–114.

———. "Inscriptions de Lydie." *Hellenica* 9 (1950): 7–39.

———. "Aphrodisias." *Hellenica* 13 (1965): 109–238.

———. *Opera Minora Selecta: Épigraphie et antiquités grecques.* 7 vols. Amsterdam, 1969–90.

———. "La titulature de Nicée et de Nicomédie: La gloire et la haine." *HSCP* 81 (1977): 1–39 (= id., *Opera Minora Selecta* 6.211–49).

———. "Décret pour un médecin de Cos." *RPhil* 52 (1978): 242–51 (= id., *Opera Minora Selecta* 6.438–47).

Robinson, O.F. "Baths: An Aspect of Roman Local Government Law." *Sodalitas* 3 (1984): 1065–82.

———. *Ancient Rome: City Planning and Administration.* London, 1992.

Roddaz, J.-M. *Marcus Agrippa.* Rome, 1984.

Rodríguez Almeida, E. Forma Urbis Marmorea: *Aggiornamento generale, 1980.* Rome, 1981.

———. "Due note marzialiane: I 'balnea quattuor in Campo' e le 'sellae Paterclianae' subcapitoline." *MEFRA* 101 (1989): 243–54.

Römer, C. "Ehrung für den Arzt Themison." *ZPE* 84 (1990): 81–88.

Rose, K.F.C. *The Date and Author of the* Satyricon. Leiden, 1971.

Roueché, C. *Performers and Partisans at Aphrodisias in the Roman and Late Roman Periods.* London, 1993.

Rowland, R.J., Jr. "Another Anachronism in the HA." *LCM* 2 (1977): 59.

Rudolph, H. *Stadt und Staat im römischen Italien.* Leipzig, 1935. Reprint, Göttingen, 1965.

Russell, J. "Mosaic Inscriptions from the Palaestra at Anemurium." *AnatSt* 24 (1974): 95–102.

———. *The Mosaic Inscriptions of Anemurium.* Vienna, 1987.

Saller, R.P. "Anecdotes as Historical Evidence for the Principate." *GaR* 27 (1980): 69–83.

Saller, R.P., and B.D. Shaw. "Tombstones and Roman Family Relations in the Principate: Civilians, Soldiers, and Slaves." *JRS* 74 (1984): 124–56.

Salles, C. "Les cachets d'oculistes." In Pelletier, *Médecine en Gaule*, 89–102.

Scarborough, J. "Roman Medicine to Galen." *ANRW* 2.37.1 (1993): 3–48.

Scobie, A. "Slums, Sanitation, and Mortality in the Roman World." *Klio* 68 (1986): 399–433.

Seager, R., comp. *The Crisis of the Roman Republic.* Cambridge, 1969.

Sgobbo, I. "L'acquedotto romano della Campania: 'Fontis Augustei Aquaeductus.'" *NSc*, 1938, 75–97.

Shatzman, I. *Senatorial Wealth and Roman Politics.* Brussels, 1975.

Shaw, B.D. "The Noblest Monuments and the Smallest Things: Wells, Walls, and Aqueducts in the Making of Roman Africa." In Hodge, *Future Currents*, 63–91.

Sherwin-White, A.N. *The Letters of Pliny: A Historical and Social Commentary.* Oxford, 1966.

———. *The Roman Citizenship*[2]. Oxford, 1973.

Shipley, F.W. "Chronology of the Building Operations in Rome from the Death of Caesar to the Death of Augustus." *MAAR* 9 (1931): 7–60.

———. *Agrippa's Building Activities in Rome.* St. Louis, 1933.

Simshäuser, W. "Untersuchungen zur Entstehung der Provinzialverfassung Italiens." *ANRW* 2.13 (1980): 401–52.

Smith R.R.R., and C. Ratté. "Archaeological Research at Aphrodisias in Caria, 1994." *AJA* 100 (1996): 5–33.

Sobel, H. *Hygieia: Die Göttin der Gesundheit.* Darmstadt, 1990.

Sommer, C.S. "Waren Frauen in der Römerzeit schmutziger als Männer? Überlegungen zur Eintrittspreisgestaltung in römishcen Thermen." *Fundberichte aus Baden-Württemberg* 21 (1996): 301–6.

Sperber, D. *The City in Roman Palestine.* Oxford, 1998.

Staccioli, R.A. "Terme minori e balnea nella documentazione della 'Forma Urbis.'" *ArchClass* 13 (1961): 92–102.

Stambaugh, J.E. *The Ancient Roman City.* Baltimore, 1988.

Stolz, S. *Die Handwerke des Körpers: Bader, Barbier, Perückenmacher, Friseur Folge und Ausdruck historischen Körperverständnisses.* Marburg, 1992.

Strong, D.E. "The Administration of Public Building in Rome during the Late Republic and Early Empire." *BICS* 15 (1968): 97–109.

Sumner, G.V. "The Family Connections of L. Aelius Seianus." *Phoenix* 19 (1965): 134–45.

Sutherland, C.H.V. *Coinage in Roman Imperial Policy.* London, 1951.

———. *The Roman Imperial Coinage.* Vol. 1[2]. London, 1982.

Sutyla, C.M. *The Finnish Sauna in Manitoba.* Ottawa, 1977.

Syme, R. "Rival Cities, Notably Tarraco and Barcino." *Ktema* 6 (1981): 271–85.

Talbert, R.J.A. "Pliny the Younger as Governor of Bithynia-Pontus." In *Studies in Latin Literature and Roman History,* vol. 2, edited by C. Deroux, 412–35. Brussels, 1980.

———. *The Senate of Imperial Rome.* Princeton, 1984.

———, ed. *Atlas of Classical History.* London, 1985.

Tamm, B. *Neros Gymnasium in Rom.* Stockholm, 1970.

Teixidor, J. "Religion und Kult in Palmyra." In *Palmyra: Geschichte, Kunst und Kultur der syrischen Oasenstadt,* 37–38. Linz, 1987.

Thomas, E., and C. Witschel. "Constructing Reconstruction: Claim and Reality of Roman Rebuilding Inscriptions from the Latin West." *BSR* 60 (1992): 135–77.

Thouvenot, R. *Volubilis.* Paris, 1949.

Thuillier, J.-P. "La nudité athlétique (Grèce, Etrurie, Rome)." *Nikephoros* 1 (1988): 29–48.

Tomlinson, R. *From Mycenae to Constantinople: The Evolution of the Ancient City.* London, 1992.

Torelli, M. *Etruria³.* Guide archeologiche Laterza. Bari, 1985.

Tortorici, E. "L'attività edilizia di Agrippa a Roma." In *Il bimillenario di Agrippa,* 19–55. Genoa, 1990.

———. "Terme Severiane, Terme 'Severiane' e Terme Septimianae." *BullCom* 95 (1993): 161–72.

Treggiari, S.M. "Domestic Staff at Rome in the Julio-Claudian Period, 27 B.C. to A.D. 68." *Histoire Sociale/Social History* 6 (1973): 241–55.

———. "Urban Labour in Rome: *Mercennarii* and *Tabernarii.*" In *Non-Slave Labour in the Greco-Roman World,* edited by P. Garnsey, 48–64. Cambridge, 1980.

———. "*Contubernales* in *CIL* 6." *Phoenix* 35 (1981): 42–69.

———. *Roman Marriage:* Iusti Coniuges *from the Time of Cicero to the Time of Ulpian.* Oxford, 1991.

Vallance, J.T. *The Lost Theory of Asclepiades of Bithynia.* Oxford, 1990.

———. "The Medical System of Asclepiades of Bithynia." *ANRW* 2.37.1 (1993): 693–727.

Vanderbroeck, P.J.J. *Popular Leadership and Collective Behavior in the Late Roman Republic (ca. 80–50 B.C.).* Amsterdam, 1987.

Varone, A. "Voices of the Ancients: A Stroll through Public and Private Pompeii." In *Rediscovering Pompeii,* 26–41. Rome, 1990.

Vassileiou, A. "Sur le date des thermes de Néron." *REA* 74 (1972): 94–106.

———. "Note sur un établissement de bains romain." *MEFRA* 97 (1985): 325–28.

Veyne, P., ed. *A History of Private Life.* Vol. 1, *From Pagan Rome to Byzantium.* Cambridge, MA, 1987.

Vigarello, G. *Concepts of Cleanliness: Changing Attitudes in France since the Middle Ages.* Cambridge, 1988.

Villard, L. "Le bain dans la médecine hippocratique." In *L'eau, la santé et la maladie dans le monde grec,* edited by R. Ginouvès, A.-M. Guimier-Sorbets, J. Jouanna, and L. Villard, 41–60. Paris, 1994.

Wallace-Hadrill, A. "The Emperor and His Virtues." *Historia* 30 (1981): 298–323.

———. *Houses and Society in Pompeii and Herculanuem.* Princeton, 1994.

———. "Public Honour and Private Shame: The Urban Texture of Pompeii." In Cornell and Lomas, *Urban Society,* 39–62.

Warden, P.G. "Bullae, Roman Custom, and Italic Tradition." *OpRom* 14 (1983): 69–75.

Ward-Perkins, J.B. "Taste, Tradition, and Technology: Some Aspects of the Architecture of Late Republican and Early Imperial Central Italy." In *Studies in Classical Art and Archaeology: A Tribute to Peter Heinrich von Blanckenhagen,* edited by G. Kopcke and M.B. Moore, 197–20. New York, 1979.

———. *Roman Imperial Architecture.* London, 1981.

———. *The Severan Buildings of Lepcis Magna: An Architectural Survey.* London, 1993.

Warmington, B.H. "The Municipal Patrons of Roman North Africa." *BSR* 22 (1954): 39–55.

Watson, G.R. *The Roman Soldier.* Ithaca, 1969.

Weaver, P.R.C. *Familia Caesaris: A Social Study of the Emperor's Freedmen and Slaves.* Cambridge, 1972.

Weaver, P.R.C., and P.I. Wilkins. "A Lost Alumna." *ZPE* 99 (1993): 241–44.

Webster, G. *The Roman Imperial Army*[3]. Totowa, 1985.

Wellmann, M. "Asklepiades aus Bithynien von einem herrschenden Vorurteil befreit." *NJbb* 21 (1908): 684–703.

Wertheimer, A.J. *Batei Midrashot*[2]. 2 vols. Jerusalem, 1954.

Wickenden, N. *Caesaromagus: A History and Description of Roman Chelmsford.* Chelmsford, 1991.

Wiedemann, T. *Emperors and Gladiators.* London, 1992.

Wierschowski, L. "AE 1980, 615 und das erste Auftreten der Formel 'omnibus honoribus in colonia sua functus' in den westlichen Provinzen." *ZPE* 64 (1986): 287–94.

Wiesner, M.E. *Working Women in Renaissance Germany.* New Brunswick, 1986.

Wikander, Ö. "Senators and Equites." Part 6, "Caius Sergius Orata and the Invention of the Hypocaust." *OpRom* 20 (1996): 177–82.

Williams, M.T. *Washing "The Great Unwashed": Public Baths in Urban America, 1840–1920.* Columbus, 1991.

Wilson, R.J.A. *Sicily under the Roman Empire: The Archaeology of a Roman Province, 36 B.C.–A.D. 535.* London, 1990.

Wiseman, T.P. *New Men in the Roman Senate, 139 B.C.–A.D. 14.* Oxford, 1971.

———. *Catullus and His World: A Reappraisal.* Cambridge, 1985.

Wissemann, M. "Das Personal des antiken römischen Bades." *Glotta* 62 (1982): 80–89.

Yavetz, Z. "The Living Conditions of the Urban Plebs in Republican Rome." *Latomus* 17 (1958): 500–517 (= Seager, *Crisis,* 162–79).

Yegül, F. "The Small City Bath in Classical Antiquity and a Reconstruction Study of Lucian's 'Baths of Hippias.'" *ArchCl* 31 (1979): 108–31.

———. *The Bath-Gymnasium Complex at Sardis.* Cambridge, MA, 1986.

———. Review of Nielsen, *AJA* 97 (1993): 185–86.

———. "The Thermo-Mineral Complex at Baiae and *De Balneis Puteolanis.*" *ArtB* 78 (1996): 137–61.

Youtie, H.C. "Records of a Roman Bath in Upper Egypt." *AJA* 53 (1949): 268–70 (= id., *Scriptiunculae,* 3 vols. [Amsterdam, 1973], 2.990–93).

Zanker, P. *The Power of Images in the Age of Augustus.* Ann Arbor, 1988.

———. *Pompei: Società, immagini e forme dell'abitare.* Turin, 1993.

Zazo, A. "Benevento romana." *Samnium* 58 (1985): 87–122.

Zienkiewicz, J.D. *The Legionary Fortress Baths at Caerleon.* Vol. 2, *The Finds.* Cardiff, 1986.

Zorzi, G. *I disegni della antichità di Andrea Palladio.* Venice, 1958.

Index of Names

Numbers in italics are references to entry numbers in the epigraphic sample. Names of famous Romans are cited under and by their familiar form ("Pompey" for "Pompeius," "Agrippa" for "Vipsanius Agrippa," and so on). The names of more obscure individuals, usually municipal magistrates or other local luminaries mentioned in the epigraphic sample, are cited as they appear in the pertinent text(s). All such names are listed with the nomen first; where names are incomplete, the first surviving letter determines its location in the index. Characters, real or imagined (e.g., Julius Cerealis, Trimalchio), appearing in purely literary contexts have not been indexed here but can be traced through the Index of Ancient Sources.

People

Acilius Aviola, M'., *174*
Acilius Granianus, L., *150*
Aedinius Julianus, M., *106*
Aeidio Victor, L., *93*
Aelia Kallituche, *324*
Aelius Alexander, T., *324*
Aelius Epaphroditus T., *324*
Aelius Gemellus, P., *180*
Aelius Julius, *120*
Aelius Sejanus, L., *159*
Aemilius Daphnus, L., *72, 242*
Aemilius Flavianus Fabius, *34*
Aemilius Fronto, *177*
Aemilius Honoratus, M., *93*
Aemilius Lepidus, M., 80n.18
Aemilius Scaurus, M., 79n.16, 80n.18
Agrippa, M. Vipsanius, *42, 50,* 81n.23, 108, 109, *123,* 123n.64, 160n.64

Agrippa Postumus, 63
Agrippina, 111
Agusius Mussus, L., *76*
Albucia Candida, *84*
Alfia Quarta, *151*
Alfius Fannius Primus, *126*
Alfius Maximus, L., *173, 174*
Alfius Maximus Numerius Avitus, P., *220*
Alleius Nigidius Maius, Cn., 64n.82, 112n.26
Ammius Namptoius, *127*
Anicius Auchenius Bassus, *37*
Aninius, P., *61*
Annaeus Hermes, L., *83*
Annaeus Thraso, T., *67*
Annius, M., *214*
Annius, P., *51*
Annius Verus, M., *195–96; 283*
Antinoos, *216*

Divinities

Geographic Index

Numbers in italics are references to entry numbers in the epigraphic sample.

Africa, 43n.11, *54*, *89*, *132*, *133*, *135*, *137*, *139*, 141, 145, 146, 148, 148n.43, 149, *150*, *152*, 152n.48, 163, 181
  Abbir Maius, 150, 165, 169; *133*
  Aubuzza, *83*
  Avitta Bibba, 227–28n.10
  Bisica, 163; *252*
  Bulla Regia, 166; *187*
  Carpis, *21*
  Carthage, 169, 192, 206–7n.53, 227–28n.10; *123*
    Antonine Baths, 121–22n.60; *42*, *86*, *231*
  Civitas Siagitana, 227–28n.10
  Colonia Vallis, 227–28n.10
  Comum, 153, 156, 163, 174, 207; *171*, *215*, *245*
  Gigthis, 209n.61
  Hippo Regius, South Baths, *94*
  Hr. Bu Auga (ancient name not known), *134*
  Hr. Faroha, 227–28n.10
  Maxula, 89n.24
  Membressa, 227–28n.10; *142*
  Mididi, *182*
  Municipium Aurelia Vina, 227–28n.10
  Municipium Tubernuc, *233*
  Schuhud el Batel, 227–28n.10
  [—]sinensium (modern Henchir-Haouli), *123*
  Thala, 227–28n.10
  Thibursicum Bure, 150, 155, 175
    Baths of Gallienus, *111*, *115*
  Thignica, 166; *237*
  Thuburbo Maius, 157, 169; *274*
    Summer Baths, *127*
    Winter Baths, *137*, *138*
  Thuburnica ad Aquas, 227–28n.10
  Thugga, 227–28n.10
    Licinian Baths, 169; *132*
  Thysdrus, 227–28n.10
  Tichilla, 227–28n.10
  Turca, 168; *114*
  Villa Magna, *183*
  Vreu, 157; *110*, *232*
Alpes. *See* Gaul
Asia, *54*, *89*, 131n.7, *137*, *139*, 186, 187
  Aphrodisias, Hadrianic Baths, 225n.4
  Beujuk Tepekeui (ancient name not known), *306*
  Byzantium (*see* Constantinople)
  Constantinople, 116, 193n.11
  Cyzicus, 100n.67
  Dorylaeum, *335*

Index of Topics

Alousia (going unwashed), 3

Amphitheaters, 18, 33, 65, 72, 76n.4, 79n.16, 208n.59. *See also* Geographic Index

Apodyterium (changing room), 67, 167n.81, 168. *See also* Appendix 3

Aqueducts, 69–74, 121n.58, 106, 122, 123, 163, 166. *See also* Water supply

Architecture, symbolism of, 104, 105–6, 121–22, 140n.26, 165–66

Arval Brethren, 22n.28, 209–10

Atrium (*thermarum;* reception hall?), 9, 169, 194. *See also* Appendix 3

Ball games, 10, 23, 24, 195–96

Balneaticum (entrance fee), 45, 51, 108, 127n.77, 160–61, 198, 202, 208. *See also under* Benefactions, free bathing

Balneator (bathman), 36, 38n.68, 45, 63, 186, 187, 202, 215

Balneum (or *balnea, balneae*), distinct from *thermae,* 14–19, 26, 31–32, 69, 76, 107–8n.11, 110–11n.21, 116, 124, 125, 127, 163, 179, 180, 193, 208

balnea meritoria, 193

See also Appendix 2; Geographic Index

Basilica (*thermarum;* entrance hall?), 9, 194

Bathers, Roman

absence of social segregation among, 206–12

annoying, 22–23, 29–30

degree of mixing among, 212–19

ill, 29, 86–87, 184–86 (*see also* Hygienic conditions; Water quality)

social identity of, 190–206

See also Commoners, as bathers; Emperors; Senators; Slaves

Bathing, public

belief in healthfulness of, 2, 3, 5, 84

social nature of, 1–5, 10, 12–13, 75

and spiritual purity, 4–5

Bathing, Roman

centrality of in daily life, 31–32, 50

"equalizing" nature of, 189, 212–19, 222

fashions in, 52, 58, 60, 68. *See also* Mixed bathing

hours of, 22, 26, 33

nature of evidence for, 7–9, 42, 54–55, 180, 202–3. *See also* Inscriptions, bath-related

perceived medical value of, 51, 84, 85–103 passim, 119, 165, 182, 184–86, 220

pleasures of, 76–77, 88, 176, 177–78

procedure, 3–4, 10, 23, 67, 82n.27, 128n.1, 182

Index of Ancient Sources

References to entry numbers in the epigraphic sample are to the notes of those entries and are set in italics.

Authors and Literary Works

Aelius Aristides (Ael. Arist.)
    13.189: 166n.76
    15.232: 41n.7, 166n.76
    23: 166n.78
    25.311: 32n.49
    27.44: 166n.78
    40.511: 197n.23
Aetius of Amidena (Aet. Amid.)
    1.P84: 187n.32
    2.3: 187n.32
Ammianus Marcellinus (Amm. Marc.)
    14.3.3: 199n.28
    26.10.5: *18*
    27.3.8: 117n.45
    28.4.8–9: 200n.35
    28.4.8–10: 195
    28.4.9: 36
    28.4.10: 20, 127n.78
    28.4.16: 199n.30
    28.4.19: 216n.82
    28.6.1–15: *35*
Anon.
    Life of Aesop
      2: 22n.28
      3: 22n.28
      28: 214–15n.80

      32: 34, 200n.36
      38: 200n.36
      38–39: 22n.28, 38n.68
      38–41: 24
      39: 32n.49
      65–67: 31, 217n.86
      66: 200n.36
      67: 22n.28, 214–15n.80
    Anthologia Palatina (Anth. Pal.)
      9.620: 26n.35
      9.624: 206–7n.53
      9.640: 210–11n.67
      9.680: 62n.75
      9.783: 26n.35
      10.112: *261*
Appian
    Bella Civilia (B Civ.)
      2.120: 82n.25
      4.53–56: *21*
    Μακεδονική *(Mac.)*
      11.9–10: 82n.25
Apuleius
    Apologia (Apol.)
      87: 170n.86
    Florida (Flor.)
      19: 97n.53
    Metamorphoses (Met.)
      1.21: 221n.1

Coins, Inscriptions, and Papyri

For entries in the epigraphic sample, see the Concordance of Inscriptions.

Inscriptions

Concordance of Inscriptions

AE	Fagan	AE	Fagan
1898.121	29	1955.287	22
1906.177/78	315/16	1957.13	325
1908.244	107	1958.141/42	94
1911.217	34	1959.9	103
1913.180	111	1960.198	4
1913.227	18	1961.109	88, 246
1914.57	138	1962.30	188
1914.196	52	1966.356	167
1916.87/88	127	1967.96	65
1916.112	274	1968.157	11
1920.16	89	1969/70.178	144
1920.33	148/49	1971.454	301
1921.45	187	1972.150	31, 155
1922.57	12	1972.202	193
1925.31	132	1974.618	324
1925.105	119	1975.873	133
1928.2	5	1975.880	110, 232
1929.7b	285	1976.175	75
1933.49	256	1977.758	120
1934.80	105	1978.217	266
1934.133	123	1979.202	209
1935.28	108, 185	1979.352	165, 243
1935.45	89	1980.900	166
1935.172	120	1981.779	287
1937.119/20	121	1981.782	322
1939.100	120	1981.834	297
1946.239	54	1984.150	22, 291
1949.27	86	1984.151	14
1949.28	42	1987.179	263
1952.19	188	1987.307	116, 181
1953.21	203	1989.420	210

AE	Fagan	CIL	Fagan
1991.1443	307	3.3047	92
1991.1619	90	3.6992	81
		3.7000	287
Bull. ép.		3.7342	60
1965.368, nos.4, 9	303	3.7380	161, 225
1967.439	304	3.7805	219
1972.461	305	3.8113	109
		3.10054	25
Cicerchia & Marinucci, *Scavi di Ostia*		3.12736	26
11.165–66 (nos. C		3.14195	29
1, 1a, b)	41	4.1136	258
11.216–19 (no. C		4.10603	276
106)	22	4.10674	277
11.219–22 (no. C		4.10675	281
107)	291	4.10676	280
CIG		4.10677	278
8622	328	4.10678	279
CIL		5.376	199
1².1473	63, 224	5.880	56
1².1529	157	5.2886	284
1².1628	62	5.3342	23
1².1635	61	5.4412	66
1².1690	64	5.5136	153, 223
1².1903a	205	5.5262	171, 245
1².2542	67	5.5279	215
1².3188	65	5.5504	57
2.191	122, 147	5.6513	84
2.1956	71, 248	5.6522	146, 200
2.3270	249	5.6668	201
2.3542	158	5.7250	135, 235
2.3361	78, 227, 241	5.7783	184
2.4112	28, 154	6.1474	220
2.4509	172, 229	6.8676	269
2.4514	218	6.8677	271
2.4610	267	6.8678	272
2.5181	282	6.8679	268
2.5354	101, 212	6.9232	273
2.5489	72, 242	6.9395/96	265
2.6102	175	6.9797	283
2.6145	172, 229	6.15258	261
3, p.1936; 7.75–		6.16740	260
66	286	8.609	182
3.324	13	8.828	114
3.352	287	8.897	183
3.1006	180	8.948	233
3.1805	189	8.1412	237

CIL	Fagan	CIL	Fagan
8.2340	150	10.819	62
8.4645	113	10.829	61
8.4878	192	10.1063	257
8.5335	130, 234	10.1707	44
8.7031	186	10.3678	239
8.8375	93	10.3714	39
8.8393	38, 236	10.3922f	143
8.8396	214	10.4559	126
8.11775	182	10.4754	253
8.12513	231	10.4792	250
8.15204	237	10.4865	40
8.16368	83	10.4884	47
8.16400	134	10.5200	125, 152
8.17938	275	10.5348	118
8.20266	38, 236	10.5349	141
8.20267	194	10.5807	157
8.21497	156	10.5917	95
8.23880	252	10.5918	179
8.24106	21	10.6312	36
9.1419	270	10.6656	37
9.1466	69	10.7004	55
9.1588	27	11.556	112
9.1596	195	11.720	1/2, 202
9.1665	10	11.721	254
9.2212	31, 155	11.3363	7
9.2338	32	11.3366	176
9.2447	33	11.3367	24
9.2660	85	11.3811	213, 221
9.3152	80, 174	11.3932	164, 228
9.3153	173	11.4090	98
9.3430	49	11.4094	136
9.3522	70	11.4095	124
9.3677	151	11.4100	198
9.4196	191	11.4781	16
9.4786	226	11.4815	99
9.4974	196	11.5939	177
9.4978	96	11.6040	50
9.5067	76	11.6167	206
9.5074	205	11.6225	73/74, 162
9.5746	3	11.6360	217
9.6261	48	11.7285	159
10.212	45	11.7298	139, 145
10.221	64	12.107	9
10.222	190	12.594	211
10.817	68	12.1357	79
10.818	160	12.1708	51

CIL	Fagan		IAM	Fagan
12.2494	82, 230		404	12
12.3165b	170		ICI	
12.3179	207		1.18	139, 145
12.4342	8		IG	
12.4388	58, 222		12.3.326	312
13.939	77		IGLS	
13.1169	100		4.1490	327
13.1376/77	97		IGRR	
13.1926	255		1.854	298
13.1983	264		1.1162	294
13.3162.I	106, 247		3.66	299, 318
13.3255	15		3.507	288
13.5257	53		3.659	289
13.5416/17	178		3.679	314
13.5661	104		3.690	293
13.5687	163		3.704	310
14.98	6		3.739	311
14.135	17		3.833	295
14.137	19		3.1155	323
14.376	87		4.216	334
14.914	262		4.228	306
14.2101	102		4.522	335
14.2112	216		4.454	333
14.2115	91		4.555	329, 332
14.2119	59		4.860	331, 338
14.2121	46		4.881	320
14.2979	204		4.1302	292, 339
14.3013	63, 224		4.1378	321
14.3015	197		4.1440	302
14.3472	208		IK	
14.3594	30		3 (Ilion) 121	334
14.4015	259		5 (Kyme) 19	292, 339
14.4717/18	41		12 (Ephesos 2)	
14.4190	251		453	325
14.5387	20		12 (Ephesos 2)	
CLE			455	309
1499	261		12 (Ephesos 2)	
1802	194		500	308
1911	194		13 (Ephesos 3)	
			661	336
EphEp			13 (Ephesos 3)	
8.456	43		672	296
			14 (Ephesos 4)	
Gerkan, von, and Krischen, *Thermen*			1314/15	29
und Palaestren			17.1 (Ephesos 7.1)	
164–66 (no. 339)	315/16		3080	296

IK	Fagan	ILPaest	Fagan
17.1 (Ephesos 7.1)		100	108, 185
3249	300	ILS	
27 (Prusias-ad-		314	81
Hypium) 20	299, 318	334	6
48 (Arykanda) 24	290	345	231
ILAfr		406	179
273	127	586	190
276	138	613	13
285	137	703	15
454a	187	739	16
506	111	1029	172, 229
573	132	1128	184
614	12	1148	23
ILAlg		1180	24
1.256	130, 234	1628	271
1.1032	113	1909	95
1.2100	128	2267	207
1.2101	129	2637	208
1.2102	131	2709	79
1.2108	140	2927	171, 245
ILCV		2943	192
229	194	4638	77
364	139, 145	5173	283
ILER		5348	157
1306	28, 154	5478	39
1417	249	5480	27
1732	203	5511	195
2040	78, 227, 241	5512	71, 248
2045	72, 242	5513	249
2046	158	5663	55
2049	122, 147	5664	47
2050	101, 212	5665	64
2054	71, 248	5666	76
5838	218	5667	63, 224
ILLRP		5668/69	49
528	157	5670	96
617	205	5671	205
575	67	5672	204
606	64	5673	206
641	62	5674	1/2, 202
648	61	5675	3
659	63, 224	5676	80, 174
1275	21	5677	250
ILM		5678	177
74	12	5679	73/74, 162

ILS	Fagan	ILS	Fagan
5680	170	5868	9
5682	161, 225	6091	287
5683	46	6198	91
5684	151	6256	197
5685	8	6356	62
5686	102	6489	270
5687	112	6583	213, 221
5688	78, 227, 241	6638	99
5689	239	6728	215
5690	31, 155	6876	93
5691	32	6891	282
5692	44	6957	218
5693	43	6988	211
5694	19	7145	219
5695	189	7212	216
5696	124	7621	273
5698	118	7718a	265
5699	122, 147	8157	261
5700	238	8158	264
5701	135, 235	8518	260
5702	37	8626f	275
5704	29	8796	293
5705	156	8996	159
5706	61	9259a, b	150
5707	59	9367	21
5708	143	*ILTG*	
5709	196	341	106, 247
5710	60	*ILTun*	
5711	50	622	123
5712	115	1500	132
5713	114	Ingholt, *Berytus* 3	
5714	113	(1936)	
5717	30	109–12 (no. 11)	317
5720	259	*InscrIt*	
5721	254	4.1.15	30
5722	255	10.3.71	199
5723	258	*IRT*	
5726	68	103a	35
5727	251	918	285
5728	214	263	119
5730	130, 234	396	90
5731	142	601b	117
5742	257		
5767	226	*ML*	
5768	82, 230	40	285
5770	164, 228	41	194

ML	Fagan	SEG	Fagan
124	283	39 (1989) 372	307
170a	261	*SIG*³	
171	262	909	328
		SuppItal	
NSc		3 (1987): 144–45	
1928, 283	168/69, 240, 244	(no. 8)	88, 246
		5 (1989): 52–53	
SEG		(no. 6)	18
14 (1957) 379	328	5 (1989): 181–82	
16 (1959) 718	325	(no. 14)	226
16 (1959) 719	309	9 (1992): 85–90	
19 (1963) 830	319	(no. 34)	121
26 (1976/77) 1474	326		
27 (1977) 842	322	*TAM*	
28 (1978) 396	337	2.396	289
28 (1978) 862	308	2.578	314
30 (1980) 1382	330	2.651	288
30 (1980) 1535	313	2.905	311
33 (1983) 773	291	5.758	324